Impaired communication, verbal, 18
Impulsive behavior, 26, 29, 85, 86, 8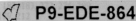
Inability to meet basic needs, 96, 121
Inappropriate/exaggerated behaviors, 19, 21, 85, 90, 117, 132, 165, 190, 232, 270, 274, 295
Inattention, 26, 41
Ineffective coping, 35–37, 50–51, 95–97, 103, 121–122, 179–180, 199–201, 211–214, 223–224, 315–319
Injury risk, 16–17, 119, 156–158, 160, 197, 278, 293
Insomnia, 75–76t, 80, 81, 82, 84, 85, 86, 87–89t, 129–130, 136, 167–168, 313, 352–355t, 364t, 367–368, 390, 395

Loose associations, 126
Loss of valued entity, recently experienced, 371
Low self-esteem, 28, 37–38, 47–48, 66–68, 98–100, 141–143, 209, 248–249, 262–264, 271, 285–287, 288, 290, 295–297, 375, 380

Manic behavior, 109, 132, 133, 153–158
Manipulative behavior, 35, 36–37, 47, 96, 156, 166, 200, 215, 275, 287, 296, 298
Memory loss, 223, 225, 353t, 390
Multiple personalities/gender dysphoria, 221, 226, 230, 242–245

Neurocognitive disorder, 462–463, 475, 479
Noncompliance, 41–42, 200, 256, 260, 330t

Orgasmic problems, 234–237
Overeating, compulsive, 252, 255

Pain, 313–315, 372, 375, 381, 392
Paraphilic behaviors, 230–233, 242
Phobias, 170–171, 174, 237, 271, 380
Physical symptoms as coping behavior, 51, 212, 213
Powerlessness, 145–147, 199, 200, 202, 204, 226, 240, 249, 307–309, 325–326, 333, 378, 400
Projection of blame, 32, 38, 99, 293, 296, 344

Regression/regressive behaviors, 27, 117, 136, 281, 304, 310, 374, 375, 381
Religiosity, 113
Repression, 102–103, 174, 221–222
Ritualistic behaviors, 21, 56, 169, 171, 174, 179–180

Seductive remarks/inappropriate sexual behaviors, 85, 270, 305
Self-image, 243, 270, 272, 304, 389
Self-mutilative behavior, 21–22, 44, 275, 276–279, 285
Sensory perception alterations, 65–66, 114, 123–124, 156, 163–165, 214–215, 227–229
Sexual abuse/assault, 185, 231, 236–237, 272, 302–303, 305, 309, 310, 338, 341, 389
Sexual behaviors, 232, 233, 241–242
Social interaction, impaired, 19–20, 27, 34–35, 45–46, 51–52, 116, 143–145, 165–166, 247–248, 282–284, 297–299, 330, 368, 382t
Social isolation, 116, 119–121, 143–145, 190, 270, 304, 326, 334–335, 373, 384
Spiritual distress (risk for), 384–385
Stealing, 28, 86
Stress from caring for chronically ill person, 68–69, 336, 402
Stress from locating to new environment, 203–204, 376
Substance abuse behaviors, 78, 96, 194, 272, 275, 288, 300, 323, 343, 390, 394, 400
Suicide, 31, 93, 117, 136–139, 194, 195–196, 197, 275, 277, 318, 349, 391, 395–396
Suspiciousness, 63, 88t, 113, 118, 121, 129, 159, 269, 343

Thought processes, disturbed, 61–63, 124–126, 135, 147–148, 155, 162–163, 396–398

Verbal communication, impaired, 18–19, 23–24, 126–128
Vomiting, excessive self-induced, 252, 254, 257–259

Withdrawn behavior, 120, 143, 213, 243, 373

Psychiatric Nursing

Assessment, Care Plans, and Medications

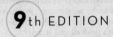

9th EDITION

Mary C. Townsend, DSN, PMHCNS-BC

Clinical Specialist/Nurse Consultant
Adult Psychiatric Mental Health Nursing

Former Assistant Professor and
Coordinator, Mental Health Nursing
Kramer School of Nursing
Oklahoma City University
Oklahoma City, Oklahoma

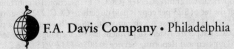

F.A. Davis Company • Philadelphia

F. A. Davis Company
1915 Arch Street
Philadelphia, PA 19103
www.fadavis.com

Printed in the United States of America

Last digit indicates print number: 10 9 8 7 6 5 4 3 2

Publisher, Nursing: Robert G. Martone
Director of Content Development: Darlene D. Pedersen
Content Project Manager: Jacalyn C. Clay
Electronic Project Editor: Katherine E. Crowley
Cover Design: Carolyn O'Brien

As new scientific information becomes available through basic and clinical research, recommended treatments and drug therapies undergo changes. The author(s) and publisher have done everything possible to make this book accurate, up to date, and in accord with accepted standards at the time of publication. The author(s), editors, and publisher are not responsible for errors or omissions or for consequences from application of the book, and make no warranty, expressed or implied, in regard to the contents of the book. Any practice described in this book should be applied by the reader in accordance with professional standards of care used in regard to the unique circumstances that may apply in each situation. The reader is advised always to check product information (package inserts) for changes and new information regarding dose and contraindications before administering any drug. Caution is especially urged when using new or infrequently ordered drugs.

Library of Congress Cataloging-in-Publication Data

Townsend, Mary C., 1941- , author.
  [Nursing diagnoses in psychiatric nursing]
  Psychiatric nursing: assessment, care plans, and medications / Mary C. Townsend. — Ninth edition.
      p. ; cm.
  Preceded by Nursing diagnoses in psychiatric nursing / Mary C. Townsend. 8th ed. c2011.
  Includes bibliographical references and indexes.
  ISBN 978-0-8036-4237-9 (alk. paper)
  I. Title.
  [DNLM: 1. Mental Disorders—nursing—Handbooks. 2. Nursing Diagnosis—Handbooks. 3. Patient Care Planning—Handbooks. 4. Psychotropic Drugs—therapeutic use—Handbooks. WY 49]
  RC440
  616.89'0231—dc23
                                    2014023510

This Book Is Dedicated:

To my husband, Jim, who encourages and supports me through-out all my writing projects, and whose love continues to nurture and sustain me, even after 53 years.

To my daughters Kerry and Tina, my grandchildren Meghan, Matthew, and Catherine, and my sons-in-law Ryan and Jonathan. You are the joys of my life.

To my faithful and beloved companion, Angel, and the granddog-gies Max, Riley, and Charlie, who make me laugh and bring pure pleasure into my life each and every day.

And finally, to the memory of my father and mother, Francis and Camalla Welsh, who reared my sister Francie and me without knowledge of psychology or developmental theories, but with the kind of unconditional love I have come to believe is so vital to the achievement and maintenance of emotional wellness.

MCT

Consultants

Maude H. Alston, RN, PhD
Assistant Professor of Nursing
University of North Carolina at Greensboro
Greensboro, North Carolina

Betty J. Carmack, RN, EdD
Assistant Professor
University of San Francisco
School of Nursing
San Francisco, California

Doris K. DeVincenzo, PhD
Professor
Pace University
Lienhard School of Nursing
Pleasantville, New York

Mary Jo Gorney-Fadiman, RN, PhD
Assistant Professor
San Jose State University
School of Nursing
San Jose, California

Mary E. Martucci, RN, PhD
Associate Professor and Chairman
Saint Mary's College
Notre Dame, Indiana

Sheridan V. McCabe, BA, BSN, MSN, PhD
Assistant Professor of Nursing
University of Virginia
School of Nursing
Charlottesville, Virginia

Elizabeth Anne Rankin, PhD
Psychotherapist and Consultant
University of Maryland
School of Nursing
Baltimore, Maryland

Judith M. Saunders, DNS, FAAN
Postdoctoral Research Fellow
University of Washington
School of Nursing
Seattle, Washington

Gail Stuart, RN, CS, PhD
Associate Professor
Medical University of South Carolina
College of Nursing
Charleston, South Carolina

Reviewers

Susan Atwood
Faculty
Antelope Valley College
Lancaster, California

Jaynee R. Boucher, MS, RN
St. Joseph's College of Nursing
Syracuse, New York

Sherry Campbell
Allegany College of Maryland
Cumberland, Maryland

Lorraine Chiappetta
Professor
Washtenaw Community College
Ann Arbor, Michigan

Ileen Craven
Instructor
Roxborough Memorial Hospital
Philadelphia, Pennsylvania

Marcy Echternacht
College of St. Mary
Omaha, Nebraska

Susan Feinstein
Instructor, Psychiatric Nursing
Cochran School of Nursing
Yonkers, New York

Mavonne Gansen
Northeast Iowa Community College
Peosta, Iowa

Diane Gardner
Assistant Professor
University of West Florida
Pensacola, Florida

Jo Anne C. Jackson, EdD, RN
Middle Georgia College
Cochran, Georgia

Elizabeth Kawecki
South University
Royal Palm Beach, Florida

Florence Keane, DNSc, MSN, BSN
Assistant Professor
Florida International University
Miami, Florida

Gayle Massie, MSN, RN
Professor
Shawne State University
Portsmouth, Ohio

Mary McClay
Walla Walla University
Portland, Oregon

Judith Nolen
Clinical Assistant Professor
University of Arizona
Tucson, Arizona

Pamela Parlocha
California State University–East Bay
Hayward, California

Joyce Rittenhouse
Burlington County College
Pemberton, New Jersey

Phyllis Rowe, DNP, RN, ANP
Riverside Community College
Riverside, California

Georgia Seward
Baptist Health Schools–Little Rock
Little Rock, Arkansas

Anna Shanks
Shoreline Community College
Seattle, Washington

Rhonda Snow
Stillman College
Tuscaloosa, Alabama

Karen Tarnow, RN, PhD
Clinical Associate Professor
University of Kansas Medical Center
Kansas City, Kansas

Shirley Weiglein
South University
Tampa, Florida

Tammie Willis
Penn Valley Community College
Kansas City, Missouri

Acknowledgments

My special thanks and appreciation:

To Bob Martone, who patiently provides assistance and guidance for all my writing projects.

To the editorial and production staffs of the F. A. Davis Company, who are always willing to provide assistance when requested and whose consistent excellence in publishing makes me proud to be associated with them.

To the gracious individuals who read and critiqued the original manuscript, providing valuable input into the final product.

And finally, a special acknowledgment to the nurses who staff the psychiatric units of the clinical agencies where nursing students go to learn about psychiatric nursing. To those of you who willingly share your knowledge and expertise with, and act as role models for, these nursing students. If this book provides you with even a small amount of nursing assistance, please acknowledge it as my way of saying "thanks."

MCT

Table of Contents

Index of DSM-5 Psychiatric Diagnoses   xix

How to Use This Book   xxix

UNIT ONE

THE FOUNDATION FOR PLANNING PSYCHIATRIC NURSING CARE

CHAPTER 1
The Nursing Process in Psychiatric/Mental Health Nursing   1

UNIT TWO

ALTERATIONS IN PSYCHOSOCIAL ADAPTATION

CHAPTER 2
Disorders Commonly Associated with Infancy, Childhood, or Adolescence   14

CHAPTER 3
Neurocognitive Disorders   54

CHAPTER 4
Substance-Related and Addictive Disorders   71

CHAPTER 5
Schizophrenia Spectrum and Other Psychotic Disorders   107

CHAPTER 6
Depressive Disorders   132

CHAPTER 7
Bipolar and Related Disorders 153

CHAPTER 8
Anxiety, Obsessive-Compulsive, and Related Disorders 169

CHAPTER 9
Trauma- and Stressor-Related Disorders 185

CHAPTER 10
Somatic Symptom and Related Disorders 206

CHAPTER 11
Dissociative Disorders 220

CHAPTER 12
Sexual Disorders and Gender Dysphoria 230

CHAPTER 13
Eating Disorders 251

CHAPTER 14
Personality Disorders 269

UNIT THREE

SPECIAL TOPICS IN PSYCHIATRIC/ MENTAL HEALTH NURSING

CHAPTER 15
Problems Related to Abuse or Neglect 302

CHAPTER 16
Premenstrual Dysphoric Disorder 312

CHAPTER 17
Homelessness 321

CHAPTER 18
Psychiatric Home Nursing Care 328

CHAPTER 19
Forensic Nursing 338

CHAPTER 20
Complementary Therapies 350

CHAPTER 21
Loss and Bereavement 371

CHAPTER 22
Military Families 386

UNIT FOUR

PSYCHOTROPIC MEDICATIONS

CHAPTER 23
Antianxiety Agents 404

CHAPTER 24
Antidepressants 416

CHAPTER 25
Mood-Stabilizing Agents 449

CHAPTER 26
Antipsychotic Agents 474

CHAPTER 27
Antiparkinsonian Agents 504

CHAPTER 28
Sedative-Hypnotics 512

CHAPTER 29
**Agents Used to Treat Attention-Deficit/
Hyperactivity Disorder** 522

APPENDICES
A. **Comparison of Developmental
   Theories** 539

B. **Ego Defense Mechanisms** 543

C. **Levels of Anxiety** 546

D. Stages of Grief 549

E. Relationship Development and Therapeutic Communication 552

F. Psychosocial Therapies 563

G. Electroconvulsive Therapy 573

H. Medication Assessment Tool 576

I. Cultural Assessment Tool 581

J. DSM-5 Classification 583

K. Mental Status Assessment 610

L. Assigning Nursing Diagnoses to Client Behaviors 618

M. Brief Mental Status Evaluation 621

N. FDA Pregnancy Categories 623

O. DEA Controlled Substances Schedules 624

P. Abnormal Involuntary Movement Scale (AIMS) 626

Q. Hamilton Depression Rating Scale (HDRS) 629

R. Hamilton Anxiety Rating Scale (HAM-A) 632

S. NANDA Nursing Diagnoses: Taxonomy II 634

Bibliography 641

Subject Index 653

Drug Index 694

Nursing Diagnoses Index 700

Index of DSM-5 Psychiatric Diagnoses

Academic or educational problem, 608

Access to medical and other health care, problems related to, 609

Acculturation difficulty, 608

Acute stress disorder, 186, 590

Adjustment disorders, 186, 590l
  with anxiety, 187, 590
  with depressed mood, 186, 590
  with disturbance of conduct, 187, 590
  with mixed anxiety and depressed mood, 187, 590
  with mixed disturbance of emotions and conduct, 187, 590
  unspecified, 187, 590

Adult antisocial behavior, 609

Adult physical abuse by nonspouse or nonpartner
  confirmed, 607
  suspected, 607

Adult psychological abuse by nonspouse or nonpartner
  confirmed, 607
  suspected, 607

Adult sexual abuse by nonspouse or nonpartner
  confirmed, 607
  suspected, 607

Agoraphobia, 589

Alcohol intoxication, 595

Alcohol use disorder, 595

Alcohol withdrawal, 595

Alzheimer's disease, 599

Anorexia nervosa, 251, 591

Antidepressant discontinuation syndrome, 604

Antisocial behavior, 609

Antisocial personality disorder, 288, 594, 602

Anxiety disorder due to another medical condition, 589

Attention-deficit/hyperactivity disorder, 26, 584

Autism spectrum disorder, 20, 583–584

Avoidant personality disorder, 602

Avoidant/restrictive food intake disorder, 591

Binge-eating disorder, 251, 591
Bipolar I disorder, 586
Bipolar II disorder, 587
Body dysmorphic disorder, 589
Borderline intellectual functioning, 609
Borderline personality disorder, 602
Brief psychotic disorder, 585
Bulimia nervosa, 251, 590

Caffeine intoxication, 595
Caffeine withdrawal, 595
Cannabis intoxication, 595
Cannabis use disorder, 595
Cannabis withdrawal, 81, 595
Catatonia associated with another mental disorder, 586
Catatonic disorder due to another medical condition, 586
Central sleep apnea, 592
Child affected by parental relationship distress, 604
Childhood-onset fluency disorder, 583
Child neglect
    confirmed, 605
    other circumstances related to, 605
    suspected, 605
Child or adolescent antisocial behavior, 609
Child physical abuse
    confirmed, 604
    other circumstances related to, 604–605
    suspected, 604
Child psychological abuse
    confirmed, 605
    other circumstances related to, 606
    suspected, 605
Child sexual abuse
    confirmed, 605
    other circumstances related to, 605
    suspected, 605
Circadian rhythm sleep-wake disorder, 592–593
Conduct disorder, 27, 594
Conversion disorder, 208, 590–591
Counseling and medical advice, other health service encounters
    for, 609
Cyclothymic disorder, 587

Delayed ejaculation, 593
Delirium, 54, 599
Delirium due to another medical condition, 54–55, 599
Delirium due to multiple etiologies, 55, 599

Delirium due to substance intoxication, 54, 599
Delirium due to substance withdrawal, 54, 599
Delusional disorder, 107, 585
Dependent personality disorder, 602
Depersonalization/derealization disorder, 590
Depressive disorder due to another medical condition, 588
Developmental coordination disorder, 584
Discord with neighbor, lodger, or landlord, 608
Discord with social service provider, including probation officer, case manager, or social services worker, 609
Disinhibited social engagement disorder, 590
Disruption of family by separation or divorce, 604
Disruptive mood dysregulation disorder, 132, 587
Dissociative amnesia, 590
Dissociative fugue, 590
Dissociative identity disorder, 590
Dysthymia, 588

Employment, other problem related to, 608
Encopresis, 591
Enuresis, 591
Erectile disorder, 593
Excoriation (skin-picking) disorder, 589
Exhibitionistic disorder, 231, 603
Exposure to disaster, war, or other hostilities, 609
Extreme poverty, 608

Factitious disorder, 591
Female orgasmic disorder, 234, 594
Female sexual interest/arousal disorder, 594
Fetishistic disorder, 231, 603
Frotteuristic disorder, 231, 603

Gambling disorder, 86, 598
Gender dysphoria, 230, 242, 594
Generalized anxiety disorder, 589
Genito-pelvic pain/penetration disorder, 594
Global developmental delay, 583

Hallucinogen intoxication, other, 596
Hallucinogen persisting perception disorder, 596
Hallucinogen use disorder, other, 596
High expressed emotion level within family, 604
Histrionic personality disorder, 270, 602
Hoarding disorder, 171, 172, 589
Homelessness, 608
Hypersomnolence disorder, 592

Illness anxiety disorder, 590
Imprisonment or other incarceration, 609
Inadequate housing, 608
Inhalant intoxication, 596
Inhalant use disorder, 596
Insomnia disorder, 592
Insufficient social insurance or welfare support, 608
Intellectual disability, 15, 583
Intermittent explosive disorder, 594

Kleptomania, 594

Lack of adequate food or safe drinking water, 608
Language disorder, 583
Learning disorders, 584
Legal circumstances, problems related to other, 609
Lifestyle, problem related to, 609
Living alone, problem related to, 608
Living in a residential institution, problem related to, 608
Low income, 608

Major depressive disorder, 587–588
Male hypoactive sexual desire disorder, 234, 594
Malingering, 609
Mathematics, impaired, 584
Medication-induced acute akathisia, 604
Medication-induced acute dystonia, 604
Medication-induced movement disorders, 603–604
Medication-induced postural tremor, 604
Mild vascular neurocognitive disorder, 600
Military deployment, personal history of, 609
Military deployment status, problem related to current, 608
Motor disorders, 584
Motor or vocal tic disorder, 584
Multiparity, problems related to, 609

Narcissistic personality disorder, 602
Narcolepsy, 592
Neglect
    of adult, 606–607
    of child, 605
Neurocognitive disorder (major or mild), 55, 599
    due to Alzheimer's disease (probable or possible), 55–56, 599
    due to another medical condition, 57, 602
    due to HIV infection, 56, 601
    due to Huntington's disease, 57, 601
    due to Parkinson's disease (probable or possible), 57, 601

due to prion disease, 56–57, 601
due to traumatic brain injury, 56, 600
frontotemporal (probable or possible), 56, 600
with Lewy bodies (probable or possible), 56, 600
substance/medication-induced, 57, 601
vascular (probable or possible), 56, 600
Neuroleptic-induced Parkinsonism, 603
Neuroleptic malignant syndrome, 603
Nightmare disorder, 594
Nonadherence to medical treatment, 609
Nonrapid eye movement sleep arousal disorders, 593

Obsessive-compulsive disorder, 589
Obsessive-compulsive personality disorder, 602
Obstructive sleep apnea hypopnea, 592
Opioid intoxication, 597
Opioid use disorder, 596
Opioid withdrawal, 597
Oppositional defiant disorder, 594
Other personal history of psychological trauma, 609
Other specified disorders
alcohol-induced disorders, 595
anxiety disorder, 589
attention-deficit/hyperactivity disorder, 584
caffeine-induced disorders, 595
cannabis-induced disorders, 596
catatonia, 586
communication disorder, 583
disruptive, impulse-control, and conduct disorders, 594
dissociative disorder, 590
elimination disorder, 592
feeding or eating disorder, 591
gender dysphoria, 594
hallucinogen-related disorders, 596
inhalant-related disorders, 596
intellectual disability, 583
neurodevelopmental disorders, 585
obsessive-compulsive and related disorder, 589
opioid-induced disorders, 597
parasomnias, 593
schizophrenia spectrum and other psychotic disorder, 586
sedative-, hypnotic-, or anxiolytic-related disorder, 597
sexual dysfunctions, 594
somatic symptom and related disorder, 591
tic disorder, 585
tobacco-induced disorders, 598
trauma- and stressor-related disorder, 590

Other specified mental disorder due to another medical condition, 603
Other (or unknown) substance-related disorders, 598
Other (or unspecified) disorders
  delirium, 599
  mental disorder, 603
  paraphilias, 603
  personality disorders, 603
Overweight or obesity, 609

Panic disorder, 588
Paranoid personality disorder, 602
Parent-child relational problem, 604
Pedophilic disorder, 231, 603
Persistent depressive disorder (dysthymia), 588
Personal history of military deployment, 609
Personal history of self-harm, 609
Personality change due to another medical condition, 602–603
Phase of life problem, 608
Phencyclidine intoxication, 596
Phencyclidine use disorder, 596
Phobias, 588
  agoraphobia, 589
  social, 588
  specific, 588
Pica, 591
Posttraumatic stress disorder, 186, 590
Poverty, extreme, 608
Premature ejaculation, 235, 594
Premenstrual dysphoric disorder, 312, 588
Provisional tic disorder, 585
Psychosocial circumstances, other problem related to, 609
Psychotic disorder due to another medical condition, 586
Pyromania, 594

Rapid eye movement sleep behavior disorder, 593
Reactive attachment disorder, 590
Relationship distress with spouse or intimate partner, 604
Release from prison, problems related to, 609
Religious or spiritual problem, 609
Restless legs syndrome, 593
Rumination disorder, 591

Schizoaffective disorder, 585
Schizoid personality disorder, 602
Schizophrenia, 585

Schizophreniform disorder, 585
Schizotypal personality disorder, 107, 602
Sedative, hypnotic, or anxiolytic intoxication, 597
Sedative, hypnotic, or anxiolytic use disorder, 597
Sedative, hypnotic, or anxiolytic withdrawal, 597
Selective mutism, 588
Self-harm, personal history of, 609
Separation anxiety disorder, 588
Sex counseling, 609
Sexual masochism disorder, 231, 603
Sexual sadism disorder, 231–232, 603
Sibling relational problem, 604
Sleep-related hypoventilation, 593
Sleep terror disorder, 593
Sleep-wake disorders, 593
Sleepwalking disorder, 593
Social anxiety disorder, 588
Social (pragmatic) communication disorder, 583
Social exclusion or rejection, 608
Somatic symptom disorder, 590
Specific learning disorder, 584
Specific phobia, 588
Speech sound disorder, 583
Spouse or partner abuse, psychological
    confirmed, 607
    other circumstances related to, 607
    suspected, 607
Spouse or partner neglect
    confirmed, 606
    other circumstances related to, 607
    suspected, 607
Spouse or partner violence
    physical
        confirmed, 606
        other circumstances related to, 606
        suspected, 606
    sexual
        confirmed, 606
        other circumstances related to, 606
        suspected, 606
Stereotypic movement disorder, 584
Stimulant intoxication, 597
Stimulant use disorder, 597–598
Stimulant withdrawal, 598
Substance/medication-induced disorders
    anxiety disorder, 172, 589
    bipolar and related disorders, 587
    obsessive-compulsive and related disorders, 589

psychotic disorders, 585
sexual dysfunctions, 594
sleep disorders, 593

Tardive akathisia, 604
Tardive dyskinesia, 604
Tardive dystonia, 604
Target of (perceived) adverse discrimination or persecution, 608
Tobacco use disorder, 598
Tobacco withdrawal, 598
Tourette's disorder, 584
Transvestic disorder, 232, 603
Trichotillomania, 171, 589

Unavailability or inaccessibility of health care facilities, 609
Unavailability or inaccessibility of other helping agencies, 609
Uncomplicated bereavement, 604
Unspecified disorders
    alcohol-induced disorders, 595
    attention-deficit/hyperactivity disorder, 584
    breathing-related sleep disorders, 593
    caffeine-induced disorders, 595
    cannabis-induced disorders, 596
    catatonia, 586
    communication disorder, 583
    delirium, 599
    disruptive, impulse-control, and conduct disorders, 594
    dissociative disorder, 590
    elimination disorder, 592
    feeding or eating disorder, 591
    gender dysphoria, 594
    hallucinogen-related disorders, 596
    inhalant-related disorders, 596
    intellectual disability, 583
    mental disorder, 603
    neurocognitive disorder, 602
    obsessive-compulsive and related disorder, 589
    opioid-induced disorders, 597
    paraphilias, 603
    parasomnias, 593
    personality disorders, 603
    schizophrenia spectrum and other psychotic
        disorder, 586
    sedative-, hypnotic-, or anxiolytic-related disorder, 597
    sexual dysfunctions, 594
    somatic symptom and related disorder, 591
    tic disorder, 585

    tobacco-induced disorders, 598
    trauma- and stressor-related disorder, 590
    unspecified anxiety disorder, 589
Unspecified housing or economic problem, 608
Unspecified mental disorder due to another medical condition, 603
Unspecified problem related to social environment, 608
Unwanted pregnancy, problems related to, 609
Upbringing away from parents, 604

Victim of crime, 608
Victim of terrorism or torture, 609
Voyeuristic disorder, 232, 603

Wandering associated with a mental disorder, 609
Written expression, impaired, 584

Introduction

■ HOW TO USE THIS BOOK

This book has been designed as a guide in the construction of care plans for various psychiatric clients. The concepts are presented in such a manner that they may be applied to various types of health-care settings: inpatient hospitalization, outpatient clinic, home health, partial hospitalization, and private practice, to name a few. Major divisions in the book are identified by psychiatric diagnostic categories as they appear in the *Diagnostic and Statistical Manual of Mental Disorders (DSM-5)* (American Psychiatric Association [APA], 2013). The nursing diagnoses used in this textbook are from the nomenclature of Taxonomy II that has been adopted by NANDA International (NANDA-I, 2012). The use of this format is not to imply that nursing diagnoses are based on, or flow from, medical diagnoses; it is meant only to enhance the usability of the book. It is valid, however, to state that certain nursing diagnoses are indeed common to individuals with specific psychiatric disorders.

In addition, I am not suggesting that those nursing diagnoses presented with each psychiatric category are all-inclusive. The diagnoses presented in this book are intended to be used as guidelines for construction of care plans that must be individualized for each client, based on the nursing assessment. The interventions can also be used in areas in which interdisciplinary treatment plans take the place of the nursing care plan.

Each chapter in Unit Two begins with an overview of information related to the psychiatric diagnostic category, which may be useful to the nurse as background assessment data. This section includes:

1. **The Disorder:** A definition and common types or categories that have been identified.
2. **Predisposing Factors:** Information regarding theories of etiology, which the nurse may use in formulating the "related to" portion of the nursing diagnosis, as it applies to the client.
3. **Symptomatology:** Subjective and objective data identifying behaviors common to the disorder. These behaviors, as they apply to the individual client, may be pertinent to the "evidenced by" portion of the nursing diagnosis.

Information presented with each nursing diagnosis includes the following:

1. **Definition:** The approved NANDA definition from the Taxonomy II nomenclature (NANDA-I, 2012).
2. **Possible Etiologies ("related to"):** This section suggests possible causes for the problem identified. Those not approved by NANDA-I are identified by brackets [ ].
3. **Related/Risk Factors** are given for diagnoses for which the client is at risk. *Note*: **Defining characteristics are replaced by "related/risk factors" for the "Risk for" diagnoses.**
4. **Defining Characteristics ("evidenced by"):** This section includes signs and symptoms that may be evident to indicate that the problem exists. Again, as with definitions and etiologies, those not approved by NANDA-I are identified by brackets [ ].
5. **Goals/Objectives:** These statements are made in client behavioral objective terminology. They are measurable short- and long-term goals, to be used in evaluating the effectiveness of the nursing interventions in alleviating the identified problem. There may be more than one short-term goal, and they may be considered "stepping stones" to fulfillment of the long-term goal. For purposes of this book, "long-term," in most instances, is designated as "by discharge from treatment," whether the client is in an inpatient or outpatient setting.
6. **Interventions with *Selected Rationales*:** Only those interventions that are appropriate to a particular nursing diagnosis within the context of the psychiatric setting are presented. Rationales for selected interventions are included to provide clarification beyond fundamental nursing knowledge, and to assist in the selection of appropriate interventions for individual clients. Important interventions related to communication may be identified by a communication icon. ☺
7. **Outcome Criteria:** These are behavioral changes that can be used as criteria to determine the extent to which the nursing diagnosis has been resolved.

To use this book in the preparation of psychiatric nursing care plans, find the section in the text applicable to the client's psychiatric diagnosis. Review background data pertinent to the diagnosis, if needed. Complete a biopsychosocial history and assessment on the client. Select and prioritize nursing diagnoses appropriate to the client. Using the list of NANDA-I approved nursing diagnoses, be sure to include those that are client-specific, and not just those that have been identified as "common" to a particular psychiatric diagnosis. Select nursing interventions and outcome criteria appropriate to the client for each nursing diagnosis identified. Include all of this information on the care plan, along with a date for evaluating the status of each problem. On the evaluation date, document success of the nursing interventions in achieving the goals of care, using the desired client outcomes as criteria. Modify the plan as required.

Unit Three addresses client populations with special psychiatric nursing needs. These include survivors of abuse or neglect, clients with premenstrual dysphoric disorder, clients who are homeless, clients who are experiencing bereavement, and military families. Topics related to forensic nursing, psychiatric home nursing care, and complementary therapies are also included.

Unit Four, Psychotropic Medications, has been updated to include new medications that have been approved by the FDA since the last edition. This information should facilitate use of the book for nurses administering psychotropic medications and also for nurse practitioners with prescriptive authority. The major categories of psychotropic medications are identified by chemical class. Information is presented related to indications, actions, contraindications and precautions, interactions, route and dosage, and adverse reactions and side effects. Examples of medications in each chemical class are presented by generic and trade name, along with information about half-life, controlled and pregnancy categories, and available forms of the medication. Therapeutic plasma level ranges are provided, where appropriate. Nursing diagnoses related to each category, along with nursing interventions, and client and family education are included in each chapter.

Another helpful feature of this text is the table in Appendix L, which lists some client behaviors commonly observed in the psychiatric setting and the most appropriate nursing diagnosis for each. It is hoped that this information will broaden the understanding of the need to use a variety of nursing diagnoses in preparing the client treatment plan.

This book helps to familiarize the nurse with the current NANDA-I approved nursing diagnoses and provides suggestions for their use within the psychiatric setting. The book is designed to be used as a quick reference in the preparation of care plans, with the expectation that additional information will be required for each nursing diagnosis as the nurse individualizes care for psychiatric clients.

MCT

 INTERNET REFERENCES

- http://www.apna.org
- http://www.nanda.org
- http://www.ispn-psych.org

THE FOUNDATION FOR PLANNING PSYCHIATRIC NURSING CARE

CHAPTER 1

The Nursing Process in Psychiatric/Mental Health Nursing

Nursing has struggled for many years to achieve recognition as a profession. Out of this struggle has emerged an awareness of the need to do the following:

1. Define the boundaries of nursing (What is nursing?).
2. Identify a scientific method for delivering nursing care.

In its statement on social policy, the American Nurses Association (ANA) presented the following definition:

> Nursing is the protection, promotion, and optimization of health and abilities, prevention of illness and injury, alleviation of suffering through the diagnosis and treatment of human response, and advocacy in the care of individuals, families, communities, and populations (ANA, 2010a, p. 10).

The nursing process has been identified as nursing's scientific methodology for the delivery of nursing care. The curricula of most nursing schools include nursing process as a component of their conceptual frameworks. The National Council of State Boards of

Nursing (NCSBN) has integrated the nursing process throughout the test plan for the National Council Licensure Examination for Registered Nurses (NCSBN, 2013). Questions that relate to nursing behaviors in a variety of client situations are presented according to the steps of the nursing process:

1. **Assessment:** Establishing a database on a client.
2. **Diagnosis:** Identifying the client's health-care needs and selecting goals of care.
3. **Outcome Identification:** Establishing criteria for measuring achievement of desired outcomes.
4. **Planning:** Designing a strategy to achieve the goals established for client care.
5. **Implementation:** Initiating and completing actions necessary to accomplish the goals.
6. **Evaluation:** Determining the extent to which the goals of care have been achieved.

By following these six steps, the nurse has a systematic framework for decision-making and problem-solving in the delivery of nursing care. The nursing process is dynamic, not static. It is an ongoing process that continues for as long as the nurse and client have interactions directed toward change in the client's physical or behavioral responses. Figure 1-1 presents a schematic of the ongoing nursing process.

Diagnosis is an integral part of the nursing process. In this step, the nurse identifies the human responses to actual or potential health problems. In some states, diagnosing is identified within

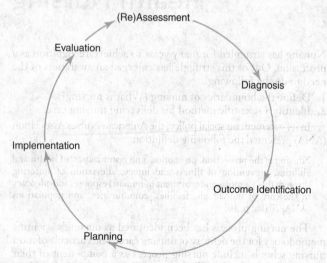

Figure 1-1: The ongoing nursing process.

the Nurse Practice Acts as a legal responsibility of the professional nurse. Nursing diagnosis provides the basis for prescribing the specific interventions for which the nurse is accountable.

As an inherent part of the nursing process, nursing diagnosis is included in the ANA Standards of Practice. These standards provide one broad basis for evaluating practice and reflect recognition of the rights of the person receiving nursing care (ANA, 2010b).

■ CONCEPT MAPPING

Concept mapping is a diagrammatic teaching and learning strategy that allows students and faculty to visualize interrelationships between medical diagnoses, nursing diagnoses, assessment data, and treatments. The concept map care plan is an innovative approach to planning and organizing nursing care. Basically, it is a diagram of client problems and interventions. Compared to the commonly used column format care plans, concept map care plans are more succinct. They are practical, realistic, and time-saving, and they serve to enhance critical-thinking skills and clinical reasoning ability.

The nursing process is foundational to developing and using the concept map care plan, just as it is with all types of nursing care plans. Client data is collected and analyzed, nursing diagnoses are formulated, outcome criteria are identified, nursing actions are planned and implemented, and the success of the interventions in meeting the outcome criteria is evaluated.

The concept map care plan may be presented in its entirety on one page, or the assessment data and nursing diagnoses may appear in diagram format on one page, with outcomes, interventions, and evaluation written on a second page. Additionally, the diagram may appear in circular format, with nursing diagnoses and interventions branching off the "client" in the center of the diagram. Or, it may begin with the "client" at the top of the diagram, with branches emanating in a linear fashion downward.

As stated previously, the concept map care plan is based on the components of the nursing process. Accordingly, the diagram is assembled in the nursing process stepwise fashion, beginning with the client and his or her reason for needing care, nursing diagnoses with subjective and objective clinical evidence for each, nursing interventions, and outcome criteria for evaluation.

Various colors may be used in the diagram to designate various components of the care plan. Lines are drawn to connect the various components to indicate any relationships that exist. For example, there may be a relationship between two nursing diagnoses (e.g., There may be a relationship between the nursing diagnoses of pain and anxiety and disturbed sleep pattern). A line between these nursing diagnoses should be drawn to show the relationship.

Concept map care plans allow for a great deal of creativity on the part of the user, and they permit viewing the "whole picture" without generating a great deal of paperwork. Because they reflect the steps of the nursing process, concept map care plans also are valuable guides for documentation of client care. Doenges, Moorhouse, & Murr (2010) state:

> As students, you are asked to develop plans of care that often contain more detail than what you see in the hospital plans of care. This is to help you learn how to apply the nursing process and create individualized client care plans. However, even though much time and energy may be spent focusing on filling the columns of traditional clinical care plan forms, some students never develop a holistic view of their clients and fail to visualize how each client need interacts with other identified needs. A new technique or learning tool [concept mapping] has been developed to assist you in visualizing the linkages, to enhance your critical thinking skills, and to facilitate the creative process of planning client care (p. 32).

An example of one format for a concept map care plan is presented in Figure 1-2.

The purpose of this book is to assist students and staff nurses as they endeavor to provide high-quality nursing care to their psychiatric clients. Following is an example of a nursing history and assessment tool that may be used to gather information about the client during the assessment phase of the nursing process.

■ NURSING HISTORY AND ASSESSMENT TOOL

I. General Information

Client name:_____   Allergies: _____
Room number:_____   Diet: _____
Doctor: _____   Height/weight: _____
Age: _____   Vital signs: TPR/BP _____
Sex: _____   Name and phone no. of
                              significant other: _____
Race: _____
Dominant language:_____   City of residence: _____
Marital status: _____ Diagnosis (admitting
                              & current): _____
Chief complaint: _____ _____
_____

II. Conditions of admission

Date: _____   Time: _____
Accompanied by: _____
Route of admission (wheelchair; ambulatory; cart): _____
Admitted from: _____

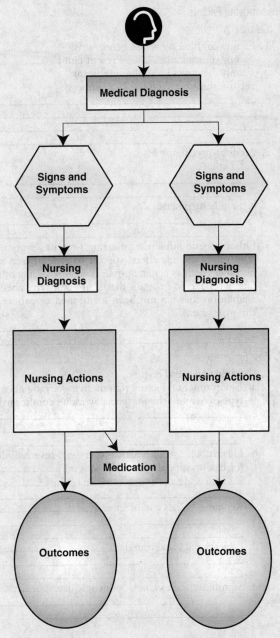

Figure 1-2: Example of a format for a concept map care plan.

III. Predisposing Factors

A. Genetic Influences

1. Family configuration (use genograms):
Family of origin: _____ Present family: _____
Family dynamics (describe significant
relationships between family members):

_____
_____
_____
_____

2. Medical/psychiatric history:
a. Client:
_____
_____

b. Family members:
_____
_____

3. Other genetic influences affecting present adaptation. This might include effects specific to gender, race, appearance, such as genetic physical defects, or any other factor related to genetics that is affecting the client's adaptation that has not been mentioned elsewhere in this assessment.

_____
_____

B. Past Experiences

1. Cultural and social history:
a. Environmental factors (family living arrangements, type of neighborhood, special working conditions):
_____
_____
_____

b. Health beliefs and practices (personal responsibility for health; special self-care practices): _____
_____
_____

c. Religious beliefs and practices: _____
_____
_____

d. Educational background: _____
_____
_____

e. Significant losses/changes (include dates): _____
_____
_____

f. Peer/friendship relationships: _____

_____

g. Occupational history: _____

_____

h. Previous pattern of coping with stress: _____

_____

i. Other lifestyle factors contributing to present adaptation: _____

_____

_____

C. *Existing Conditions*

1. Stage of development (Erikson):
   a. Theoretically: _____
   b. Behaviorally: _____
   c. Rationale: _____

   _____

   _____

2. Support systems: _____

   _____

3. Economic security: _____

   _____

4. Avenues of productivity/contribution:
   a. Current job status: _____

   _____

   b. Role contributions and responsibility for others:

   _____

IV. Precipitating Event

Describe the situation or events that precipitated this illness/hospitalization: _____

_____

_____

V. Client's Perception of the Stressor

Client's or family member's understanding or description of stressor/illness and expectations of hospitalization: _____

_____

_____

_____

VI. Adaptation Responses

A. Psychosocial

1. Anxiety level (circle level, and check the behaviors that apply):

   Mild   Moderate   Severe   Panic

   Calm _____ Friendly _____ Passive _____

   Alert _____ Perceives environment correctly _____

   Cooperative _____ Impaired attention _____

   "Jittery" _____ Unable to concentrate _____

   Hypervigilant ____ Tremors ____ Rapid speech _____

   Withdrawn _____ Confused _____

   Disoriented ____ Fearful _____ Hyperventilating _____

   Misinterpreting the environment
   (hallucinations or delusions) _____

   Depersonalization _____ Obsessions _____

   Compulsions _____ Somatic complaints _____

   Excessive hyperactivity _____ Other _____

2. Mood/affect (circle as many as apply):

   Happiness   Sadness   Dejection   Despair

   Elation   Euphoria   Suspiciousness

   Apathy (little emotional tone)   Anger/hostility

3. Ego defense mechanisms (describe how used by client):

   Projection _____

   Suppression _____

   Undoing _____

   Displacement _____

   Intellectualization _____

   Rationalization _____

   Denial _____

   Repression _____

   Isolation _____

   Regression _____

   Reaction formation _____

   Splitting _____

   Religiosity _____

   Sublimation _____

   Compensation _____

4. Level of self-esteem (circle one):

   Low   Moderate   High

   Things client likes about self: _____

   _____

   Things client would like to change about self: _____

   Nurse's objective assessment of self-esteem:

   _____

   Eye contact _____

General appearance _____

_____

Personal hygiene _____
Participation in group activities and interactions with others _____

5. Stage and manifestations of grief (circle one):
Denial   Anger   Bargaining   Depression
Acceptance
Describe the client's behaviors that are associated with this stage of grieving in response to loss or change. _____

_____

6. Thought processes (circle as many as apply):
Clear   Logical   Easy to follow   Relevant
Confused   Blocking   Delusional   Rapid flow of thoughts

Slowness in thought association   Suspicious
Recent memory: Loss   Intact
Remote memory: Loss   Intact
Other: _____

_____

7. Communication patterns (circle as many as apply):

Clear	Coherent	Slurred speech	Incoherent
Neologisms	Loose associations	Flight of ideas	
Aphasic	Perseveration	Rumination	
Tangential speech	Loquaciousness		

Slow, impoverished speech
Speech impediment (describe): _____
Other: _____

8. Interaction patterns (describe client's pattern of interpersonal interactions with staff and peers on the unit; e.g., manipulative, withdrawn, isolated, verbally or physically hostile, argumentative, passive, assertive, aggressive, passive-aggressive, other): _____

_____

9. Reality orientation (check those that apply): _____
Oriented to: Time _____   Person _____
                Place _____   Situation _____

10. Ideas of destruction to self/others?   Yes   No
    If yes, consider plan; available means: _____
    _____
    _____
    _____

B. Physiological

1. Psychosomatic manifestations (describe any somatic complaints that may be stress-related): _____
   _____
   _____
   _____

2. Drug history and assessment:
   Use of prescribed drugs:

NAME	DOSAGE	PRESCRIBED FOR	RESULTS

   Use of over-the-counter drugs:

NAME	DOSAGE	USED FOR	RESULTS

   Use of street drugs or alcohol:

NAME	AMOUNT USED	HOW OFTEN USED	WHEN LAST USED	EFFECTS PRODUCED

3. Pertinent physical assessments:
   a. Respirations: Normal _____ Labored _____
      Rate _____ Rhythm _____
   b. Skin: Warm _____ Dry _____ Moist _____
      Cool _____ Clammy _____ Pink _____
      Cyanotic _____ Poor turgor _____ Edematous _____
      Evidence of: Rash _____ Bruising _____
      Needle tracts _____ Hirsutism _____ Loss of hair _____
      Other _____
      _____
   c. Musculoskeletal status: Weakness _____
      Tremors _____

Degree of range of motion (describe limitations)
_____
_____

Pain (describe) _____
_____

Skeletal deformities (describe) _____
Coordination (describe limitations) _____

d. Neurological status:
   History of (check all that apply):
   Seizures (describe method of control) _____
   _____
   Headaches (describe location and frequency) _____
   Fainting spells _____ Dizziness _____
   Tingling/numbness (describe location) _____

e. Cardiovascular: B/P_____ Pulse _____
   History of (check all that apply):
   Hypertension _____ Palpitations _____
   Heart murmur _____ Chest pain _____
   Shortness of breath _____ Pain in legs _____
   Phlebitis _____ Ankle/leg edema _____
   Numbness/tingling in extremities _____
   Varicose veins _____

f. Gastrointestinal:
   Usual diet pattern _____
   Food allergies _____
   Dentures? Upper _____ Lower _____
   Any problems with chewing or swallowing? _____
   Any recent change in weight? _____
   Any problems with:
   Indigestion/heartburn? _____
   Relieved by _____
   Nausea/vomiting? _____
   Relieved by _____
   History of ulcers? _____
   Usual bowel pattern _____
   Constipation? _____ Diarrhea? _____
   Type of self-care assistance provided for either of
   the above problems _____
   _____

g. Genitourinary/Reproductive:
   Usual voiding pattern _____
   Urinary hesitancy? _____
   Frequency? _____
   Nocturia? _____ Pain/burning? _____
   Incontinence? _____

Any genital lesions? _____

Discharge? _____ Odor? _____

History of sexually transmitted disease? _____

If yes, please explain: _____
_____

Any concerns about sexuality/sexual activity? _____
_____

Method of birth control used _____

Females:

Date of last menstrual cycle _____

Length of cycle _____

Problems associated with menstruation? _____
_____

Breasts: Pain/tenderness? _____

Swelling? _____ Discharge? _____

Lumps? _____ Dimpling? _____

Practice breast self-examination? _____

Frequency? _____

Males:

Penile discharge? _____

Prostate problems? _____

h. Eyes:

	Yes	No	Explain
Glasses?	____	____	_____
Contacts?	____	____	_____
Swelling?	____	____	_____
Discharge?	____	____	_____
Itching?	____	____	_____
Blurring?	____	____	_____
Double vision?	____	____	_____

i. Ears:

	Yes	No	Explain
Pain?	____	____	_____
Drainage?	____	____	_____
Difficulty hearing?	____	____	_____
Hearing aid?	____	____	_____
Tinnitus?	____	____	_____

j. Medication side effects:

What symptoms is the client experiencing that may be attributed to current medication usage?
_____
_____

k. Altered lab values and possible significance: _____
_____
_____

l. Activity/rest patterns:
  Exercise (amount, type, frequency) _____
  _____

  Leisure time activities: _____
  _____

  Patterns of sleep: Number of hours per night _____
  Use of sleep aids? _____
  Pattern of awakening during the night? _____
  Feel rested upon awakening? _____

m. Personal hygiene/activities of daily living:
  Patterns of self-care: Independent _____
  Requires assistance with: Mobility _____
                              Hygiene _____
                              Toileting _____
                              Feeding _____
                              Dressing _____
                              Other _____
  Statement describing personal hygiene and
  general appearance: _____
  _____

n. Other pertinent physical assessments: _____
  _____
  _____

VII. Summary of Initial Psychosocial/Physical Assessment:

Knowledge Deficits Identified: _____
Nursing Diagnoses Indicated: _____

ALTERATIONS IN PSYCHOSOCIAL ADAPTATION

CHAPTER **2**

Disorders Commonly Associated With Infancy, Childhood, or Adolescence

■ BACKGROUND ASSESSMENT DATA

Several common psychiatric disorders may arise or become evident during infancy, childhood, or adolescence. Essential features of many disorders are identical, regardless of the age of the individual. Examples include the following:

Neurocognitive disorders
Schizophrenia
Schizophreniform disorder
Adjustment disorder
Sexual disorders

Personality disorders
Substance-related disorders
Mood disorders
Somatic symptom disorders
Psychological factors affecting
    medical condition

There are, however, several disorders that appear during the early developmental years and are identified according to the child's ability or inability to perform age-appropriate tasks or intellectual

14

functions. Selected disorders are presented here. It is essential that the nurse working with these clients understands normal behavior patterns characteristic of the infant, childhood, and adolescent years.

■ INTELLECTUAL DISABILITY (INTELLECTUAL DEVELOPMENTAL DISORDER)

Defined

The *Diagnostic and Statistical Manual of Mental Disorders, Fifth Edition (DSM-5*, American Psychiatric Association [APA], 2013) defines intellectual disability as a "disorder with onset during the developmental period that includes both intellectual and adaptive functioning deficits in conceptual, social, and practical domains" (p. 33). Onset of intellectual and adaptive deficits occurs during the developmental period. Level of severity (mild, moderate, severe, or profound) is based on adaptive functioning within the three domains.

Predisposing Factors

1. Physiological
   a. About 5% of cases of intellectual disability are caused by genetic factors, such as Tay-Sachs disease, phenylketonuria, and hyperglycinemia. Chromosomal disorders, such as Down syndrome and Klinefelter syndrome, have also been implicated.
   b. Events that occur during the prenatal period (e.g., fetal malnutrition, viral and other infections, maternal ingestion of alcohol or other drugs, and uncontrolled diabetes) and perinatal period (e.g., birth trauma or premature separation of the placenta) can result in intellectual disability.
   c. Intellectual disability can occur as an outcome of childhood illnesses, such as encephalitis or meningitis, or be the result of poisoning or physical trauma in childhood.
2. Sociocultural Factors and Other Mental Disorders
   a. An estimated 15% to 20% of cases of intellectual disability may be attributed to deprivation of nurturance and social stimulation and to impoverished environments associated with poor prenatal and perinatal care and inadequate nutrition. Additionally, severe mental disorders, such as autism spectrum disorder, can result in intellectual disability.

Symptomatology (Subjective and Objective Data)

1. At the mild level (IQ in the range of 50 to 70), the individual can live independently but with some assistance. He or she is capable of work at the sixth grade level and can learn a vocational skill. Social skills are possible, but the individual functions best in a structured, sheltered setting. Coordination may be slightly affected.

2. At the moderate level (IQ in the range of 35 to 49), the individual can perform some activities independently but requires supervision. Academic skill can be achieved to about the second grade level. The individual may experience some limitation in speech communication and in interactions with others. Motor development may be limited to gross motor ability.

3. The severe level of intellectual disability (IQ in the range of 20 to 34) is characterized by the need for complete supervision. Systematic habit training may be accomplished, but the individual does not have the ability for academic or vocational training. Verbal skills are minimal and psychomotor development is poor.

4. The individual with profound intellectual disability (IQ commonly less than 20) has no capacity for independent living. Constant aid and supervision are required. No ability exists for academic or vocational training. There is a lack of ability for speech development, socialization skills, or fine or gross motor movements. The individual requires constant supervision and care.

Common Nursing Diagnoses and Interventions for the Client With Intellectual Disability

(Interventions are applicable to various health-care settings, such as inpatient and partial hospitalization, community outpatient clinic, home health, and private practice.)

■ RISK FOR INJURY

Definition: *At risk of injury as a result of environmental conditions interacting with the individual's adaptive and defensive resources* (NANDA International [NANDA-I], 2012, p. 430)

Risk Factors ("related to")

Altered physical mobility
[Aggressive behavior]
[Developmental immaturity]

Goals/Objectives

Short-/Long-term Goal

Client will not experience injury.

Interventions With *Selected Rationales*

1. *To ensure client safety:*
   a. Create a safe environment for the client. Remove small items from the area where the client will be ambulating and move sharp items out of his or her reach.

b. Store items that client uses frequently within easy reach.
c. Pad side rails and headboard of client who has a history of seizures.
d. Prevent physical aggression and acting out behaviors by learning to recognize signs that client is becoming agitated.

Outcome Criteria

1. Client has experienced no physical harm.
2. Client responds to attempts to inhibit agitated behavior.

▥ SELF-CARE DEFICIT

Definition: *Impaired ability to perform or complete [activities of daily living] for self* (NANDA-I, 2012, pp. 250–253)

Possible Etiologies ("related to")

Musculoskeletal impairment
Cognitive impairment

Defining Characteristics ("evidenced by")

Inability to wash body
Inability to put on clothing
Inability to bring food from receptacle to the mouth
[Inability to toilet self without assistance]

Goals/Objectives

Short-term Goal
Client will be able to participate in aspects of self-care.

Long-term Goal
Client will have all self-care needs met.

Interventions With *Selected Rationales*

1. Identify aspects of self-care that may be within the client's capabilities. Work on one aspect of self-care at a time. Provide simple, concrete explanations. *Because clients' capabilities vary so widely, it is important to know each client individually and to ensure that no client is set up to fail.*
2. Offer positive feedback for efforts at assisting with own self-care. *Positive reinforcement enhances self-esteem and encourages repetition of desirable behaviors.*
3. When one aspect of self-care has been mastered to the best of the client's ability, move on to another. Encourage independence, but intervene when client is unable to perform. *Client comfort and safety are nursing priorities.*

Outcome Criteria

1. Client assists with self-care activities to the best of his or her ability.
2. Client's self-care needs are being met.

■ IMPAIRED VERBAL COMMUNICATION

Definition: *Decreased, delayed, or absent ability to receive, process, transmit, and/or use a system of symbols [to communicate]* (NANDA-I, 2012, p. 275)

Possible Etiologies ("related to")

[Developmental alteration]

Defining Characteristics ("evidenced by")

Speaks or verbalizes with difficulty
Difficulty forming words or sentences
Difficulty expressing thought verbally
Inappropriate verbalization
Does not or cannot speak

Goals/Objectives

Short-term Goal

Client will establish trust with caregiver and a means of communicating needs.

Long-term Goals

1. Client's needs are being met through established means of communication.
2. If client cannot speak or communicate by other means, needs are met by caregiver's anticipation of client's needs.

Interventions With *Selected Rationales*

1. Maintain consistency of staff assignment over time. *This facilitates trust and the ability to understand client's actions and communication.*
2. Anticipate and fulfill client's needs until satisfactory communication patterns are established. Learn (from family, if possible) special words client uses that are different from the norm.
3. Identify nonverbal gestures or signals that client may use to convey needs if verbal communication is absent. Practice these communication skills repeatedly. *Some children with intellectual disability, particularly at the severe level, can only learn by systematic habit training.*

Outcome Criteria

1. Client is able to communicate with consistent caregiver.
2. For client who is unable to communicate: Client's needs, as anticipated by caregiver, are being met.

■ IMPAIRED SOCIAL INTERACTION

Definition: *Insufficient or excessive quantity or ineffective quality of social exchange* (NANDA-I, 2012, p. 320)

Possible Etiologies ("related to")

[Speech deficiencies]
[Difficulty adhering to conventional social behavior (because of delayed maturational development)]

Defining Characteristics ("evidenced by")

Use of unsuccessful social interaction behaviors
Dysfunctional interaction with others
[Observed] discomfort in social situations

Goals/Objectives

Short-term Goal

Client will attempt to interact with others in the presence of trusted caregiver.

Long-term Goal

Client will be able to interact with others using behaviors that are socially acceptable and appropriate to developmental level.

Interventions With *Selected Rationales*

1. Remain with client during initial interactions with others. *The presence of a trusted individual provides a feeling of security*.
2. Explain to other clients the meaning of some of the client's nonverbal gestures and signals. *Others may be more accepting of the client's differentness if they have a better understanding of his or her behavior*.
3. Use simple language to explain to client which behaviors are acceptable and which are not. Establish a procedure for behavior modification that offers rewards for appropriate behaviors and renders an aversive reinforcement in response to the use of inappropriate behaviors. *Positive, negative, and aversive reinforcements can contribute to desired changes in behavior. The privileges and penalties are individually determined as caregiver learns the likes and dislikes of the client.*

Outcome Criterion

Client interacts with others in a socially appropriate manner.

■ AUTISM SPECTRUM DISORDER

Defined

Autism spectrum disorder (ASD) is characterized by a withdrawal of the child into the self and into a fantasy world of his or her own creation. Activities and interests are restricted and may be considered somewhat bizarre. In 2012, the Centers for Disease Control and Prevention reported the prevalence of ASD in the United States to be about 11.3 per 1000 (1 in 88) children. ASD includes a spectrum of symptoms based on level of severity. ASD occurs about 4.5 times more often in boys than in girls. Onset of the disorder occurs in early childhood, and, in most cases, it runs a chronic course with symptoms persisting into adulthood.

Predisposing Factors

1. **Physiological**
   a. *Genetic*. Studies have shown that parents who have one child with ASD are at increased risk for having more than one child with the disorder. Other studies with both monozygotic and dizygotic twins have also provided evidence of a genetic involvement.
   b. *Neurological*. Abnormalities in brain structures or functions have been correlated with ASD. In one study, the investigators found a disproportionate enlargement in temporal lobe white matter and an increase in surface area in the temporal, frontal, and parieto-occipital lobes (Hazlett et al., 2011). Certain developmental problems, such as postnatal neurological infections, congenital rubella, phenylketonuria, and fragile X syndrome, also have been implicated.
2. **Environmental**
   a. The *DSM-5* reports that "a variety of nonspecific risk factors, such as advanced parental age, low birth weight, or fetal exposure to valproate, may contribute to risk of ASD" (p. 56).

Symptomatology (Subjective and Objective Data)

1. Failure to form interpersonal relationships, characterized by unresponsiveness to people; lack of eye contact and facial responsiveness; indifference or aversion to affection and physical contact. In early childhood, there is a failure to develop cooperative play and friendships.
2. Impairment in communication and imaginative activity. Language may be totally absent or characterized by immature grammatical structure, incorrect use of words, echolalia, or inability

to use abstract terms. Accompanying nonverbal expressions may be inappropriate or absent.
3. Bizarre responses to the environment, characterized by resistance or extreme behavioral reactions to minor occurrences; abnormal, obsessive attachment to peculiar objects; ritualistic behaviors.
4. Extreme fascination for objects that move (e.g., fans, trains). Special interest in music, playing with water, buttons, or parts of the body.
5. Unreasonable insistence on following routines in precise detail (e.g., insisting that exactly the same route always be followed when shopping).
6. Marked distress over changes in trivial aspects of environment (e.g., when a vase is moved from its usual position).
7. Stereotyped body movements (e.g., hand flicking or clapping, rocking, or whole-body swaying).
8. Behaviors that are self-injurious, such as head banging or biting the hands or arms, may be evident.

Common Nursing Diagnoses and Interventions for the Client With ASD

(Interventions are applicable to various health-care settings, such as inpatient and partial hospitalization, community outpatient clinic, home health, and private practice.)

■ RISK FOR SELF-MUTILATION

Definition: *At risk for deliberate self-injurious behavior causing tissue damage with the intent of causing nonfatal injury to attain relief of tension* (NANDA-I, 2012, p. 451)

Risk Factors ("related to")

[Neurological alterations]
[History of self-mutilative behaviors in response to increasing anxiety]
[Obvious indifference to environment or hysterical reactions to changes in the environment]

Goals/Objectives

Short-term Goal

Client will demonstrate alternative behavior (e.g., initiating interaction between self and nurse) in response to anxiety within specified time. (Length of time required for this objective will depend on severity and chronicity of the disorder.)

Long-term Goal
Client will not harm self.

Interventions With *Selected Rationales*

1. Intervene to protect child when self-mutilative behaviors, such as head banging or other hysterical behaviors, become evident. *The nurse is responsible for ensuring client safety.*
2. A helmet may be used to protect against head banging, hand mitts to prevent hair pulling, and appropriate padding to protect extremities from injury during hysterical movements.
3. Try to determine if self-mutilative behaviors occur in response to increasing anxiety, and if so, to what the anxiety may be attributed. *Mutilative behaviors may be averted if the cause can be determined.*
4. Work on one-to-one basis with child *to establish trust.*
5. Offer self to child during times of increasing anxiety, *in order to decrease need for self-mutilative behaviors and provide feelings of security.*

Outcome Criteria

1. Anxiety is maintained at a level at which client feels no need for self-mutilation.
2. When feeling anxious, client initiates interaction between self and nurse.

■ IMPAIRED SOCIAL INTERACTION

Definition: *Insufficient or excessive quantity or ineffective quality of social exchange* (NANDA-I, 2012, p. 320)

Possible Etiologies ("related to")

Self-concept disturbance
Absence of [available] significant others
[Unfulfilled tasks of trust versus mistrust]
[Neurological alterations]

Defining Characteristics ("evidenced by")

[Lack of responsiveness to, or interest in, people]
[Failure to cuddle]
[Lack of eye contact and facial responsiveness]
[Indifference or aversion to affection and physical contact]
[Failure to develop cooperative play and peer friendships]

Goals/Objectives

Short-term Goal

Client will demonstrate trust in one caregiver (as evidenced by facial responsiveness and eye contact) within specified time (depending on severity and chronicity of disorder).

Long-term Goal

Client will initiate social interactions (physical, verbal, nonverbal) with caregiver by discharge from treatment.

Interventions With *Selected Rationales*

1. Assign a limited number of caregivers to the child. Ensure that warmth, acceptance, and availability are conveyed. *Warmth, acceptance, and availability, along with consistency of staff assignment, enhance the establishment and maintenance of a trusting relationship.*
2. Provide child with familiar objects (favorite toys, blanket). *These items will offer security during times when the child feels distressed.* Go slowly. Do not force interactions. Begin with positive reinforcement for eye contact.
3. Gradually introduce touch, smiling, hugging. *The client with ASD may feel threatened by an onslaught of stimuli to which he or she is unaccustomed.*
4. Support client with your presence as he or she endeavors to relate to others in the environment. *The presence of an individual with whom a trusting relationship has been established provides a feeling of security.*

Outcome Criteria

1. Client initiates interactions between self and others.
2. Client uses eye contact, facial responsiveness, and other nonverbal behaviors in interactions with others.
3. Client does not withdraw from physical contact.

▧ IMPAIRED VERBAL COMMUNICATION

Definition: *Decreased, delayed, or absent ability to receive, process, transmit, and/or use a system of symbols [to communicate]* (NANDA-I, 2012, p. 275)

Possible Etiologies ("related to")

[Inability to trust]
[Withdrawal into the self]
[Neurological alterations]

Defining Characteristics ("evidenced by")

Does not or cannot speak.
[Immature grammatical structure]
[Echolalia]
[Pronoun reversal]
[Inability to name objects]
[Inability to use abstract terms]
[Absence of nonverbal expression (e.g., eye contact, facial responsiveness, gestures)]

Goals/Objectives

Short-term Goal

Client will establish trust with one caregiver (as evidenced by facial responsiveness and eye contact) by specified time (depending on severity and chronicity of disorder).

Long-term Goal

Client will establish a means of communicating needs and desires to others by time of discharge from treatment.

Interventions With *Selected Rationales*

1. Maintain consistency in assignment of caregivers. ***Consistency facilitates trust and enhances the caregiver's ability to understand the child's attempts to communicate.***
2. Anticipate and fulfill client's needs until satisfactory communication patterns are established. ***Anticipating needs helps to minimize frustration as the child is learning communication skills.***
3. ◉ Use the techniques of *consensual validation* and *seeking clarification* to decode communication patterns. (Examples: "I think you must have meant . . ." or "Did you mean to say that . . . ?"). (See Appendix E.) ***These techniques work to verify the accuracy of the message received or to clarify any hidden meanings within the message. Take caution not to "put words into the client's mouth."***
4. Give positive reinforcement when eye contact is used to convey nonverbal expressions. ***Positive reinforcement increases self-esteem and encourages repetition of the behavior.***

Outcome Criteria

1. Client is able to communicate in a manner that is understood by others.
2. Client's nonverbal messages are congruent with verbalizations.
3. Client initiates verbal and nonverbal interaction with others.

▓ DISTURBED PERSONAL IDENTITY

Definition*: Inability to maintain an integrated and complete perception of self* (NANDA-I, 2012, p. 282)

Possible Etiologies ("related to")

[Unfulfilled tasks of trust versus mistrust]
[Neurological alterations]
[Inadequate sensory stimulation]

Defining Characteristics ("evidenced by")

[Inability to separate own physiological and emotional needs from those of others]
[Increased levels of anxiety resulting from contact with others]
[Inability to differentiate own body boundaries from those of others]
[Repeating words he or she hears others say or mimicking movements of others]
Unable to distinguish between inner and outer stimuli

Goals/Objectives

Short-term Goal

Client will name own body parts as separate and individual from those of others (within specified time, depending on severity and chronicity of disorder).

Long-term Goal

Client will develop ego identity (evidenced by ability to recognize physical and emotional self as separate from others) by time of discharge from treatment.

Interventions With *Selected Rationales*

1. Function in a one-to-one relationship with the child. ***Consistency of staff-client interaction enhances the establishment of trust.***
2. Assist child to recognize separateness during self-care activities, such as dressing and feeding. ***These activities increase child's awareness of self as separate from others.***
3. Point out and assist child in naming own body parts. ***This activity may increase the child's awareness of self as separate from others.***
4. Gradually increase amount of physical contact, using touch to point out differences between client and nurse. Be cautious with touch until trust is established, ***because this gesture may be interpreted by the client as threatening.***

5. Use mirrors and drawings or pictures of the child to reinforce the child's learning of body parts and boundaries.

Outcome Criteria

1. Client is able to differentiate own body parts from those of others.
2. Client communicates ability to separate self from environment by discontinuing use of echolalia (repeating words heard) and echopraxia (imitating movements seen).

■ DISRUPTIVE BEHAVIOR DISORDERS

Attention-Deficit/Hyperactivity Disorder

Defined

Attention-deficit/hyperactivity disorder (ADHD) is characterized by a "persistent pattern of inattention and/or hyperactivity-impulsivity that interferes with functioning or development" (APA, 2013, p. 61). The disorder often is not diagnosed until the child begins school because, prior to that time, childhood behavior is much more variable than that of older children. ADHD is more common in boys than in girls by a ratio of approximately 3 to 1 and may occur in as many as 9% of school-age children (CDC, 2011). The course can be chronic, persisting into adulthood. The *DSM-5* further categorizes the disorder according to current clinical presentation. These subtypes include a combined presentation (meeting the criteria for both inattention and hyperactivity/impulsivity), a predominantly inattentive presentation, and a predominantly hyperactive/impulsive presentation.

Predisposing Factors

1. **Physiological**
   a. *Genetic.* A number of studies have indicated that hereditary factors may be implicated in the predisposition to ADHD. Siblings of hyperactive children are more likely than normal children to have the disorder. Results of some studies have indicated that a large number of parents of hyperactive children showed signs of hyperactivity during their own childhood.
   b. ***Biochemical.*** Abnormal levels of the neurotransmitters dopamine, norepinephrine, and possibly serotonin have been suggested as a causative factor.
   c. ***Prenatal, Perinatal, and Postnatal.*** Maternal smoking during pregnancy has been linked to ADHD in offspring (Linnet et al., 2005; Rizwan, Manning, & Brabin, 2007). Intrauterine exposure to toxic substances, including alcohol, can produce effects on behavior. Premature birth, fetal distress, precipitated or prolonged labor, and perinatal asphyxia have also been implicated. Postnatal factors include

cerebral palsy, epilepsy, and other central nervous system abnormalities resulting from trauma, infections, or other neurological disorders.

2. **Psychosocial**
    a. *Environmental Influences.* Disorganized or chaotic environments or a disruption in family equilibrium may predispose some individuals to ADHD. A high degree of psychosocial stress, maternal mental disorder, paternal criminality, low socioeconomic status, poverty, growing up in an institution, and unstable foster care are factors that have been implicated (Dopheide & Pliszka, 2009; Voeller, 2004).

Symptomatology (Subjective and Objective Data)

1. Difficulties in performing age-appropriate tasks.
2. Highly distractible.
3. Extremely limited attention span.
4. Shifts from one uncompleted activity to another.
5. Impulsivity, or deficit in inhibitory control, is common.
6. Difficulty forming satisfactory interpersonal relationships.
7. Disruptive and intrusive behaviors inhibit acceptable social interaction.
8. Difficulty complying with social norms.
9. Some children with ADHD are very aggressive or oppositional. Others exhibit more regressive and immature behaviors.
10. Low frustration tolerance and outbursts of temper are common.
11. Boundless energy, exhibiting excessive levels of activity, restlessness, and fidgeting.
12. Often described as "perpetual motion machines," continuously running, jumping, wiggling, or squirming.
13. They experience a greater than average number of accidents, from minor mishaps to more serious incidents that may lead to physical injury or the destruction of property.

Conduct Disorder

Defined

The *DSM-5* describes the essential feature of this disorder as a "repetitive and persistent pattern of behavior in which the basic rights of others or major age-appropriate societal norms or rules are violated" (APA, 2013, p. 472). The behavior is more serious than the ordinary mischief and pranks of children and adolescents. The disorder is more common in boys than in girls, and the behaviors may continue into adulthood, often meeting the criteria for antisocial personality disorder. Conduct disorder is divided into two subtypes based on the age at onset: childhood-onset type (onset of symptoms before age 10 years) and adolescent-onset type (absence of symptoms before age 10 years).

Predisposing Factors

1. **Physiological**
   a. ***Birth Temperament.*** The term temperament refers to personality traits that become evident very early in life and may be present at birth. Evidence suggests a genetic component in temperament and an association between temperament and behavioral problems later in life.
   b. ***Genetics.*** Family, twin, and adoptive studies have revealed a significantly higher number of conduct disorders among those who have family members with the disorder.
2. **Psychosocial**
   a. ***Peer Relationships.*** Social groups have a significant impact on a child's development. Peers play an essential role in the socialization of interpersonal competence, and skills acquired in this manner affect the child's long-term adjustment. Studies have shown that poor peer relations during childhood were consistently implicated in the etiology of later deviance (Ladd, 1999). Aggression was found to be the principal cause of peer rejection, thus contributing to a cycle of maladaptive behavior.
   b. ***Theory of Family Dynamics.*** The following factors related to family dynamics have been implicated as contributors in the predisposition to this disorder (Foley et al., 2004; Sadock & Sadock, 2007; Ursano et al., 2008):
      • Parental rejection
      • Inconsistent management with harsh discipline
      • Early institutional living
      • Frequent shifting of parental figures
      • Large family size
      • Absent father
      • Parents with antisocial personality disorder and/or alcohol dependence
      • Marital conflict and divorce
      • Inadequate communication patterns
      • Parental permissiveness

Symptomatology (Subjective and Objective Data)

1. Uses physical aggression in the violation of the rights of others.
2. The behavior pattern manifests itself in virtually all areas of the child's life (home, school, with peers, and in the community).
3. Stealing, fighting, lying, and truancy are common problems.
4. There is an absence of feelings of guilt or remorse.
5. The use of tobacco, liquor, or nonprescribed drugs, as well as the participation in sexual activities, occurs earlier than the peer group's expected age.
6. Projection is a common defense mechanism.
7. Low self-esteem is manifested by a "tough guy" image. Often threatens and intimidates others.

8. Characteristics include poor frustration tolerance, irritability, and frequent temper outbursts.
9. Symptoms of anxiety and depression are not uncommon.
10. Level of academic achievement may be low in relation to age and IQ.
11. Manifestations associated with ADHD (e.g., attention difficulties, impulsiveness, and hyperactivity) are very common in children with conduct disorder.

Oppositional Defiant Disorder

Defined

Oppositional defiant disorder (ODD) is characterized by a pattern of angry mood and defiant behavior that occurs more frequently than is usually observed in individuals of comparable age and developmental level and interferes with social, occupational, or other important areas of functioning (APA, 2013). The disorder typically begins by 8 years of age and usually not later than early adolescence. The disorder is more prevalent in boys than in girls before puberty, but the rates are more closely equal after puberty. In some cases of ODD, there may be a progression to conduct disorder (Lubit, 2013).

Predisposing Factors

1. **Physiological**
   a. Refer to this section under Conduct Disorder.
2. **Psychosocial**
   a. *Theory of Family Dynamics*. It is thought that some parents interpret average or increased levels of developmental oppositionalism as hostility and a deliberate effort on the part of the child to be in control. If power and control are issues for parents or if they exercise authority for their own needs, a power struggle can be established between the parents and the child that sets the stage for the development of ODD.

Symptomatology (Subjective and Objective Data)

1. Characterized by passive-aggressive behaviors such as stubbornness, procrastination, disobedience, carelessness, negativism, testing of limits, resistance to directions, deliberately ignoring the communication of others, and unwillingness to compromise.
2. Other symptoms that may be evident are running away, school avoidance, school underachievement, temper tantrums, fighting, and argumentativeness.
3. In severe cases, there may be elective mutism, enuresis, encopresis, or eating and sleeping problems.
4. Blames others for mistakes and misbehavior.
5. Has poor peer relationships.

Common Nursing Diagnoses and Interventions for Clients
With Disruptive Behavior Disorders

(Interventions are applicable to various health-care settings, such as in-patient and partial hospitalization, community outpatient clinic, home health, and private practice.)

■ RISK FOR SELF-DIRECTED OR OTHER-DIRECTED VIOLENCE

Definition: *At risk for behaviors in which an individual demonstrates that he or she can be physically, emotionally, and/or sexually harmful [either to self or to others]* (NANDA-I, 2012, p. 447–448)

Risk Factors ("related to")

[Unsatisfactory parent-child relationship]
[Neurological alteration related to premature birth, fetal distress, precipitated or prolonged labor]
[Dysfunctional family system]
[Disorganized or chaotic environments]
[Child abuse or neglect]
[Birth temperament]
Body language (e.g., rigid posture, clenching of fists and jaw, hyperactivity, pacing, breathlessness, threatening stances)
[History or threats of violence toward self or others or of destruction to the property of others]
Impulsivity
[History of] cruelty to animals
Suicidal ideation, plan, [available means]

Goals/Objectives

Short-term Goals

1. Client will seek out staff at any time if thoughts of harming self or others should occur.
2. Client will not harm self or others.

Long-term Goal

Client will not harm self or others.

Interventions With *Selected Rationales*

1. Observe client's behavior frequently. Do this through routine activities and interactions to avoid appearing watchful and suspicious. ***Clients at high risk for violence require close observation to prevent harm to self or others.***

2. Observe for suicidal behaviors: Verbal statements, such as "I'm going to kill myself," or "Very soon my mother won't have to worry herself about me any longer," or nonverbal behaviors, such as giving away cherished items or mood swings. *Most clients who attempt suicide have communicated their intent, either verbally or nonverbally.*

3. Determine suicidal intent and available means. Ask, "Do you plan to kill yourself?" and "How do you plan to do it?" *Direct, closed-ended questions are appropriate in this instance. The client who has a usable plan is at higher risk than one who does not.*

4. Obtain verbal or written contract from client agreeing not to harm self and agreeing to seek out staff in the event that such ideation occurs. *Discussion of suicidal feelings with a trusted individual provides a degree of relief to the client. A contract gets the subject out in the open and places some of the responsibility for his or her safety with the client. An attitude of acceptance of the client as a worthwhile individual is conveyed.*

5. Help client to recognize when anger occurs and to accept those feelings as his or her own. Have client keep an "anger notebook," in which a record of anger experienced on a 24-hour basis is kept. Information regarding source of anger, behavioral response, and client's perception of the situation should also be noted. Discuss entries with client, suggesting alternative behavioral responses for those identified as maladaptive.

6. Act as a role model for appropriate expression of angry feelings and give positive reinforcement to client for attempting to conform. *It is vital that the client express angry feelings, because suicide and other self-destructive behaviors are often viewed as a result of anger turned inward on the self.*

7. Remove all dangerous objects from client's environment. *The client's physical safety is a nursing priority.*

8. Try to redirect violent behavior with physical outlets for the client's anxiety (e.g., punching bag, jogging, volleyball). *Anxiety and tension can be relieved safely and with benefit to the client in this manner.*

9. Be available to stay with client as anxiety level and tensions begin to rise. *The presence of a trusted individual provides a feeling of security.*

10. Staff should maintain and convey a calm attitude to client. Anxiety is contagious and can be communicated from staff to client and vice versa. *A calm attitude conveys a sense of control and a feeling of security to the client.*

11. Have sufficient staff available to indicate a show of strength to client if it becomes necessary. *This conveys to the client an evidence of control over the situation and provides some physical security for staff.*

12. Administer tranquilizing medications as ordered by physician, or obtain an order if necessary. Monitor medication for effectiveness and for adverse side effects. *Short-term use of antianxiety medications (e.g., chlordiazepoxide, alprazolam, lorazepam) provide relief from the immobilizing effects of anxiety and facilitate client's cooperation with therapy.*

13. Mechanical restraints or isolation room may be required if less restrictive interventions are unsuccessful. *It is the client's right to expect the use of techniques that ensure safety of the client and others by the least restrictive means.*

Outcome Criteria

1. Anxiety is maintained at a level at which client feels no need for aggression.
2. Client seeks out staff to discuss true feelings.
3. Client recognizes, verbalizes, and accepts possible consequences of own maladaptive behaviors.
4. Client does not harm self or others.

■ DEFENSIVE COPING

Definition: *Repeated projection of falsely positive self-evaluation based on a self-protective pattern that defends against underlying perceived threats to positive self-regard* (NANDA-I, 2012, p. 346)

Possible Etiologies ("related to")

[Low self-esteem]
[Negative role models]
[Lack of positive feedback]
[Repeated negative feedback, resulting in feelings of diminished self-worth]
[Unsatisfactory parent-child relationship]
[Disorganized or chaotic environments]
[Child abuse or neglect]
[Dysfunctional family system]
[Neurological alteration related to premature birth, fetal distress, precipitated or prolonged labor]

Defining Characteristics ("evidenced by")

Denial of obvious problems or weaknesses
Projection of blame or responsibility
Rationalization of failures
Hypersensitivity to criticism
Grandiosity
Superior attitude toward others

Difficulty establishing or maintaining relationships
Hostile laughter or ridicule of others
Difficulty in perception of reality testing
Lack of follow-through or participation in treatment or therapy

Goals/Objectives

Short-term Goal

Client will verbalize personal responsibility for difficulties experienced in interpersonal relationships.

Long-term Goal

Client will demonstrate ability to interact with others without becoming defensive, rationalizing behaviors, or expressing grandiose ideas.

Interventions With *Selected Rationales*

1. Recognize and support basic ego strengths. *Focusing on positive aspects of the personality may help to improve self-concept.*
2. Encourage client to recognize and verbalize feelings of inadequacy and need for acceptance from others and to recognize how these feelings provoke defensive behaviors, such as blaming others for own behaviors. *Recognition of the problem is the first step in the change process toward resolution.*
3. Provide immediate, matter-of-fact, nonthreatening feedback for unacceptable behaviors. *Client may not realize how these behaviors are being perceived by others. Providing this information in a nonthreatening manner may help to eliminate these undesirable behaviors.*

CLINICAL PEARL ☺ Say to the client, "When you say those things to people, they don't like it, and they don't want to be around you. Try to think how you would feel if someone said those things to you."

4. Help client identify situations that provoke defensiveness and practice through role play more appropriate responses. *Role playing provides confidence to deal with difficult situations when they actually occur.*
5. Provide immediate positive feedback for acceptable behaviors. *Positive feedback enhances self-esteem and encourages repetition of desirable behaviors.*
6. Help client set realistic, concrete goals and determine appropriate actions to meet those goals. *Success increases self-esteem.*
7. With client, evaluate the effectiveness of the new behaviors and discuss any modifications for improvement. *Because of limited problem-solving ability, assistance may be required to reassess and develop new strategies in the event that some new coping methods prove ineffective.*

Outcome Criteria

1. Client verbalizes and accepts responsibility for own behavior.
2. Client verbalizes correlation between feelings of inadequacy and the need to defend the ego through rationalization and grandiosity.
3. Client does not ridicule or criticize others.
4. Client interacts with others in group situations without taking a defensive stance.

■ IMPAIRED SOCIAL INTERACTION

Definition: *Insufficient or excessive quantity or ineffective quality of social exchange* (NANDA-I, 2012, p. 320)

Possible Etiologies ("related to")

Self-concept disturbance
[Neurological alterations related to premature birth, fetal distress, precipitated or prolonged labor]
[Dysfunctional family system]
[Disorganized or chaotic environments]
[Child abuse or neglect]
[Unsatisfactory parent-child relationship]
[Negative role models]

Defining Characteristics ("evidenced by")

[Verbalized or observed] discomfort in social situations
[Verbalized or observed] inability to receive or communicate a satisfying sense of belonging, caring, interest, or shared history
[Observed] use of unsuccessful social interaction behaviors
Dysfunctional interaction with others
[Behavior unacceptable for appropriate age by dominant cultural group]

Goals/Objectives

Short-term Goal

Client will interact in age-appropriate manner with nurse in one-to-one relationship within 1 week.

Long-term Goal

By time of discharge from treatment, client will be able to interact with staff and peers using age-appropriate, acceptable behaviors.

Interventions With *Selected Rationales*

1. Develop trusting relationship with client. Be honest; keep all promises; convey acceptance of the person, separate from

unacceptable behaviors ("It is not *you*, but *your behavior*, that is unacceptable.") *Acceptance of the client increases his or her feelings of self-worth.*

2. Offer to remain with client during initial interactions with others. *Presence of a trusted individual provides a feeling of security.*

3. Provide constructive criticism and positive reinforcement for client's efforts. *Positive feedback enhances self-esteem and encourages repetition of desirable behaviors.*

4. Confront client and withdraw attention when interactions with others are manipulative or exploitative. *Attention to the unacceptable behavior may reinforce it.*

5. Act as a role model for client through appropriate interactions with other clients and staff members.

6. Provide group situations for client. *It is through these group interactions that client will learn socially acceptable behavior, with positive and negative feedback from his or her peers.*

Outcome Criteria

1. Client seeks out staff member for social, as well as therapeutic interaction.

2. Client has formed and satisfactorily maintained one interpersonal relationship with another client.

3. Client willingly and appropriately participates in group activities.

4. Client verbalizes reasons for past inability to form close interpersonal relationships.

▨ INEFFECTIVE COPING

Definition: *Inability to form a valid appraisal of the stressors, inadequate choices of practiced responses, and/or inability to use available resources* (NANDA-I, 2012, p. 348)

Possible Etiologies ("related to")

Situational crisis
Maturational crisis
[Inadequate support systems]
[Inadequate coping strategies]
[Negative role models]
[Neurological alteration related to premature birth, fetal distress, precipitated or prolonged labor]
[Low self-esteem]
[Dysfunctional family system]
[Disorganized or chaotic environments]
[Child abuse or neglect]

Defining Characteristics ("evidenced by")

Inability to meet [age-appropriate] role expectations
Inadequate problem solving
Poor concentration
Risk taking
[Manipulation of others in the environment for purposes of fulfilling own desires]
[Verbal hostility toward staff and peers]
[Hyperactivity, evidenced by excessive motor activity, easily distracted, short attention span]
[Unable to delay gratification]
[Oppositional and defiant responses to adult requests or rules]

Goals/Objectives

Short-term Goal

Within 7 days, client will demonstrate ability and willingness to follow rules of the treatment setting.

Long-term Goal

By discharge from treatment, client will develop and utilize, age-appropriate, socially acceptable coping skills.

Interventions With *Selected Rationales*

1. If client is hyperactive, make environment safe for continuous large muscle movement. Rearrange furniture and other objects to prevent injury. *Client physical safety is a nursing priority.*
2. Provide large motor activities in which client may participate. Nurse may join in some of these activities *to facilitate relationship development. Tension is released safely and with benefit to the client through physical activities.*
3. Provide frequent, nutritious snacks that client may "eat on the run" *to ensure adequate calories to offset client's excessive use of energy.*

CLINICAL PEARL ◉ Set limits on manipulative behavior. Say, "I understand why you are saying these things (or doing these things) and I will not tolerate these behaviors from you." Take caution not to reinforce manipulative behaviors by providing desired attention.

4. Identify for the client the consequences of manipulative behavior. All staff must follow through and be consistent. *Client may try to play one staff member against another, so consistency is vital if intervention is to be successful. Aversive reinforcement may work to decrease unacceptable behaviors.*
5. Do not debate, argue, rationalize, or bargain with the client. *Ignoring these attempts may work to decrease manipulative behaviors.*

6. Caution should be taken to avoid reinforcing manipulative behaviors by providing desired attention. *Attention provides positive reinforcement and encourages repetition of the undesirable behavior.*

7. Confront client's use of manipulative behaviors and explore their damaging effects on interpersonal relationships. *Manipulative clients often deny responsibility for their behaviors.*

8. Encourage discussion of angry feelings. Help client identify the true object of the hostility. *Dealing with the feelings honestly and directly will discourage displacement of the anger onto others.*

9. Explore with client alternative ways of handling frustration that would be most suited to his or her lifestyle. Provide support and positive feedback to client as new coping strategies are tried. *Positive feedback encourages use of the acceptable behaviors.*

Outcome Criteria

1. Client is able to delay gratification without resorting to manipulation of others.
2. Client is able to express anger in a socially acceptable manner.
3. Client is able to verbalize alternative, socially acceptable, and lifestyle-appropriate coping skills he or she plans to use in response to frustration.

■ LOW SELF-ESTEEM

Definition: *Negative self-evaluating/feelings about self or self-capabilities* (NANDA-I, 2012, pp. 285–287)

Possible Etiologies ("related to")

[Negative role models]
Lack of approval
Repeated negative reinforcement
[Unsatisfactory parent-child relationship]
[Disorganized or chaotic environments]
[Child abuse or neglect]
[Dysfunctional family system]

Defining Characteristics ("evidenced by")

Lack of eye contact
Exaggerates negative feedback about self
Expressions of shame or guilt
Evaluation of self as unable to deal with events
Rejects positive feedback about self

Hesitant to try new things or situations
[Denial of problems obvious to others]
[Projection of blame or responsibility for problems]
[Rationalization of personal failures]
[Hypersensitivity to criticism]
[Grandiosity]

Goals/Objectives

Short-term Goal

Client will independently direct own care and activities of daily living within 1 week.

Long-term Goal

By time of discharge from treatment, client will exhibit increased feelings of self-worth as evidenced by verbal expression of positive aspects about self, past accomplishments, and future prospects.

Interventions With *Selected Rationales*

1. Ensure that goals are realistic. It is important for client to achieve something, so plan for activities in which the possibility for success is likely. *Success enhances self-esteem.*
2. Convey unconditional positive regard for client. *Communication of your acceptance of him or her as a worthwhile human being increases self-esteem.*
3. Spend time with client, both on a one-to-one basis and in group activities. *This conveys to client that you feel he or she is worth your time.*
4. Assist client in identifying positive aspects of self and in developing plans for changing the characteristics he or she views as negative.
5. Help client decrease use of denial as a defense mechanism. Give positive reinforcement for problem identification and development of more adaptive coping behaviors. *Positive reinforcement enhances self-esteem and increases client's use of acceptable behaviors.*
6. Encourage and support client in confronting the fear of failure by having client attend therapy activities and undertake new tasks. Offer recognition of successful endeavors and positive reinforcement for attempts made. *Recognition and positive reinforcement enhance self-esteem.*

Outcome Criteria

1. Client verbalizes positive perception of self.
2. Client participates in new activities without exhibiting extreme fear of failure.

■ ANXIETY (Moderate to Severe)

Definition: *Vague uneasy feeling of discomfort or dread accompanied by an autonomic response (the source often nonspecific or unknown to the individual); a feeling of apprehension caused by anticipation of danger. It is an alerting signal that warns of impending danger and enables the individual to take measures to deal with threat* (NANDA-I, 2012, p. 344)

Possible Etiologies ("related to")

Situational and maturational crises
Threat to self-concept [perceived or real]
Threat of death
Unmet needs
[Fear of failure]
[Dysfunctional family system]
[Unsatisfactory parent-child relationship]
[Innately, easily agitated temperament since birth]

Defining Characteristics ("evidenced by")

Overexcited
Fearful
Feelings of inadequacy
Fear of unspecified consequences
Restlessness
Insomnia
Poor eye contact
Focus on self
[Continuous attention-seeking behaviors]
Difficulty concentrating
Impaired attention
Increased respiration and pulse

Goals/Objectives

Short-term Goals

1. Within 7 days, client will be able to verbalize behaviors that become evident as anxiety starts to rise.
2. Within 7 days, client will be able to verbalize strategies to interrupt escalation of anxiety.

Long-term Goal

By time of discharge from treatment, client will be able to maintain anxiety below the moderate level as evidenced by absence of disabling behaviors in response to stress.

Interventions With *Selected Rationales*

1. Establish a trusting relationship with client. Be honest, consistent in responses, and available. Show genuine positive regard. *Honesty, availability, and acceptance promote trust in the nurse-client relationship.*
2. Provide activities geared toward reduction of tension and decreasing anxiety (walking or jogging, volleyball, musical exercises, housekeeping chores, group games). *Tension and anxiety are released safely and with benefit to the client through physical activities.*
3. Encourage client to identify true feelings and to acknowledge ownership of those feelings. *Anxious clients often deny a relationship between emotional problems and their anxiety. Use of the defense mechanisms of projection and displacement is exaggerated.*
4. The nurse must maintain an atmosphere of calmness; *anxiety is easily transmitted from one person to another.*
5. Offer support during times of elevated anxiety. Reassure client of physical and psychological safety. *Client safety is a nursing priority.*
6. Use of touch is comforting to some clients. However, the nurse must be cautious with its use, *because anxiety may foster suspicion in some individuals who might misinterpret touch as aggression.*
7. As anxiety diminishes, assist client to recognize specific events that preceded its onset. Work on alternative responses to future occurrences. *A plan of action provides the client with a feeling of security for handling a difficult situation more successfully should it recur.*
8. Help client recognize signs of escalating anxiety and explore ways client may intervene before behaviors become disabling.
9. Administer tranquilizing medication, as ordered. Assess for effectiveness and instruct client regarding possible adverse side effects. *Short-term use of antianxiety medications (e.g., lorazepam, chlordiazepoxide, alprazolam) provides relief from the immobilizing effects of anxiety and facilitates client's cooperation with therapy.*

Outcome Criteria

1. Client is able to verbalize behaviors that become evident when anxiety starts to rise and takes appropriate action to interrupt progression of the condition.
2. Client is able to maintain anxiety at a manageable level.

■ NONCOMPLIANCE

Definition: *Behavior of person and/or caregiver that fails to coincide with a health-promoting or therapeutic plan agreed on by the person [or caregiver] and health-care professional. In the presence of an agreed-upon, health-promoting, or therapeutic plan, person's or caregiver's behavior is fully or partially nonadherent and may lead to clinically ineffective or partially ineffective outcomes* (NANDA-I, 2012, p. 400)

Possible Etiologies ("related to")

[Biochemical alteration]
[Neurological alteration related to premature birth, fetal distress, precipitated, or prolonged labor]
[Negative temperament]
[Dysfunctional family system]
[Negative role models]
[Retarded ego development]
[Low frustration tolerance and short attention span]
[Denial of problems]

Defining Characteristics ("evidenced by")

Behavior indicative of failure to adhere [to treatment regimen]
[Inability to sit still long enough to complete a task]
[Expression of opposition to requests for participation]
[Refusal to follow directions or suggestions of treatment team]

Goals/Objectives

Short-term Goal

Client will participate in and cooperate during therapeutic activities.

Long-term Goal

Client will complete assigned tasks willingly and independently or with a minimum of assistance.

Interventions With *Selected Rationales*

For the client with inattention and hyperactivity:

1. Provide an environment for task efforts that is as free of distractions as possible. ***Client is highly distractible and is unable to perform in the presence of even minimal stimulation.***
2. Provide assistance on a one-to-one basis, beginning with simple, concrete instructions. ***Client lacks the ability to assimilate information that is complicated or has abstract meaning.***
3. Ask that instructions be repeated ***to determine client's level of comprehension.***

4. Establish goals that allow client to complete a part of the task, rewarding completion of each step with a break for physical activity. ***Short-term goals are not so overwhelming to the client with such a short attention span. The positive reinforcement (physical activity) increases self-esteem and provides incentive for client to pursue the task to completion.***

5. Gradually decrease the amount of assistance given to task performance, while assuring the client that assistance is still available if deemed necessary. ***This encourages the client to perform independently while providing a feeling of security with the presence of a trusted individual.***

For the client with oppositional tendencies:

6. Set forth a structured plan of therapeutic activities. Start with minimum expectations and increase as client begins to manifest evidence of compliance. ***Structure provides security, and one or two activities may not seem as overwhelming as the whole schedule of activities presented at one time.***

7. Establish a system of rewards for compliance with therapy and consequences for noncompliance. Ensure that the rewards and consequences are concepts of value to the client. ***Positive and negative reinforcements can contribute to desired changes in behavior.***

8. Convey acceptance of the client separate from the undesirable behaviors being exhibited. ("It is not *you*, but *your behavior*, that is unacceptable.") ***Unconditional acceptance enhances self-worth and may contribute to a decrease in the need for passive-aggressive behavior toward others.***

Outcome Criteria

1. Client cooperates with staff in an effort to complete assigned tasks.
2. Client complies with treatment by participating in therapies without negativism.
3. Client takes direction from staff without becoming defensive.

■ TOURETTE'S DISORDER

Defined

Tourette's disorder is characterized by the presence of multiple motor tics and one or more vocal tics, which may appear simultaneously or at different periods during the illness (APA, 2013). Onset of the disorder can be as early as 2 years, but it occurs most commonly during childhood (around age 6 to 7 years). Tourette's disorder is more common in boys than in girls. Although the disorder can be lifelong, the symptoms usually diminish during adolescence and adulthood and, in some cases, disappear altogether by early adulthood.

Predisposing Factors

1. **Physiological**
   a. *Genetic*. Family studies have shown that Tourette's disorder is more common in relatives of individuals with the disorder than in the general population. It may be transmitted in an autosomal pattern intermediate between dominant and recessive (Sadock & Sadock, 2007).
   b. *Brain Alterations*. Altered levels of neurotransmitters and dysfunction in the area of the basal ganglia have been implicated in the etiology of Tourette's disorder.
   c. *Biochemical*. Abnormalities in levels of dopamine, serotonin, dynorphin, gamma-aminobutyric acid (GABA), acetylcholine, and norepinephrine have been associated with Tourette's disorder (Popper et al., 2003).

2. **Environmental**
   a. The genetic predisposition to Tourette's disorder may be reinforced by certain factors in the environment, such as complications of pregnancy (e.g., severe nausea and vomiting or excessive stress), low birth weight, head trauma, carbon monoxide poisoning, and encephalitis.

Symptomatology (Subjective and Objective Data)

Signs and symptoms of Tourette's disorder are as follows (APA, 2013; Popper et al., 2003):

1. The disorder may begin with a single motor tic, such as eye blinking, neck jerking, shoulder shrugging, facial grimacing, or coughing.
2. Complex motor tics may follow and include touching, squatting, hopping, skipping, deep knee bends, retracing steps, and twirling when walking.
3. Vocal tics include various words or sounds such as clicks, grunts, yelps, barks, sniffs, snorts, coughs, and, in rare instances, a complex vocal tic involving uttering obscenities.
4. Vocal tics may include repeating certain words or phrases out of context, repeating one's own sounds or words (palilalia), or repeating what others say (echolalia).
5. The movements and vocalizations are experienced as compulsive and irresistible, but they can be suppressed for varying lengths of time.
6. Tics are exacerbated by stress and attenuated during periods in which the individual becomes totally absorbed by an activity.
7. Tics are markedly diminished during sleep.

Common Nursing Diagnoses and Interventions for the Client With Tourette's Disorder

(Interventions are applicable to various health-care settings, such as inpatient and partial hospitalization, community outpatient clinic, home health, and private practice.)

■ RISK FOR SELF-DIRECTED OR OTHER-DIRECTED VIOLENCE

Definition: *At risk for behaviors in which an individual demonstrates that he or she can be physically, emotionally, and/or sexually harmful [either to self or to others]* (NANDA-I, 2012, pp. 447–448)

Risk Factors ("related to")

[Low tolerance for frustration]
[Abnormalities in brain neurotransmitters]
Body language (e.g., rigid posture, clenching of fists and jaw, hyperactivity, pacing, breathlessness, and threatening stances)
[History or threats of violence toward self or others or of destruction to the property of others]
Impulsivity
Suicidal ideation, plan, [available means]

Goals/Objectives

Short-term Goals

1. Client will seek out staff or support person at any time if thoughts of harming self or others should occur.
2. Client will not harm self or others.

Long-term Goal

Client will not harm self or others.

Interventions With *Selected Rationales*

1. Observe client's behavior frequently through routine activities and interactions. Become aware of behaviors that indicate a rise in agitation. *Stress commonly increases tic behaviors. Recognition of behaviors that precede the onset of aggression may provide the opportunity to intervene before violence occurs.*
2. Monitor for self-destructive behavior and impulses. A staff member may need to stay with the client to prevent self-mutilation. *Client safety is a nursing priority.*
3. Provide hand coverings and other restraints that prevent the client from self-mutilative behaviors. *Provides immediate external controls against self-aggressive behaviors.*
4. Redirect violent behavior with physical outlets for frustration. *Excess energy is released through physical activities and a feeling of relaxation is induced.*
5. Administer medication as ordered by the physician. Several medications have been used to treat Tourette's disorder. The most common ones include the following:
   a. **Haloperidol (Haldol)**. Haloperidol has been the drug of choice for Tourette's disorder. Children on this medication

must be monitored for adverse effects associated with most antipsychotic medications (see Chapter 26). Because of the potential for adverse effects, haloperidol should be reserved for children with severe symptoms or with symptoms that interfere with their ability to function. Usual dosage for children 3 to 12 years of age is 0.05 to 0.075 mg/kg/day given in two to three divided doses.

b. **Pimozide (Orap).** The response rate and side effect profile of pimozide are similar to haloperidol. It is used in the management of severe motor or vocal tics that have failed to respond to more conventional treatment. It is not recommended for children younger than age 12 years. Dosage is initiated at 0.05 mg/kg at bedtime; dosage may be increased every third day to a maximum of 0.2 mg/kg, not to exceed 10 mg/day.

c. **Clonidine (Catapres).** Clonidine is an antihypertensive medication, the efficacy of which in the treatment of Tourette's disorder has been mixed. Some physicians like it and use it as a drug of first choice because of its relative safety and few side effects. Recommended dosage is 150 to 200 mcg/day.

d. **Atypical Antipsychotics.** Atypical antipsychotics are less likely to cause extrapyramidal side effects than the older antipsychotics (e.g., haloperidol and pimozide). Risperidone, the most studied atypical antipsychotic in Tourette's disorder, has been shown to reduce symptoms by 21% to 61% when compared to placebo (results which are similar to that of pimozide and clonidine) (Dion et al., 2002). Both olanzapine and ziprasidone have demonstrated effectiveness in decreasing tic symptoms of Tourette's disorder. However, weight gain and abnormal glucose tolerance may be troublesome side effects, and ziprasidone has been associated with increased risk of QTc interval prolongation (Zinner, 2004).

Outcome Criteria

1. Anxiety is maintained at a level at which client feels no need for aggression.
2. Client seeks out staff or support person for expression of true feelings.
3. Client has not harmed self or others.

▓ IMPAIRED SOCIAL INTERACTION

Definition: *Insufficient or excessive quantity or ineffective quality of social exchange* (NANDA-I, 2012, p. 320)

Possible Etiologies ("related to")

Self-concept disturbance
[Low tolerance for frustration]
[Impulsiveness]
[Oppositional behavior]
[Aggressive behavior]

Defining Characteristics ("evidenced by")

[Verbalized or observed] discomfort in social situations
[Verbalized or observed inability] to receive or communicate a satisfying sense of belonging, caring, interest, or shared history
[Observed] use of unsuccessful social interaction behaviors
Dysfunctional interaction with others

Goals/Objectives

Short-term Goal

Client will develop a one-to-one relationship with a nurse or support person within 1 week.

Long-term Goal

Client will be able to interact with staff and peers using age-appropriate, acceptable behaviors.

Interventions With *Selected Rationales*

1. Develop a trusting relationship with the client. Convey acceptance of the person separate from the unacceptable behavior. *Unconditional acceptance increases feelings of self-worth.*
2. Discuss with client which behaviors are and are not acceptable. Describe in matter-of-fact manner the consequences of unacceptable behavior. Follow through. *Aversive reinforcement can alter undesirable behaviors.*
3. Provide group situations for client. *Appropriate social behavior is often learned from the positive and negative feedback of peers.*
4. Act as a role model for client through appropriate interactions with others. *Role modeling of a respected individual is one of the strongest forms of learning.*

Outcome Criteria

1. Client seeks out staff or support person for social as well as for therapeutic interaction.
2. Client verbalizes reasons for past inability to form close interpersonal relationships.
3. Client interacts with others using age-appropriate, acceptable behaviors.

■ LOW SELF-ESTEEM

Definition: *Negative self-evaluating/feelings about self or self-capabilities* (NANDA-I, 2012, pp. 285–287)

Possible Etiologies ("related to")

[Embarrassment associated with tic behaviors]

Defining Characteristics ("evidenced by")

Lack of eye contact
Self-negating verbalizations
[Expressions] of shame or guilt
Hesitant to try new things or situations
[Manipulation of others]

Goals/Objectives

Short-term Goal

Client will verbalize positive aspects about self not associated with tic behaviors.

Long-term Goal

Client will exhibit increased feeling of self-worth as evidenced by verbal expression of positive aspects about self, past accomplishments, and future prospects.

Interventions With *Selected Rationales*

1. Convey unconditional acceptance and positive regard. *Communication of client as worthwhile human being may increase self-esteem.*
2. Set limits on manipulative behavior. Take caution not to reinforce manipulative behaviors by providing desired attention. Identify the consequences of manipulation. Administer consequences matter-of-factly when manipulation occurs. *Aversive reinforcement may work to decrease unacceptable behaviors.*
3. Help client understand that he or she uses manipulation in order to try to increase own self-esteem. Interventions should reflect other actions to accomplish this goal. *When client feels better about self, the need to manipulate others will diminish.*
4. If client chooses to suppress tics in the presence of others, provide a specified "tic time," during which client "vents" tics, feelings, and behaviors (alone or with staff). *Allows for release of tics and assists in sense of control and management of symptoms.*
5. Ensure that client has regular one-to-one time with staff or support person. *One-to-one time gives the nurse the opportunity to provide the client with information about the illness*

and healthy ways to manage it. Exploring feelings about the illness helps the client incorporate the illness into a healthy sense of self.

Outcome Criteria

1. Client verbalizes positive perception of self.
2. Client willingly participates in new activities and situations.

■ SEPARATION ANXIETY DISORDER

Defined

The APA (2013) defines separation anxiety disorder as "excessive fear or anxiety concerning separation from home or attachment figures (p. 191)." Onset may occur anytime before age 18 years but is most commonly diagnosed around age 5 or 6, when the child goes to school. The disorder is more common in girls than in boys. Most children grow out of it, but in some instances, the symptoms can persist into adulthood.

Predisposing Factors

1. **Physiological**
   a. *Genetics.* The results of studies indicate that a greater number of children with relatives who manifest anxiety problems develop anxiety disorders themselves than do children with no such family patterns.
   b. *Temperament.* Studies have shown that differences in temperamental characteristics at birth may be correlated to the acquisition of fear and anxiety disorders in childhood. This may denote an inherited vulnerability or predisposition toward developing these disorders.
2. **Psychosocial**
   a. *Stressful Life Events.* Studies indicate that children who are predisposed to anxiety disorders may be affected significantly by stressful life events.
   b. *Family Influences.* Several theories exist that relate the development of separation anxiety to the following dynamics within the family:
      • An overattachment to the mother (primary caregiver)
      • Separation conflicts between parent and child
      • Enmeshment of members within a family
      • Overprotection of the child by the parents
      • Transfer of parents' fears and anxieties to the children through role modeling

Symptomatology (Subjective and Objective Data)

Symptoms of separation anxiety disorder include the following:

1. In most cases the child has difficulty separating from the mother, although occasionally the separation reluctance is

directed toward the father, siblings, or other significant individual to whom the child is attached.
2. Anticipation of separation may result in tantrums, crying, screaming, complaints of physical problems, and clinging behaviors.
3. Reluctance or refusal to attend school is especially common in adolescence.
4. Younger children may "shadow" or follow around the person from whom they are afraid to be separated.
5. During middle childhood or adolescence, they may refuse to sleep away from home (e.g., at a friend's house or at camp).
6. Worrying is common and relates to the possibility of harm coming to self or to the attachment figure. Younger children may have nightmares to this effect.
7. Specific phobias may be present.
8. Depressed mood is frequently present and often precedes the onset of the anxiety symptoms, which commonly occur following a major stressor.

Common Nursing Diagnoses and Interventions for the Client With Separation Anxiety Disorder

(Interventions are applicable to various health-care settings, such as inpatient and partial hospitalization, community outpatient clinic, home health, and private practice.)

ANXIETY (SEVERE)

Definition: *Vague uneasy feeling of discomfort or dread accompanied by an autonomic response (the source is often nonspecific or unknown to the individual); a feeling of apprehension caused by anticipation of danger. It is an alerting signal that warns of impending danger and enables the individual to take measures to deal with threat (NANDA-I, 2012, p. 344).*

Possible Etiologies ("related to")

Heredity
[Birth temperament]
[Overattachment to parent]
[Negative role modeling]

Defining Characteristics ("evidenced by")

[Excessive distress when separated from attachment figure]
[Fear or anticipation of separation from attachment figure]
[Fear of being alone or without attachment figure]
[Reluctance or refusal to go to school or anywhere else without attachment figure]

[Nightmares about being separated from attachment figure]
[Somatic symptoms occurring as a result of fear of separation]

Goals/Objectives

Short-term Goal

Client will discuss fears of separation with trusted individual.

Long-term Goal

Client will maintain anxiety at no higher than moderate level in the face of events that formerly have precipitated panic.

Interventions With *Selected Rationales*

1. Establish an atmosphere of calmness, trust, and genuine positive regard. *Trust and unconditional acceptance are necessary for satisfactory nurse-client relationship. Calmness is important because anxiety is easily transmitted from one person to another.*
2. Assure client of his or her safety and security. *Symptoms of panic anxiety are very frightening.*
3. Explore the child's or adolescent's fears of separating from the parents. Explore with the parents possible fears they may have of separation from the child. *Some parents may have an underlying fear of separation from the child, of which they are unaware and which they are unconsciously transferring to the child.*
4. Help parents and child initiate realistic goals (e.g., child to stay with sitter for 2 hours with minimal anxiety; or, child to stay at friend's house without parents until 9 p.m. without experiencing panic anxiety). *Parents may be so frustrated with the child's clinging and demanding behaviors that assistance with problem solving may be required.*
5. Give and encourage parents to give positive reinforcement for desired behaviors. *Positive reinforcement encourages repetition of desirable behaviors.*

Outcome Criteria

1. Client and parents are able to discuss their fears regarding separation.
2. Client experiences no somatic symptoms from fear of separation.
3. Client maintains anxiety at moderate level when separation occurs or is anticipated.

■ INEFFECTIVE COPING

Definition: *Inability to form a valid appraisal of the stressors, inadequate choices of practiced responses, and/or inability to use available resources* (NANDA-I, 2012, p. 348)

Possible Etiologies ("related to")

[Unresolved separation conflicts]
[Inadequate coping skills]

Defining Characteristics ("evidenced by")

[Somatic complaints in response to occurrence or anticipation of separation from attachment figure]

Goals/Objectives

Short-term Goal

Client will verbalize correlation of somatic symptoms to fear of separation.

Long-term Goal

Client will demonstrate use of more adaptive coping strategies (than physical symptoms) in response to stressful situations.

Interventions With *Selected Rationales*

1. Encourage child or adolescent to discuss specific situations in life that produce the most distress and describe his or her response to these situations. Include parents in the discussion. *Client and family may be unaware of the correlation between stressful situations and the exacerbation of physical symptoms.*
2. Help the child or adolescent who is perfectionistic to recognize that self-expectations may be unrealistic. Connect times of unmet self-expectations to the exacerbation of physical symptoms. *Recognition of maladaptive patterns is the first step in the change process.*
3. Encourage parents and child to identify more adaptive coping strategies that the child could use in the face of anxiety that feels overwhelming. Practice through role play. *Practice facilitates the use of the desired behavior when the individual is actually faced with the stressful situation.*

Outcome Criteria

1. Client and family verbalize the correlation between separation anxiety and somatic symptoms.
2. Client verbalizes the correlation between unmet self-expectations and somatic symptoms.
3. Client responds to stressful situations without exhibiting physical symptoms.

■ IMPAIRED SOCIAL INTERACTION

Definition: *Insufficient or excessive quantity or ineffective quality of social exchange* (NANDA-I, 2012, p. 320)

Possible Etiologies ("related to")

[Reluctance to be away from attachment figure]

Defining Characteristics ("evidenced by")

[Symptoms of severe anxiety]
[Verbalized or observed] discomfort in social situations
[Verbalized or observed] inability to receive or communicate a
    satisfying sense of belonging, caring, interest, or shared history
[Observed] use of unsuccessful social interaction behaviors
Dysfunctional interaction with others

Goals/Objectives

Short-term Goal

Client will spend time with staff or other support person (without
    presence of attachment figure) without excessive anxiety.

Long-term Goal

Client will be able to spend time with others (without presence of
    attachment figure) without excessive anxiety.

Interventions With *Selected Rationales*

1. Develop a trusting relationship with client. *This is the first step
   in helping the client learn to interact with others.*
2. Attend groups with the child and support efforts to interact
   with others. Give positive feedback. *Presence of a trusted individual provides security during times of distress. Positive
   feedback encourages repetition.*
3. Convey to the child the acceptability of his or her not participating in group in the beginning. Gradually encourage small
   contributions until client is able to participate more fully. *Small
   successes will gradually increase self-confidence and decrease
   self-consciousness, so that client will feel less anxious in the
   group situation.*
4. Help client set small personal goals (e.g., "Today I will speak
   to one person I don't know."). *Simple, realistic goals provide
   opportunities for success that increase self-confidence and may
   encourage the client to attempt more difficult objectives in the
   future.*

Outcome Criteria

1. Client spends time with others using acceptable, age-appropriate
   behaviors.
2. Client is able to interact with others away from the attachment
   figure without excessive anxiety.

@ INTERNET REFERENCES

- Additional information about ADHD may be located at the following Web sites:
  a. www.chadd.org
  b. www.nimh.nih.gov/health/topics/attention-deficit-hyperactivity-disorder-adhd/index.shtml
- Additional information about ASD may be located at the following Web sites:
  a. www.autism-society.org
  b. www.nimh.nih.gov/health/topics/autism-spectrum-disorders-pervasive-developmental-disorders/index.shtml
- Additional information about medications to treat ADHD and Tourette's disorder may be located at the following Web sites:
  a. www.drugs.com
  b. http://www.nlm.nih.gov/medlineplus/druginformation.html

Movie Connections

Bill (Intellectual disability) • *Bill, On His Own* (Intellectual disability) • *Sling Blade* (Intellectual disability) • *Forrest Gump* (Intellectual disability) • *Rain Man* (ASD) • *Mercury Rising* (ASD) • *Niagara, Niagara* (Tourette's Disorder) • *Toughlove* (Conduct Disorder)

CHAPTER 3

Neurocognitive Disorders

■ BACKGROUND ASSESSMENT DATA

Delirium

Defined

The American Psychiatric Association (APA, 2013) *Diagnostic and Statistical Manual of Mental Disorders, Fifth Edition (DSM-5)* defines "delirium" as a disturbance in attention and awareness and a change in cognition that develop rapidly over a short period of time (usually hours to a few days). Duration is usually brief (e.g., 1 week; rarely more than 1 month), and the disorder subsides completely on recovery from the underlying determinant. If the underlying condition persists, the delirium may gradually progress to stupor, coma, seizures, or death (APA, 2013).

Predisposing Factors to Delirium

The *DSM-5* differentiates among the disorders of delirium by their etiology, although they share a common symptom presentation. Categories of delirium include the following:

1. **Substance Intoxication Delirium**. Delirium symptoms can occur in response to taking high doses of cannabis, cocaine, hallucinogens, alcohol, anxiolytics, or narcotics.

2. **Substance Withdrawal Delirium.** Reduction or termination of long-term, high-dose use of certain substances, such as alcohol, sedatives, hypnotics, or anxiolytics, can result in withdrawal delirium symptoms.

3. **Medication-Induced Delirium**. The symptoms of delirium can occur as a side effect of a medication taken as prescribed. Medications that have been known to precipitate delirium include anticholinergics, antihypertensives, corticosteroids, anticonvulsants, cardiac glycosides, analgesics, anesthetics, antineoplastic agents, antiparkinson drugs, H2-receptor antagonists (e.g., cimetidine), and others (Puri & Treasaden, 2012; Sadock & Sadock, 2007).

4. **Delirium Due to Another Medical Condition**. Certain medical conditions, such as systemic infections, metabolic

disorders, fluid and electrolyte imbalances, liver or kidney disease, thiamine deficiency, postoperative states, hypertensive encephalopathy, postictal states, and sequelae of head trauma, can cause the symptoms of delirium.

5. **Delirium Due to Multiple Etiologies**. Symptoms of delirium may be related to more than one medical condition or to the combined effects of another medical condition and substance use or medication side effects.

Symptomatology (Subjective and Objective Data)

The following symptoms have been identified with the syndrome of delirium:

1. Alteration in awareness (reduced orientation to the environment).
2. Extreme distractibility with difficulty focusing attention.
3. Disorientation to time and place.
4. Impaired reasoning ability and goal-directed behavior.
5. Disturbance in the sleep-wake cycle.
6. Emotional instability as manifested by fear, anxiety, depression, irritability, anger, euphoria, or apathy.
7. Misperceptions of the environment, including illusions and hallucinations.
8. Autonomic manifestations, such as tachycardia, sweating, flushed face, dilated pupils, and elevated blood pressure.
9. Incoherent speech.
10. Impairment of recent memory.

Neurocognitive Disorder

Defined

Neurocognitive disorder (NCD) is defined by the *DSM-5* as "evidence of significant cognitive decline from a previous level of performance in one or more cognitive domains (complex attention, executive function, learning and memory, language, perceptual-motor, or social cognition)" (APA, 2013, p. 602). The disorder is identified as *Major NCD* or *Mild NCD*, according to the degree of impairment. The symptoms usually have a slow, insidious onset and are chronic, progressive, and irreversible.

Predisposing Factors to NCD

Following are major etiological categories for the syndrome of NCD:

1. **NCD due to Alzheimer's Disease.** The exact cause of Alzheimer's disease is unknown, but several theories have been proposed, such as reduction in brain acetylcholine, the formation of plaques and tangles, serious head trauma, and genetic factors. Pathological changes in the brain include atrophy, enlarged ventricles, and the presence of numerous neurofibrillary

plaques and tangles. Definitive diagnosis is by biopsy or autopsy examination of brain tissue, although refinement of diagnostic criteria and discriminating diagnostic instruments now enable clinicians to use specific clinical features to identify the disease at a high rate of accuracy.

2. **Vascular NCD**. This type of NCD is caused by significant cerebrovascular disease. The client suffers the equivalent of small strokes caused by arterial hypertension or cerebral emboli or thrombi, which destroy many areas of the brain. The onset of symptoms is more abrupt than in Alzheimer's disease and runs a highly variable course, progressing in steps rather than as a gradual deterioration.

3. **Frontotemporal NCD**. Symptoms from frontotemporal NCD occur as a result of shrinking of the frontal and temporal anterior lobes of the brain. The cause is unknown, but a genetic factor appears to be involved. Symptoms may include behavioral and personality changes, speech and language problems, or both. Apathy, a decline in social cognition, and compulsive/ritualistic behaviors are common. The disease progresses steadily and often rapidly, ranging from less than 2 years in some individuals to more than 10 years in others.

4. **NCD with Lewy Bodies.** Clinically, Lewy body NCD is fairly similar to Alzheimer's disease; however, it tends to progress more rapidly, and there is an earlier appearance of visual hallucinations and parkinsonian features (Rabins, 2006). This disorder is distinctive by the presence of Lewy bodies—eosinophilic inclusion bodies—seen in the cerebral cortex and brainstem (Andreasen & Black, 2011).

5. **NCD due to Traumatic Brain Injury.** *DSM-5* criteria states that this disorder "is caused by an impact to the head or other mechanisms of rapid movement or displacement of the brain within the skull, with one or more of the following: loss of consciousness, posttraumatic amnesia, disorientation and confusion, or neurological signs (e.g., positive neuroimaging demonstrating injury, a new onset of seizures or a marked worsening of a preexisting seizure disorder, visual field cuts, anosmia, hemiparesis)" (APA, 2013, p. 624). Depending on the severity of the injury, the symptoms may eventually subside or may become permanent (Smith, 2011).

6. **NCD Due to HIV Infection**. The immune dysfunction associated with human immunodeficiency virus (HIV) disease can lead to brain infections by other organisms. HIV also appears to cause NCD directly.

7. **NCD Due to Prion Disease.** This disorder is identified by its insidious onset, rapid progression, and manifestations of motor features of prion disease, such as myoclonus or ataxia, or biomarker evidence (APA, 2013). The clinical presentation

is typical of the syndrome of mild or major NCD, along with involuntary movements, muscle rigidity, and ataxia. The clinical course is extremely rapid, with progression from diagnosis to death in less than 2 years.

8. **NCD Due to Parkinson's Disease.** Parkinson's disease is caused by a loss of nerve cells in the substantia nigra of the basal ganglia. NCD is observed in as many as 60% of clients with Parkinson's disease. The symptoms of NCD associated with Parkinson's disease often closely resemble those of Alzheimer's disease.

9. **NCD Due to Huntington's Disease.** This disease is transmitted as a Mendelian dominant gene, and damage occurs in the areas of the basal ganglia and the cerebral cortex. The average duration of the disease is based on age at onset. One study concluded that juvenile-onset and late-onset clients have the shortest duration (Foroud et al., 1999). In this study, the median duration of the disease was 21.4 years.

10. **NCD Due to Another Medical Condition.** A number of other general medical conditions can cause NCD. Some of these include hypothyroidism, hyperparathyroidism, pituitary insufficiency, uremia, encephalitis, brain tumor, pernicious anemia, thiamine deficiency, pellagra, uncontrolled epilepsy, cardiopulmonary insufficiency, fluid and electrolyte imbalances, central nervous system and systemic infections, systemic lupus erythematosus, and multiple sclerosis (Black & Andreasen, 2011; Puri & Treasaden, 2011).

11. **Substance/Medication-Induced NCD.** NCD can occur as the result of substance reactions, overuse, or abuse (Davis, 2012). Symptoms are consistent with major or mild NCD, and persist beyond the usual duration of intoxication and acute withdrawal (APA, 2013). Substances that have been associated with the development of NCDs include alcohol, sedatives, hypnotics, anxiolytics, and inhalants. Drugs that cause anticholinergic side effects and toxins such as lead and mercury, have also been implicated.

Symptomatology (Subjective and Objective Data)

The following symptoms have been identified with the syndrome of NCD:

1. Memory impairment (impaired ability to learn new information or to recall previously learned information).

2. Impairment in abstract thinking, judgment, and impulse control.

3. Impairment in language ability, such as difficulty naming objects. In some instances, the individual may not speak at all (aphasia).

4. Personality changes.
5. Impaired ability to perform motor activities despite intact motor abilities (apraxia).
6. Disorientation.
7. Wandering.
8. Delusions (particularly delusions of persecution).

Common Nursing Diagnoses and Interventions for Delirium and NCD

(Interventions are applicable to various health-care settings, such as inpatient and partial hospitalization, community outpatient clinic, home health, and private practice.)

■ RISK FOR TRAUMA

Definition: At risk of accidental tissue injury (e.g., wound, burn, fracture) (NANDA International [NANDA-I], 2012, p. 444)

Risk Factors ("related to")

[Chronic alteration in structure or function of brain tissue, secondary to the aging process, multiple infarcts, HIV disease, head trauma, chronic substance abuse, or progressively dysfunctional physical condition resulting in the following symptoms:
  Disorientation; confusion
  Weakness
  Muscular incoordination
  Seizures
  Memory impairment
  Poor vision
  Extreme psychomotor agitation observed in the late stages of delirium]
[Frequent shuffling of feet and stumbling]
[Falls, caused by muscular incoordination or seizures]
[Bumping into furniture]
[Exposing self to frigid conditions with insufficient protective clothing]
[Cutting self when using sharp instruments]
[History of attempting to light burner or oven and leaving gas on in house]
[Smoking and leaving burning cigarettes in various places; smoking in bed; falling asleep sitting on couch or chair with lighted cigarette in hand]
[Purposeless, thrashing movements; hyperactivity that is out of touch with the environment]

Goals/Objectives

Short-term Goals

1. Client will call for assistance when ambulating or carrying out other activities.
2. Client will not experience physical injury.

Long-term Goal

Client will not experience physical injury.

Interventions With *Selected Rationales*

1. Assess client's level of disorientation and confusion to determine specific requirements for safety. ***Knowledge of client's level of functioning is necessary to formulate appropriate plan of care.***
2. Institute appropriate safety measures, such as the following:
   a. Place furniture in the room in an arrangement that best accommodates client's disabilities.
   b. Observe client behaviors frequently; assign staff on one-to-one basis if condition warrants; accompany and assist client when ambulating; use wheelchair for transporting long distances.
   c. Store items that client uses frequently within easy access.
   d. Remove potentially harmful articles from client's room: cigarettes, matches, lighters, and sharp objects.
   e. Remain with client when he or she smokes.
   f. Pad side rails and headboard of client with seizure disorder. Institute seizure precautions as described in procedure manual of individual institution.
   g. If client is prone to wander, provide an area within which wandering can be carried out safely.
3. Frequently orient client to reality and surroundings. ***Disorientation may endanger client safety if he or she unknowingly wanders away from safe environment.***
4. Use tranquilizing medications and soft restraints, as prescribed by physician, for client's protection during periods of excessive hyperactivity. ***Use restraints judiciously, because they can increase agitation. They may be required, however, to provide for client safety.***
5. Teach prospective caregivers methods that have been successful in preventing client injury. ***These caregivers will be responsible for client's safety after discharge from the hospital. Sharing successful interventions may be helpful.***

Outcome Criteria

1. Client is able to accomplish daily activities within the environment without experiencing injury.
2. Prospective caregivers are able to verbalize means of providing safe environment for client.

▨ RISK FOR SELF-DIRECTED OR OTHER-DIRECTED VIOLENCE

Definition: *At risk for behaviors in which an individual demonstrates that he or she can be physically, emotionally, and/or sexually harmful [either to self or to others]* (NANDA-I, 2012, p. 447–448)

Risk Factors ("related to")

[Chronic alteration in structure or function of brain tissue, secondary to the aging process, multiple infarcts, HIV disease, head trauma, chronic substance abuse, or progressively dysfunctional physical condition resulting in the following symptoms:
    Delusional thinking
    Suspiciousness of others
    Hallucinations
    Illusions
    Disorientation or confusion
    Impairment of impulse control]
[Inaccurate perception of the environment]
Body language—rigid posture, clenching of fists and jaw, hyperactivity, pacing, breathlessness, and threatening stances.
Suicidal ideation, plan, available means
Cognitive impairment
[Depressed mood]

Goals/Objectives

Short-term Goals

1. Client will maintain agitation at manageable level so as not to become violent.
2. Client will not harm self or others.

Long-term Goal

Client will not harm self or others.

Interventions With *Selected Rationales*

1. Assess client's level of anxiety and behaviors that indicate the anxiety is increasing. ***Recognizing these behaviors, the nurse may be able to intervene before violence occurs.***
2. Maintain low level of stimuli in client's environment (low lighting, few people, simple decor, low noise level). ***Anxiety increases in a highly stimulating environment.***
3. Remove all potentially dangerous objects from client's environment. ***In a disoriented, confused state, the client may use these objects to harm self or others.***
4. Have sufficient staff available to execute a physical confrontation, if necessary. ***Assistance may be required from***

others to provide for physical safety of client or primary nurse or both.

5. Maintain a calm manner with client. Attempt to prevent frightening the client unnecessarily. Provide continual reassurance and support. *Anxiety is contagious and can be transferred to the client.*

6. Interrupt periods of unreality and reorient. *Client safety is jeopardized during periods of disorientation. Correcting misinterpretations of reality enhances client's feelings of self-worth and personal dignity.*

7. Use tranquilizing medications and soft restraints, as prescribed by physician, *for protection of client and others during periods of elevated anxiety.* Use restraints judiciously, *because agitation sometimes increases; however, they may be required to ensure client safety.*

8. Sit with client and provide one-to-one observation if assessed to be actively suicidal. *Client safety is a nursing priority, and one-to-one observation may be necessary to prevent a suicidal attempt.*

9. Teach relaxation exercises *to intervene in times of increasing anxiety.*

10. Teach prospective caregivers to recognize client behaviors that indicate anxiety is increasing and ways to intervene before violence occurs.

Outcome Criteria

1. Prospective caregivers are able to verbalize behaviors that indicate an increasing anxiety level and ways they may assist client to manage the anxiety before violence occurs.

2. With assistance from caregivers, client is able to control impulse to perform acts of violence against self or others.

■ CHRONIC CONFUSION

Definition: *Irreversible, longstanding, and/or progressive deterioration of intellect and personality characterized by decreased ability to interpret environmental stimuli and decreased capacity for intellectual thought processes, and manifested by disturbances of memory, orientation, and behavior* (NANDA-I, 2012, p. 265)

Possible Etiologies ("related to")

[Alteration in structure/function of brain tissue, secondary to the following conditions:

    Advanced age

    Vascular disease

    Hypertension

Cerebral hypoxia
Long-term abuse of mood- or behavior-altering substances
Exposure to environmental toxins
Various other physical disorders that predispose to cerebral abnormalities (see Predisposing Factors)]

Defining Characteristics ("evidenced by")

Altered interpretation
Altered personality
Altered response to stimuli
Clinical evidence of organic impairment
Impaired long-term memory
Impaired short-term memory
Impaired socialization
Long-standing cognitive impairment
No change in level of consciousness
Progressive cognitive impairment

Goals/Objectives

Short-term Goal

Client will accept explanations of inaccurate interpretations within the environment.

Long-term Goal

With assistance from caregiver, client will be able to interrupt nonreality-based thinking.

Interventions With *Selected Rationales*

1. Frequently orient client to reality and surroundings. Allow client to have familiar objects around him or her. Use other items, such as clock, calendar, and daily schedules, to assist in maintaining reality orientation. *Client safety is jeopardized during periods of disorientation. Maintaining reality orientation enhances client's sense of self-worth and personal dignity.*

2. Teach prospective caregivers how to orient client to time, person, place, and circumstances as required. *These caregivers will be responsible for client safety after discharge from the hospital. Sharing successful interventions may be helpful.*

3. Give positive feedback when thinking and behavior are appropriate, or when client verbalizes that certain ideas expressed are not based in reality. *Positive feedback increases self-esteem and enhances desire to repeat appropriate behaviors.*

4. Use simple explanations and face-to-face interaction when communicating with client. Do not shout message into client's ear. *Speaking slowly and in a face-to-face position is most effective when communicating with an elderly individual*

experiencing a hearing loss. Visual cues facilitate understanding. Shouting causes distortion of high-pitched sounds and in some instances creates a feeling of discomfort for the client.

5. Express reasonable doubt if client relays suspicious beliefs in response to delusional thinking. Discuss with client the potential personal negative effects of continued suspiciousness of others. Reinforce accurate perception of people and situations. *Expressions of doubt by a trusted individual may foster similar uncertainties about the delusion on the part of the client.*

6. Do not permit rumination of false ideas. When this begins, talk to client about real people and real events. *Reality orientation increases client's sense of self-worth and personal dignity.*

7. Close observation of client's behavior is indicated if delusional thinking reveals an intention for violence. *Client safety is a nursing priority.*

CLINICAL PEARL Medications for Alzheimer's disease. Cholinesterase inhibitors are used for mild to moderate cognitive impairment in clients with Alzheimer's disease. Examples include *donepezil (Aricept), rivastigmine (Exelon),* and *galantamine (Razadyne).* (Higher dose donepezil has also been approved for moderate to severe AD.) Common side effects include dizziness, headache, and gastrointestinal upset. *Memantine (Namenda),* a NMDA receptor antagonist, is used for treatment of moderate to severe cognitive impairment in clients with Alzheimer's disease. Common side effects of memantine include dizziness, headache, and constipation. These medications do not stop or reverse the disease process, but may slow down the progression of the decline in functionality.

Outcome Criteria

1. With assistance from caregiver, client is able to distinguish between reality-based and nonreality-based thinking.

2. Prospective caregivers are able to verbalize ways in which to orient client to reality, as needed.

■ SELF-CARE DEFICIT

Definition: *Impaired ability to perform or complete [activities of daily living (ADLs)] for self* (NANDA-I, 2012, p. 250–253)

Possible Etiologies ("related to")

Cognitive impairment

Defining Characteristics ("evidenced by")

Inability to wash body
Inability to put on clothing
Inability to bring food from receptacle to the mouth
[Inability to toilet self without assistance]

Goals/Objectives

Short-term Goal

Client will participate in ADLs with assistance from caregiver.

Long-term Goal

Client will accomplish ADLs to the best of his or her ability. Unfulfilled needs will be met by caregiver.

Interventions With *Selected Rationales*

1. Provide a simple, structured environment *to minimize confusion:*
   a. Identify self-care deficits and provide assistance as required.
   b. Allow plenty of time for client to perform tasks.
   c. Provide guidance and support for independent actions by talking the client through the task one step at a time.
   d. Provide a structured schedule of activities that does not change from day to day.
   e. Ensure that ADLs follow home routine as closely as possible.
   f. Provide for consistency in assignment of daily caregivers.
2. In planning for discharge:
   a. Perform ongoing assessment of client's ability to fulfill nutritional needs, ensure personal safety, follow medication regimen, and communicate need for assistance with those activities that he or she cannot accomplish independently. *Client safety and security are nursing priorities.*
   b. Assess prospective caregivers' ability to anticipate and fulfill client's unmet needs. Provide information to assist caregivers with this responsibility. Ensure that caregivers are aware of available community support systems from which they can seek assistance when required. *This will facilitate transition to discharge from treatment center*.
   c. National support organizations can provide information:

   National Parkinson Foundation Inc.
   1501 NW 9th Ave.
   Miami, FL 33136-1494
   1-800-327-4545

   Alzheimer's Association
   225 N. Michigan Ave., Floor 17
   Chicago, IL 60601-7633
   1-800-272-3900

Outcome Criteria

1. Client willingly participates in ADLs.
2. Client accomplishes ADLs to the best of his or her ability.
3. Client's unfulfilled needs are met by caregivers.

■ DISTURBED SENSORY PERCEPTION (Specify)

Definition: *Change in the amount or patterning of incoming stimuli [either internally or externally initiated] accompanied by a diminished, exaggerated, distorted, or impaired response to such stimuli* (Note: This diagnosis has been resigned by NANDA-I, but is retained in this text because of its appropriateness in describing these specific behaviors.)

Possible Etiologies ("related to")

[Alteration in structure/function of brain tissue, secondary to the following conditions:
    Advanced age
    Vascular disease
    Hypertension
    Cerebral hypoxia
    Abuse of mood- or behavior-altering substances
    Exposure to environmental toxins
    Various other physical disorders that predispose to cerebral abnormalities (see Predisposing Factors)]

Defining Characteristics ("evidenced by")

Poor concentration
Sensory distortions
Hallucinations
[Disorientation to time, place, person, or circumstances]
[Inappropriate responses]
[Talking and laughing to self]
[Suspiciousness]

Goals/Objectives

Short-term Goal

With assistance from caregiver, client will maintain orientation to time, place, person, and circumstances for specified period of time.

Long-term Goal

Client will demonstrate accurate perception of the environment by responding appropriately to stimuli indigenous to the surroundings.

Interventions With *Selected Rationales*

1. Decrease the amount of stimuli in the client's environment (e.g., low noise level, few people, simple decor). *This decreases the possibility of client's forming inaccurate sensory perceptions.*

2. Do not reinforce the hallucination. Let client know that you do not share the perception. Maintain reality through reorientation and focus on real situations and people. *Reality orientation decreases false sensory perceptions and enhances client's sense of self-worth and personal dignity.*
3. Provide reassurance of safety if client responds with fear to inaccurate sensory perception. *Client safety and security are nursing priorities.*
4. Correct client's description of inaccurate perception, and describe the situation as it exists in reality. *Explanation of and participation in real situations and real activities interferes with the ability to respond to hallucinations.*
5. Allow for care to be given by same personnel on a regular basis, if possible, *to provide a feeling of security and stability in the client's environment.*
6. Teach prospective caregivers how to recognize signs and symptoms of client's inaccurate sensory perceptions. Explain techniques they may use to restore reality to the situation.

Outcome Criteria

1. With assistance from caregiver, client is able to recognize when perceptions within the environment are inaccurate.
2. Prospective caregivers are able to verbalize ways in which to correct inaccurate perceptions and restore reality to the situation.

■ LOW SELF-ESTEEM

Definition: *Negative self-evaluating/feelings about self or self-capabilities* (NANDA-I, 2012, p. 285)

Possible Etiologies ("related to")

[Loss of independent functioning]
[Loss of capacity for remembering]
[Loss of capability for effective verbal communication]

Defining Characteristics ("evidenced by")

[Withdraws into social isolation]
Lack of eye contact
[Excessive crying alternating with expressions of anger]
[Refusal to participate in therapies]
[Refusal to participate in own self-care activities]
[Becomes increasingly dependent on others to perform ADLs]
Expressions of shame or guilt

Goals/Objectives

Short-term Goal

Client will voluntarily spend time with staff and peers in dayroom activities (time dimension to be individually determined).

Long-term Goal

Client will exhibit increased feelings of self-worth as evidenced by voluntary participation in own self-care and interaction with others (time dimension to be individually determined).

Interventions With *Selected Rationales*

1. Encourage client to express honest feelings in relation to loss of prior level of functioning. Acknowledge pain of loss. Support client through process of grieving. *Client may be fixed in anger stage of grieving process, which is turned inward on the self, resulting in diminished self-esteem.*
2. Devise methods for assisting client with memory deficit. *These aids may assist client to function more independently, thereby increasing self-esteem.* Examples follow:
   a. Name sign on door identifying client's room.
   b. Identifying sign on outside of dining room door.
   c. Identifying sign on outside of restroom door.
   d. Large clock, with oversized numbers and hands, appropriately placed.
   e. Large calendar, indicating one day at a time, with month, day, and year identified in bold print.
   f. Printed, structured daily schedule, with one copy for client and one posted on unit wall.
   g. "News board" on unit wall on which current national and local events may be posted.
3. Encourage client's attempts to communicate. If verbalizations are not understandable, express to client what you think he or she intended to say. It may be necessary to reorient client frequently. *The ability to communicate effectively with others may enhance self-esteem.*
4. Encourage reminiscence and discussion of life review. Also discuss present-day events. Sharing picture albums, if possible, is especially good. *Reminiscence and life review help the client resume progression through the grief process associated with disappointing life events and increase self-esteem as successes are reviewed.*
5. Encourage participation in group activities. Caregiver may need to accompany client at first, until he or she feels secure that the group members will be accepting, regardless of limitations in verbal communication. *Positive feedback from group members will increase self-esteem.*

6. Offer support and empathy when client expresses embarrassment at inability to remember people, events, and places. Focus on accomplishments *to lift self-esteem.*
7. Encourage client to be as independent as possible in self-care activities. Provide written schedule of tasks to be performed. Intervene in areas in which client requires assistance. *The ability to perform independently preserves self-esteem.*

Outcome Criteria

1. Client initiates own self-care according to written schedule and willingly accepts assistance as needed.
2. Client interacts with others in group activities, maintaining anxiety at minimal level in response to difficulties with verbal communication.

■ CAREGIVER ROLE STRAIN

Definition: *Difficulty in performing family/significant other caregiver role* (NANDA-I, 2012, p. 298)

Possible Etiologies ("related to")

Severity of the care receiver's illness
Chronicity of the care receiver's illness
[Lack of respite and recreation for the caregiver]
Caregiver's competing role commitments
Inadequate physical environment for providing care
Family or caregiver isolation
Complexity and amount of caregiving activities

Defining Characteristics ("evidenced by")

Apprehension about possible institutionalization of care receiver
Apprehension about future regarding care receiver's health and caregiver's ability to provide care
Difficulty performing and/or completing required tasks
Apprehension about care receiver's care if caregiver unable to provide care

Goals/Objectives

Short-term Goal

Caregivers will verbalize understanding of ways to facilitate the caregiver role.

Long-term Goal

Caregivers will demonstrate effective problem-solving skills and develop adaptive coping mechanisms to regain equilibrium.

Interventions With *Selected Rationales*

1. Assess caregivers' ability to anticipate and fulfill client's unmet needs. Provide information to assist caregivers with this responsibility. *Caregivers may be unaware of what client will realistically be able to accomplish. They may be unaware of the progressive nature of the illness.*
2. Ensure that caregivers are aware of available community support systems from which they can seek assistance when required. Examples include adult day-care centers, housekeeping and homemaker services, respite-care services, and a local chapter of the Alzheimer's Association. This organization sponsors a nationwide 24-hour hotline to provide information and link families who need assistance with nearby chapters and affiliates. The hotline number is 1-800-272-3900. *Caregivers require relief from the pressures and strain of providing 24-hour care for their loved one. Studies show that elder abuse arises out of caregiving situations that place overwhelming stress on caregivers.*
3. Encourage caregivers to express feelings, particularly anger. *Release of these emotions can serve to prevent psychopathology, such as depression or psychophysiological disorders, from occurring.*
4. Encourage participation in support groups composed of members with similar life situations. *Hearing others who are experiencing the same problems discuss ways in which they have coped may help caregiver adopt more adaptive strategies. Individuals who are experiencing similar life situations provide empathy and support for each other.*

Outcome Criteria

1. Caregivers are able to problem solve effectively regarding care of elderly client.
2. Caregivers demonstrate adaptive coping strategies for dealing with stress of caregiver role.
3. Caregivers express feelings openly.
4. Caregivers express desire to join support group of other caregivers.

@ INTERNET REFERENCES

- Additional information about Alzheimer's Disease may be located at the following Web sites:
    a. www.alz.org
    b. www.nia.nih.gov/
    c. www.ninds.nih.gov/health_and_medical/disorders/alzheimers-disease_doc.htm

- Information on caregiving can be located at the following Web site:
  a. www.aarp.org/home-family/caregiving/
- Additional information about medications to treat Alzheimer's disease may be located at the following Web sites:
  a. www.nlm.nih.gov/medlineplus/druginformation.html
  b. www.drugs.com/condition/alzheimer-s-disease.html

 Movie Connections

The Notebook (Alzheimer's disease) • *Away From Her* (Alzheimer's disease) • *Iris* (Alzheimer's disease)

CHAPTER 4

Substance-Related and Addictive Disorders

■ BACKGROUND ASSESSMENT DATA

The substance-related disorders are composed of two groups: the substance use disorders (addiction) and the substance-induced disorders (intoxication and withdrawal). Other substance-induced disorders (delirium, neurocognitive disorder, psychotic disorders, bipolar disorders, depressive disorders, anxiety disorders, obsessive-compulsive and related disorders, and sexual dysfunctions) are included in the chapters with which they share symptomatology (e.g., substance-induced anxiety disorder is included in Chapter 8; substance-induced sexual dysfunction is included in Chapter 12, etc.). Also included in this chapter is a discussion of gambling disorder, a nonsubstance addiction disorder.

■ SUBSTANCE USE DISORDERS
Substance Addiction
Defined

The *Diagnostic and Statistical Manual of Mental Disorders, Fifth Edition (DSM-5)* (American Psychiatric Association [APA], 2013) lists diagnostic criteria for addiction to specific substances, including alcohol, cannabis, hallucinogens, inhalants, opioids, sedative/hypnotics/anxiolytics, stimulants, and tobacco. Individuals are considered to have a substance use disorder when use of the substance interferes with their ability to fulfill role obligations, such as at work, school, or home. Often the individual would like to cut down or control use of the substance, but attempts fail, and use of the substance continues to increase. There is an intense craving for the substance, and an excessive amount of time is spent trying to procure more of the substance or recover from the effects of its use. Use of the substance causes problems with interpersonal relationships, and the individual may become socially isolated. Individuals with substance use disorders often participate in hazardous activities when they are impaired by the substance, and continue to use the substance despite knowing that its use is contributing to a physical or psychological problem. Addiction is evident when tolerance develops and the amount required to achieve the desired effect continues to increase. A syndrome of symptoms, characteristic of the specific substance, occurs when the individual with the addiction attempts to discontinue use of the substance.

■ SUBSTANCE-INDUCED DISORDERS
Substance Intoxication
Defined

Intoxication is defined as a physical and mental state of exhilaration and emotional frenzy or lethargy and stupor (Townsend, 2015). With substance intoxication, the individual experiences a reversible syndrome of symptoms that occur with ingestion of a substance and that are specific to the substance ingested. The behavior changes can be attributed to the physiological effects of the substance on the central nervous system (CNS).

Substance Withdrawal
Defined

Withdrawal is defined as the physiological and mental readjustment that accompanies the discontinuation of an addictive substance (Townsend, 2015). The symptoms of withdrawal are specific to the substance that has been ingested and occur after prolonged or heavy use of the substance. The effects are of sufficient significance to interfere with usual role performance.

■ CLASSIFICATION OF SUBSTANCES
Alcohol

Although alcohol is a CNS depressant, it is considered separately because of the complex effects and widespread nature of its use. Low to moderate consumption produces a feeling of well-being and reduced inhibitions. At higher concentrations, both motor and intellectual functioning are impaired, mood becomes very labile, and behaviors characteristic of depression, euphoria, and aggression are exhibited. The only medical use for alcohol (with the exception of its inclusion in a number of pharmacological concentrates) is as an antidote for methanol consumption.

Examples: *Beer, wine, bourbon, scotch, gin, vodka, rum, tequila, liqueurs.*

Common substances containing alcohol and used by some dependent individuals to satisfy their need include liquid cough medications, liquid cold preparations, mouthwashes, isopropyl rubbing alcohol, nail polish removers, colognes, aftershave and preshave preparations.

Opioids

Opioids have a medical use as analgesics, antitussives, and antidiarrheals. They produce the effects of analgesia and euphoria by stimulating the opiate receptors in the brain, thereby mimicking the naturally occurring endorphins.

Examples: *Opioids of natural origin (opium, morphine, codeine); opioid derivatives (heroin, hydromorphone, hydrocodone, oxycodone); synthetic opiate-like drugs (meperidine, methadone, pentazocine, fentanyl).*

Common Street Names: *Horse, junk, H (heroin); black stuff, poppy, big O (opium); M, white stuff, Miss Emma (morphine); dollies (methadone); terp (terpin hydrate or cough syrup with codeine); oxy, O.C. (oxycodone); Vike (hydrocodone); doctors (meperidine); Apache, China girl, goodfella (fentanyl).*

CNS Depressants

CNS depressants have a medical use as antianxiety agents, sedatives, hypnotics, anticonvulsants, and anesthetics. They depress the action of the CNS, resulting in an overall calming, relaxing effect on the individual. At higher dosages they can induce sleep.

Examples: *Benzodiazepines; barbiturates; nonbarbiturate hypnotics (e.g., chloral hydrate, eszopiclone, ramelteon, zaleplon, zolpidem); meprobamate; club drugs (e.g., flunitrazepam, gamma-hydroxybutyrate [GHB])*

Common Street Names: *Peter, Mickey (chloral hydrate); green and whites, roaches (Librium); blues (Valium, 10 mg); yellows (Valium, 5 mg); candy, tranks (other benzodiazepines); red birds, red devils (secobarbital); downers (barbiturates; tranquilizers); rophies, forget-me pill, R2 (flunitrazepam [Rohypnol]); G, liquid X, grievous bodily harm, easy lay (GHB).*

CNS Stimulants

CNS stimulants have a medical use in the management of hyperactivity disorders, narcolepsy, and weight control. They stimulate the action of the CNS, resulting in increased alertness, excitation, euphoria, increased pulse rate and blood pressure, insomnia, and loss of appetite. Recent research indicates that their effectiveness in the treatment of hyperactivity disorders is based on the activation of dopamine D4 receptors in the basal ganglia and thalamus, which depress, rather than enhance, motor activity (Erlij et al, 2012).

Examples: *Amphetamines (e.g., dextroamphetamine; methamphetamine; 3,4-methylenedioxyamphetamine [MDMA]); nonamphetamine stimulants (e.g., phendimetrazine, benzphetamine, methylphenidate, dexmethylphenidate, modafinil); synthetic stimulants (e.g., mephedrone, methylone); cocaine; caffeine; tobacco. (Note: MDMA, mephedrone, and methylone are cross-listed with the hallucinogens.)*

Common Street Names: *Dexies, pep pills, uppers, speed (amphetamines); coke, snow, gold dust, girl (cocaine); crack, rock (hydrochloride cocaine); speedball (mixture of heroin and cocaine); Adam, Ecstasy, XTC (MDMA); bath salts (mephedrone, methylone).*

Hallucinogens

Hallucinogens act as sympathomimetic agents, producing effects resembling those resulting from stimulation of the sympathetic nervous system (e.g., excitation, increased energy, distortion of the senses). Therapeutic medical uses for lysergic acid diethylamide (LSD) have been proposed in the treatment of chronic alcoholism and in the reduction of intractable pain, such as terminal malignant disease and phantom limb sensations. At this time, there is no real evidence of the safety and efficacy of the drug in humans.

Examples: *Naturally occurring hallucinogens (e.g., mescaline, psilocybin, ololiuqui); synthetic compounds (e.g., LSD; 2,5-dimethoxy-4-methylamphetamine [DOM]; phencyclidine [PCP]; ketamine; 3,4-methylenedioxyamphetamine [MDMA]; mephedrone; methylone)*

Common Street Names: *Cactus, mesc (mescaline); magic mushroom, shrooms (psilocybin); heavenly blue, pearly gates (ololiuqui); Acid, cube, California sunshine (LSD); serenity, tranquility, peace; STP (DOM); angel dust (PCP); vitamin K (ketamine); XTC, ecstasy, Adam (MDMA); mephedrone, methylone (bath salts). (Note: MDMA, mephedrone, and methylone are cross-listed with the CNS stimulants.)*

Cannabinoids

Cannabinoids depress higher centers in the brain and consequently release lower centers from inhibitory influence. They produce an anxiety-free state of relaxation characterized by a feeling of extreme well-being. Large doses of the drug can produce hallucinations. Marijuana has been used therapeutically in the relief of nausea and vomiting associated with antineoplastic chemotherapy and in the relief of chronic pain.

Examples: *Marijuana, hashish.*

Common Street Names: *Joints, reefers, pot, grass, Mary Jane (marijuana); hash, bhang, ganja (hashish).*

Inhalants

Inhalant disorders are induced by inhaling the aliphatic and aromatic hydrocarbons found in substances such as fuels, solvents, adhesives, aerosol propellants, and paint thinners. Inhalants are absorbed through the lungs and reach the CNS very rapidly. Inhalants generally act as a CNS depressant. The effects are relatively brief, lasting from several minutes to a few hours, depending on the specific substance and amount consumed.

Examples: *Gasoline, varnish remover, lighter fluid, airplane glue, rubber cement, cleaning fluid, spray paint, shoe conditioner, typewriter correction fluid.*

A profile summary of these psychoactive substances is presented in Table 4-1.

TABLE 4–1   Psychoactive Substances: A Profile Summary

Class of Drugs	Symptoms of Use	Therapeutic Uses	Symptoms of Overdose	Trade Names	Common Names
CNS Depressants					
Alcohol	Relaxation, loss of inhibitions, lack of concentration, drowsiness, slurred speech, sleep	Antidote for methanol consumption; ingredient in many pharmacological concentrates	Nausea, vomiting; shallow respirations; cold, clammy skin; weak, rapid pulse; coma; possible death	Ethyl alcohol, beer, gin, rum, vodka, bourbon, whiskey, liqueurs, wine, brandy, sherry, champagne	Booze, alcohol, liquor, drinks, cocktails, highballs, nightcaps, moonshine, white lightening, firewater
Other (barbiturates and nonbarbiturates)	Same as alcohol	Relief from anxiety and insomnia; as anticonvulsants and anesthetics	Anxiety, fever, agitation, hallucinations, disorientation, tremors, delirium, convulsions, possible death	Seconal, Amytal, Nembutal Valium Librium Noctec Miltown	Red birds, yellow birds, blue birds Blues/yellows Green & whites Mickies Downers
CNS Stimulants					
Amphetamines and related drugs	Hyperactivity, agitation, euphoria, insomnia, loss of appetite	Management of narcolepsy, hyperkinesia, and weight control	Cardiac arrhythmias, headache, convulsions, hypertension, rapid heart rate, coma, possible death	Dexedrine, Didrex, Tenuate, Bontril, Ritalin, Focalin, Meridia, Provigil	Uppers, pep pills, wakeups, bennies, eye-openers, speed, black beauties, sweet As

(Continued)

TABLE 4–1 Psychoactive Substances: A Profile Summary—cont'd

Class of Drugs	Symptoms of Use	Therapeutic Uses	Symptoms of Overdose	Trade Names	Common Names
Cocaine	Euphoria, hyperactivity, restlessness, talkativeness, increased pulse, dilated pupils, rhinitis		Hallucinations, convulsions, pulmonary edema, respiratory failure, coma, cardiac arrest, possible death	Cocaine hydrochloride	Coke, flake, snow, dust, happy dust, gold dust, girl, cecil, C, toot, blow, crack
Synthetic stimulants	Agitation, insomnia, irritability, dizziness, decreased ability to think clearly, increased heart rate, chest pains		Depression, paranoia, delusions, suicidal thoughts, seizures, panic attacks, nausea, vomiting, heart attack, stroke, hallucinations, aggressive behavior	Mephedrone, MDPV (3-4 methylene-dioxypyrovalerone)	Bath salts, bliss, vanilla sky, ivory wave purple wave
Opioids	Euphoria, lethargy, drowsiness, lack of motivation, constricted pupils	As analgesics; antidiarrheals, and antitussives; methadone in substitution therapy; heroin has no therapeutic use	Shallow breathing, slowed pulse, clammy skin, pulmonary edema, respiratory arrest, convulsions, coma, possible death	Heroin Morphine Codeine Dilaudid Demerol Dolophine	Snow, stuff, H, harry, horse M, morph, Miss Emma Schoolboy Lords Doctors Dollies

Category	Pharmacological Name	Street Names	Symptoms	Therapeutic Uses
	Percodan	Perkies		
	Talwin	Ts		
	Opium	Big O, black stuff		
Hallucinogens	LSD	Acid, cube, big D	Agitation, extreme hyperactivity, violence, hallucinations, psychosis, convulsions, possible death	LSD has been proposed in the treatment of chronic alcoholism, and in the reduction of intractable pain
	PCP	Angel dust, hog, peace pill		
	Mescaline	Mesc		
	DMT	Businessman's trip		
	STP, DOM	Serenity and peace	Visual hallucinations, disorientation, confusion, paranoid delusions, euphoria, anxiety, panic, increased pulse	
	MDMA	Ecstasy, XTC		
	Ketamine	Special K, vitamin K, kit kat		
	MDPV	Bath Salts		
Cannabinoids	Cannabis	Marijuana, pot, grass, joint, Mary Jane, MJ	Fatigue, paranoia, delusions, hallucinations, possible psychosis	Marijuana has been used for relief of nausea and vomiting associated with antineoplastic chemotherapy and to reduce eye pressure in glaucoma
	Hashish	Hash, rope, Sweet Lucy	Relaxation, talkativeness, lowered inhibitions, euphoria, mood swings	

■ PREDISPOSING FACTORS ASSOCIATED WITH SUBSTANCE-RELATED DISORDERS

1. **Physiological**
   a. *Genetic.* A genetic link may be involved in the development of substance-related disorders. This is especially evident with alcoholism, less so with other substances. Children of alcoholics are four times more likely than other children to become alcoholics (American Academy of Child and Adolescent Psychiatry, 2011). Studies with monozygotic and dizygotic twins have also supported the genetic hypothesis.
   b. *Biochemical.* A second physiological hypothesis relates to the possibility that alcohol may produce morphine-like substances in the brain that are responsible for alcohol addiction. This occurs when the products of alcohol metabolism react with biologically active amines.
2. **Psychosocial**
   a. *Psychodynamic Theory.* The psychodynamic approach to the etiology of substance abuse focuses on a punitive superego and fixation at the oral stage of psychosexual development (Sadock & Sadock, 2007). Individuals with punitive superegos turn to alcohol to diminish unconscious anxiety and increase feelings of power and self-worth. Sadock and Sadock (2007) state, "As a form of self-medication, alcohol may be used to control panic, opioids to diminish anger, and amphetamines to alleviate depression" (p. 386).
   b. *Social Learning Theory.* The effects of modeling, imitation, and identification on behavior can be observed from early childhood onward. In relation to drug consumption, the family appears to be an important influence. Various studies have shown that children and adolescents are more likely to use substances if they have parents who provide a model for substance use. Peers often exert a great deal of influence in the life of the child or adolescent who is being encouraged to use substances for the first time. Modeling may continue to be a factor in the use of substances once the individual enters the work force. This is particularly true in the work setting that provides plenty of leisure time with coworkers and in which drinking is valued and is used to express group cohesiveness.

■ COMMON PATTERNS OF USE IN SUBSTANCE-RELATED DISORDERS

Symptomatology (Subjective and Objective Data)

Alcohol Use Disorder

1. Begins with social drinking that provides feeling of relaxation and well-being, which soon requires more and more to produce the same effects.

2. Drinks in secret; hides bottles of alcohol; drinks first thing in the morning (to "steady my nerves") and at any other opportunity that arises during the day.

3. As the disease progresses, the individual may drink in binges. During a binge, drinking continues until the individual is too intoxicated or too sick to consume any more. Behavior borders on the psychotic, with the individual wavering in and out of reality.

4. Begins to have blackouts. Periods of amnesia occur (in the absence of intoxication or loss of consciousness) during which the individual is unable to remember periods of time or events that have occurred.

5. Experiences multisystem physiological impairments from chronic use that include (but are not limited to) the following:

   a. *Peripheral Neuropathy:* Numbness, tingling, pain in extremities (caused by thiamine deficiency).

   b. *Wernicke-Korsakoff Syndrome:* Mental confusion, agitation, diplopia (caused by thiamine deficiency). Without immediate thiamine replacement, rapid deterioration to coma and death will occur.

   c. *Alcoholic Cardiomyopathy:* Enlargement of the heart caused by an accumulation of excess lipids in myocardial cells. Symptoms of tachycardia, dyspnea, and arrhythmias may be evident.

   d. *Esophagitis:* Inflammation of, and pain in, the esophagus.

   e. *Esophageal Varices:* Distended veins in the esophagus, with risk of rupture and subsequent hemorrhage.

   f. *Gastritis:* Inflammation of lining of stomach caused by irritation from the alcohol, resulting in pain, nausea, vomiting, and possibility of bleeding because of erosion of blood vessels.

   g. *Pancreatitis:* Inflammation of the pancreas, resulting in pain, nausea and vomiting, and abdominal distention. With progressive destruction to the gland, symptoms of diabetes mellitus could occur.

   h. *Alcoholic Hepatitis:* Inflammation of the liver, resulting in enlargement, jaundice, right upper quadrant pain, and fever.

   i. *Cirrhosis of the Liver:* Fibrous and degenerative changes occurring in response to chronic accumulation of large amounts of fatty acids in the liver. In cirrhosis, symptoms of alcoholic hepatitis progress to include the following:

      • **Portal Hypertension**: Elevation of blood pressure through the portal circulation resulting from defective blood flow through the cirrhotic liver.

      • **Ascites**: An accumulation of serous fluid in the peritoneal cavity.

      • **Hepatic Encephalopathy**: Liver disorder caused by inability of the liver to convert ammonia to urea (the body's natural method of discarding excess ammonia); as serum ammonia levels rise, confusion occurs, accompanied by restlessness, slurred speech, fever, and without intervention, an eventual progression to coma and death.

Alcohol Intoxication

1. Symptoms of alcohol intoxication include disinhibition of sexual or aggressive impulses, mood lability, impaired judgment, impaired social or occupational functioning, slurred speech, incoordination, unsteady gait, nystagmus, and flushed face.
2. Physical and behavioral impairment based on blood alcohol concentrations differ according to gender, body size, physical condition, and level of tolerance.
3. The legal definition of intoxication in the United States is a blood alcohol concentration of 80 mg ethanol per deciliter of blood (mg/dL), which is also measured as 0.08 g/dL.
4. Nontolerant individuals with blood alcohol concentrations greater than 300 mg/dL are at risk for respiratory failure, coma, and death (Sadock & Sadock, 2007).

Alcohol Withdrawal

1. Occurs within 4 to 12 hours of cessation of, or reduction in, heavy and prolonged alcohol use.
2. Symptoms include coarse tremor of hands, tongue, or eyelids; nausea or vomiting; malaise or weakness; tachycardia; sweating; elevated blood pressure; anxiety; depressed mood or irritability; transient hallucinations or illusions; headache; seizures; and insomnia.
3. Without aggressive intervention, the individual may progress to *alcohol withdrawal delirium* about the second or third day following cessation of, or reduction in, prolonged, heavy alcohol use. Symptoms include those described under the syndrome of delirium (see Chapter 3).

Amphetamine (or Amphetamine-type) Use Disorder

1. The use of amphetamines is often initiated for their appetite-suppressant effect in an attempt to lose or control weight.
2. Amphetamines are also taken for the initial feeling of well-being and confidence.
3. They are typically taken orally, intravenously, or by nasal inhalation.
4. Chronic daily (or almost daily) use usually results in an increase in dosage over time to produce the desired effect.
5. Episodic use often takes the form of binges, followed by an intense and unpleasant "crash" in which the individual experiences anxiety, irritability, and feelings of fatigue and depression.
6. Continued use appears to be related to a "craving" for the substance, rather than to prevention or alleviation of withdrawal symptoms.

Amphetamine (or Amphetamine-type) Intoxication

1. Amphetamine intoxication usually begins with a "high" feeling, followed by the development of symptoms of affective blunting; changes in sociability; hypervigilance; interpersonal sensitivity; anxiety, tension, or anger; stereotyped behaviors; and impaired judgment.
2. Physical signs and symptoms that occur with amphetamine intoxication include tachycardia or bradycardia, pupillary dilation, elevated or lowered blood pressure, perspiration or chills, nausea or vomiting, weight loss, psychomotor retardation or agitation, muscular weakness, respiratory depression, chest pain or cardiac arrhythmias, confusion, seizures, dyskinesias, dystonia, or coma (APA, 2013).

Amphetamine (or Amphetamine-type) Withdrawal

1. Amphetamine withdrawal symptoms occur after cessation of (or reduction in) amphetamine (or a related substance) use that has been heavy and prolonged.
2. Symptoms of amphetamine withdrawal develop within a few hours to several days and include fatigue and depression; vivid, unpleasant dreams; insomnia or hypersomnia; increased appetite; headache; profuse sweating; and muscle cramps.

Cannabis Use Disorder

1. Cannabis preparations are almost always smoked but may also be taken orally.
2. It is commonly regarded incorrectly to be a substance without potential for addiction.
3. Tolerance to the substance may result in increased frequency of its use.
4. Abuse is evidenced by participation in hazardous activities when motor coordination is impaired from cannabis use.

Cannabis Intoxication

1. Cannabis intoxication is characterized by impaired motor coordination, euphoria, anxiety, sensation of slowed time, impaired judgment, and social withdrawal that develop during or shortly after cannabis use.
2. Physical symptoms of cannabis intoxication include conjunctival injection, increased appetite, dry mouth, and tachycardia (APA, 2013).
3. The impairment of motor skills lasts for 8 to 12 hours.

Cannabis Withdrawal

1. The *DSM-5* (APA, 2013) describes a syndrome of symptoms that occur upon cessation of cannabis use that has been heavy and prolonged. Symptoms occur within a week following cessation of use and may include any of the following: irritability, anger, or aggression; nervousness or anxiety; sleep difficulty

(e.g., insomnia, disturbing dreams); decreased appetite or weight loss; restlessness; depressed mood.
2. Physical symptoms of cannabis withdrawal may include abdominal pain, tremors, sweating, fever, chills, or headache.

Cocaine Use Disorder

1. Various forms are smoked, inhaled, injected, or taken orally.
2. Chronic daily (or almost daily) use usually results in an increase in dosage over time to produce the desired effect.
3. Episodic use often takes the form of binges, followed by an intense and unpleasant "crash" in which the individual experiences anxiety, irritability, and feelings of fatigue and depression.
4. The drug user often abuses, or is dependent on, a CNS depressant to relieve the residual effects of cocaine.
5. Regular, prolonged use of cocaine leads to tolerance of the substance and subsequent use of increasing doses.
6. Continued use appears to be related to a "craving" for the substance, rather than to prevention or alleviation of withdrawal symptoms.

Cocaine Intoxication

1. Symptoms of cocaine intoxication develop during, or shortly after, use of cocaine.
2. Symptoms of cocaine intoxication include euphoria, fighting, grandiosity, hypervigilance, psychomotor agitation, and impaired judgment.
3. Physical symptoms of cocaine intoxication include tachycardia, elevated blood pressure, papillary dilation, perspiration or chills, nausea/vomiting, chest pain, cardiac arrhythmias, hallucinations, seizures, and delirium.

Cocaine Withdrawal

1. Symptoms of withdrawal occur after cessation of, or reduction in, cocaine use that has been heavy and prolonged.
2. Symptoms of cocaine withdrawal include depression, anxiety, irritability, fatigue, insomnia or hypersomnia, psychomotor agitation, paranoid or suicidal ideation, apathy, and social withdrawal.

Hallucinogen Use Disorder

1. Hallucinogenic substances are taken orally.
2. The cognitive and perceptual impairment may last for up to 12 hours, so use is generally episodic, because the individual must organize time during the daily schedule for its use.
3. Frequent use results in tolerance to the effects of the substance.
4. Addiction is rare, and most people are able to resume their previous lifestyle, following a period of hallucinogen use, without much difficulty.

5. Flashbacks may occur following cessation of hallucinogen use. These episodes consist of visual or auditory misperceptions usually lasting only a few seconds, but sometimes lasting up to several hours.
6. Hallucinogens are highly unpredictable in the effects they may induce each time they are used.

Hallucinogen Intoxication

1. Symptoms of intoxication develop during or shortly after hallucinogen use.
2. Symptoms include marked anxiety or depression, ideas of reference, fear of losing one's mind, paranoid ideation, and impaired judgment.
3. Other symptoms include subjective intensification of perceptions, depersonalization, derealization, illusions, hallucinations, and synesthesia.
4. Because hallucinogens are sympathomimetics, they can cause tachycardia, hypertension, sweating, blurred vision, pupillary dilation, and tremors (Black & Andreasen, 2011).

Inhalant Use Disorder

1. Effects are induced by inhaling the vapors of volatile substances through the nose or mouth.
2. Examples of substances include glue, gasoline, paint, paint thinners, various cleaning chemicals, and typewriter correction fluid.
3. Use of inhalants often begins in childhood, and considerable family dysfunction is characteristic.
4. Use may be daily or episodic, and chronic use may continue into adulthood.
5. Tolerance has been reported among individuals with heavy use, but a withdrawal syndrome from these substances has not been well documented.

Inhalant Intoxication

1. Symptoms of intoxication develop during, or shortly after, use of, or exposure to, volatile inhalants.
2. Symptoms of inhalant intoxication include euphoria, excitation, disinhibition, belligerence, impaired judgment, and impaired social or occupational functioning.
3. Physical symptoms of inhalant intoxication include dizziness, ataxia, nystagmus, blurred vision, slurred speech, hypoactive reflexes, psychomotor retardation, lethargy, generalized muscular weakness, stupor, or coma (at higher doses) (APA, 2013).

Tobacco Use Disorder

1. The effects of tobacco are induced through inhaling the smoke of cigarettes, cigars, or pipe tobacco, and orally through the use of snuff or chewing tobacco.
2. Continued use results in a "craving" for the substance.

3. Tobacco is commonly used to relieve or to avoid withdrawal symptoms that occur when the individual has been in a situation in which use is restricted.
4. Continued use despite knowledge of medical problems related to smoking is a particularly important health problem.

Tobacco Withdrawal

1. Symptoms of withdrawal develop within 24 hours after abrupt cessation of (or reduction in) prolonged tobacco use.
2. Symptoms of tobacco withdrawal include dysphoric or depressed mood, insomnia, irritability, frustration, anger, anxiety, difficulty concentrating, restlessness, decreased heart rate, and increased appetite (APA, 2013).

Opioid Use Disorder

1. Various forms are taken orally, intravenously, by nasal inhalation, and by smoking.
2. Dependence occurs after recreational use of the substance "on the street," or after prescribed use of the substance for relief of pain or cough.
3. Chronic use leads to remarkably high levels of tolerance.
4. Once addiction is established, substance procurement often comes to dominate the person's life.
5. Cessation or decreased consumption results in a "craving" for the substance and produces a specific syndrome of withdrawal.

Opioid Intoxication

1. Symptoms of intoxication develop during or shortly after opioid use.
2. Symptoms of opioid intoxication include euphoria (initially) followed by apathy, dysphoria, psychomotor agitation or retardation, impaired judgment, and impaired social or occupational functioning.
3. Physical symptoms of opioid intoxication include pupillary constriction (or dilation due to anoxia from severe overdose), drowsiness, slurred speech, and impairment in attention or memory (APA, 2013).
4. Severe opioid intoxication can lead to respiratory depression, coma, and death.

Opioid Withdrawal

1. Symptoms of opioid withdrawal occur after cessation of (or reduction in) heavy and prolonged opioid use.
2. Symptoms of opioid withdrawal include dysphoric mood, nausea or vomiting, muscle aches, lacrimation or rhinorrhea, pupillary dilation, piloerection, sweating, diarrhea, yawning, fever, and insomnia (APA, 2013).
3. Withdrawal symptoms are consistent with the half-life of the drug that is used. Withdrawal from the ultra-short-acting

drugs such as meperidine begins quickly (within minutes to hours). With longer-acting drugs such as methadone, withdrawal begins within 1 to 3 days and may last for as long as 3 weeks.

Phencyclidine (PCP) Use Disorder

1. Phencyclidine is taken orally, intravenously, or by smoking or inhaling.
2. Use can be on a chronic daily basis, but more often is taken episodically in binges that can last several days.
3. Physical addiction does not occur with PCP; however, psychological addiction, characterized by craving for the drug, has been reported in chronic users, as has the development of tolerance.
4. Tolerance apparently develops quickly with frequent use.

Phencyclidine Intoxication

1. Symptoms of intoxication develop during or shortly after PCP use.
2. Symptoms of PCP intoxication include belligerence, assaultiveness, impulsiveness, unpredictability, psychomotor agitation, and impaired judgment.
3. Physical symptoms occur within an hour or less of PCP use and include vertical or horizontal nystagmus, hypertension, tachycardia, numbness or diminished responsiveness to pain, ataxia, muscle rigidity, and seizures.

Sedative, Hypnotic, or Anxiolytic Use Disorder

1. Effects are produced through oral intake of these substances.
2. Dependence can occur following recreational use of the substance "on the street" or after prescribed use of the substance for relief of anxiety or insomnia.
3. Chronic use leads to remarkably high levels of tolerance.
4. Once dependence develops, there is evidence of strong substance-seeking behaviors (obtaining prescriptions from several physicians or resorting to illegal sources to maintain adequate supplies of the substance).
5. Abrupt cessation of these substances can result in life-threatening withdrawal symptoms.

Sedative, Hypnotic, or Anxiolytic Intoxication

1. Symptoms of intoxication develop during or shortly after intake of sedatives, hypnotics, or anxiolytics.
2. Symptoms of intoxication include inappropriate sexual or aggressive behavior, mood lability, impaired judgment, and impaired social or occupational functioning.
3. Physical symptoms of sedative, hypnotic, or anxiolytic intoxication include slurred speech, incoordination, unsteady gait, nystagmus, impairment in attention or memory, stupor, or coma.

Sedative, Hypnotic, or Anxiolytic Withdrawal

1. Withdrawal symptoms occur after cessation of (or reduction in) heavy and prolonged use of sedatives, hypnotics, or anxiolytics.
2. Symptoms of withdrawal occur within several hours to a few days after abrupt cessation or reduction in use of the drug (depending on the half-life of the drug).
3. Symptoms of withdrawal include autonomic hyperactivity (e.g., sweating or pulse rate greater than 100); increased hand tremor; insomnia; nausea or vomiting; transient visual, tactile, or auditory hallucinations or illusions; psychomotor agitation; anxiety; or grand mal seizures.

A summary of symptoms associated with the syndromes of intoxication and withdrawal is presented in Table 4-2.

■ NONSUBSTANCE-RELATED DISORDERS

Gambling Disorder

This disorder is defined by the *DSM-5* as persistent and recurrent problematic gambling behavior leading to clinically significant impairment or distress (APA, 2013). The preoccupation with and impulse to gamble often intensifies when the individual is under stress. Many impulsive gamblers describe a physical sensation of restlessness and anticipation that can only be relieved by placing a bet. Often, the individual exhibits characteristics associated with narcissism and grandiosity and has difficulties with intimacy, empathy, and trust.

As the need to gamble increases, the individual is forced to obtain money by any means available. This may include borrowing money from illegal sources or pawning personal items (or items that belong to others). As gambling debts accrue or out of a need to continue gambling, the individual may desperately resort to forgery, theft, or even embezzlement. Family relationships are disrupted, and impairment in occupational functioning may occur because of absences from work in order to gamble.

Gambling behavior usually begins in adolescence; however, compulsive behaviors rarely occur before young adulthood. The disorder generally runs a chronic course, with periods of waxing and waning, largely dependent on periods of psychosocial stress. Prevalence estimates for pathological gambling range from 1.2% to 3.4% (Hollander, Berlin, & Stein, 2008). It is more common among men than women.

Predisposing Factors Associated With Gambling Disorder

1. **Biological**
   a. Genetic. Familial and twin studies show an increased prevalence of pathological gambling in family members of individuals diagnosed with the disorder. Hollander, Berlin, and Stein (2008) report the results of research that indicates a

TABLE 4-2 Summary of Symptoms Associated With the Syndromes of Intoxication and Withdrawal

Class of Drugs	Intoxication	Withdrawal	Comments
Alcohol	Aggressiveness, impaired judgment, impaired attention, irritability, euphoria, depression, emotional lability, slurred speech, incoordination, unsteady gait, nystagmus, flushed face	Tremors, nausea/vomiting, malaise, weakness, tachycardia, sweating, elevated blood pressure, anxiety, depressed mood, irritability, hallucinations, headache, insomnia, seizures	Alcohol withdrawal begins within 4–6 hr after last drink. May progress to delirium tremens on 2nd or 3rd day. Use of Librium or Serax is common for substitution therapy.
Amphetamines and related substances	Fighting, grandiosity, hypervigilance, psychomotor agitation, impaired judgment, tachycardia, pupillary dilation, elevated blood pressure, perspiration or chills, nausea and vomiting	Anxiety, depressed mood, irritability, craving for the substance, fatigue, insomnia or hypersomnia, psychomotor agitation, paranoid and suicidal ideation	Withdrawal symptoms usually peak within 2–4 days, although depression and irritability may persist for months. Antidepressants may be used.
Caffeine	Restlessness, nervousness, excitement, insomnia, flushed face, diuresis, gastrointestinal complaints, muscle twitching, rambling flow of thought and speech, cardiac arrhythmia, periods of inexhaustibility, psychomotor agitation	Headache	Caffeine is contained in coffee, tea, colas, cocoa, chocolate, some over-the-counter analgesics, "cold" preparations, and stimulants.

(Continued)

TABLE 4–2 Summary of Symptoms Associated With the Syndromes of Intoxication and Withdrawal—cont'd

Class of Drugs	Intoxication	Withdrawal	Comments
Cannabis	Euphoria, anxiety, suspiciousness, sensation of slowed time, impaired judgment, social withdrawal, tachycardia, conjunctival redness, increased appetite, hallucinations	Restlessness, irritability, insomnia, loss of appetite	Intoxication occurs immediately and lasts about 3 hours. Oral ingestion is more slowly absorbed and has longer-lasting effects.
Cocaine	Euphoria, fighting, grandiosity, hypervigilance, psychomotor agitation, impaired judgment, tachycardia, elevated blood pressure, pupillary dilation, perspiration or chills, nausea/vomiting, hallucinations, delirium	Depression, anxiety, irritability, fatigue, insomnia or hypersomnia, psychomotor agitation, paranoid or suicidal ideation, apathy, social withdrawal	Large doses of the drug can result in convulsions or death from cardiac arrhythmias or respiratory paralysis.
Inhalants	Belligerence, assaultiveness, apathy, impaired judgment, dizziness, nystagmus, slurred speech, unsteady gait, lethargy, depressed reflexes, tremor, blurred vision, stupor or coma, euphoria, irritation around eyes, throat, and nose		Intoxication occurs within 5 minutes of inhalation. Symptoms last 60–90 min. Large doses can result in death from CNS depression or cardiac arrhythmia.
Tobacco		Craving for the drug, irritability, anger, frustration, anxiety, difficulty concentrating, restlessness,	Symptoms of withdrawal begin within 24 hours of last drug use and decrease in intensity

Substance	Intoxication/Effects	Withdrawal Symptoms	Course/Timing
		decreased heart rate, increased appetite, weight gain, tremor, headaches, insomnia	over days, weeks, or sometimes longer.
Opioids	Euphoria, lethargy, somnolence, apathy, dysphoria, impaired judgment, pupillary constriction, drowsiness, slurred speech, constipation, nausea, decreased respiratory rate and blood pressure	Craving for the drug, nausea/vomiting, muscle aches, lacrimation or rhinorrhea, pupillary dilation, piloerection or sweating, diarrhea, yawning, fever, insomnia	Withdrawal symptoms appear within 6-8 hours after last dose, reach a peak in the 2nd or 3rd day, and subside in 5-10 days. Times are shorter with meperidine and longer with methadone.
Phencyclidine and related substances	Belligerence, assaultiveness, impulsiveness, psychomotor agitation, impaired judgment, nystagmus, increased heart rate and blood pressure, diminished pain response, ataxia, dysarthria, muscle rigidity, seizures, hyperacusis, delirium		Delirium can occur within 24 hours after use of phencyclidine, or may occur up to a week following recovery from an overdose of the drug.
Sedatives, hypnotics, and anxiolytics	Disinhibition of sexual or aggressive impulses, mood lability, impaired judgment, slurred speech, incoordination, unsteady gait, impairment in attention or memory, disorientation, confusion	Nausea/vomiting, malaise, weakness, tachycardia, sweating, anxiety, irritability, orthostatic hypotension, tremor, insomnia, seizures	Withdrawal may progress to delirium, usually within 1 week of last use. Long-acting barbiturates or benzodiazepines may be used in withdrawal substitution therapy.

common genetic vulnerability for pathological gambling and alcohol addiction in men.

b. ***Physiological.*** Hodgins, Stea, and Grant (2011) suggest a correlation between pathological gambling and abnormalities in the serotonergic, noradrenergic, and dopaminergic neurotransmitter systems. They stated:

Dopamine is implicated in learning, motivation, and the salience of stimuli, including rewards. Alterations in dopaminergic pathways might underlie the seeking of rewards (i.e., gambling) that trigger the release of dopamine and produce feelings of pleasure (p. 1878).

Other studies have indicated alterations in the electroencephalographic patterns of pathologic gamblers (Regard, Knoch, Gutling, & Landis, 2003).

2. **Psychological**

Sadock and Sadock (2007) report that the following may be predisposing factors to the development of pathological gambling: "loss of a parent by death, separation, divorce, or desertion before the child is 15 years of age; inappropriate parental discipline (absence, inconsistency, or harshness); exposure to and availability of gambling activities for the adolescent; a family emphasis on material and financial symbols; and a lack of family emphasis on saving, planning, and budgeting" (p. 779).

The early psychoanalytical view attempted to explain compulsive gambling in terms of psychosexual maturation. In this theory, the gambling is compared to masturbation; both of these activities derive motive force from a build-up of tension that is released through repetitive actions or the anticipation of them. Another view suggests a masochistic component to pathological gambling and the gambler's inherent need for punishment, which is then achieved through losing (Moreyra, Ibanez, Saiz-Ruiz, Nissenson, & Blanco, 2000).

Common Nursing Diagnoses and Interventions for Clients With Substance-Related and Addictive Disorders

(Interventions are applicable to various health-care settings, such as inpatient and partial hospitalization, community outpatient clinic, home health, and private practice.)

■ RISK FOR INJURY

Definition: *At risk for injury as a result of [internal or external] environmental conditions interacting with the individual's adaptive and defensive resources* (NANDA International [NANDA-I], 2012, p. 430)

Risk Factors ("related to")

[Substance intoxication]
[Substance withdrawal]
[Disorientation]
[Seizures]
[Hallucinations]
[Psychomotor agitation]
[Unstable vital signs]
[Delirium]
[Flashbacks]
[Panic level of anxiety]

Goals/Objectives

Short-term Goal
Client's condition will stabilize within 72 hours.

Long-term Goal
Client will not experience physical injury.

Interventions With Selected Rationales

1. Assess client's level of disorientation to determine specific requirements for safety. *Knowledge of client's level of functioning is necessary to formulate appropriate plan of care.*
2. Obtain a drug history, if possible, to determine the following:
   a. Type of substance(s) used.
   b. Time of last ingestion and amount consumed.
   c. Length and frequency of consumption.
   d. Amount consumed on a daily basis.
3. Obtain urine sample for laboratory analysis of substance content. *Subjective history is often not accurate. Knowledge regarding substance ingestion is important for accurate assessment of client condition.*
4. Place client in quiet, private room. *Excessive stimuli increase client agitation.*
5. Institute necessary safety precautions *(Client safety is a nursing priority.)*:
   a. Observe client behaviors frequently; assign staff on one-to-one basis if condition is warranted; accompany and assist client when ambulating; use wheelchair for transporting long distances.
   b. Be sure that side rails are up when client is in bed.
   c. Pad headboard and side rails of bed with thick towels to protect client in case of seizure.
   d. Use mechanical restraints as necessary to protect client if excessive hyperactivity accompanies the disorientation.

6. Ensure that smoking materials and other potentially harmful objects are stored away from client's access. *Client may harm self or others in disoriented, confused state.*

7. Frequently orient client to reality and surroundings. *Disorientation may endanger client safety if he or she unknowingly wanders away from safe environment.*

8. Monitor client's vital signs every 15 minutes initially and less frequently as acute symptoms subside. *Vital signs provide the most reliable information about client condition and need for medication during acute detoxification period.*

9. Follow medication regimen, as ordered by physician. Common medical intervention for detoxification from the following substances includes:

   a. **Alcohol.** Benzodiazepines are the most widely used group of drugs for substitution therapy in alcohol withdrawal. They are administered in decreasing doses until withdrawal is complete. Commonly used agents include chlordiazepoxide (Librium), oxazepam (Serax), diazepam (Valium) and alprazolam (Xanax). In clients with liver disease, accumulation of the longer-acting agents, such as chlordiazepoxide (Librium), may be problematic, and the use of shorter-acting benzodiazepines, such as oxazepam (Serax), is more appropriate. Some physicians may order anticonvulsant medication to be used prophylactically; however, this is not a universal intervention. Multivitamin therapy, in combination with daily thiamine (either orally or by injection), is common protocol.

   b. **Narcotics.** Narcotic antagonists, such as naloxone (Narcan), naltrexone (ReVia), or nalmefene (Revex), are administered intravenously for narcotic overdose. Withdrawal is managed with rest and nutritional therapy. Substitution therapy may be instituted to decrease withdrawal symptoms using methadone (Dolophine) or buprenorphine (Subutex). Clonidine (Catapres) also has been used to suppress opiate withdrawal symptoms. As monotherapy, it is not as effective as substitution with methadone, but it is nonaddicting and serves effectively as a bridge that enables the client to stay opiate free long enough to facilitate termination of methadone maintenance.

   c. **Depressants.** Substitution therapy may be instituted to decrease withdrawal symptoms using a long-acting barbiturate, such as phenobarbital (Luminal). The dosage required to suppress withdrawal symptoms is administered. When stabilization has been achieved, the dose is gradually decreased by 30 mg/day until withdrawal is complete. Long-acting benzodiazepines are commonly used for substitution therapy when the abused substance is a nonbarbiturate CNS depressant.

d. **Stimulants.** Treatment of stimulant intoxication usually begins with minor tranquilizers such as chlordiazepoxide (Librium) and progresses to major tranquilizers such as haloperidol (Haldol). Antipsychotics should be administered with caution because of their propensity to lower seizure threshold. Repeated seizures are treated with intravenous diazepam. Withdrawal treatment is usually aimed at reducing drug craving and managing severe depression. The client is placed in a quiet atmosphere and allowed to sleep and eat as much as is needed or desired. Suicide precautions may need to be instituted. Antidepressant therapy may be helpful in treating symptoms of depression. Desipramine has been especially successful with symptoms of cocaine withdrawal and abstinence (Mack, Franklin, & Frances, 2003).

e. **Hallucinogens and Cannabinoids.** Substitution therapy is not required with these drugs. When adverse reactions, such as anxiety or panic, occur, benzodiazepines (e.g., diazepam or chlordiazepoxide) may be prescribed to prevent harm to the client or others. Psychotic reactions may be treated with antipsychotic medications.

Outcome Criteria

1. Client is no longer exhibiting any signs or symptoms of substance intoxication or withdrawal.
2. Client shows no evidence of physical injury obtained during substance intoxication or withdrawal.

■ INEFFECTIVE DENIAL

Definition: *Conscious or unconscious attempt to disavow the knowledge or meaning of an event to reduce anxiety/fear, leading to the detriment of health [or other aspects of the individual's life]* (NANDA-I, 2012, p. 358)

Possible Etiologies ("related to")

[Weak, underdeveloped ego]
[Underlying fears and anxieties]
[Low self-esteem]
[Fixation in early level of development]

Defining Characteristics ("evidenced by")

[Denies substance-related or other addictions]
[Denies that substance use or gambling creates problems in his or her life]

[Continues to use substance or gamble, knowing it contributes to impairment in functioning, exacerbation of physical symptoms, or disruption on interpersonal relationships]

[Uses substance(s) in physically hazardous situations]

[Use of rationalization and projection to explain maladaptive behaviors]

Unable to admit impact of [the disorder] on life pattern

Goals/Objectives

Short-term Goal

Client will divert attention away from external issues and focus on behavioral outcomes associated with substance-related or addictive disorder.

Long-term Goal

Client will verbalize acceptance of responsibility for own behavior and acknowledge association between substance use or gambling and personal problems.

Interventions With *Selected Rationales*

1. Begin by working to develop a trusting nurse-client relationship. Be honest. Keep all promises. ***Trust is the basis of a therapeutic relationship.***

2. Convey an attitude of acceptance to the client. Ensure that he or she understands, "It is not *you* but your *behavior* that is unacceptable." ***An attitude of acceptance promotes feelings of dignity and self-worth.***

3. Provide information to correct misconceptions about the substance use or gambling behavior. Client may rationalize his or her behavior with statements such as, "I'm not addicted. I can stop drinking (or gambling) any time I want." or "I only smoke pot to relax before class. So what? I know lots of people who do. Besides, you can't get hooked on pot." ***Many myths abound regarding addictions. Factual information presented in a matter-of-fact, nonjudgmental way explaining what behaviors constitute substance-related and addictive disorders may help the client focus on his or her own behaviors as an illness that requires help.***

4. Identify recent maladaptive behaviors or situations that have occurred in the client's life, and discuss how use of substances or gambling behavior may have been a contributing factor. ***The first step in decreasing use of denial is for client to see the relationship between substance use (or gambling) and personal problems.***

5. Use confrontation with caring. Do not allow client to fantasize about his or her lifestyle. ***Confrontation interferes with client's ability to use denial; a caring attitude preserves self-esteem and avoids putting the client on the defensive.***

CLINICAL PEARL It is important to speak objectively and nonjudgmentally to a person in denial. Examples: "It is my understanding that the last time you drank alcohol (gambled), you . . ." or "The lab report shows that your blood alcohol level was 250 when you were involved in that automobile accident" or "Your family is being evicted from their home because you lost the rent money when you bet on the horses."

6. Do not accept the use of rationalization or projection as client attempts to make excuses for or blame his or her behavior on other people or situations. *Rationalization and projection prolong the stage of denial that problems exist in the client's life because of substance use or gambling.*
7. Encourage participation in group activities. *Peer feedback is often more accepted than feedback from authority figures. Peer pressure can be a strong factor as well as the association with individuals who are experiencing or who have experienced similar problems.*
8. Offer immediate positive recognition of client's expressions of insight gained regarding illness and acceptance of responsibility for own behavior. *Positive reinforcement enhances self-esteem and encourages repetition of desirable behaviors.*

Outcome Criteria

1. Client verbalizes understanding of the relationship between personal problems and the use of substances or gambling behaviors.
2. Client verbalizes acceptance of responsibility for own behavior.
3. Client verbalizes understanding of substance (or gambling) addiction as an illness requiring ongoing support and treatment.

■ INEFFECTIVE COPING

Definition: *Inability to form a valid appraisal of the stressors, inadequate choices of practiced responses, and/or inability to use available resources* (NANDA-I, 2012, P. 348)

Possible Etiologies ("related to")

[Inadequate support systems]
[Inadequate coping skills]
[Underdeveloped ego]
[Possible hereditary factor]
[Dysfunctional family system]
[Negative role modeling]
[Personal vulnerability]

Defining Characteristics ("evidenced by")

[Low self-esteem]
[Chronic anxiety]

[Chronic depression]
Inability to meet role expectations
[Alteration in societal participation]
Inability to meet basic needs
[Inappropriate use of defense mechanisms]
Substance abuse
[Pathological gambling behaviors]
[Low frustration tolerance]
[Need for immediate gratification]
[Manipulative behavior]

Goals/Objectives

Short-term Goal

Client will express true feelings associated with gambling or the use of substances as a method of coping with stress.

Long-term Goal

Client will be able to verbalize adaptive coping mechanisms to use, instead of gambling or substance abuse, in response to stress.

Interventions With *Selected Rationales*

1. Establish trusting relationship with client (be honest; keep appointments; be available to spend time). *The therapeutic nurse-client relationship is built on trust.*
2. Set limits on manipulative behavior. Be sure that the client knows what is acceptable, what is not, and the consequences for violating the limits set. Ensure that all staff maintains consistency with this intervention. *Client is unable to establish own limits, so limits must be set for him or her. Unless administration of consequences for violation of limits is consistent, manipulative behavior will not be eliminated.*
3. Encourage client to verbalize feelings, fears, and anxieties. Answer any questions he or she may have regarding the disorder. *Verbalization of feelings in a nonthreatening environment may help client come to terms with long-unresolved issues.*
4. Explain the effects of substance abuse on the body. Emphasize that prognosis is closely related to abstinence. *Many clients lack knowledge regarding the deleterious effects of substance abuse on the body.*
5. Explore with client the options available to assist with stressful situations rather than resorting to gambling or use of substances (e.g., contacting various members of Alcoholics Anonymous, Narcotics Anonymous, or Gamblers Anonymous; physical exercise; relaxation techniques; or meditation). *Client may have persistently resorted to addictive behaviors and thus may possess little or no knowledge of adaptive responses to stress.*

6. Provide positive reinforcement for evidence of gratification delayed appropriately. ***Positive reinforcement enhances self-esteem and encourages client to repeat acceptable behaviors.***
7. Encourage client to be as independent as possible in own self-care. Provide positive feedback for independent decision-making and effective use of problem-solving skills.

Outcome Criteria

1. Client is able to verbalize adaptive coping strategies as alternatives to use of addictive behaviors in response to stress.
2. Client is able to verbalize the names of support people from whom he or she may seek help when the desire to gamble or use substances is intense.

■ IMBALANCED NUTRITION: LESS THAN BODY REQUIREMENTS

Definition: *Intake of nutrients insufficient to meet metabolic needs* (NANDA-I, 2012, p. 174)

Possible Etiologies ("related to")

[Drinking alcohol instead of eating nourishing food]
[Eating only "junk food"]
[Eating nothing (or very little) while on a "binge"]
[No money for food (having spent what is available on substances)]
[Problems with malabsorption caused by chronic alcohol abuse]

Defining Characteristics ("evidenced by")

Loss of weight
Pale conjunctiva and mucous membranes
Poor muscle tone
[Poor skin turgor]
[Edema of extremities]
[Electrolyte imbalances]
[Cheilosis (cracks at corners of mouth)]
[Scaly dermatitis]
[Weakness]
[Neuropathies]
[Anemia]
[Ascites]

Goals/Objectives

Short-term Goals

1. Client will gain 2 lb during next 7 days.
2. Client's electrolytes will be restored to normal within 1 week.

Long-term Goal

Client will exhibit no signs or symptoms of malnutrition by discharge. (This is not a realistic goal for a chronic alcoholic in the end stages of the disease. For such a client, it is more appropriate to establish short-term goals as realistic step objectives to use in the evaluation of care given.)

Interventions With *Selected Rationales*

1. In collaboration with dietitian, determine number of calories required to provide adequate nutrition and realistic (according to body structure and height) weight gain.
2. Strict documentation of intake, output, and calorie count. *This information is necessary to make an accurate nutritional assessment and maintain client safety.*
3. Weigh daily. *Weight loss or gain is important assessment information.*
4. Determine client's likes and dislikes and collaborate with dietitian to provide favorite foods. *Client is more likely to eat foods that he or she particularly enjoys.*
5. Ensure that client receives small, frequent feedings, including a bedtime snack, rather than three larger meals. *Large amounts of food may be objectionable, or even intolerable, to the client.*
6. Administer vitamin and mineral supplements, as ordered by physician, *to improve nutritional state.*
7. If appropriate, ask family members or significant others to bring in special foods that client particularly enjoys.
8. Monitor laboratory work, and report significant changes to physician.
9. Explain the importance of adequate nutrition. *Client may have inadequate or inaccurate knowledge regarding the contribution of good nutrition to overall wellness.*

Outcome Criteria

1. Client has achieved and maintained at least 90% of normal body weight.
2. Client's vital signs, blood pressure, and laboratory serum studies are within normal limits.
3. Client is able to verbalize importance of adequate nutrition.

■ CHRONIC LOW SELF-ESTEEM

Definition: *Longstanding negative self-evaluating/feelings about self or self-capabilities* (NANDA-I, 2012, p. 285)

Possible Etiologies ("related to")

[Retarded ego development]
[Dysfunctional family system]
[Lack of positive feedback]
[Perceived failures]

Defining Characteristics ("evidenced by")

[Difficulty accepting positive reinforcement]
[Failure to take responsibility for self-care]
[Self-destructive behavior (substance use or pathological gambling)]
Lack of eye contact
[Withdraws into social isolation]
[Highly critical and judgmental of self and others]
[Sense of worthlessness]
[Fear of failure]
[Unable to recognize own accomplishments]
[Setting up self for failure by establishing unrealistic goals]
[Unsatisfactory interpersonal relationships]
[Negative or pessimistic outlook]
[Denial of problems obvious to others]
[Projection of blame or responsibility for problems]
[Rationalizing personal failures]
[Hypersensitivity to slight criticism]
[Grandiosity]

Goals/Objectives

Short-term Goal

Client will accept responsibility for personal failures and verbalize the role substances or gambling behaviors played in those failures.

Long-term Goal

By time of discharge, client will exhibit increased feelings of self-worth as evidenced by verbal expression of positive aspects about self, past accomplishments, and future prospects.

Interventions With *Selected Rationales*

1. Be accepting of client and his or her negativism. *An attitude of acceptance enhances feelings of self-worth.*
2. Spend time with client *to convey acceptance and contribute toward feelings of self-worth.*
3. Help client to recognize and focus on strengths and accomplishments. Discuss past (real or perceived) failures, but minimize amount of attention devoted to them beyond client's need to accept responsibility for them. *Client must*

accept responsibility for own behavior before change in behavior can occur. Minimizing attention to past failures may help to eliminate negative ruminations and increase client's sense of self-worth.

4. Encourage participation in group activities *from which client may receive positive feedback and support from peers.*

5. Help client identify areas he or she would like to change about self and assist with problem-solving toward this effort. *Low self-worth may interfere with client's perception of own problem-solving ability. Assistance may be required.*

6. Ensure that client is not becoming increasingly dependent and that he or she is accepting responsibility for own behaviors. *Client must be able to function independently if he or she is to be successful within the less-structured community environment.*

7. Ensure that therapy groups offer client simple methods of achievement. Offer recognition and positive feedback for actual accomplishments. *Successes and recognition increase self-esteem.*

8. Provide instruction in assertiveness techniques: the ability to recognize the difference among passive, assertive, and aggressive behaviors and the importance of respecting the human rights of others while protecting one's own basic human rights. *Self-esteem is enhanced by the ability to interact with others in an assertive manner.*

9. Teach effective communication techniques, such as the use of "I" messages and placing emphasis on ways to avoid making judgmental statements.

Outcome Criteria

1. Client is able to verbalize positive aspects about self.
2. Client is able to communicate assertively with others.
3. Client expresses an optimistic outlook for the future.

■ DEFICIENT KNOWLEDGE (Effects of Substance Use on the Body)

Definition: *Absence or deficiency of cognitive information related to [the effects of substance abuse on the body and its interference with achievement and maintenance of optimal wellness]* (NANDA-I, 2012, p. 271)

Possible Etiologies ("related to")

Lack of interest in learning
[Low self-esteem]
[Denial of need for information]

[Denial of risks involved with substance abuse]
Unfamiliarity with information resources

Defining Characteristics ("evidenced by")

[Abuse of substances]
[Statement of lack of knowledge]
[Statement of misconception]
[Request for information]
Verbalization of the problem

Goals/Objectives

Short-term Goal

Client will be able to verbalize effects of [substance used] on the body following implementation of teaching plan.

Long-term Goal

Client will verbalize the importance of abstaining from use of [substance] to maintain optimal wellness.

Interventions With *Selected Rationales*

1. Assess client's level of knowledge regarding effects of [substance] on body. *Baseline assessment of knowledge is required to develop appropriate teaching plan for client.*
2. Assess client's level of anxiety and readiness to learn. *Learning does not take place beyond moderate level of anxiety.*
3. Determine method of learning most appropriate for client (e.g., discussion, question and answer, use of audio or visual aids, oral or written method). *Level of education and development are important considerations as to methodology selected.*
4. Develop teaching plan, including measurable objectives for the learner. *Measurable objectives provide criteria on which to base evaluation of the teaching experience.*
5. Include significant others, if possible. *Lifestyle changes often affect all family members.*
6. Implement teaching plan at a time that facilitates and in a place that is conducive to optimal learning (e.g., in the evening when family members visit, in an empty, quiet classroom or group therapy room). *Learning is enhanced by an environment with few distractions.*
7. Begin with simple concepts and progress to the more complex. *Retention is increased if introductory material presented is easy to understand.*
8. Include information on physical effects of [substance]: substance's capacity for physiological and psychological addiction; its effects on family functioning; its effects on a fetus (and the importance of contraceptive use until abstinence has been

achieved); and the importance of regular participation in an appropriate treatment program.

9. Provide activities for client and significant others in which to participate actively during the learning exercise. *Active participation increases retention.*

10. Ask client and significant others to demonstrate knowledge gained by verbalizing information presented. *Verbalization of knowledge gained is a measurable method of evaluating the teaching experience.*

11. Provide positive feedback for participation as well as for accurate demonstration of knowledge acquired. *Positive feedback enhances self-esteem and encourages repetition of desired behaviors.*

12. Evaluate teaching plan. Identify strengths and weaknesses, as well as any changes that may enhance the effectiveness of the plan.

Outcome Criteria

1. Client is able to verbalize effects of [substance] on the body.
2. Client verbalizes understanding of risks involved in use of [substance].
3. Client is able to verbalize community resources for obtaining knowledge and support with substance-related problems.

■ DYSFUNCTIONAL FAMILY PROCESSES

Definition: *Psychosocial, spiritual, and physiological functions of the family unit are chronically disorganized, which leads to conflict, denial of problems, resistance to change, ineffective problem-solving, and a series of self-perpetuating crises* (NANDA-I, 2012, p. 308)

Possible Etiologies ("related to")

Substance abuse
Genetic predisposition [to addictions]
Lack of problem-solving skills
Inadequate coping skills
Family history of substance abuse
Biochemical influences
Addictive personality
[Pathological gambling]

Defining Characteristics ("evidenced by")

Anxiety, anger/suppressed rage; shame and embarrassment
Emotional isolation/loneliness; vulnerability; repressed emotions

Disturbed family dynamics; closed communication systems, ineffective spousal communication and marital problems

Altered role function/disruption of family roles

Manipulation; dependency; blaming/criticizing; rationalization/denial of problems

Enabling to maintain [addiction]; refusal to get help/inability to accept and receive help appropriately

Goals/Objectives

Short-term Goals

1. Family members will participate in individual family programs and support groups.
2. Family members will identify ineffective coping behaviors and consequences.
3. Family will initiate and plan for necessary lifestyle changes.

Long-term Goal

Family members will take action to change self-destructive behaviors and alter behaviors that contribute to client's addiction.

Interventions With *Selected Rationales*

1. Review family history; explore roles of family members, circumstances involving the addictive behavior, strengths, areas of growth. *This information determines areas for focus and potential for change.*
2. Explore how family members have coped with the client's addiction (e.g., denial, repression, rationalization, hurt, loneliness, projection). *Persons who enable also suffer from the same feelings as the client and use ineffective methods for dealing with the situation, necessitating help in learning new and effective coping skills.*
3. Determine understanding of current situation and previous methods of coping with life's problems. *Provides information on which to base present plan of care.*
4. Assess current level of functioning of family members. *Affects individual's ability to cope with the situation.*
5. Determine extent of enabling behaviors being evidenced by family members; explore with each individual and client. *Enabling is doing for the client what he or she needs to do for self (rescuing). People want to be helpful and do not want to feel powerless to help their loved one to stop substance use or gambling and change the behavior that is so destructive. However, the addicted person often relies on others to cover up own inability to cope with daily responsibilities.*
6. Provide information about enabling behavior and addictive disease characteristics for both the user and nonuser. *Awareness*

and knowledge of behaviors (e.g., avoiding and shielding, taking over responsibilities, rationalizing, and subserving) provide opportunity for individuals to begin the process of change.

7. Identify and discuss sabotage behaviors of family members. *Even though family member(s) may verbalize a desire for the individual to become addiction-free, the reality of interactive dynamics is that they may unconsciously not want the individual to recover, as this would affect the family members' own role in the relationship. Additionally, they may receive sympathy or attention from others (secondary gain).*

8. Encourage participation in therapeutic writing, e.g., journaling (narrative), guided or focused. *Serves as a release for feelings (e.g., anger, grief, stress); helps move individual(s) forward in the treatment process.*

9. Provide factual information to client and family about the effects of addictive behaviors on the family and what to expect after discharge. *Many people are unaware of the nature of addiction. If client is using legally obtained drugs, he or she may believe this does not constitute abuse.*

10. Encourage family members to be aware of their own feelings, to look at the situation with perspective and objectivity. They can ask themselves: "Am I being conned? Am I acting out of fear, shame, guilt, or anger? Do I have a need to control?" *When the enabling family members become aware of their own actions that perpetuate the client's problems, they need to decide to change themselves. If they change, the client can then face the consequences of own actions and may choose to get well.*

11. Provide support for enabling family members. *For change to occur, families need support as much as the person who has the problem with the addiction.*

12. Assist the client's partner to become aware that the client's behavior is not the partner's responsibility. *Partners need to learn that the client's gambling or use of substances may or may not change despite partner's involvement in treatment.*

13. Help a recovering (formerly addicted) partner who is enabling to distinguish between destructive aspects of own behavior and genuine motivation to aid the client. *Enabling behavior can be a recovering individual's attempts at personal survival.*

14. Note how the partner relates to the treatment team and staff. *Determines enabling style. A parallel exists between how partner relates to client and to staff, based on the partner's feelings about self and situation.*

15. Explore conflicting feelings the enabling partner may have about treatment (e.g., feelings similar to those of the person with the addiction [blend of anger, guilt, fear, exhaustion, embarrassment, loneliness, distrust, grief, and possibly relief]). *This is useful in establishing the need for therapy for the partner. This individual's own identity may have been lost— he or she may fear self-disclosure to staff and may have difficulty giving up the dependent relationship.*

16. Involve family in discharge referral plans. *Addiction is a family illness. Because the family has been so involved in dealing with the addictive behavior, family members need help adjusting to the new behavior of sobriety/abstinence. Incidence of recovery is almost doubled when the family is treated along with the client.*

17. Encourage involvement with self-help associations, such as 12-step programs for clients, partners, and children, and professional family therapy. *Puts client and family in direct contact with support systems necessary for continued sobriety/abstinence and assists with problem resolution.*

Outcome Criteria

1. Family verbalizes understanding of dynamics of enabling behaviors.
2. Family members demonstrate patterns of effective communication.
3. Family members regularly participate in self-help support programs.
4. Family members demonstrate behaviors required to change destructive patterns of behavior that contribute to and enable dysfunctional family process.

@ INTERNET REFERENCES

- Additional information on addictions may be located at the following Web sites:
  a. www.samhsa.gov/index.aspx
  b. www.well.com/user/woa
  c. www.addictions.org
  d. www.ccsa.ca/Eng/Pages/Home.aspx
- Additional information on self-help organizations may be located at the following Web sites:
  a. www.ca.org (Cocaine Anonymous)
  b. www.aa.org (Alcoholics Anonymous)
  c. www.na.org (Narcotics Anonymous)
  d. www.al-anon.org
  e. www.gamblersanonymous.org/ga

- Additional information about medications for treatment of alcohol and drug addiction may be located at the following Web sites:
  a. www.medicinenet.com/medications/article.htm
  b. www.nlm.nih.gov/medlineplus
  c. www.drugs.com/condition/alcoholism.html

Movie Connections

Affliction (Alcoholism) • *Days of Wine and Roses* (Alcoholism) • *I'll Cry Tomorrow* (Alcoholism) • *When a Man Loves a Woman* (Alcoholism) • *Clean and Sober* (Addiction-cocaine) • *28 Days* (Alcoholism) • *Lady Sings the Blues* (Addiction-heroin) • *I'm Dancing as Fast as I Can* (Addiction-sedatives) • *The Rose* (Polysubstance addiction) • *The Gambler* (Gambling disorder)

CHAPTER 5

Schizophrenia Spectrum and Other Psychotic Disorders

■ BACKGROUND ASSESSMENT DATA

The syndrome of symptoms associated with schizophrenia and other psychotic disorders reveals alterations in content and organization of thoughts, perception of sensory input, affect or emotional tone, sense of identity, volition, psychomotor behavior, and ability to establish satisfactory interpersonal relationships.

The *Diagnostic and Statistical Manual of Mental Disorders, Fifth Edition (DSM-5)* (American Psychiatric Association, APA, 2013) identifies a spectrum of psychotic disorders that are organized to reflect gradient of psychopathology from least to most severe. Degree of severity is determined by the level, number, and duration of psychotic signs and symptoms.

Several of the disorders may carry the additional specification of *With Catatonic Features*, the criteria for which are described under the category of *Catatonia Associated With Another Mental Disorder*. The disorders to which this specifier may be applied include brief psychotic disorder, schizophreniform disorder, schizophrenia, schizoaffective disorder, and substance induced psychotic disorder. It may also be applied to neurodevelopmental disorder, major depressive disorder, and bipolar disorders I and II (APA, 2013).

The *DSM-5* initiates the spectrum of disorders with Schizotypal Personality Disorder. For purposes of this textbook, this disorder is presented in Chapter 15, *Personality Disorders*.

Categories

Delusional Disorder

Delusional disorder is characterized by the presence of delusions that have been experienced by the individual for at least 1 month (APA, 2013). Hallucinatory activity is not prominent, and behavior is not bizarre. The subtype of delusional disorder is based on the predominant delusional theme. The *DSM-5* states that a specifier may be added to denote if the delusions are considered *bizarre*, (i.e., if the thought is "clearly implausible, not understandable, and not derived from ordinary life experiences" [p. 91]). Subtypes include the following:

1. **Erotomanic Type.** Delusions that another person of higher status is in love with him or her.
2. **Grandiose Type.** Delusions of inflated worth, power, knowledge, special identity, or special relationship to a deity or famous person.
3. **Jealous Type.** Delusions that one's sexual partner is unfaithful.
4. **Persecutory Type.** Delusions that one is being malevolently treated in some way.
5. **Somatic Type.** Delusions that the person has some physical defect, disorder, or disease.
6. **Mixed Type.** When the disorder is *mixed*, delusions are prominent, but no single theme is predominant.

Brief Psychotic Disorder

This disorder is identified by the sudden onset of psychotic symptoms that may or may not be preceded by a severe psychosocial stressor. These symptoms last at least 1 day but less than 1 month, and there is an eventual full return to the premorbid level of functioning (APA, 2013). The individual experiences emotional turmoil or overwhelming perplexity or confusion. Evidence of impaired reality testing may include incoherent speech, delusions, hallucinations, bizarre behavior, and disorientation. Individuals with preexisting personality disorders (most commonly, histrionic, narcissistic, paranoid, schizotypal, and borderline personality disorders) appear to be susceptible to this disorder (Sadock & Sadock, 2007). Catatonic features may also be associated with this disorder.

Schizophreniform Disorder

The essential features of schizophreniform disorder are identical to those of schizophrenia, with the exception that the duration is at least 1 month but less than 6 months. The diagnosis is termed "provisional" if a diagnosis must be made prior to recovery.

Schizophrenia

Characteristic symptoms of schizophrenia include dysfunctions in perception, inferential thinking, language, memory, and executive functions (Black & Andreasen, 2011). There is evidence of deterioration in social, occupational, and interpersonal relationships. Symptoms of schizophrenia are commonly described as positive or negative. Positive symptoms tend to reflect an alteration or distortion of normal mental functions (e.g., delusions, hallucinations), whereas negative symptoms reflect a diminution or loss of normal functions (e.g., apathy, anhedonia). Most clients exhibit a mixture of both types of symptoms. Signs of the disturbance have been continuous for at least 6 months.

Schizoaffective Disorder

Schizoaffective disorder refers to behaviors characteristic of schizophrenia, in addition to those indicative of disorders of mood, such as depression or mania. The decisive factor in the diagnosis of schizoaffective disorder is the presence of hallucinations and/or delusions that occur for at least 2 weeks in the absence of a major mood episode (APA, 2013). However, prominent mood disorder symptoms must be evident for a majority of the time.

Substance/Medication-Induced Psychotic Disorder

The prominent hallucinations and delusions associated with this disorder are found to be directly attributable to substance intoxication or withdrawal or after exposure to a medication or toxin. This diagnosis is made when the symptoms are more excessive and more severe than those usually associated with the intoxication or withdrawal syndrome (APA, 2013). The medical history, physical examination, or laboratory findings provide evidence that the appearance of the symptoms occurred in association with a substance intoxication or withdrawal or exposure to a medication or toxin. Substances that are believed to induce psychotic disorders are presented in Table 5-1. Catatonic features may also be associated with this disorder.

Psychotic Disorder Due to Another Medical Condition

The essential features of this disorder are prominent hallucinations and delusions that can be directly attributed to another medical condition (APA, 2013). The diagnosis is not made if the symptoms occur during the course of a delirium. A number of medical conditions that can cause psychotic symptoms are presented in Table 5-1.

Catatonia Associated With Another Mental Disorder (Catatonia Specifier)

The characteristics of catatonia are identified by symptoms such as stupor; waxy flexibility; mutism; negativism; posturing; stereotypical, repetitive movements; agitation; grimacing; echolalia (mimicking another's speech); and echopraxia (mimicking another's movements) (APA, 2013). As previously stated, catatonia may be associated with brief psychotic disorder, schizophreniform disorder, schizophrenia, schizoaffective disorder, substance-induced psychotic disorder, neurocognitive disorder, depressive disorder, and bipolar disorder.

Catatonic Disorder Due to Another Medical Condition

Catatonic disorder is identified by the symptoms described in the previous section. This diagnosis is made when the symptomatology

| TABLE 5–1 | Substances and Medical Conditions That May Precipitate Psychotic Symptoms |

Substances	Medical Conditions
Drugs of abuse	Acute intermittent porphyria
Alcohol	Cerebrovascular disease
Amphetamines and related substances	CNS infections
Cannabis	CNS trauma
Cocaine	Deafness
Hallucinogens	Fluid or electrolyte imbalances
Inhalants	Hepatic disease
Opioids	Herpes encephalitis
Phencyclidine and related substances	Huntington's disease
Sedatives, hypnotics, and anxiolytics	Hypoadrenocorticism
	Hypo- or Hyperparathyroidism
Medications	Hypo- or Hyperthyroidism
Anesthetics and analgesics	Metabolic conditions (e.g.,
Anticholinergic agents	hypoxia; hypercarbia;
Anticonvulsants	hypoglycemia)
Antidepressant medication	Migraine headache
Antihistamines	Neoplasms
Antihypertensive agents	Neurosyphilis
Cardiovascular medications	Normal pressure hydrocephalus
Antimicrobial medications	Renal disease
Antineoplastic medications	Systemic lupus erythematosus
Antiparkinsonian agents	Temporal lobe epilepsy
Corticosteroids	Vitamin deficiency (e.g., B_{12})
Disulfiram	Wilson's disease
Gastrointestinal medications	
Muscle relaxants	
Nonsteroidal anti-inflammatory agents	
Toxins	
Anticholinesterase	
Organophosphate insecticides	
Nerve gases	
Carbon dioxide	
Carbon monoxide	
Volatile substances (e.g., fuel, paint, gasoline, toluene)	

Sources: APA (2013); Black & Andreasen (2011); Eisendrath & Lichtmacher (2012); Fohrman & Stein (2006); Freudenreich (2010); Sadock & Sadock (2007).

is evidenced from medical history, physical examination, or laboratory findings to be directly attributable to the physiological consequences of another medical condition (APA, 2013). Types of medical conditions that have been associated with catatonic disorder include metabolic disorders (e.g. hepatic encephalopathy, hypo- and hyperthyroidism, hypo- and hyperadrenalism, and vitamin B_{12} deficiency) and neurological conditions (e.g., epilepsy, tumors, cerebrovascular disease, head trauma, and encephalitis) (Levenson, 2009).

Predisposing Factors

1. **Physiological**
   a. *Genetics.* Studies show that relatives of individuals with schizophrenia have a much higher probability of developing the disease than does the general population. Whereas the lifetime risk for developing schizophrenia is about 1% in most population studies, the siblings of an identified client have a 10% risk of developing schizophrenia, and offspring with one parent who has schizophrenia have a 5% to 6% chance of developing the disorder (Black & Andreasen, 2011). Twin and adoption studies add additional evidence for the genetic basis of schizophrenia.
   b. *Histological Changes.* Jonsson and associates (1997) have suggested that schizophrenic disorders may in fact be a birth defect, occurring in the hippocampus region of the brain, and related to an influenza virus encountered by the mother during the second trimester of pregnancy. The studies have shown a "disordering" of the pyramidal cells in the brains of individuals with schizophrenia, but the cells in the brains of individuals without the disorder appeared to be arranged in an orderly fashion. Further research is required to determine the possible link between this birth defect and the development of schizophrenia.
   c. *Biochemical.* This theory suggests that schizophrenia (or schizophrenia-like symptoms) may be caused by an excess of dopamine-dependent neuronal activity in the brain. This excess activity may be related to increased production or release of the substance at nerve terminals, increased receptor sensitivity, too many dopamine receptors, or a combination of these mechanisms (Sadock & Sadock, 2007). Various other biochemicals have also been implicated in the predisposition to schizophrenia. Abnormalities in the neurotransmitters norepinephrine, serotonin, acetylcholine, and gamma-aminobutyric acid and in the neuroregulators, such as prostaglandins and endorphins, have been suggested.
   d. *Anatomical Abnormalities.* With the use of neuroimaging technologies, structural brain abnormalities have been observed in individuals with schizophrenia. Ventricular enlargement is the most consistent finding; however, sulci enlargement and cerebellar atrophy are also reported.

2. **Environmental**
   a. *Sociocultural.* Many studies have been conducted that have attempted to link schizophrenia to social class. Indeed, epidemiological statistics have shown that greater numbers of

individuals from the lower socioeconomic classes experience symptoms associated with schizophrenia than do those from the higher socioeconomic groups (Puri & Treasaden, 2011). This may occur as a result of the conditions associated with living in poverty, such as congested housing accommodations, inadequate nutrition, absence of prenatal care, few resources for dealing with stressful situations, and feelings of hopelessness for changing one's lifestyle of poverty.

An alternative view is that of the *downward drift hypothesis*. This hypothesis suggests that, because of the characteristic symptoms of the disorder, individuals with schizophrenia have difficulty maintaining gainful employment and "drift down" to a lower socioeconomic level (or fail to rise out of a lower socioeconomic group). Proponents of this notion view poor social conditions as a consequence rather than a cause of schizophrenia.

b. **Stressful Life Events.** Studies have been conducted in an effort to determine whether psychotic episodes may be precipitated by stressful life events. There is no scientific evidence to indicate that stress causes schizophrenia. It is very probable, however, that stress may contribute to the severity and course of the illness. It is known that extreme stress can precipitate psychotic episodes. Stress may indeed precipitate symptoms in an individual who possesses a genetic vulnerability to schizophrenia. Stressful life events may be associated with exacerbation of schizophrenic symptoms and increased rates of relapse.

Symptomatology–Positive Symptoms (Subjective/Objective Data)
Content of Thought

1. **Delusions.** Delusions are false personal beliefs that are inconsistent with the person's intelligence or cultural background. The individual continues to have the belief in spite of obvious proof that it is false or irrational. Delusions are subdivided according to their content. Some of the more common ones are listed here.
   - **Delusion of Persecution.** The individual feels threatened and believes that others intend harm or persecution toward him or her in some way (e.g., "The FBI has 'bugged' my room and intends to kill me." "I can't take a shower in this bathroom; the nurses have put a camera in there so that they can watch everything I do").
   - **Delusion of Grandeur.** The individual has an exaggerated feeling of importance, power, knowledge, or identity (e.g., "I am Jesus Christ").
   - **Delusion of Reference.** All events within the environment are referred by the psychotic person to him- or herself (e.g.,

"Someone is trying to get a message to me through the articles in this magazine [or newspaper or TV program]; I must break the code so that I can receive the message"). *Ideas* of reference are less rigid than delusions of reference. An example of an idea of reference is irrationally assuming that, when in the presence of others, one is the object of their discussion or ridicule.

- **Delusion of Control or Influence.** The individual believes certain objects or persons have control over his or her behavior (e.g., "The dentist put a filling in my tooth; I now receive transmissions through the filling that control what I think and do").
- **Somatic Delusion.** The individual has a false idea about the functioning of his or her body (e.g., "I'm 70 years old and I will be the oldest person ever to give birth. The doctor says I'm not pregnant, but I know I am.").
- **Nihilistic Delusion.** The individual has a false idea that the self, a part of the self, others, or the world is nonexistent (e.g., "The world no longer exists." "I have no heart.").

2. **Religiosity.** Religiosity is an excessive demonstration of or obsession with religious ideas and behavior. Because individuals vary greatly in their religious beliefs and level of spiritual commitment, religiosity is often difficult to assess. The individual with schizophrenia may use religious ideas in an attempt to provide rational meaning and structure to his or her behavior. Religious preoccupation in this vein may therefore be considered a manifestation of the illness. However, clients who derive comfort from their religious beliefs should not be discouraged from employing this means of support. An example of religiosity is the individual who believes the voice he or she hears is God and incessantly searches the Bible for interpretation.

3. **Paranoia.** Individuals with paranoia have extreme suspiciousness of others and of their actions or perceived intentions (e.g., "I won't eat this food. I know it has been poisoned.").

4. **Magical Thinking.** With magical thinking, the person believes that his or her thoughts or behaviors have control over specific situations or people (e.g., the mother who believed if she scolded her son in any way he would be taken away from her). Magical thinking is common in children (e.g., "It's raining; the sky is sad." "It snowed last night because I wished very, very hard that it would.").

Form of Thought

1. **Associative Looseness.** Thinking is characterized by speech in which ideas shift from one unrelated subject to another. With associative looseness, the individual is unaware that the topics are unconnected. When the condition is severe, speech may be incoherent. (e.g., "We wanted to take the bus, but the

airport took all the traffic. Driving is the ticket when you want to get somewhere. No one needs a ticket to heaven. We have it all in our pockets.")

2. **Neologisms.** The psychotic person invents new words, or neologisms, that are meaningless to others but have symbolic meaning to the psychotic person (e.g., "She wanted to give me a ride in her new *uniphorum*.").

3. **Concrete Thinking.** Concreteness, or literal interpretations of the environment, represents a regression to an earlier level of cognitive development. Abstract thinking is very difficult. For example, the client with schizophrenia would have great difficulty describing the abstract meaning of sayings such as "I'm climbing the walls," or "It's raining cats and dogs."

4. **Clang Associations.** Choice of words is governed by sounds. Clang associations often take the form of rhyming. For instance "It is very cold. I am cold and bold. The gold has been sold."

5. **Word Salad.** A word salad is a group of words that are put together randomly, without any logical connection (e.g., "Most forward action grows life double plays circle uniform.").

6. **Circumstantiality.** With circumstantiality, the individual delays in reaching the point of a communication because of unnecessary and tedious details. The point or goal is usually met but only with numerous interruptions by the interviewer to keep the person on track of the topic being discussed.

7. **Tangentiality.** Tangentiality differs from circumstantiality in that the person never really gets to the point of the communication. Unrelated topics are introduced, and the focus of the original discussion is lost.

8. **Mutism.** Mutism is an individual's inability or refusal to speak.

9. **Perseveration.** The individual who exhibits perseveration persistently repeats the same word or idea in response to different questions.

Perception

1. **Hallucinations.** Hallucinations, or false sensory perceptions not associated with real external stimuli, may involve any of the five senses. Types of hallucinations include the following:
   - **Auditory.** Auditory hallucinations are false perceptions of sound. Most commonly they are of voices, but the individual may report clicks, rushing noises, music, and other noises. Command hallucinations may place the individual or others in a potentially dangerous situation. "Voices" that issue commands for violence to self or others may or may not be heeded by the psychotic person. Auditory hallucinations are the most common type in psychiatric disorders.
   - **Visual.** These are false visual perceptions. They may consist of formed images, such as of people, or of unformed images, such as flashes of light.

- **Tactile.** Tactile hallucinations are false perceptions of the sense of touch, often of something on or under the skin. One specific tactile hallucination is formication, the sensation that something is crawling on or under the skin.
- **Gustatory.** This type is a false perception of taste. Most commonly, gustatory hallucinations are described as unpleasant tastes.
- **Olfactory.** Olfactory hallucinations are false perceptions of the sense of smell.

2. **Illusions.** Illusions are misperceptions or misinterpretations of real external stimuli.

Sense of Self

Sense of self describes the uniqueness and individuality a person feels. Because of extremely weak ego boundaries, the individual with schizophrenia lacks this feeling of uniqueness and experiences a great deal of confusion regarding his or her identity.

1. **Echolalia.** The client with schizophrenia may repeat words that he or she hears, which is called echolalia. This is an attempt to identify with the person speaking. (For instance, the nurse says, "John, it's time for lunch." The client may respond, "It's time for lunch, it's time for lunch" or sometimes, "Lunch, lunch, lunch, lunch").
2. **Echopraxia.** The client who exhibits echopraxia may purposelessly imitate movements made by others.
3. **Identification and Imitation.** Identification, which occurs on an unconscious level, and imitation, which occurs on a conscious level, are ego defense mechanisms used by individuals with schizophrenia and reflect their confusion regarding self-identity. Because they have difficulty knowing where their ego boundaries end and another person's begins, their behavior often takes on the form of that which they see in the other person.
4. **Depersonalization.** The unstable self-identity of an individual with schizophrenia may lead to feelings of unreality (e.g., feeling that one's extremities have changed in size; or a sense of seeing oneself from a distance).

Symptomatology–Negative Symptoms (Subjective/Objective Data)

Affect

Affect describes the behavior associated with an individual's feeling state or emotional tone.

1. **Inappropriate Affect.** Affect is inappropriate when the individual's emotional tone is incongruent with the circumstances (e.g., a young woman who laughs when told of the death of her mother).

2. **Bland or Flat Affect.** Affect is described as bland when the emotional tone is very weak. The individual with flat affect appears to be void of emotional tone (or overt expression of feelings).
3. **Apathy.** The client with schizophrenia often demonstrates an indifference to or disinterest in the environment. The bland or flat affect is a manifestation of the emotional apathy.

Volition

Impaired volition has to do with the inability to initiate goal-directed activity. In the individual with schizophrenia, this may take the form of inadequate interest, motivation, or ability to choose a logical course of action in a given situation.

1. **Emotional Ambivalence.** Ambivalence in the client with schizophrenia refers to the coexistence of opposite emotions toward the same object, person, or situation. These opposing emotions may interfere with the person's ability to make even a very simple decision (e.g., whether to have coffee or tea with lunch). Underlying the ambivalence is the difficulty the client with schizophrenia has in fulfilling a satisfying human relationship. This difficulty is based on the *need-fear dilemma*—the simultaneous need for and fear of intimacy.
2. **Deteriorated Appearance.** Personal grooming and self-care activities may be neglected. The client with schizophrenia may appear disheveled and untidy and may need to be reminded of the need for personal hygiene.

Interpersonal Functioning and Relationship to the External World

Impairment in social functioning may be reflected in social isolation, emotional detachment, and lack of regard for social convention.

1. **Impaired Social Interaction.** Some clients with acute schizophrenia cling to others and intrude on the personal space of others, exhibiting behaviors that are not socially and culturally acceptable.
2. **Social Isolation.** Individuals with schizophrenia sometimes focus inward on themselves to the exclusion of the external environment.

Psychomotor Behavior

1. **Anergia.** Anergia is a deficiency of energy. The individual with schizophrenia may lack sufficient energy to carry out activities of daily living or to interact with others.
2. **Waxy Flexibility.** Waxy flexibility describes a condition in which the client with schizophrenia allows body parts to be placed in bizarre or uncomfortable positions. Once placed in position, the arm, leg, or head remains in that position for long periods, regardless of how uncomfortable it is for the client.

For example, the nurse may position the client's arm in an outward position to take a blood pressure measurement. When the cuff is removed, the client may maintain the arm in the position in which it was placed to take the reading.

3. **Posturing.** This symptom is manifested by the voluntary assumption of inappropriate or bizarre postures.

4. **Pacing and Rocking.** Pacing back and forth and body rocking (a slow, rhythmic, backward-and-forward swaying of the trunk from the hips, usually when sitting) are common psychomotor behaviors of the client with schizophrenia.

Associated Features

1. **Anhedonia.** Anhedonia is the inability to experience pleasure. This is a particularly distressing symptom that compels some clients to attempt suicide.

2. **Regression.** Regression is the retreat to an earlier level of development. Regression, a primary defense mechanism of schizophrenia, is a dysfunctional attempt to reduce anxiety. It provides the basis for many of the behaviors associated with schizophrenia.

Common Nursing Diagnoses and Interventions for Individuals with Schizophrenia and other Psychotic Disorders

(Interventions are applicable to various health-care settings, such as inpatient and partial hospitalization, community outpatient clinic, home health, and private practice.)

▨ RISK FOR SELF-DIRECTED OR OTHER-DIRECTED VIOLENCE

Definition: *At risk for behaviors in which an individual demonstrates that he or she can be physically, emotionally, and/or sexually harmful [either to self or to others]* (NANDA International [NANDA-I], 2012, pp. 447–448)

Risk Factors ("related to")

[Lack of trust (suspiciousness of others)]
[Panic level of anxiety]
[Negative role modeling]
[Rage reactions]
[Command hallucinations]
[Delusional thinking]
Body language—rigid posture, clenching of fists and jaw, hyperactivity, pacing, breathlessness, and threatening stances
[History or threats of violence toward self or others or of destruction to the property of others]

Impulsivity
Suicidal ideation, plan, available means
[Perception of the environment as threatening]
[Receiving auditory or visual commands of a threatening nature]

Goals/Objectives

Short-term Goals

1. Within [a specified time], client will recognize signs of increasing anxiety and agitation and report to staff (or other care provider) for assistance with intervention.
2. Client will not harm self or others.

Long-term Goal

Client will not harm self or others.

Interventions With *Selected Rationales*

1. Maintain low level of stimuli in client's environment (low lighting, few people, simple decor, low noise level). *Anxiety level rises in a stimulating environment. A suspicious, agitated client may perceive individuals as threatening.*
2. Observe client's behavior frequently (every 15 minutes). Do this when carrying out routine activities *so as to avoid creating suspiciousness in the individual. Close observation is necessary so that intervention can occur if required to ensure client (and others') safety.*
3. Remove all dangerous objects from client's environment *so that in his or her agitated, confused state client may not use them to harm self or others.*

CLINICAL PEARL Intervene at the first sign of increased anxiety, agitation, or verbal or behavioral aggression. Offer empathetic response to client's feelings: "You seem anxious (or frustrated, or angry) about this situation. How can I help?" Validation of the client's feelings conveys a caring attitude and offering assistance reinforces trust.

---

4. Try to redirect the violent behavior with physical outlets for the client's anxiety (e.g., punching bag). *Physical exercise is a safe and effective way of relieving pent-up tension.*
5. Staff should maintain and convey a calm attitude toward client. *Anxiety is contagious and can be transmitted from staff to client.*
6. Have sufficient staff available to indicate a show of strength to client if it becomes necessary. *This shows the client evidence of control over the situation and provides some physical security for staff.*
7. Administer tranquilizing medications as ordered by physician. Monitor medication for its effectiveness and for any adverse side effects. *The avenue of the "least restrictive alternative" must be selected when planning interventions for a psychiatric client.*

8. If client is not calmed by "talking down" or by medication, use of mechanical restraints may be necessary. Restraints should be used only as a last resort, after all other interventions have been unsuccessful, and the client is clearly at risk of harm to self or others. Be sure to have sufficient staff available to assist.

   Follow protocol established by the institution. The Joint Commission (formerly the Joint Commission on Accreditation of Healthcare Organizations [JCAHO]) requires that an in-person evaluation by a physician or other licensed independent practitioner (LIP) be conducted within 1 hour of the initiation of the restraint or seclusion (The Joint Commission, 2010). The physician or LIP must reissue a new order for restraints every 4 hours for adults and every 1 to 2 hours for children and adolescents.

9. The Joint Commission requires that the client in restraints be observed at least every 15 minutes to ensure that circulation to extremities is not compromised (check temperature, color, pulses); to assist the client with needs related to nutrition, hydration, and elimination; and to position client so that comfort is facilitated and aspiration is prevented. Continuous one-to-one monitoring may be necessary for the client who is highly agitated or for whom there is a high risk of self- or accidental injury. *Client safety is a nursing priority.*

10. As agitation decreases, assess client's readiness for restraint removal or reduction. Remove one restraint at a time while assessing client's response. *This minimizes risk of injury to client and staff.*

Outcome Criteria

1. Anxiety is maintained at a level at which client feels no need for aggression.
2. Client demonstrates trust of others in his or her environment.
3. Client maintains reality orientation.
4. Client causes no harm to self or others.

■ SOCIAL ISOLATION

Definition: *Aloneness experienced by the individual and perceived as imposed by others and as a negative or threatening state* (NANDA-I, 2012, p. 480)

Possible Etiologies ("related to")

[Lack of trust]
[Panic level of anxiety]
[Regression to earlier level of development]
[Delusional thinking]

[Past experiences of difficulty in interactions with others]
[Repressed fears]
Unaccepted social behavior
Alterations in mental status

Defining Characteristics ("evidenced by")

[Staying alone in room]
Uncommunicative, withdrawn, no eye contact
Sad, dull affect
[Lying on bed in fetal position with back to door]
[Inappropriate or immature interests and activities for developmental age or stage]
Preoccupation with own thoughts; repetitive, meaningless actions
[Approaching staff for interaction, then refusing to respond to staff's acknowledgment]
Expression of feelings of rejection or of aloneness imposed by others

Goals/Objectives

Short-term Goal

Client will willingly attend therapy activities accompanied by trusted staff member within 1 week.

Long-term Goal

Client will voluntarily spend time with other clients and staff members in group activities.

Interventions With *Selected Rationales*

1. Convey an accepting attitude by making brief, frequent contacts. *An accepting attitude increases feelings of self-worth and facilitates trust.*
2. Show unconditional positive regard. *This conveys your belief in the client as a worthwhile human being.*
3. Be with the client to offer support during group activities that may be frightening or difficult for him or her. *The presence of a trusted individual provides emotional security for the client.*
4. Be honest and keep all promises. *Honesty and dependability promote a trusting relationship.*
5. Orient client to time, person, and place, as necessary.
6. Be cautious with touch. Allow client extra space and an avenue for exit if he or she becomes too anxious. *A suspicious client may perceive touch as a threatening gesture.*
7. Administer tranquilizing medications as ordered by physician. Monitor for effectiveness and for adverse side effects. *Antipsychotic medications help to reduce psychotic symptoms in some individuals, thereby facilitating interactions with others.*
8. Discuss with client the signs of increasing anxiety and techniques to interrupt the response (e.g., relaxation exercises,

thought stopping). *Maladaptive behaviors such as withdrawal and suspiciousness are manifested during times of increased anxiety.*

9. Give recognition and positive reinforcement for client's voluntary interactions with others. *Positive reinforcement enhances self-esteem and encourages repetition of acceptable behaviors.*

Outcome Criteria

1. Client demonstrates willingness and desire to socialize with others.
2. Client voluntarily attends group activities.
3. Client approaches others in appropriate manner for one-to-one interaction.

▨ INEFFECTIVE COPING

Definition: *Inability to form a valid appraisal of the stressors, inadequate choices of practiced responses, and/or inability to use available resources* (NANDA-I, 2012, p. 348)

Possible Etiologies ("related to")

[Inability to trust]
[Panic level of anxiety]
[Personal vulnerability]
[Low self-esteem]
[Inadequate support systems]
[Negative role model]
[Repressed fears]
[Possible hereditary factor]
[Dysfunctional family system]

Defining Characteristics ("evidenced by")

[Suspiciousness of others, resulting in:
 • Alteration in societal participation
 • Inability to meet basic needs
 • Inappropriate use of defense mechanisms]

Goals/Objectives

Short-term Goal

Client will develop trust in at least one staff member within 1 week.

Long-term Goal

Client will demonstrate use of more adaptive coping skills as evidenced by appropriateness of interactions and willingness to participate in the therapeutic community.

Interventions With *Selected Rationales*

1. Encourage same staff to work with client as much as possible *in order to promote development of trusting relationship.*
2. Avoid physical contact. *Suspicious clients may perceive touch as a threatening gesture.*
3. Avoid laughing, whispering, or talking quietly where client can see but not hear what is being said. *Suspicious clients often believe others are discussing them, and secretive behaviors reinforce the paranoid feelings.*
4. Be honest and keep all promises. *Honesty and dependability promote a trusting relationship.*
5. A creative approach may have to be used to encourage food intake (e.g., canned food and own can opener or family-style meals). *Suspicious clients may believe they are being poisoned and refuse to eat food from the individually prepared tray.*
6. Mouth checks may be necessary following medication administration *to verify whether client is swallowing the tablets or capsules. Suspicious clients may believe they are being poisoned with their medication and attempt to discard the pills.*
7. Activities should never include anything competitive. Activities that encourage a one-to-one relationship with the nurse or therapist are best. *Competitive activities are very threatening to suspicious clients.*
8. Encourage client to verbalize true feelings. The nurse should avoid becoming defensive when angry feelings are directed at him or her. *Verbalization of feelings in a nonthreatening environment may help client come to terms with long-unresolved issues.*
9. An assertive, matter-of-fact, yet genuine approach is least threatening and most therapeutic. *A suspicious person does not have the capacity to relate to an overly friendly, overly cheerful attitude.*

Outcome Criteria

1. Client is able to appraise situations realistically and refrain from projecting own feelings onto the environment.
2. Client is able to recognize and clarify possible misinterpretations of the behaviors and verbalizations of others.
3. Client eats food from tray and takes medications without evidence of mistrust.
4. Client appropriately interacts and cooperates with staff and peers in therapeutic community setting.

■ DISTURBED SENSORY PERCEPTION: AUDITORY/VISUAL

Definition: *Change in the amount or patterning of incoming stimuli [either internally or externally initiated] accompanied by a diminished, exaggerated, distorted, or impaired response to such stimuli* (Note: This diagnosis has been retired by NANDA-I, but is retained in this text because of its appropriateness in describing these specific behaviors.)

Possible Etiologies ("related to")

[Panic level of anxiety]
[Withdrawal into the self]
[Stress sufficiently severe to threaten an already weak ego]

Defining Characteristics ("evidenced by")

[Talking and laughing to self]
[Listening pose (tilting head to one side as if listening)]
[Stops talking in middle of sentence to listen]
[Rapid mood swings]
[Disordered thought sequencing]
[Inappropriate responses]
Disorientation
Poor concentration
Sensory distortions

Goals/Objectives

Short-term Goal

Client will discuss content of hallucinations with nurse or therapist within 1 week.

Long-term Goal

Client will be able to define and test reality, eliminating the occurrence of hallucinations.

(This goal may not be realistic for the individual with chronic illness who has experienced auditory hallucinations for many years.) A more realistic goal may be: Client will verbalize understanding that the voices are a result of his or her illness and demonstrate ways to interrupt the hallucination.

Interventions With *Selected Rationales*

1. Observe client for signs of hallucinations (listening pose, laughing or talking to self, stopping in mid-sentence). ***Early intervention may prevent aggressive responses to command hallucinations.***

2. Avoid touching the client before warning him or her that you are about to do so. *Client may perceive touch as threatening and respond in an aggressive manner.*
3. An attitude of acceptance will encourage the client to share the content of the hallucination with you. Ask, "What do you hear the voices saying to you?" *This is important in order to prevent possible injury to the client or others from command hallucinations.*
4. Do not reinforce the hallucination. Use words such as "the voices" instead of "they" when referring to the hallucination. *Words like "they" validate that the voices are real.*

CLINICAL PEARL Let the client who is "hearing voices" know that you do not share the perception. Say, "Even though I realize that the voices are real to you, I do not hear any voices speaking." The nurse must be honest with the client so that he or she may realize that the hallucinations are not real.

---

5. Help the client to understand the connection between increased anxiety and the presence of hallucinations. *If client can learn to interrupt escalating anxiety, hallucinations may be prevented.*
6. Try to distract the client away from the hallucination. *Involvement in interpersonal activities and explanation of the actual situation will help bring the client back to reality.*
7. For some clients, auditory hallucinations persist after the acute psychotic episode has subsided. Listening to the radio or watching television helps distract some clients from attention to the voices. Others have benefited from an intervention called *voice dismissal*. With this technique, the client is taught to say loudly, "Go away!" or "Leave me alone!" thereby exerting some conscious control over the behavior.

Outcome Criteria

1. Client is able to recognize that hallucinations occur at times of extreme anxiety.
2. Client is able to recognize signs of increasing anxiety and employ techniques to interrupt the response.

■ DISTURBED THOUGHT PROCESSES

Definition: *Disruption in cognitive operations and activities* (Note: This diagnosis has been retired by NANDA-I, but is retained in this text because of its appropriateness in describing these specific behaviors.)

Possible Etiologies ("related to")

[Inability to trust]
[Panic level of anxiety]

[Repressed fears]
[Stress sufficiently severe to threaten an already weak ego]
[Possible hereditary factor]

Defining Characteristics ("evidenced by")

[Delusional thinking (false ideas)]
[Inability to concentrate]
Hypervigilance
[Altered attention span]—distractibility
Inaccurate interpretation of the environment
[Impaired ability to make decisions, problem-solve, reason, abstract
or conceptualize, calculate]
[Inappropriate social behavior (reflecting inaccurate thinking)]
Inappropriate [nonreality-based] thinking

Goals/Objectives

Short-term Goal

[By specified time deemed appropriate], client will recognize and
verbalize that false ideas occur at times of increased anxiety.

Long-term Goal

Depending on chronicity of disease process, choose the most realistic long-term goal for the client:
1. By time of discharge from treatment, client's verbalizations
   will reflect reality-based thinking with no evidence of delusional ideation.
2. By time of discharge from treatment, the client will be able
   to differentiate between delusional thinking and reality.

Interventions With *Selected Rationales*

1. Convey your acceptance of client's need for the false belief, but
   indicate that you do not share the belief. *It is important to communicate to the client that you do not view the idea as real.*
2. Do not argue or deny the belief. *Arguing with the client or
   denying the belief serves no useful purpose, because delusional
   ideas are not eliminated by this approach, and the development
   of a trusting relationship may be impeded.*

CLINICAL PEARL 👁 Use *reasonable doubt* as a therapeutic technique: "I understand that you believe this is true, but I personally find it hard to accept."

---

3. Help the client try to connect the false beliefs to times of increased anxiety. Discuss techniques that could be used to control
   anxiety (e.g., deep breathing exercises, other relaxation exercises,
   thought-stopping techniques). *If the client can learn to interrupt escalating anxiety, delusional thinking may be prevented.*

4. Reinforce and focus on reality. Discourage long ruminations about the irrational thinking. Talk about real events and real people. *Discussions that focus on the false ideas are purposeless and useless, and may even aggravate the psychosis.*
5. Assist and support client in his or her attempt to verbalize feelings of anxiety, fear, or insecurity. *Verbalization of feelings in a nonthreatening environment may help client come to terms with long-unresolved issues.*

Outcome Criteria

1. Verbalizations reflect thinking processes oriented in reality.
2. Client is able to maintain activities of daily living (ADLs) to his or her maximal ability.
3. Client is able to refrain from responding to delusional thoughts, should they occur.

■ IMPAIRED VERBAL COMMUNICATION

Definition: *Decreased, delayed, or absent ability to receive, process, transmit, and use a system of symbols [to communicate]* (NANDA-I, 2012, p. 275)

Possible Etiologies ("related to")

Altered perceptions
[Inability to trust]
[Panic level of anxiety]
[Regression to earlier level of development]
[Withdrawal into the self]
[Disordered, unrealistic thinking]

Defining Characteristics ("evidenced by")

[Loose association of ideas]
[Use of words that are symbolic to the individual (neologisms)]
[Use of words in a meaningless, disconnected manner (word salad)]
[Use of words that rhyme in a nonsensical fashion (clang association)]
[Repetition of words that are heard (echolalia)]
[Does not speak (mutism)]
[Verbalizations reflect concrete thinking (inability to think in abstract terms)]
[Poor eye contact (either no eye contact or continuous staring into the other person's eyes)]

Goals/Objectives

Short-term Goal

Client will demonstrate ability to remain on one topic, using appropriate, intermittent eye contact for 5 minutes with nurse or therapist.

Long-term Goal

By time of discharge from treatment, client will demonstrate ability to carry on a verbal communication in a socially acceptable manner with health care providers and peers.

Interventions With *Selected Rationales*

1. Maintain consistency of staff assignment as much as possible. In a nonthreatening manner, explain to the client how his or her behavior and verbalizations are viewed by and may alienate others. *Consistency of staff assignment helps to facilitate trust and the ability to understand client's actions and communication.*

> **CLINICAL PEARL** 🕊 Attempt to decode incomprehensible communication patterns. Seek validation and clarification by stating, "Is it that you mean . . . ?" or "I don't understand what you mean by that. Would you please explain it to me?" These techniques reveal to the client how he or she is being perceived by others, and the responsibility for not understanding is accepted by the nurse.

2. Anticipate and fulfill the client's needs until functional communication has been established. *Client safety and comfort are nursing priorities.*
3. Orient the client to reality as required. Call the client by name. Validate those aspects of communication that help differentiate between what is real and not real. *These techniques may facilitate restoration of functional communication patterns in the client.*

> **CLINICAL PEARL** 🕊 If the client is unable or unwilling to speak (mutism), using the technique of verbalizing the implied is therapeutic. (Example: "That must have been a very difficult for you when your mother left. You must have felt very alone.") This approach conveys empathy, facilitates trust, and eventually may encourage the client to discuss painful issues.

4. Abstract phrases and clichés must be avoided, and explanations must be provided at the client's level of comprehension. *Because concrete thinking prevails, misinterpretations are more likely to occur.*

Outcome Criteria

1. Client is able to communicate in a manner that is understood by others.
2. Client's nonverbal messages are congruent with verbalizations.
3. Client is able to recognize that disorganized thinking and impaired verbal communication occur at times of increased anxiety and intervene to interrupt the process.

■ SELF-CARE DEFICIT (Identify Specific Area)

Definition: *Impaired ability to perform or complete [activities of daily living (ADLs)]* (NANDA-I, 2012, pp. 250–253)

Possible Etiologies ("related to")

[Withdrawal into the self]
[Regression to an earlier level of development]
[Panic level of anxiety]
Perceptual or cognitive impairment
[Inability to trust]

Defining Characteristics ("evidenced by")

[Difficulty in bringing or] inability to bring food from receptacle to mouth
Inability [or refusal] to wash body
[Impaired ability or lack of interest in selecting appropriate clothing to wear, dressing, grooming, or maintaining appearance at a satisfactory level]
[Inability or unwillingness to carry out toileting procedures without assistance]

Goals/Objectives

Short-term Goal

Client will verbalize a desire to perform ADLs by end of 1 week.

Long-term Goal

By time of discharge from treatment, client will be able to perform ADLs in an independent manner and demonstrate a willingness to do so.

Interventions With *Selected Rationales*

1. Encourage client to perform normal ADLs to his or her level of ability. *Successful performance of independent activities enhances self-esteem.*

2. Encourage independence, but intervene when client is unable to perform. *Client comfort and safety are nursing priorities.*
3. Offer recognition and positive reinforcement for independent accomplishments. (Example: "Mrs. J., I see you have put on a clean dress and combed your hair.") *Positive reinforcement enhances self-esteem and encourages repetition of desirable behaviors.*

CLINICAL PEARL 👁 Show client, on a concrete level, how to perform activities with which he or she is having difficulty. For example, if the client is not eating, place a spoon in his or her hand, scoop some food into it, and say, "Now, eat a bite of mashed potatoes (or other food)." Speak plainly and clearly in words that cannot be misinterpreted.

---

4. Keep strict records of food and fluid intake. *This information is necessary to acquire an accurate nutritional assessment.*
5. Offer nutritious snacks and fluids between meals. *Client may be unable to tolerate large amounts of food at mealtimes and may therefore require additional nourishment at other times during the day to receive adequate nutrition.*
6. If client is not eating because of suspiciousness and fears of being poisoned, provide canned foods and allow client to open them; or, if possible, suggest that food be served family-style *so that client may see everyone eating from the same servings.*
7. If client is soiling self, establish routine schedule for toileting needs. Assist client to bathroom on hourly or bi-hourly schedule, as need is determined, until he or she is able to fulfill this need without assistance.

Outcome Criteria

1. Client feeds self without assistance.
2. Client selects appropriate clothing, dresses, and grooms self daily without assistance.
3. Client maintains optimal level of personal hygiene by bathing daily and carrying out essential toileting procedures without assistance.

▓ INSOMNIA

Definition: *A disruption in amount and quality of sleep that impairs functioning* (NANDA-I, 2012, p. 217)

Possible Etiologies ("related to")

[Panic level of anxiety]
[Repressed fears]

[Hallucinations]
[Delusional thinking]

Defining Characteristics ("evidenced by")

[Difficulty falling asleep]
[Awakening very early in the morning]
[Pacing; other signs of increasing irritability caused by lack of sleep]
[Frequent yawning, nodding off to sleep]

Goals/Objectives

Short-term Goal

Within first week of treatment, client will fall asleep within 30 minutes of retiring and sleep 5 hours without awakening, with use of sedative if needed.

Long-term Goal

By time of discharge from treatment, client will be able to fall asleep within 30 minutes of retiring and sleep 6 to 8 hours without a sleeping aid.

Interventions With Selected Rationales

1. Keep strict records of sleeping patterns. *Accurate baseline data are important in planning care to assist client with this problem.*
2. Discourage sleep during the day *to promote more restful sleep at night.*
3. Administer antipsychotic medication at bedtime *so client does not become drowsy during the day.*
4. Assist with measures that promote sleep, such as warm, nonstimulating drinks, light snacks, warm baths, and back rubs.
5. Performing relaxation exercises to soft music may be helpful prior to sleep.
6. Limit intake of caffeinated drinks such as tea, coffee, and colas. *Caffeine is a CNS stimulant and may interfere with the client's achievement of rest and sleep.*

Outcome Criteria

1. Client is able to fall asleep within 30 minutes after retiring.
2. Client sleeps at least 6 consecutive hours without waking.
3. Client does not require a sedative to fall asleep.

@ INTERNET REFERENCES

- Additional information about schizophrenia may be located at the following Web sites:
  a. www.schizophrenia.com
  b. www.nimh.nih.gov

c. www.nami.org
d. http://mentalhealth.com
e. http://bbrfoundation.org
• Additional information about medications to treat schizophrenia may be located at the following Web sites:
a. www.medicinenet.com/medications/article.htm
b. www.drugs.com
c. www.nlm.nih.gov/medlineplus

Movie Connections

I Never Promised You a Rose Garden (Schizophrenia) • *A Beautiful Mind* (Schizophrenia) • *The Fisher King* (Schizophrenia) • *Bennie & Joon* (Schizophrenia) • *Out of Darkness* (Schizophrenia) • *Conspiracy Theory* (Delusional disorder) • *The Fan* (Delusional disorder)

CHAPTER 6

Depressive Disorders

■ BACKGROUND ASSESSMENT DATA

Depression is defined as an alteration in mood that is expressed by feelings of sadness, despair, and pessimism. There is a loss of interest in usual activities, and somatic symptoms may be evident. Changes in appetite and sleep patterns are common. Depression is likely the oldest and still one of the most frequently diagnosed psychiatric illnesses. It is so common in our society as to sometimes be called "the common cold of psychiatric disorders."

■ TYPES OF DEPRESSIVE DISORDERS

Disruptive Mood Dysregulation Disorder

Disruptive mood dysregulation disorder is a new diagnostic category in the *Diagnostic and Statistical Manual of Mental Disorders, Fifth Edition* (*DSM-5;* American Psychiatric Association [APA], 2013). This disorder is characterized by chronic, severe, and persistent irritability. Clinical manifestations include frequent, developmentally inappropriate temper outbursts and persistently angry mood that is present between the severe temper outbursts. The behavior has been present for 12 or more months, and occurs in more than one setting. Onset of the disorder occurs before age 10 years, but the diagnosis is not applied to children younger than 6 years.

Major Depressive Disorder

Major depressive disorder (MDD) is described as a disturbance of mood involving depression or loss of interest or pleasure in usual activities and pastimes. There is evidence of interference in social and occupational functioning for at least 2 weeks. There is no history of manic behavior and the symptoms cannot be attributed to use of substances or another medical condition. The diagnosis of MDD is specified according to whether it is a *single episode* (the individual's first encounter with a major depressive episode) or *recurrent* (the individual has a history of previous major depressive episodes). The diagnosis will also identify the degree of severity of symptoms (mild, moderate, or severe) and whether the disorder is in partial or full remission.

Additionally, the following specifiers may be used to further describe the depressive episode:

1. **With Anxious Distress:** Feelings of restlessness, anxiety, and worry accompany the depressed mood.
2. **With Mixed Features:** The depression is accompanied by intermittent symptoms of mania or hypomania.
3. **With Melancholic Features:** The depressed mood is characterized by profound despondency and despair. There is an absence of the ability to experience pleasure and expression of feelings of excessive or inappropriate guilt. Psychomotor agitation or retardation and anorexia or weight loss are evident.
4. **With Atypical Features:** Includes the ability for cheerful mood when presented with positive events. There may be increased appetite or weight gain and hypersomnia. Additional symptoms include long-standing sensitivity to interpersonal rejection and heavy, leaden feelings in the arms or legs.
5. **With Psychotic Features:** Depressive symptoms include the presence of delusions and/or hallucinations.
6. **With Catatonia:** Depressive symptoms are accompanied by additional symptoms associated with catatonia (e.g., stupor, waxy flexibility, mutism, posturing).
7. **With Peripartum Onset:** This specifier is used when symptoms of major depressive disorder occur during pregnancy or in the 4 weeks following delivery.
8. **With Seasonal Pattern:** This diagnosis indicates the presence of depressive episodes that occur at characteristic times of the year. Commonly, the episodes occur during the fall or winter months, and remit in the spring. Less commonly, there may be recurrent summer depressive episodes (APA, 2013).

Persistent Depressive Disorder (Dysthymia)

Persistent depressive disorder is a mood disturbance with characteristics similar to, if somewhat milder than, those ascribed to major depressive disorder. There is no evidence of psychotic symptoms. The essential feature of the disorder is "a depressed mood that occurs for most of the day, for more days than not, for at least 2 years, or at least 1 year in children and adolescents" (APA, 2013, p. 169). Intermittent symptoms of MDD may or may not occur with this disorder. The same diagnostic specifiers described for MDD may also apply to persistent depressive disorder.

Premenstrual Dysphoric Disorder

The essential features of premenstrual dysphoric disorder include markedly depressed mood, excessive anxiety, mood swings, and decreased interest in activities during the week prior to menses, improving shortly after the onset of menstruation, and becoming minimal or absent in the week postmenses (APA, 2013) (See Chapter 16).

Substance/Medication-Induced Depressive Disorder

The depressed mood associated with this disorder is considered to be the direct result of the physiological effects of a substance (e.g., a drug of abuse, a medication, or toxin exposure) and causes clinically significant distress or impairment in social, occupational, or other important areas of functioning.

Depressive Disorder Due to Another Medical Condition

This disorder is characterized by symptoms associated with a major depressive episode that are the direct physiological conse-quence of another medical condition (APA, 2013). The depression causes clinically significant distress or impairment in social, occu-pational, or other important areas of functioning.

■ PREDISPOSING FACTORS TO DEPRESSIVE DISORDER

1. **Physiological**
   a. *Genetic:* Numerous studies have been conducted that support the involvement of heredity in depressive illness. First-degree relatives of individuals with MDD have a two-to fourfold higher risk for the disorder than that of the general population (APA, 2013).
   b. *Biochemical:* A biochemical theory implicates the biogenic amines norepinephrine, dopamine, and serotonin. The lev-els of these chemicals have been found to be deficient in individuals with depressive illness.
   c. *Neuroendocrine Disturbances:* Elevated levels of serum cortisol and decreased levels of thyroid stimulating hor-mone have been associated with depressed mood in some individuals.
   d. *Substance Intoxication and Withdrawal:* Depressed mood may be associated with intoxication or withdrawal from substances such as alcohol, amphetamines, cocaine, hallu-cinogens, opioids, phencyclidine-like substances, sedatives, hypnotics, or anxiolytics.
   e. *Medication Side Effects:* A number of drugs can produce a depressive syndrome as a side effect. Common ones include anxiolytics, antipsychotics, and sedative-hypnotics. Antihy-pertensive medications such as propranolol and reserpine have been known to produce depressive symptoms. Others include steroids, hormones, antineoplastics, analgesics, and antiulcer medications.
   f. *Other Physiological Conditions:* Depressive symptoms may occur in the presence of electrolyte disturbances, hormonal

disturbances, nutritional deficiencies, and with certain physical disorders, such as cardiovascular accident, systemic lupus erythematosus, hepatitis, and diabetes mellitus.

2. **Psychosocial**

a. *Psychoanalytical Theory:* Freud observed that melancholia occurs after the loss of a loved object, either actually by death or emotionally by rejection, or the loss of some other abstraction of value to the individual. Freud indicated that in clients with melancholia, the depressed person's rage is internally directed because of identification with the lost object (Sadock & Sadock, 2007).

b. *Cognitive Theory:* Beck and colleagues (1979) proposed that depressive illness occurs as a result of impaired cognition. Disturbed thought processes foster a negative evaluation of self by the individual. The perceptions are of inadequacy and worthlessness. Outlook for the future is one of pessimism and hopelessness.

c. *Learning Theory:* The learning theory (Seligman, 1973) proposes that depressive illness is predisposed by the individual's belief that there is a lack of control over his or her life situation. It is thought that this belief arises out of experiences that result in failure (either perceived or real). Following numerous failures, the individual feels helpless to succeed at any endeavor and therefore gives up trying. This "learned helplessness" is viewed as a predisposition to depressive illness.

d. *Object Loss Theory:* The theory of object loss suggests that depressive illness occurs as a result of having been abandoned by, or otherwise separated from, a significant other during the first 6 months of life. Because during this period the mother represents the child's main source of security, she is the "object." The response occurs not only with a physical loss. This absence of attachment, which may be either physical or emotional, leads to feelings of helplessness and despair that contribute to lifelong patterns of depression in response to loss.

■ SYMPTOMATOLOGY (SUBJECTIVE AND OBJECTIVE DATA)

1. The affect of a depressed person is one of sadness, dejection, helplessness, and hopelessness. The outlook is gloomy and pessimistic. A feeling of worthlessness prevails.

2. Thoughts are slowed and concentration is difficult. Obsessive ideas and rumination of negative thoughts are common. In severe depression, psychotic features such as hallucinations and delusions may be evident, reflecting misinterpretations of the environment.

3. Physically, there is evidence of weakness and fatigue—very little energy to carry on activities of daily living (ADLs). The individual may express an exaggerated concern over bodily functioning, seemingly experiencing heightened sensitivity to somatic sensations.

4. Some individuals may be inclined toward excessive eating and drinking, whereas others may experience anorexia and weight loss. In response to a general slowdown of the body, digestion is often sluggish, constipation is common, and urinary retention is possible.

5. Sleep disturbances are common, either insomnia or hypersomnia.

6. At the less severe level (dysthymia), individuals tend to feel their best early in the morning, then continually feel worse as the day progresses. The opposite is true of persons experiencing severe depression. The exact cause of this phenomenon is unknown, but it is thought to be related to the circadian rhythm of the hormones and their effects on the body.

7. A general slowdown of motor activity commonly accompanies depression (called *psychomotor retardation*). At the severe level, energy is depleted, movements are lethargic, and performance of daily activities is extremely difficult. Regression is common, evidenced by withdrawal into the self and retreat to the fetal position. Conversely, severely depressed persons may manifest psychomotor activity through symptoms of agitation. These are constant, rapid, purposeless movements, out of touch with the environment.

8. Verbalizations are limited. When depressed persons do speak, the content may be either ruminations regarding their own life regrets or, in psychotic clients, a reflection of their delusional thinking.

9. Social participation is diminished. The depressed client has an inclination toward egocentrism and narcissism—an intense focus on the self. This discourages others from pursuing a relationship with the individual, which increases his or her feelings of worthlessness and penchant for isolation.

Common Nursing Diagnoses and Interventions for Depression

(Interventions are applicable to various health-care settings, such as inpatient and partial hospitalization, community outpatient clinic, home health, and private practice.)

▦ RISK FOR SUICIDE

Definition: *At risk for self-inflicted, life-threatening injury* (NANDA International [NANDA-I], 2012, p. 452)

Risk Factors ("related to")

[Depressed mood]
Grief; hopelessness; social isolation
History of prior suicide attempt
[Has a suicide plan and means to carry it out]
Widowed or divorced
Chronic or terminal illness
Psychiatric illness or substance abuse
States desire to die
Threats of killing self

Goals/Objectives

Short-term Goals

1. Client will seek out staff when feeling urge to harm self.
2. Client will make short-term verbal (or written) contract with nurse not to harm self.
3. Client will not harm self.

Long-term Goal

Client will not harm self.

Interventions With *Selected Rationales*

1. Create a safe environment for the client. Remove all potentially harmful objects from client's access (sharp objects, straps, belts, ties, glass items). Supervise closely during meals and medication administration. Perform room searches as deemed necessary. *Client safety is a nursing priority.*

> **CLINICAL PEARL** 🕾 Ask the client directly, "Have you thought about killing yourself?" or "Have you thought about harming yourself in any way?" "If so, what do you plan to do? Do you have the means to carry out this plan?" The risk of suicide is greatly increased if the client has developed a plan and particularly if means exist for the client to execute the plan.

2. Formulate a short-term verbal or written contract with the client that he or she will not harm self during specific time period. When that contract expires, make another, and so forth. *Discussion of suicidal feelings with a trusted individual provides some relief to the client. A contract gets the subject out in the open and places some of the responsibility for the client's safety with the client. An attitude of acceptance of the client as a worthwhile individual is conveyed.*

NOTE: Some clinicians believe that suicide prevention contracting is not helpful (Knoll, 2011). Obviously, the contract for safety comes with no guarantee, and it holds no legal credibility. It should never be used as a single intervention, but can be viewed as one among many that serve to ensure the client's safety.

3. Secure promise from client that he or she will seek out a staff member or support person if thoughts of suicide emerge. *Suicidal clients are often very ambivalent about their feelings. Discussion of feelings with a trusted individual may provide assistance before the client experiences a crisis situation.*

4. Maintain close observation of client. Depending on level of suicide precaution, provide one-to-one contact, constant visual observation, or 15-minute checks. Place in room close to nurse's station; do not assign to private room. Accompany to off-unit activities if attendance is indicated. May need to accompany to bathroom. *Close observation is necessary to ensure that client does not harm self in any way. Remaining alert for suicidal and escape attempts facilitates ability to prevent or interrupt harmful behavior.*

5. Maintain special care in administration of medications. *Prevents saving up to overdose or discarding and not taking.*

6. Make rounds at frequent, *irregular* intervals (especially at night, toward early morning, at change of shift, or other predictably busy times for staff). *Prevents staff surveillance from becoming predictable. To be aware of client's location is important, especially when staff is busy, unavailable, or less observable.*

7. Encourage verbalizations of honest feelings. Through exploration and discussion, help client to identify symbols of hope in his or her life.

8. Encourage client to express angry feelings within appropriate limits. Provide safe method of hostility release. Help client to identify true source of anger and to work on adaptive coping skills for use outside the treatment setting. *Depression and suicidal behaviors may be viewed as anger turned inward on the self. If this anger can be verbalized in a nonthreatening environment, the client may be able to eventually resolve these feelings.*

9. Identify community resources that client may use as support system and from whom he or she may request help if feeling suicidal. *Having a concrete plan for seeking assistance during a crisis may discourage or prevent self-destructive behaviors.*

10. Orient client to reality, as required. Point out sensory misperceptions or misinterpretations of the environment. Take care not to belittle client's fears or indicate disapproval of verbal expressions.

11. Most important, spend time with client. *This provides a feeling of safety and security, while also conveying the message, "I want to spend time with you because I think you are a worthwhile person."*

Outcome Criteria

1. Client verbalizes no thoughts of suicide.
2. Client commits no acts of self-harm.
3. Client is able to verbalize names of resources outside the hospital from whom he or she may request help if feeling suicidal.

■ COMPLICATED GRIEVING

Definition: *A disorder that occurs after the death of a significant other [or any other loss of significance to the individual], in which the experience of distress accompanying bereavement fails to follow normative expectations and manifests in functional impairment* (NANDA-I, 2012, p. 365)

Possible Etiologies ("related to")

[Real or perceived loss of any entity of value to the individual]
[Bereavement overload (cumulative grief from multiple unresolved losses)]
[Thwarted grieving response to a loss]
[Absence of anticipatory grieving]
[Feelings of guilt generated by ambivalent relationship with the lost entity]

Defining Characteristics ("evidenced by")

[Idealization of the lost entity]
[Denial of loss]
[Excessive anger, expressed inappropriately]
[Obsessions with past experiences]
[Ruminations of guilt feelings, excessive and exaggerated out of proportion to the situation]
[Developmental regression]
[Difficulty in expressing loss]
[Prolonged difficulty coping following a loss]
[Reliving of past experiences with little or no reduction of intensity of the grief]
[Prolonged interference with life functioning, with onset or exacerbation of somatic or psychosomatic responses]
[Labile affect]
[Alterations in eating habits, sleep patterns, dream patterns, activity level, libido]

Goals/Objectives

Short-term Goals

1. Client will express anger regarding the loss.
2. Client will verbalize behaviors associated with normal grieving.

Long-term Goal

Client will be able to recognize his or her position in the grief process, while progressing at own pace toward resolution.

Interventions With *Selected Rationales*

1. Determine the stage of grief in which the client is fixed. Identify behaviors associated with this stage. *Accurate baseline assessment data are necessary to effectively plan care for the grieving client.*

2. Develop trusting relationship with the client. Show empathy, concern, and unconditional positive regard. Be honest and keep all promises. *Trust is the basis for a therapeutic relationship.*

3. Convey an accepting attitude, and encourage the client to express feelings openly. *An accepting attitude conveys to the client that you believe he or she is a worthwhile person. Trust is enhanced.*

4. Encourage the client to express anger. Do not become defensive if the initial expression of anger is displaced on the nurse or therapist. Help the client to explore angry feelings so that they may be directed toward the intended person or situation. *Verbalization of feelings in a nonthreatening environment may help the client come to terms with unresolved issues.*

5. Help the client to discharge pent-up anger through participation in large motor activities (e.g., brisk walks, jogging, physical exercises, volleyball, punching bag, exercise bike). *Physical exercise provides a safe and effective method for discharging pent-up tension.*

6. Teach the normal stages of grief and behaviors associated with each stage. Help client to understand that feelings such as guilt and anger toward the lost entity are appropriate and acceptable during the grief process and should be expressed rather than held inside. *Knowledge of acceptability of the feelings associated with normal grieving may help to relieve some of the guilt that these responses generate.*

7. Encourage the client to review relationship with the lost entity. With support and sensitivity, point out the reality of the situation in areas where misrepresentations are expressed. *The client must give up an idealized perception and be able to accept both positive and negative aspects about the lost entity before the grief process is complete.*

8. Communicate to the client that crying is acceptable. The use of touch is therapeutic and appropriate with most clients. Knowledge of cultural influences specific to the client is important before using this technique.

9. Assist client in problem solving as he or she attempts to determine methods for more adaptive coping with the experienced

loss. Provide positive feedback for strategies identified and decisions made. ***Positive feedback increases self-esteem and encourages repetition of desirable behaviors.***

10. Encourage the client to reach out for spiritual support during this time in whatever form is desirable to him or her. Assess spiritual needs of client and assist as necessary in the fulfillment of those needs.

11. Encourage the client to attend a support group of individuals who are experiencing life situations similar to his or her own. Help the client to locate a group of this type.

Outcome Criteria

1. Client is able to verbalize normal stages of the grief process and behaviors associated with each stage.
2. Client is able to identify own position within the grief process and express honest feelings related to the lost entity.
3. Client is no longer manifesting exaggerated emotions and behaviors related to complicated grieving and is able to carry out ADLs independently.

■ LOW SELF-ESTEEM

Definition: *Negative self-evaluation/feelings about self or self-capabilities* (NANDA-I, 2012, p. 285)

Possible Etiologies ("related to")

[Lack of positive feedback]
[Feelings of abandonment by significant other]
[Numerous failures (learned helplessness)]
[Underdeveloped ego and punitive superego]
[Impaired cognition fostering negative view of self]

Defining Characteristics ("evidenced by")

[Difficulty accepting positive reinforcement]
[Withdrawal into social isolation]
[Being highly critical and judgmental of self and others]
[Expressions of worthlessness]
[Fear of failure]
[Inability to recognize own accomplishments]
[Setting up self for failure by establishing unrealistic goals]
[Unsatisfactory interpersonal relationships]
[Negative, pessimistic outlook]
[Hypersensitive to slight or criticism]
[Grandiosity]

Goals/Objectives

Short-term Goals

1. Within reasonable time period, client will discuss fear of failure with nurse.
2. Within reasonable time period, client will verbalize things he or she likes about self.

Long-term Goals

1. By time of discharge from treatment, client will exhibit increased feelings of self-worth as evidenced by verbal expression of positive aspects of self, past accomplishments, and future prospects.
2. By time of discharge from treatment, client will exhibit increased feelings of self-worth by setting realistic goals and trying to reach them, thereby demonstrating a decrease in fear of failure.

Interventions With *Selected Rationales*

1. Be accepting of the client and his or her negativism. *An attitude of acceptance enhances feelings of self-worth.*
2. Spend time with client *to convey acceptance and contribute toward feelings of self-worth.*
3. Help client to recognize and focus on strengths and accomplishments. Minimize attention given to past (real or perceived) failures. *Lack of attention may help to eliminate negative ruminations.*
4. Encourage participation in group activities *from which client may receive positive feedback and support from peers.*
5. Help client identify areas he or she would like to change about self, and assist with problem solving toward this effort. *Low self-worth may interfere with client's perception of own problem-solving ability. Assistance may be required.*
6. Ensure that client is not becoming increasingly dependent and that he or she is accepting responsibility for own behaviors. *Client must be able to function independently if he or she is to be successful within the less-structured community environment.*
7. Ensure that therapy groups offer client simple methods of achievement. Offer recognition and positive feedback for actual accomplishments. *Successes and recognition increase self-esteem.*
8. Teach assertiveness techniques: the ability to recognize the differences among passive, assertive, and aggressive behaviors, and the importance of respecting the human rights of others while protecting one's own basic human rights. *Self-esteem is enhanced by the ability to interact with others in an assertive manner.*

9. ◉ Teach effective communication techniques, such as the use of "I" messages. "I-statements" can be used to take ownership for one's feelings rather than saying they are caused by the other person. *Example*: "I feel angry when you criticize me in front of other people, and I would prefer that you stop doing that." "You-statements" put the other individual on the defensive. *Example*: "You are a jerk for criticizing me in front of other people!"

10. Assist client in performing aspects of self-care when required. Offer positive feedback for tasks performed independently. ***Positive feedback enhances self-esteem and encourages repetition of desirable behaviors.***

Outcome Criteria

1. Client is able to verbalize positive aspects about self.
2. Client is able to communicate assertively with others.
3. Client expresses some optimism and hope for the future.
4. Client sets realistic goals for self and demonstrates willing attempt to reach them.

■ SOCIAL ISOLATION/IMPAIRED SOCIAL INTERACTION

Definition: *Social isolation is the condition of aloneness experienced by the individual and perceived as imposed by others and as a negative or threatened state (NANDA-I, 2012, p. 480). Impaired social interaction is an insufficient or excessive quantity or ineffective quality of social exchange (NANDA-I, 2012, p. 320).*

Possible Etiologies ("related to")

[Developmental regression]
[Egocentric behaviors (which offend others and discourage relationships)]
Disturbed thought processes [delusional thinking]
[Fear of rejection or failure of the interaction]
[Impaired cognition fostering negative view of self]
[Unresolved grief]
Absence of significant others

Defining Characteristics ("evidenced by")

Sad, dull affect
Being uncommunicative, withdrawn; lacking eye contact
Preoccupation with own thoughts; performance of repetitive, meaningless actions

Seeking to be alone
[Assuming fetal position]
Expression of feelings of aloneness or rejection
Discomfort in social situations
Dysfunctional interaction with others

Goals/Objectives

Short-term Goal

Client will develop trusting relationship with nurse or counselor within time period to be individually determined.

Long-term Goals

1. Client will voluntarily spend time with other clients and nurse or therapist in group activities by time of discharge from treatment.
2. Client will refrain from using egocentric behaviors that offend others and discourage relationships by time of discharge from treatment.

Interventions With *Selected Rationales*

1. Spend time with the client. This may mean just sitting in silence for a while. *Your presence may help improve client's perception of self as a worthwhile person.*
2. Develop a therapeutic nurse-client relationship through frequent, brief contacts and an accepting attitude. Show unconditional positive regard. *Your presence, acceptance, and conveyance of positive regard enhance the client's feelings of self-worth.*
3. After client feels comfortable in a one-to-one relationship, encourage attendance in group activities. May need to attend with client the first few times to offer support. Accept client's decision to remove self from group situation if anxiety becomes too great. *The presence of a trusted individual provides emotional security for the client.*
4. Verbally acknowledge client's absence from any group activities. *Knowledge that his or her absence was noticed may reinforce the client's feelings of self-worth.*
5. Teach assertiveness techniques. Interactions with others may be discouraged by client's use of passive or aggressive behaviors. *Knowledge of the use of assertive techniques could improve client's relationships with others.*
6. Provide direct feedback about client's interactions with others. Do this in a nonjudgmental manner. Help client learn how to respond more appropriately in interactions with others. Teach client skills that may be used to approach others in a more socially acceptable manner. Practice these skills through role-play. *Client may not realize how he or she is*

being perceived by others. Direct feedback from a trusted individual may help to alter these behaviors in a positive manner. Having practiced these skills in role-play facilitates their use in real situations.

7. The depressed client must have lots of structure in his or her life because of the impairment in decision-making and problem-solving ability. Devise a plan of therapeutic activities and provide client with a written time schedule. *Remember:* The client who is moderately depressed feels best early in the day, whereas later in the day is a better time for the severely depressed individual to participate in activities. *It is important to plan activities at a time when the client has more energy and is more likely to gain from the experience.*

8. Provide positive reinforcement for client's voluntary interactions with others. *Positive reinforcement enhances self-esteem and encourages repetition of desirable behaviors.*

Outcome Criteria

1. Client demonstrates willingness and desire to socialize with others.
2. Client voluntarily attends group activities.
3. Client approaches others in appropriate manner for one-to-one interaction.

■ POWERLESSNESS

Definition: *The lived experience of lack of control over a situation, including a perception that one's actions do not significantly affect an outcome* (NANDA-I, 2012, p. 370)

Possible Etiologies ("related to")

[Lifestyle of helplessness]
[Healthcare] environment
[Complicated grieving process]
[Lack of positive feedback]
[Consistent negative feedback]

Defining Characteristics ("evidenced by")

Reports lack of control [e.g., over self-care, situation, outcome]
Nonparticipation in care
Reports doubt regarding role performance
[Reluctance to express true feelings]
[Apathy]
Dependence on others
[Passivity]

Goals/Objectives

Short-term Goal

Client will participate in decision making regarding own care within 5 days.

Long-term Goal

Client will be able to effectively solve problems in ways to take control of his or her life situation by time of discharge from treatment, thereby decreasing feelings of powerlessness.

Interventions With *Selected Rationales*

1. Encourage the client to take as much responsibility as possible for own self-care practices. ***Providing the client with choices will increase his or her feelings of control***.
   Examples:
   a. Include the client in setting the goals of care he or she wishes to achieve.
   b. Allow the client to establish own schedule for self-care activities.
   c. Provide the client with privacy as need is determined.
   d. Provide positive feedback for decisions made. Respect the client's right to make those decisions independently, and refrain from attempting to influence him or her toward those that may seem more logical.
2. Help the client set realistic goals. ***Unrealistic goals set the client up for failure and reinforce feelings of powerlessness***.
3. Help the client identify areas of his or her life situation that can be controlled. ***Client's emotional condition interferes with his or her ability to solve problems. Assistance is required to perceive the benefits and consequences of available alternatives accurately***.
4. Help client identify areas of life situation that are not within his or her ability to control. Encourage verbalization of feelings related to this inability ***in an effort to deal with unresolved issues and accept what cannot be changed***.
5. Identify ways in which client can achieve. Encourage participation in these activities, and provide positive reinforcement for participation, as well as for achievement. ***Positive reinforcement enhances self-esteem and encourages repetition of desirable behaviors***.

Outcome Criteria

1. Client verbalizes choices made in a plan to maintain control over his or her life situation.
2. Client verbalizes honest feelings about life situations over which he or she has no control.

3. Client is able to verbalize system for problem solving as required for adequate role performance.

■ DISTURBED THOUGHT PROCESSES

Definition: *Disruption in cognitive operations and activities* (Note: This diagnosis has been retired by NANDA-I but is retained in this text because of its appropriateness in describing these specific behaviors.)

Possible Etiologies ("related to")

[Withdrawal into the self]
[Underdeveloped ego; punitive superego]
[Impaired cognition fostering negative perception of self and the environment]

Defining Characteristics ("evidenced by")

[Inaccurate interpretation of environment]
[Delusional thinking]
[Altered attention span—distractibility]
[Egocentricity]
[Impaired ability to make decisions, problem-solve, reason]
[Negative ruminations]

Goals/Objectives

Short-term Goal

Client will recognize and verbalize when interpretations of the environment are inaccurate within 1 week.

Long-term Goal

By time of discharge from treatment, client's verbalizations will reflect reality-based thinking with no evidence of delusional or distorted ideation.

Interventions With *Selected Rationales*

1. Convey your acceptance of client's need for the false belief, while letting him or her know that you do not share the delusion. *A positive response would convey to the client that you accept the delusion as reality.*

2. Do not argue or deny the belief. Use *reasonable doubt* as a therapeutic technique: "I understand that you believe this is true, but I personally find it hard to accept." *Arguing with the client or denying the belief serves no useful purpose as delusional ideas are not eliminated by this approach, and the development of a trusting relationship may be impeded.*

3. 👁 Use the techniques of *consensual validation* and *seeking clarification* when communication reflects alteration in thinking. (Examples: "Is it that you mean ...?" or "I don't understand what you mean by that. Would you please explain?") *These techniques reveal to the client how he or she is being perceived by others, while the responsibility for not understanding is accepted by the nurse.*

4. Reinforce and focus on reality. Talk about real events and real people. Use real situations and events to divert client away from long, purposeless, repetitive verbalizations of false ideas.

5. Give positive reinforcement as client is able to differentiate between reality-based and nonreality-based thinking. *Positive reinforcement enhances self-esteem and encourages repetition of desirable behaviors.*

6. Teach client to intervene, using thought-stopping techniques, when irrational or negative thoughts prevail. *Thought stopping* involves using the command "stop!" or a loud noise (such as hand clapping) to interrupt unwanted thoughts. *This noise or command distracts the individual from the undesirable thinking that often precedes undesirable emotions or behaviors.*

7. Use touch cautiously, particularly if thoughts reveal ideas of persecution. *Clients who are suspicious may perceive touch as threatening and may respond with aggression.*

Outcome Criteria

1. Client's thinking processes reflect accurate interpretation of the environment.

2. Client is able to recognize negative or irrational thoughts and intervene to "stop" their progression.

■ IMBALANCED NUTRITION, LESS THAN BODY REQUIREMENTS

Definition: *Intake of nutrients insufficient to meet metabolic needs* (NANDA-I, 2012, p. 174)

Possible Etiologies ("related to")

Inability to ingest food because of:

    [Depressed mood]
    [Loss of appetite]
    [Energy level too low to meet own nutritional needs]
    [Regression to lower level of development]
    [Ideas of self-destruction]

Defining Characteristics ("evidenced by")

Loss of weight
Lack of interest in food
Pale mucous membranes
Poor muscle tone
[Amenorrhea]
[Poor skin turgor]
[Edema of extremities]
[Electrolyte imbalances]
[Weakness]
[Constipation]
[Anemia]

Goals/Objectives

Short-term Goal

Client will gain 2 lb per week for the next 3 weeks.

Long-term Goal

Client will exhibit no signs or symptoms of malnutrition by time of discharge from treatment (e.g., electrolytes and blood counts will be within normal limits; a steady weight gain will be demonstrated; constipation will be corrected; client will exhibit increased energy in participation in activities).

Interventions With *Selected Rationales*

1. In collaboration with dietitian, determine number of calories required to provide adequate nutrition and realistic (according to body structure and height) weight gain.
2. To prevent constipation, ensure that diet includes foods high in fiber content. Encourage client to increase fluid consumption and physical exercise to promote normal bowel functioning. *Depressed clients are particularly vulnerable to constipation because of psychomotor retardation. Constipation is also a common side effect of many antidepressant medications.*
3. Keep strict documentation of intake, output, and calorie count. *This information is necessary to make an accurate nutritional assessment and maintain client safety.*
4. Weigh client daily. *Weight loss or gain is important assessment information.*
5. Determine client's likes and dislikes and collaborate with dietitian to provide favorite foods. *Client is more likely to eat foods that he or she particularly enjoys.*
6. Ensure that client receives small, frequent feedings, including a bedtime snack, rather than three larger meals. *Large amounts of food may be objectionable, or even intolerable, to the client.*

7. Administer vitamin and mineral supplements and stool softeners or bulk extenders, as ordered by physician.
8. If appropriate, ask family members or significant others to bring in special foods that client particularly enjoys.
9. Stay with the client during meals *to assist as needed and to offer support and encouragement.*
10. Monitor laboratory values, and report significant changes to physician. *Laboratory values provide objective data regarding nutritional status.*
11. Explain the importance of adequate nutrition and fluid intake. *Client may have inadequate or inaccurate knowledge regarding the contribution of good nutrition to overall wellness.*

Outcome Criteria

1. Client has shown a slow, progressive weight gain during hospitalization.
2. Vital signs, blood pressure, and laboratory serum studies are within normal limits.
3. Client is able to verbalize importance of adequate nutrition and fluid intake.

▓ DISTURBED SLEEP PATTERN

Definition: *Time-limited interruptions of sleep amount and quality due to [internal or] external factors* (NANDA-I, 2012, p. 221)

Possible Etiologies ("related to")

[Depression]
[Repressed fears]
[Feelings of hopelessness]
[Anxiety]
[Hallucinations]
[Delusional thinking]

Defining Characteristics ("evidenced by")

[Verbal complaints of difficulty falling asleep]
[Awakening earlier or later than desired]
[Interrupted sleep]
Reports not feeling well rested
[Awakening very early in the morning and being unable to go back to sleep]
[Excessive yawning and desire to nap during the day]
[Hypersomnia; using sleep as an escape]

Goals/Objectives

Short-term Goal

Client will be able to sleep 4 to 6 hours with the aid of a sleeping medication within 5 days.

Long-term Goal

Client will be able to fall asleep within 30 minutes of retiring and obtain 6 to 8 hours of uninterrupted sleep each night without medication by time of discharge from treatment.

Interventions With *Selected Rationales*

1. Keep strict records of sleeping patterns. *Accurate baseline data are important in planning care to assist client with this problem.*
2. Discourage sleep during the day *to promote more restful sleep at night.*
3. Administer antidepressant medication at bedtime *so client does not become drowsy during the day.*
4. Assist with measures that may promote sleep, such as warm, nonstimulating drinks, light snacks, warm baths, and back rubs.
5. Performing relaxation exercises to soft music may be helpful prior to sleep.
6. Limit intake of caffeinated drinks, such as tea, coffee, and colas. *Caffeine is a central nervous system (CNS) stimulant that may interfere with the client's achievement of rest and sleep.*
7. Administer sedative medications, as ordered, *to assist client to achieve sleep until normal sleep pattern is restored.*
8. Some depressed clients may use excessive sleep as an escape. For the client experiencing hypersomnia, set limits on time spent in room. Plan stimulating diversionary activities on a structured, daily schedule. Explore fears and feelings that sleep is helping to suppress.

Outcome Criteria

1. Client is sleeping 6 to 8 hours per night without medication.
2. Client is able to fall asleep within 30 minutes of retiring.
3. Client is dealing with fears and feelings rather than escaping from them through excessive sleep.

@ INTERNET REFERENCES

Additional information about depressive disorders, including psychosocial and pharmacological treatment of these disorders, may be located at the following Web sites:

a. www.ndmda.org
b. www.mentalhealth.com/

c. www.mental-health-matters.com/
d. www.mentalhelp.net
e. www.nlm.nih.gov/medlineplus/
f. www.nami.org/
g. www.medicinenet.com/medications/article.htm
h. www.drugs.com

Movie Connections

Prozac Nation (Depression) • *The Butcher Boy* (Depression) •
Night, Mother (Depression) • *The Prince of Tides* (Depression/suicide)

Bipolar and Related Disorders

■ BACKGROUND ASSESSMENT DATA

Bipolar disorders are manifested by cycles of mania and depression. Mania is an alteration in mood that is expressed by feelings of elation, inflated self-esteem, grandiosity, hyperactivity, agitation, and accelerated thinking and speaking. A somewhat milder degree of this clinical symptom picture is called *hypomania*. Bipolar disorder affects approximately 5.7 million American adults, or about 2.6% of the U.S. population age 18 and older in a given year (National Institute of Mental Health [NIMH], 2013). In terms of gender, the incidence of bipolar disorder is roughly equal, with a ratio of women to men of about 1.2 to 1. The average age of onset for bipolar disorder is the early twenties, and following the first manic episode, the disorder tends to be recurrent.

Types of Bipolar and Related Disorders

Bipolar I Disorder

Bipolar I disorder is the diagnosis given to an individual who is experiencing or has a history of one or more manic episodes. The client may also have experienced episodes of depression. This diagnosis is further specified by the current or most recent behavioral episode experienced. For example, the specifier might be *single manic episode* (to describe individuals having a first episode of mania) or *current* (or most recent) *episode manic, hypomanic, mixed,* or *depressed* (to describe individuals who have had recurrent mood episodes). Psychotic or catatonic features and level of severity of symptoms may also be specified.

Bipolar II Disorder

Bipolar II disorder is characterized by recurrent bouts of major depression with the episodic occurrence of hypomania. The individual who is assigned this diagnosis may present with symptoms (or history) of depression or hypomania. The client has never experienced a full manic episode. The diagnosis may specify whether the current or most recent episode is hypomanic, depressed, or with mixed features. If the current syndrome is a major depressive episode, psychotic or catatonic features may be noted.

Cyclothymic Disorder

The essential feature is a chronic mood disturbance with a duration of at least 2 years, involving numerous periods of elevated mood that do not meet the criteria for a hypomanic episode and numerous periods of depressed mood of insufficient severity or duration to meet the criteria for major depressive episode. The individual is never without the symptoms for more than 2 months.

Substance/Medication-Induced Bipolar Disorder

The disturbance of mood associated with this disorder is considered to be the direct result of physiological effects of a substance (e.g., ingestion of or withdrawal from a drug of abuse or a medication). The mood disturbance may involve elevated, expansive, or irritable mood, with inflated self-esteem, decreased need for sleep, and distractibility. The disorder causes clinically significant distress or impairment in social, occupational, or other important areas of functioning.

Bipolar Disorder Due to Another Medical Condition

This disorder is characterized by an abnormally and persistently elevated, expansive, or irritable mood and excessive activity or energy that is judged to be the result of direct physiological consequence of another medical condition (APA, 2013). The mood disturbance causes clinically significant distress or impairment in social, occupational, or other important areas of functioning.

■ PREDISPOSING FACTORS TO BIPOLAR DISORDER

1. **Biological**
   a. ***Genetic:*** Twin studies have indicated a concordance rate for bipolar disorder among monozygotic twins at 60% to 80% compared to 10% to 20% in dizygotic twins. Family studies have shown that if one parent has bipolar disorder, the risk that a child will have the disorder is around 28% (Dubovsky, Davies, & Dubovsky, 2003). If both parents have the disorder, the risk is two to three times as great. Increasing evidence continues to support the role of genetics in the predisposition to bipolar disorder.
   b. ***Biochemical:*** Just as there is an indication of lowered levels of norepinephrine and dopamine during an episode of depression, the opposite appears to be true of an individual experiencing a manic episode. Thus, the behavioral responses of elation and euphoria may be caused by an excess of these biogenic amines in the brain. It has also been suggested that manic individuals have increased intracellular sodium and calcium. These electrolyte imbalances may be related to abnormalities in cellular membrane function in bipolar disorder.

2. **Physiological**
   a. *Neuroanatomical:* Right-sided lesions in the limbic system, temporobasal areas, basal ganglia, and thalamus have been shown to induce secondary mania. Magnetic resonance imaging studies have revealed enlarged third ventricles and subcortical white matter and periventricular hyperintensities in clients with bipolar disorder (Dubovsky, Davies, & Dubovsky, 2003).
   b. *Medication Side Effects:* Certain medications used to treat somatic illnesses have been known to trigger a manic response. The most common of these are the steroids frequently used to treat chronic illnesses such as multiple sclerosis and systemic lupus erythematosus. Some clients whose first episode of mania occurred during steroid therapy have reported spontaneous recurrence of manic symptoms years later. Amphetamines, antidepressants, and high doses of anticonvulsants and narcotics also have the potential for initiating a manic episode (Dubovsky, Davies, & Dubovsky, 2003).
   c. *Substance Intoxication and Withdrawal:* Mood disturbances may be associated with intoxication from substances such as alcohol, amphetamines, cocaine, hallucinogens, inhalants, opioids, phencyclidine, sedatives, hypnotics, and anxiolytics. Symptoms can occur with withdrawal from substances such as alcohol, amphetamines, cocaine, sedatives, hypnotics, and anxiolytics.

■ SYMPTOMATOLOGY (SUBJECTIVE AND OBJECTIVE DATA)

(**NOTE:** The symptoms and treatment of Bipolar Depression are comparable to those of Major Depression that are addressed in Chapter 6. This chapter will focus on the symptoms and treatment of Bipolar Mania.)

1. The affect of an individual experiencing a manic episode is one of elation and euphoria—a continuous "high." However, the affect is very labile and may change quickly to hostility (particularly in response to attempts at limit setting) or to sadness, ruminating about past failures.
2. Alterations in thought processes and communication patterns are manifested by the following:
   a. *Flight of Ideas.* There is a continuous, rapid shift from one topic to another.
   b. *Loquaciousness.* The pressure of the speech is so forceful and strong that it is difficult to interrupt maladaptive thought processes.
   c. *Delusions of Grandeur.* The individual believes he or she is all important, all powerful, with feelings of greatness and magnificence.

    d. ***Delusions of Persecution.*** The individual believes some-
      one or something desires to harm or violate him or her
      in some way.
3. Motor activity is constant. The individual is literally moving
   at all times.
4. Dress is often inappropriate: bright colors that do not match;
   clothing inappropriate for age or stature; excessive makeup
   and jewelry.
5. The individual has a meager appetite, despite excessive activity level. He or she is unable or unwilling to stop moving in
   order to eat.
6. Sleep patterns are disturbed. Client becomes oblivious to feelings of fatigue, and rest and sleep are abandoned for days or
   weeks.
7. Spending sprees are common. The individual spends large
   amounts of money, which is not available, on numerous items,
   which are not needed.
8. Usual inhibitions are discarded in favor of sexual and behavioral indiscretions.
9. Manipulative behavior and limit testing are common in the
   attempt to fulfill personal desires. Verbal or physical hostility
   may follow failure in these attempts.
10. Projection is a major defense mechanism. The individual re-
    fuses to accept responsibility for the negative consequences
    of personal behavior.
11. There is an inability to concentrate because of a limited at-
    tention span. The individual is easily distracted by even the
    slightest stimulus in the environment.
12. Alterations in sensory perception may occur, and the individ-
    ual may experience hallucinations.
13. As agitation increases, symptoms intensify. Unless the client
    is placed in a protective environment, death can occur from
    exhaustion or injury.

■ COMMON NURSING DIAGNOSES AND INTERVENTIONS FOR MANIA

*(Interventions are applicable to various health-care settings, such as in-
patient and partial hospitalization, community outpatient clinic, home
health, and private practice.)*

▨ RISK FOR INJURY

Definition: *At risk of injury as a result of environmental conditions interacting with the individual's adaptive and defensive resources* (NANDA-I,
2012, p. 430)

Risk Factors ("related to")

Biochemical dysfunction
Psychological (affective orientation)
[Extreme hyperactivity]
[Destructive behaviors]
[Anger directed at the environment]
[Hitting head (hand, arm, foot, etc.) against wall when angry]
[Temper tantrums—becomes destructive of inanimate objects]
[Increased agitation and lack of control over purposeless, and potentially injurious, movements]

Goals/Objectives

Short-term Goal

Client will no longer exhibit potentially injurious movements after 24 hours with administration of tranquilizing medication.

Long-term Goal

Client will experience no physical injury.

Interventions With *Selected Rationales*

1. Reduce environmental stimuli. Assign private room, if possible, with soft lighting, low noise level, and simple room decor. *In hyperactive state, client is extremely distractible, and responses to even the slightest stimuli are exaggerated.*
2. Assign to quiet unit, if possible. *Milieu unit may be too distracting.*
3. Limit group activities. Help client try to establish one or two close relationships. *Client's ability to interact with others is impaired. He or she feels more secure in a one-to-one relationship that is consistent over time.*
4. Remove hazardous objects and substances from client's environment (including smoking materials). *Client's rationality is impaired, and he or she may harm self inadvertently. Client safety is a nursing priority.*
5. Stay with the client to offer support and provide a feeling of security as agitation grows and hyperactivity increases.
6. Provide structured schedule of activities that includes established rest periods throughout the day. *A structured schedule provides a feeling of security for the client.*
7. Provide physical activities as a substitution for purposeless hyperactivity. (Examples: brisk walks, housekeeping chores, dance therapy, aerobics.) *Physical exercise provides a safe and effective means of relieving pent-up tension.*
8. Administer tranquilizing medication, as ordered by physician. Antipsychotic drugs are commonly prescribed for rapid relief of agitation and hyperactivity. Atypical forms commonly used

include olanzapine, ziprasidone, quetiapine, risperidone, ase-napine, and aripiprazole. Chlorpromazine is a typical antipsychotic that is indicated in the treatment of bipolar mania. Observe for effectiveness and evidence of adverse side effects (see Chapter 26).

Outcome Criteria

1. Client is no longer exhibiting signs of physical agitation.
2. Client exhibits no evidence of physical injury obtained while experiencing hyperactive behavior.

■ RISK FOR SELF-DIRECTED OR OTHER-DIRECTED VIOLENCE

Definition: *At risk for behaviors in which an individual demonstrates that he or she can be physically, emotionally, and/or sexually harmful [either to self or to others]* (NANDA-I, 2012, p. 447–448)

Risk Factors ("related to")

[Manic excitement]
[Biochemical alterations]
[Threat to self-concept]
[Suspicion of others]
[Paranoid ideation]
[Delusions]
[Hallucinations]
[Rage reactions]
Body language (e.g., rigid posture, clenching of fists and jaw, hyperactivity, pacing, breathlessness, threatening stances)
[History or threats of violence toward self or others or of destruction to the property of others]
Impulsivity
Suicidal ideation, plan, available means
[Repetition of verbalizations (continuous complaints, requests, and demands)]

Goals/Objectives

Short-term Goals

1. Client's agitation will be maintained at manageable level with the administration of tranquilizing medication during first week of treatment (decreasing risk of violence to self or others).
2. Within [a specified time], client will recognize signs of increasing anxiety and agitation and report to staff (or other care provider) for assistance with intervention.
3. Client will not harm self or others.

Long-term Goal

Client will not harm self or others.

Interventions With *Selected Rationales*

1. Maintain low level of stimuli in client's environment (low lighting, few people, simple decor, low noise level). *Anxiety and agitation rise in a stimulating environment. A suspicious, agitated client may perceive others as threatening.*

2. Observe client's behavior frequently. Do this while carrying out routine activities so as to avoid creating suspiciousness in the individual. *Close observation is required so that intervention can occur if needed to ensure client's (and others') safety.*

3. Remove all dangerous objects from client's environment (sharp objects, glass or mirrored items, belts, ties, smoking materials) *so that in his or her agitated, hyperactive state, client may not use them to harm self or others.*

4. Try to redirect the violent behavior with physical outlets for the client's hostility (e.g., punching bag). *Physical exercise is a safe and effective way of relieving pent-up tension.*

5. Intervene at the first sign of increased anxiety, agitation, or verbal or behavioral aggression. Offer empathetic response to client's feelings: "You seem anxious (or frustrated, or angry) about this situation. How can I help?" *Validation of the client's feelings conveys a caring attitude and offering assistance reinforces trust.*

6. It is important to maintain a calm attitude toward the client. Respond in a matter-of-fact manner to verbal hostility. *Anxiety is contagious and can be transmitted from staff to client.*

7. As the client's anxiety increases, offer some alternatives: participating in a physical activity (e.g., punching bag, physical exercise), talking about the situation, taking some antianxiety medication. *Offering alternatives to the client gives him or her a feeling of some control over the situation.*

8. Have sufficient staff available to indicate a show of strength to client if it becomes necessary. *This conveys to the client evidence of control over the situation and provides some physical security for staff.*

9. Administer tranquilizing medications as ordered by physician. Monitor medication for effectiveness and for adverse side effects.

10. If the client is not calmed by "talking down" or by medication, use of mechanical restraints may be necessary. The avenue of the "least restrictive alternative" must be selected when planning interventions for a violent client. Restraints should be used only as a last resort, after all other interventions have

been unsuccessful, and the client is clearly at risk of harm to self or others.

11. If restraint is deemed necessary, ensure that sufficient staff is available to assist. Follow protocol established by the institution. The Joint Commission (formerly the Joint Commission on Accreditation of Healthcare Organizations [JCAHO]) requires that an in-person evaluation by a physician or other licensed independent practitioner (LIP) be conducted within 1 hour of the initiation of the restraint or seclusion (The Joint Commission, 2010). The physician or LIP must reissue a new order for restraints every 4 hours for adults and every 1 to 2 hours for children and adolescents.

12. The Joint Commission requires that the client in restraints be observed at least every 15 minutes to ensure that circulation to extremities is not compromised (check temperature, color, pulses); to assist client with needs related to nutrition, hydration, and elimination; and to position client so that comfort is facilitated and aspiration can be prevented. Some institutions may require continuous one-to-one monitoring of restrained clients, particularly those who are highly agitated, and for whom there is a high risk of self- or accidental injury. *Client safety is a nursing priority.*

13. As agitation decreases, assess the client's readiness for restraint removal or reduction. Remove one restraint at a time, while assessing client's response. *This procedure minimizes the risk of injury to client and staff.*

Outcome Criteria

1. Client is able to verbalize anger in an appropriate manner.
2. There is no evidence of violent behavior to self or others.
3. Client is no longer exhibiting hyperactive behaviors.

■ IMBALANCED NUTRITION, LESS THAN BODY REQUIREMENTS

Definition: *Intake of nutrients insufficient to meet metabolic needs* (NANDA-I, 2012, p. 174)

Possible Etiologies ("related to")

[Refusal or inability to sit still long enough to eat meals]
[Lack of appetite]
[Excessive physical agitation]
[Physical exertion in excess of energy produced through caloric intake]
[Lack of interest in food]

Defining Characteristics ("evidenced by")

Loss of weight
Pale mucous membranes
Poor muscle tone
[Amenorrhea]
[Poor skin turgor]
[Anemia]
[Electrolyte imbalances]

Goals/Objectives

Short-term Goal

Client will consume sufficient finger foods and between-meal snacks to meet recommended daily allowances of nutrients.

Long-term Goal

Client will exhibit no signs or symptoms of malnutrition.

Interventions With *Selected Rationales*

1. 🐾 In collaboration with dietitian, determine number of calories required to provide adequate nutrition for maintenance or realistic (according to body structure and height) weight gain.
2. Provide client with high-protein, high-calorie, nutritious finger foods and drinks that can be consumed "on the run." *Because of hyperactive state, client has difficulty sitting still long enough to eat a meal. The likelihood is greater that he or she will consume food and drinks that can be carried around and eaten with little effort.*
3. Have juice and snacks available on the unit at all times. *Nutritious intake is required on a regular basis to compensate for increased caloric requirements due to hyperactivity.*
4. Maintain accurate record of intake, output, and calorie count. *This information is necessary to make an accurate nutritional assessment and maintain client's safety.*
5. Weigh client daily. *Weight loss or gain is important nutritional assessment information.*
6. Determine client's likes and dislikes, and collaborate with dietitian to provide favorite foods. *Client is more likely to eat foods that he or she particularly enjoys.*
7. Administer vitamin and mineral supplements, as ordered by physician, *to improve nutritional state.*
8. Pace or walk with client as finger foods are taken. As agitation subsides, sit with client during meals. Offer support and encouragement. Assess and record amount consumed. *Presence of a trusted individual may provide feeling of security and decrease agitation. Encouragement and positive reinforcement increase self-esteem and foster repetition of desired behaviors.*

9. Monitor laboratory values, and report significant changes to physician. *Laboratory values provide objective nutritional assessment data.*

10. Explain the importance of adequate nutrition and fluid intake. *Client may have inadequate or inaccurate knowledge regarding the contribution of good nutrition to overall wellness.*

Outcome Criteria

1. Client has gained (maintained) weight during hospitalization.
2. Vital signs, blood pressure, and laboratory serum studies are within normal limits.
3. Client is able to verbalize importance of adequate nutrition and fluid intake.

■ DISTURBED THOUGHT PROCESSES

Definition: *Disruption in cognitive operations and activities* (Note: This diagnosis has been retired by NANDA-I but is retained in this text because of its appropriateness in describing these specific behaviors.)

Possible Etiologies ("related to")

[Biochemical alterations]
[Electrolyte imbalance]
[Psychotic process]
[Sleep deprivation]

Defining Characteristics ("evidenced by")

[Inaccurate interpretation of environment]
[Hypervigilance]
[Altered attention span—distractibility]
[Egocentricity]
[Decreased ability to grasp ideas]
[Impaired ability to make decisions, solve problems, reason]
[Delusions of grandeur]
[Delusions of persecution]
[Suspiciousness]

Goals/Objectives

Short-term Goal

Within 1 week, client will be able to recognize and verbalize when thinking is not reality-based.

Long-term Goal

By time of discharge from treatment, client's verbalizations will reflect reality-based thinking with no evidence of delusional ideation.

Interventions With *Selected Rationales*

1. Convey acceptance of client's need for the false belief, while letting him or her know that you do not share the delusion. *A positive response would convey to the client that you accept the delusion as reality.*

2. 🐾 Do not argue or deny the belief. Use *reasonable doubt* as a therapeutic technique: "I understand that you believe this is true, but I personally find it hard to accept." *Arguing with the client or denying the belief serves no useful purpose because delusional ideas are not eliminated by this approach, and the development of a trusting relationship may be impeded.*

3. 🐾 Use the techniques of *consensual validation* and *seeking clarification* when communication reflects alteration in thinking. (Examples: "Is it that you mean . . . ?" or "I don't understand what you mean by that. Would you please explain?") *These techniques reveal to the client how he or she is being perceived by others, and the responsibility for not understanding is accepted by the nurse.*

4. Reinforce and focus on reality. Talk about real events and real people. Use real situations and events to divert client away from long, tedious, repetitive verbalizations of false ideas.

5. Give positive reinforcement as client is able to differentiate between reality-based and nonreality-based thinking. *Positive reinforcement enhances self-esteem and encourages repetition of desirable behaviors.*

6. Teach client to intervene, using thought-stopping techniques, when irrational thoughts prevail. Thought stopping involves using the command "Stop!" or a loud noise (such as hand clapping) to interrupt unwanted thoughts. *This noise or command distracts the individual from the undesirable thinking, which often precedes undesirable emotions or behaviors.*

7. Use touch cautiously, particularly if thoughts reveal ideas of persecution. *Clients who are suspicious may perceive touch as threatening and may respond with aggression.*

Outcome Criteria

1. Thought processes reflect an accurate interpretation of the environment.

2. Client is able to recognize thoughts that are not based in reality and intervene to stop their progression.

▓ DISTURBED SENSORY PERCEPTION

Definition: *Change in the amount or patterning of incoming stimuli [either internally or externally initiated] accompanied by a diminished, exaggerated, distorted, or impaired response to such stimuli* (Note: This diagnosis has been retired by NANDA-I but is retained in this text because of its appropriateness in describing these specific behaviors.)

Possible Etiologies ("related to")

[Biochemical imbalance]
[Electrolyte imbalance]
[Sleep deprivation]
[Psychotic process]

Defining Characteristics ("evidenced by")

[Change in usual response to stimuli]
[Hallucinations]
[Disorientation]
[Inappropriate responses]
[Rapid mood swings]
[Exaggerated emotional responses]
[Visual and auditory distortions]
[Talking and laughing to self]
[Listening pose (tilting head to one side as if listening)]
[Stops talking in middle of sentence to listen]

Goals/Objectives

Short-term Goal

Client will be able to recognize and verbalize when he or she is interpreting the environment inaccurately.

Long-term Goal

Client will be able to define and test reality, eliminating the occurrence of sensory misperceptions.

Interventions With *Selected Rationales*

1. Observe client for signs of hallucinations (listening pose, laughing or talking to self, stopping in midsentence). *Early intervention may prevent aggressive responses to command hallucinations.*
2. Avoid touching the client before warning him or her that you are about to do so. *Client may perceive touch as threatening and respond in an aggressive manner.*
3. An attitude of acceptance will encourage the client to share the content of the hallucination with you. *This is important in order to prevent possible injury to the client or others from command hallucinations.*
4. Do not reinforce the hallucination. Use words such as "the voices" instead of "they" when referring to the hallucination. *Words like "they" validate that the voices are real.*

CLINICAL PEARL Let the client who is "hearing voices" know that you do not share the perception. Say, "Even though I realize that the voices are real to you, I do not hear any voices speaking." The nurse must be honest with the client so that he or she may realize that the hallucinations are not real.

5. Try to connect the times of the misperceptions to times of increased anxiety. Help client to understand this connection. *If client can learn to interrupt the escalating anxiety, reality orientation may be maintained.*

6. Try to distract the client away from the misperception. *Involvement in interpersonal activities and explanation of the actual situation may bring the client back to reality.*

Outcome Criteria

1. Client is able to differentiate between reality and unrealistic events or situations.
2. Client is able to refrain from responding to false sensory perceptions.

■ IMPAIRED SOCIAL INTERACTION

Definition: *Insufficient or excessive quantity or ineffective quality of social exchange* (NANDA-I, 2012, p. 320)

Possible Etiologies ("related to")

Disturbed thought processes
[Delusions of grandeur]
[Delusions of persecution]
Self-concept disturbance

Defining Characteristics ("evidenced by")

Discomfort in social situations
Inability to receive or communicate a satisfying sense of social engagement (e.g., belonging, caring, interest, or shared history)
Use of unsuccessful social interaction behaviors
Dysfunctional interaction with others
[Excessive use of projection—does not accept responsibility for own behavior]
[Verbal manipulation]
[Inability to delay gratification]

Goals/Objectives

Short-term Goal

Client will verbalize which of his or her interaction behaviors are appropriate and which are inappropriate within 1 week.

Long-term Goal

Client will demonstrate use of appropriate interaction skills as evidenced by lack of or marked decrease in manipulation of others to fulfill own desires.

Interventions With *Selected Rationales*

1. Recognize the purpose these behaviors serve for the client: to reduce feelings of insecurity by increasing feelings of power and control. *Understanding the motivation behind the manipulation may facilitate acceptance of the individual and his or her behavior.*

2. Set limits on manipulative behaviors. Explain to client what you expect and what the consequences are if the limits are violated. Terms of the limitations must be agreed on by all staff who will be working with the client. *Client is unable to establish own limits, so this must be done for him or her. Unless administration of consequences for violation of limits is consistent, manipulative behavior will not be eliminated.*

3. Do not argue, bargain, or try to reason with the client. Merely state the limits and expectations. Individuals with mania can be very charming in their efforts to fulfill their own desires. Confront the client as soon as possible when interactions with others are manipulative or exploitative. Follow through with established consequences for unacceptable behavior. *Because of the strong id influence on the client's behavior,* he or she should receive immediate feedback when behavior is unacceptable. *Consistency in enforcing the consequences is essential if positive outcomes are to be achieved. Inconsistency creates confusion and encourages testing of limits.*

4. Provide positive reinforcement for nonmanipulative behaviors. Explore feelings, and help the client seek more appropriate ways of dealing with them. *Positive reinforcement enhances self-esteem and promotes repetition of desirable behaviors.*

5. Help the client recognize that he or she must accept the consequences of own behaviors and refrain from attributing them to others. *Client must accept responsibility for own behaviors before adaptive change can occur.*

6. Help the client identify positive aspects about self, recognize accomplishments, and feel good about them. *As self-esteem is increased, client will feel less need to manipulate others for own gratification.*

Outcome Criteria

1. Client is able to verbalize positive aspects of self.
2. Client accepts responsibility for own behaviors.
3. Client does not manipulate others for gratification of own needs.

■ INSOMNIA

Definition: *A disruption in amount and quality of sleep that impairs functioning* (NANDA-I, 2012, p. 217)

Possible Etiologies ("related to")

[Excessive hyperactivity]
[Agitation]
[Biochemical alterations]

Defining Characteristics ("evidenced by")

Reports difficulty falling asleep
[Pacing in hall during sleeping hours]
[Sleeping only short periods at a time]
[Numerous periods of wakefulness during the night]
[Awakening and rising extremely early in the morning; exhibiting signs of restlessness]

Goals/Objectives

Short-term Goal

Within 3 days, with the aid of a sleeping medication, client will sleep 4 to 6 hours without awakening.

Long-term Goal

By time of discharge from treatment, client will be able to acquire 6 to 8 hours of uninterrupted sleep without sleeping medication.

Interventions With *Selected Rationales*

1. Provide a quiet environment, with a low level of stimulation. *Hyperactivity increases and ability to achieve sleep and rest are hindered in a stimulating environment.*
2. Monitor sleep patterns. Provide structured schedule of activities that includes established times for naps or rest. *Accurate baseline data are important in planning care to help client with this problem. A structured schedule, including time for naps, will help the hyperactive client achieve much-needed rest.*
3. Assess client's activity level. Client may ignore or be unaware of feelings of fatigue. Observe for signs such as increasing restlessness, fine tremors, slurred speech, and puffy, dark circles under eyes. *Client can collapse from exhaustion if hyperactivity is uninterrupted and rest is not achieved.*
4. Before bedtime, provide nursing measures that promote sleep, such as back rub; warm bath; warm, nonstimulating drinks; soft music; and relaxation exercises.

5. Prohibit intake of caffeinated drinks, such as tea, coffee, and colas. *Caffeine is a CNS stimulant and may interfere with the client's achievement of rest and sleep.*
6. Administer sedative medications, as ordered, to assist client achieve sleep until normal sleep pattern is restored.

Outcome Criteria

1. Client is sleeping 6 to 8 hours per night without sleeping medication.
2. Client is able to fall asleep within 30 minutes of retiring.
3. Client is dealing openly with fears and feelings rather than manifesting denial of them through hyperactivity.

@ INTERNET REFERENCES

Additional information about bipolar disorders, including psychosocial and pharmacological treatment of these disorders, may be located at the following Web sites:

a. www.ndmda.org
b. www.mentalhealth.com
c. www.nami.org
d. www.mental-health-matters.com
e. www.mentalhelp.net
f. www.nlm.nih.gov/medlineplus
g. www.drugs.com

Movie Connections

Lust for Life (Bipolar disorder) • *Call Me Anna* (Bipolar disorder) • *Blue Sky* (Bipolar disorder) • *A Woman Under the Influence* (Bipolar disorder)

CHAPTER 8

Anxiety, Obsessive-Compulsive, and Related Disorders

■ BACKGROUND ASSESSMENT DATA

Anxiety may be defined as apprehension, tension, or uneasiness from anticipation of danger, the source of which is largely unknown or unrecognized. Anxiety may be regarded as pathological when it interferes with social and occupational functioning, achievement of desired goals, or emotional comfort (Black & Andreasen, 2011). Anxiety disorders are among the most common of all psychiatric illnesses. They are more common in women than in men by about 2 to 1.

The manifestations of obsessive-compulsive disorder (OCD) include the presence of obsessions, compulsions, or both, the severity of which is significant enough to cause distress or impairment in social, occupational, or other important areas of functioning (APA, 2013). Obsessions are defined as recurrent and persistent thoughts, impulses, or images experienced as intrusive and stressful. Compulsions are identified as repetitive, ritualistic behaviors that the individual feels compelled and driven to perform, in an effort to decrease feelings of anxiety and discomfort. Related disorders (OCD-types) include body dysmorphic disorder, hoarding disorder, trichotillomania (hair-pulling disorder), and excoriation (skin-picking) disorder.

Selected types of anxiety, obsessive-compulsive, and related disorders are presented in the following sections.

Panic Disorder

Panic disorder is characterized by recurrent panic attacks, the onset of which are unpredictable, and manifested by intense apprehension, fear, or terror, often associated with feelings of impending doom, and accompanied by intense physical discomfort. The symptoms come on unexpectedly; that is, they do not occur immediately before or on exposure to a situation that usually causes anxiety (as in specific phobia). They are not triggered by situations in which the person is the focus of others' attention (as in social anxiety disorder). The attacks usually last minutes, or more rarely, hours. The individual often experiences varying degrees of nervousness and apprehension between attacks. Symptoms of depression are common.

Generalized Anxiety Disorder

This disorder is characterized by persistent, unrealistic, and excessive anxiety and worry, which have occurred more days than not for at least 6 months. The symptoms cause clinically significant distress or impairment in social, occupational, or other important areas of functioning. The anxiety and worry are associated with muscle tension, restlessness, or feeling "keyed up" or "on edge" (APA, 2013).

Agoraphobia

The individual with agoraphobia experiences fear of being in places or situations from which escape might be difficult or in which help might not be available in the event that panic symptoms should occur. It is possible that the individual may have experienced the symptom(s) in the past and is preoccupied with fears of their recurrence. Black and Andreasen (2011) suggest that "their true fear is being separated from a source of security" (p. 171). Impairment can be severe. In extreme cases, the individual is unable to leave his or her home without being accompanied by a friend or relative. If this is not possible, the person may become totally confined to his or her home.

Social Anxiety Disorder (Social Phobia)

Social anxiety disorder is an excessive fear of situations in which a person might do something embarrassing or be evaluated negatively by others. The individual has extreme concerns about being exposed to possible scrutiny by others and fears social or performance situations in which embarrassment may occur (APA, 2013). In some instances, the fear may be quite defined, such as the fear of speaking or eating in a public place, fear of using a public restroom, or fear of writing in the presence of others. In other cases, the social phobia may involve general social situations, such as saying things or answering questions in a manner that would provoke laughter on the part of others. Exposure to the phobic situation usually results in feelings of panic anxiety, with sweating, tachycardia, and dyspnea.

Specific Phobia

Specific phobia is identified by fear of specific objects or situations that could conceivably cause harm (e.g., snakes, heights), but the person's reaction to them is excessive, unreasonable, and inappropriate.

Exposure to the phobic stimulus produces overwhelming symptoms of panic, including palpitations, sweating, dizziness, and difficulty breathing. A diagnosis of specific phobia is made only when the irrational fear restricts the individual's activities and interferes with his or her daily living.

Obsessive-Compulsive Disorder

OCD is characterized by involuntary recurring thoughts or images that the individual is unable to ignore and by the recurring impulse to perform a seemingly purposeless, ritualistic activity. These obsessions and compulsions serve to prevent extreme anxiety on the part of the individual. The disorder is equally common among men and women. It may begin in childhood but more often begins in adolescence or early adulthood. The course is usually chronic and may be complicated by depression or substance abuse.

Body Dysmorphic Disorder

Body dysmorphic disorder is characterized by the exaggerated belief that the body is deformed or defective in some specific way. The most common complaints involve imagined or slight flaws of the face or head, such as wrinkles or scars, the shape of the nose, excessive facial hair, and facial asymmetry (Puri & Treasaden, 2011). Other complaints may have to do with some aspect of the ears, eyes, mouth, lips, or teeth. Some clients may present with complaints involving other parts of the body, and in some instances, a true defect is present. The significance of the defect is unrealistically exaggerated, however, and the person's concern is grossly excessive.

Trichotillomania (Hair-Pulling Disorder)

The *DSM-5* defines this disorder as the recurrent pulling out of one's hair, which results in hair loss (APA, 2013). The impulse is preceded by an increasing sense of tension and results in a sense of release or gratification from pulling out the hair. The most common sites for hair pulling are the scalp, eyebrows, and eyelashes but may occur in any area of the body on which hair grows. These areas of hair loss are often found on the opposite side of the body from the dominant hand. Pain is seldom reported to accompany the hair pulling, although tingling and pruritus in the area are not uncommon. The disorder is relatively rare but occurs more often in women than it does in men.

Hoarding Disorder

The *DSM-5* defines the essential feature of hoarding disorder as "persistent difficulties discarding or parting with possessions, regardless of their actual value"(APA, 2013, p. 248) Additionally, the diagnosis may be specified as "with excessive acquisition," which identifies the excessive need for continual acquiring of items (either by buying them or by other means). In previous editions of the *DSM*, hoarding was considered a symptom of OCD. However, in the *DSM-5*, it has been reclassified as a diagnostic disorder.

Individuals with this disorder collect items until virtually all surfaces within the home are covered. There may be only narrow pathways, winding through stacks of clutter, in which to walk. Some individuals also hoard food and animals, keeping dozens or hundreds of pets, often in unsanitary conditions (The Mayo Clinic, 2011).

Hoarding disorder affects an estimated 700,000 to 1.4 million Americans, but few receive adequate treatment (Symonds & Janney, 2013). More men than women are diagnosed with the disorder, and it is almost three times more prevalent in older adults (ages 55 to 94) compared with younger adults (ages 34 to 44) (APA, 2013). The severity of the symptoms, regardless of when they begin, appears to become more severe with each decade of life. Associated symptoms include perfectionism, indecisiveness, anxiety, depression, distractibility, and difficulty planning and organizing tasks (APA, 2013; Symonds & Janney, 2013).

Anxiety Disorder Due to Another Medical Condition

The symptoms of this disorder are judged to be the direct physiological consequence of another medical condition. Symptoms may include prominent generalized anxiety symptoms, panic attacks, or obsessions or compulsions. Medical conditions that have been known to cause anxiety disorders include endocrine, cardiovascular, respiratory, metabolic, and neurological disorders.

Substance/Medication-Induced Anxiety Disorder

The *DSM-5* describes the essential features of this disorder as prominent anxiety symptoms that are judged to be caused by the direct physiological effects of a substance (i.e., a drug of abuse, a medication, or toxin exposure). The symptoms may occur during substance intoxication or withdrawal from alcohol, amphetamines, cocaine, hallucinogens, sedatives, hypnotics, anxiolytics, caffeine, cannabis, or other substances (APA, 2013).

■ PREDISPOSING FACTORS TO ANXIETY, OCD, AND RELATED DISORDERS

1. **Physiological**
   a. ***Biochemical:*** Increased levels of norepinephrine have been noted in panic and generalized anxiety disorders. Abnormal elevations of blood lactate have also been noted in clients with panic disorder. Decreased levels of serotonin have been implicated in the etiology of obsessive-compulsive

disorder. Alterations in the serotonin and endogenous opi-oid systems have been noted with trichotillomania. The serotonergic system may also be a factor in the etiology of body dysmorphic disorder. This can be reflected in a high incidence of comorbidity with major mood disorder and anxiety disorder and the positive responsiveness of the con-dition to the serotonin-specific drugs.

b. *Genetic:* Studies suggest that anxiety disorders are prevalent within the general population. It has been shown that they are more common among first-degree biological relatives of people with the disorders than among the general popu-lation. Trichotillomania has commonly been associated with obsessive-compulsive disorders among first-degree relatives, leading researchers to conclude that the disorder has a possible hereditary or familial predisposition.

c. *Neuroanatomical:* Structural brain imaging studies in patients with panic disorder have implicated pathological involvement in the temporal lobes, particularly the hippocampus (Sadock & Sadock, 2007). Functional neuroimaging techniques have shown abnormal metabolic rates in the basal ganglia and or-bitofrontal cortex of individuals with OCD (Hollander & Simeon, 2008). In individuals with hoarding disorder, neu-roimaging studies have indicated less activity in the cingulate cortex, the area of the brain that connects the emotional part of the brain with the parts that control higher-level thinking (Saxena, 2013).

d. *Medical or Substance-Induced:* Anxiety disorders may be caused by a variety of medical conditions or the ingestion of various substances. (Refer to previous section on cate-gories of anxiety disorders.)

2. **Psychosocial**

a. *Psychodynamic Theory:* The psychodynamic view focuses on the inability of the ego to intervene when conflict occurs between the id and the superego, producing anxiety. For various reasons (unsatisfactory parent-child relationship, conditional love, or provisional gratification), ego develop-ment is delayed. If developmental defects in ego functions compromise the capacity to modulate anxiety, the individual resorts to unconscious mechanisms to resolve the conflict. Overuse or ineffective use of ego defense mechanisms results in maladaptive responses to anxiety.

b. *Cognitive Theory:* The main thesis of the cognitive view is that faulty, distorted, or counterproductive thinking pat-terns accompany or precede maladaptive behaviors and emotional disorders (Sadock & Sadock, 2007). If there is a disturbance in this central mechanism of cognition, there is a consequent disturbance in feeling and behavior. Because of distorted thinking, anxiety is maintained by erroneous or dysfunctional appraisal of a situation. There is a loss of ability to reason regarding the problem, whether it is physical or interpersonal. The individual feels vulnerable in a given situation, and the distorted thinking results in an irrational appraisal, fostering a negative outcome.

c. *Learning Theory:* Phobias may be acquired by direct learning or imitation (modeling) (e.g., a mother who exhibits fear toward an object will provide a model for the child, who may also develop a phobia of the same object). They may be maintained as conditioned responses when reinforcements occur. In the case of phobias, when the individual avoids the phobic object, he or she escapes fear, which is indeed a powerful reinforcement.

d. *Life Experiences:* Certain early experiences may set the stage for phobic reactions later in life. Some researchers believe that phobias, particularly specific phobias, are symbolic of original anxiety-producing objects or situations that have been repressed.

Examples include:

- A child who is punished by being locked in a closet develops a phobia for elevators or other closed places.
- A child who falls down a flight of stairs develops a phobia for high places.
- A young woman who, as a child, survived a plane crash in which both her parents were killed has a phobia of airplanes.

Some studies have shown a possible correlation between trichotillomania and body dysmorphic disorder and a history of childhood abuse (e.g., physical, emotional, or sexual) or emotional neglect (Lochner et al., 2002; Phillips, 2009).

■ SYMPTOMATOLOGY (SUBJECTIVE AND OBJECTIVE DATA)

An individual may experience a panic attack under any of the following conditions:

- As the predominant disturbance, with no apparent precipitant
- When exposed to a phobic stimulus
- When attempts are made to curtail ritualistic behavior
- Following a psychologically stressful event

Symptoms of a panic attack include the following (APA, 2013):

- Palpitations, pounding heart, or accelerated heart rate
- Sweating
- Trembling or shaking
- Sensations of shortness of breath or smothering
- Feelings of choking
- Chest pain or discomfort
- Nausea or abdominal distress
- Feeling dizzy, unsteady, light-headed, or faint

- Chills or heat sensations
- Paresthesia (numbness or tingling sensations)
- Derealization (feelings of unreality) or depersonalization (feelings of being detached from oneself)
- Fear of losing control or going crazy
- Fear of dying

Other symptoms of anxiety, OCD, or related disorders include the following:

1. Restlessness, feeling "on edge," excessive worry, being easily fatigued, difficulty concentrating, irritability, and sleep disturbances (generalized anxiety disorder).
2. Repetitive, obsessive thoughts, common ones being related to violence, contamination, and doubt; repetitive, compulsive performance of purposeless activity, such as hand washing, counting, checking, touching (obsessive-compulsive disorder).
3. Marked and persistent fears of specific objects or situations (specific phobia), social or performance situations (social anxiety disorder), or being in a situation from which one has difficulty escaping (agoraphobia).
4. Repetitive pulling out of one's own hair (trichotillomania).
5. Persistent difficulty discarding or parting with possessions (hoarding disorder).
6. Having the exaggerated belief that the body is deformed or defective in some specific way (body dysmorphic disorder).

Common Nursing Diagnoses and Interventions

(Interventions are applicable to various health-care settings, such as inpatient and partial hospitalization, community outpatient clinic, home health, and private practice.)

■ ANXIETY (PANIC)

Definition: *Vague uneasy feeling of discomfort or dread accompanied by an autonomic response (the source often nonspecific or unknown to the individual); a feeling of apprehension caused by anticipation of danger. It is an alerting signal that warns of impending danger and enables the individual to take measures to deal with threat* (NANDA International [NANDA-I], 2012, p. 344).

Possible Etiologies ("related to")

Unconscious conflict about essential values and goals of life
Situational and maturational crises
[Real or perceived] threat to self-concept
[Real or perceived] threat of death
Unmet needs
[Being exposed to a phobic stimulus]
[Attempts at interference with ritualistic behaviors]

Defining Characteristics ("evidenced by")

Increased respiration
Increased pulse
Decreased or increased blood pressure
Nausea
Confusion
Increased perspiration
Faintness
Trembling or shaking
Restlessness
Insomnia
[Fear of dying, going crazy, or doing something uncontrolled during an attack]

Goals/Objectives

Short-term Goal

Client will verbalize ways to intervene in escalating anxiety within 1 week.

Long-term Goal

By time of discharge from treatment, client will be able to recognize symptoms of onset of anxiety and intervene before reaching panic stage.

Interventions With *Selected Rationales*

1. Maintain a calm, nonthreatening manner while working with client. *Anxiety is contagious and may be transferred from staff to client or vice versa. Client develops feeling of security in presence of calm staff person.*
2. Reassure client of his or her safety and security. This can be conveyed by physical presence of nurse. Do not leave client alone at this time. *Client may fear for his or her life. Presence of a trusted individual provides client with feeling of security and assurance of personal safety.*
3. Use simple words and brief messages, spoken calmly and clearly, to explain hospital experiences to client. *In an intensely anxious situation, client is unable to comprehend anything but the most elementary communication.*
4. Hyperventilation may occur during periods of extreme anxiety. Hyperventilation causes the amount of carbon dioxide (CO_2) in the blood to decrease, possibly resulting in light-headedness, rapid heart rate, shortness of breath, numbness or tingling in the hands or feet, and syncope. If hyperventilation occurs, assist the client to breathe into a small paper bag held over the mouth and nose. The client should take 6 to 12 natural breaths, alternating with short periods of diaphragmatic breathing. This

technique should not be used with clients who have coronary or respiratory disorders, such as coronary artery disease, asthma, or chronic obstructive pulmonary disease.

5. Keep the immediate surroundings low in stimuli (dim lighting, few people, simple decor). *A stimulating environment may increase level of anxiety.*

6. Administer tranquilizing medication, as ordered by physician. Assess medication for effectiveness and for adverse side effects.

7. When level of anxiety has been reduced, explore with the client possible reasons for occurrence. *Recognition of precipitating factor(s) is the first step in teaching the client to interrupt escalation of the anxiety.*

8. Teach the client signs and symptoms of escalating anxiety and ways to interrupt its progression (e.g., relaxation techniques, deep-breathing exercises, physical exercises, brisk walks, jogging, meditation). The client will determine which method is most appropriate for him or her. *Relaxation techniques result in a physiological response opposite that of the anxiety response, and physical activities discharge excess energy in a healthful manner.*

Outcome Criteria

1. Client is able to maintain anxiety at level in which problem solving can be accomplished.

2. Client is able to verbalize signs and symptoms of escalating anxiety.

3. Client is able to demonstrate techniques for interrupting the progression of anxiety to the panic level.

■ FEAR

Definition: *Response to perceived threat that is consciously recognized as a danger* (NANDA-I, 2012, p. 361)

Possible Etiologies ("related to")

Phobic stimulus
[Being in place or situation from which escape might be difficult]
[Causing embarrassment to self in front of others]

Defining Characteristics ("evidenced by")

[Refuses to leave own home alone]
[Refuses to eat in public]
[Refuses to speak or perform in public]
[Refuses to expose self to (specify phobic object or situation)]
Identifies object of fear
[Symptoms of apprehension or sympathetic stimulation in presence of phobic object or situation]

Goals/Objectives

Short-term Goal

Client will discuss the phobic object or situation with the health-care provider within (time specified).

Long-term Goal

By time of discharge from treatment, client will be able to function in the presence of the phobic object or situation without experiencing panic anxiety.

Interventions With *Selected Rationales*

1. Reassure client of his or her safety and security. *At panic level of anxiety, client may fear for own life.*
2. Explore the client's perception of threat to physical integrity or threat to self-concept. *It is important to understand the client's perception of the phobic object or situation in order to assist with the desensitization process.*
3. Discuss reality of the situation with client in order to recognize aspects that can be changed and those that cannot. *Client must accept the reality of the situation (aspects that cannot change) before the work of reducing the fear can progress.*
4. Include client in making decisions related to selection of alternative coping strategies. (Example: Client may choose either to avoid the phobic stimulus or attempt to eliminate the fear associated with it.) *Encouraging the client to make choices promotes feelings of empowerment and serves to increase feelings of self-worth.*
5. If the client elects to work on elimination of the fear, the techniques of desensitization may be employed. This is a systematic plan of behavior modification, designed to expose the individual gradually to the situation or object (either in reality or through fantasizing) until the fear is no longer experienced. This is also sometimes accomplished through implosion therapy, in which the individual is "flooded" with stimuli related to the phobic situation or object (rather than in gradual steps) until anxiety is no longer experienced in relation to the object or situation. *Fear is decreased as the physical and psychological sensations diminish in response to repeated exposure to the phobic stimulus under nonthreatening conditions.*
6. Encourage client to explore underlying feelings that may be contributing to irrational fears. Help client to understand how facing these feelings, rather than suppressing them, can result in more adaptive coping abilities. *Verbalization of feelings in a nonthreatening environment may help client come to terms with unresolved issues.*

Outcome Criteria

1. Client does not experience disabling fear when exposed to phobic object or situation.
   or
2. Client verbalizes ways in which he or she will be able to avoid the phobic object or situation with minimal change in lifestyle.
3. Client is able to demonstrate adaptive coping techniques that may be used to maintain anxiety at a tolerable level.

■ INEFFECTIVE COPING

Definition: *Inability to form a valid appraisal of the stressors, inadequate choices of practiced responses, and/or inability to use available resources* (NANDA-I, 2012, p. 348)

Possible Etiologies ("related to")

[Underdeveloped ego; punitive superego]
[Fear of failure]
Situational crises
Maturational crises
[Personal vulnerability]
[Inadequate support systems]
[Unmet dependency needs]

Defining Characteristics ("evidenced by")

[Ritualistic behavior]
[Obsessive thoughts]
Inability to meet basic needs
Inability to meet role expectations
Inadequate problem-solving
[Alteration in societal participation]

Goals/Objectives

Short-term Goal

Within 1 week, client will decrease participation in ritualistic behavior by half.

Long-term Goal

By time of discharge from treatment, client will demonstrate ability to cope effectively without resorting to obsessive-compulsive behaviors or increased dependency.

Interventions With *Selected Rationales*

1. Assess client's level of anxiety. Try to determine the types of situations that increase anxiety and result in ritualistic behaviors.

Recognition of precipitating factors is the first step in teaching the client to interrupt the escalating anxiety.

2. Initially meet client's dependency needs as required. Encourage independence and give positive reinforcement for independent behaviors. *Sudden and complete elimination of all avenues for dependency would create intense anxiety on the part of the client. Positive reinforcement enhances self-esteem and encourages repetition of desired behaviors.*

3. In the beginning of treatment, allow plenty of time for rituals. Do not be judgmental or verbalize disapproval of the behavior. *To deny client this activity may precipitate panic level of anxiety.*

4. Support client's efforts to explore the meaning and purpose of the behavior. *Client may be unaware of the relationship between emotional problems and compulsive behaviors. Knowledge and recognition of this fact is important before change can occur.*

5. Provide structured schedule of activities for the client, including adequate time for completion of rituals. *Structure provides a feeling of security for the anxious client.*

6. Gradually begin to limit amount of time allotted for ritualistic behavior as client becomes more involved in other activities. *Anxiety is minimized when client is able to replace ritualistic behaviors with more adaptive ones.*

7. Give positive reinforcement for nonritualistic behaviors. *Positive reinforcement enhances self-esteem and encourages repetition of desired behaviors.*

8. Encourage recognition of situations that provoke obsessive thoughts or ritualistic behaviors. Explain ways of interrupting these thoughts and patterns of behavior (e.g., thought-stopping techniques, relaxation techniques, physical exercise, or other constructive activity with which client feels comfortable). *Knowledge and practice of coping techniques that are more adaptive will help the client change and let go of maladaptive responses to anxiety.*

Outcome Criteria

1. Client is able to verbalize signs and symptoms of increasing anxiety and intervene to maintain anxiety at manageable level.

2. Client demonstrates ability to interrupt obsessive thoughts and refrain from ritualistic behaviors in response to stressful situations.

■ DISTURBED BODY IMAGE

Definition: *Confusion in mental picture of one's physical self* (NANDA-I, 2012, p. 291)

Possible Etiologies ("related to")

[Severe level of anxiety, repressed]
[Low self-esteem]
[Unmet dependency needs]

Defining Characteristics ("evidenced by")

[Preoccupation with real or imagined change in bodily structure
     or function]
[Verbalizations about physical appearance that are out of propor-
     tion to any actual physical abnormality that may exist]
Reports fear of reaction by others
Reports negative feelings about body
Change in social involvement

Goals/Objectives

Short-term Goal

Client will verbalize understanding that changes in bodily struc-
     ture or function are exaggerated out of proportion to the change
     that actually exists. (Time frame for this goal must be deter-
     mined according to individual client's situation.)

Long-term Goal

Client will verbalize perception of own body that is realistic to ac-
     tual structure or function by time of discharge from treatment.

Interventions With *Selected Rationales*

1. Establish trusting relationship with client. ***Trust enhances
   therapeutic interactions between nurse and client.***
2. If there is actual change in structure or function, encourage
   client to progress through stages of grieving. Assess level of
   knowledge and provide information regarding normal grieving
   process and associated feelings. ***Knowledge of acceptable feelings facilitates progression through the grieving process.***
3. Identify misperceptions or distortions client has regarding body
   image. Correct inaccurate perceptions in a matter-of-fact, nonthreatening manner. Withdraw attention when preoccupation
   with distorted image persists. ***Lack of attention may encourage
   elimination of undesirable behaviors.***
4. Help client recognize personal body boundaries. ***Use of touch
   may help him or her recognize acceptance of the individual by
   others and reduce fear of rejection because of changes in bodily
   structure or function.***
5. Encourage independent self-care activities, providing assistance
   as required. ***Self-care activities accomplished independently***

enhance self-esteem and also create the necessity for client to confront reality of his or her bodily condition.

6. Provide positive reinforcement for client's expressions of realistic bodily perceptions. *Positive reinforcement enhances self-esteem and encourages repetition of desired behaviors.*

Outcome Criteria

1. Client verbalizes realistic perception of body.
2. Client demonstrates acceptance of changes in bodily structure or function (if they exist), as evidenced by expression of positive feelings about body, ability or willingness to perform self-care activities independently, and a focus on personal achievements rather than preoccupation with distorted body image.

■ INEFFECTIVE IMPULSE CONTROL

Definition: *A pattern of performing rapid, unplanned reactions to internal or external stimuli without regard for the negative consequences of these reactions to the impulsive individual or to others* (NANDA-I, 2012, p. 269)

Possible Etiologies ("related to")

Stress vulnerability
Ineffective coping
Disorder of personality
[Genetic vulnerability]
[Possible childhood abuse or neglect]

Defining Characteristics ("evidenced by")

[Inability to control impulse to pull out own hair]

Goals/Objectives

Short-term Goal

Client will verbalize adaptive ways to cope with stress by means other than pulling out own hair (time dimension to be individually determined).

Long-term Goal

Client will be able to demonstrate adaptive coping strategies in response to stress and a discontinuation of pulling out own hair (time dimension to be individually determined).

Interventions With *Selected Rationales*

1. Support client in his or her effort to stop hair pulling. Help client understand that it is possible to discontinue the behavior. Client realizes that the behavior is maladaptive but feels helpless to stop. *Support from the nurse builds trust.*

2. Ensure that a nonjudgmental attitude is conveyed, and criticism of the behavior is avoided. *An attitude of acceptance promotes feelings of dignity and self-worth.*
3. Assist the client with Habit Reversal Training (HRT), *which has been shown to be an effective tool in treatment of hair-pulling disorder.* Three components of HRT include the following:
    a. *Awareness training.* Help the client become aware of times when the hair-pulling most often occurs (e.g., client learns to recognize urges, thoughts, or sensations that precede the behavior; the therapist points out to the client each time the behavior occurs). *This helps the client identify situations in which the behavior occurs, or is most likely to occur. Awareness gives the client a feeling of increased self-control.*
    b. *Competing response training.* In this step, the client learns to substitute another response to the urge to pull his or her hair. For example, when a client experiences a hair-pulling urge, suggest that the individual ball up his or her hands into fists, tightening arm muscles, and "locking" his or her arms so as to make hair pulling impossible at that moment (Golomb et al., 2011). *Substituting an incompatible behavior may help to extinguish the undesirable behavior.*
    c. *Social support.* Encourage family members to participate in the therapy process and to offer positive feedback for attempts at habit reversal. *Positive feedback enhances self esteem and increases the client's desire to continue with the therapy. It also provides cues for family members to use in their attempts to help the client in treatment.*
4. Once the client has become aware of hair-pulling times, suggest that client hold something (a ball, paperweight, or other item) in his or her hand at the times when hair pulling is anticipated. *This would help to prevent behaviors occurring without client being aware that they are happening.*
5. Practice stress management techniques: deep breathing, meditation, stretching, physical exercise, listening to soft music. *Hair pulling is thought to occur at times of increased anxiety.*
6. Offer support and encouragement when setbacks occur. Help client to understand the importance of not quitting when it seems that change is not happening as quickly as he or she would like. Although some people see a decrease in behavior within a few days, most will take several months to notice the greatest change.

@ INTERNET REFERENCES

- Additional information about anxiety disorders and medications to treat these disorders may be located at the following Web sites:
    a. www.adaa.org
    b. www.mentalhealth.com
    c. www.nlm.nih.gov/medlineplus

d. www.nami.org
e. www.mental-health-matters.com/disorders
f. www.drugs.com

Movie Connections

As Good As It Gets (OCD) • *The Aviator* (OCD) • *What About Bob?* (Phobias) • *Copycat* (Agoraphobia) • *Analyze This* (Panic disorder) • *Vertigo* (Specific phobia)

CHAPTER 9

Trauma- and Stressor-Related Disorders

■ BACKGROUND ASSESSMENT DATA

Puri and Treasaden (2011) describe Posttraumatic Stress Disorder (PTSD) as "a reaction to an extreme trauma, which is likely to cause pervasive distress to almost anyone, such as natural or man-made disasters, combat, serious accidents, witnessing the violent death of others, being the victim of torture, terrorism, rape, or other crimes" (p. 197). These symptoms are not related to common experiences such as uncomplicated bereavement, marital conflict, or chronic illness but are associated with events that would be markedly distressing to almost anyone. The individual may experience the trauma alone or in the presence of others.

About 60% of men and 50% of women are exposed to a traumatic event in their lifetime (Department of Veterans Affairs, 2012). Women are more likely to experience sexual assault and childhood sexual abuse, whereas men are more likely to experience accidents, physical assaults, combat, or to witness death or injury. Although the exposure to trauma is high, less than 10% of trauma victims develop PTSD (Breslau, 2009). The disorder appears to be more common in women than in men.

As previously stated, historically, individuals who experienced stress reactions that followed exposure to an extreme traumatic event were given the diagnosis of PTSD. Accordingly, stress reactions from "normal" daily events (e.g., divorce, failure, rejection) were characterized as adjustment disorders rather than PTSD. An adjustment disorder is characterized by a maladaptive reaction to an identifiable stressor or stressors that results in the development of clinically significant emotional or behavioral symptoms (APA, 2013). The response occurs within 3 months after onset of the stressor and has persisted for no longer than 6 months after the stressor or its consequences have ended.

A number of studies have indicated that adjustment disorders are probably quite common. Sadock and Sadock (2007) report:

Adjustment disorders are one of the most common psychiatric diagnoses for disorders of patients hospitalized for medical and surgical problems. In one study, 5 percent of people admitted to a hospital over a 3-year period were classified as having an adjustment disorder (p. 786).

Adjustment disorders are more common in women, unmarried persons, and younger people (Black & Andreasen, 2011). It can occur at any age, from childhood to senescence.

■ TYPES OF TRAUMA- AND STRESSOR-RELATED DISORDERS

Posttraumatic Stress Disorder

The *Diagnostic and Statistical Manual of Mental Disorders, Fifth Edition (DSM-5)* describes the essential feature of PTSD as "the development of characteristic symptoms following exposure to one or more traumatic events" (APA, 2013, p. 274). The trauma may be experienced by the individual or witnessed as it occurred to others, or the symptoms may be in response to having learned about a traumatic event having occurred to a significant other. Symptoms of the disturbance have been endured for more than 1 month; or, in the event of delayed expression, the full diagnostic criteria may not have occurred until at least 6 months after the trauma.

Acute Stress Disorder

Acute stress disorder (ASD) is described by the *DSM-5* as a trauma-related disorder similar to PTSD. The similarities between the two disorders occur in terms of precipitating traumatic events and symptomatology; however, in ASD, the symptoms are time limited, up to 1 month following the trauma. By definition, if the symptoms last longer than 1 month, the diagnosis would be PTSD.

Adjustment Disorder

An adjustment disorder is characterized by a maladaptive reaction to an identifiable stressor or stressors that results in the development of clinically significant emotional or behavioral symptoms (APA, 2013). The response occurs within 3 months after onset of the stressor and has persisted for no longer than 6 months after the stressor or its consequences have ended. A number of clinical presentations are associated with adjustment disorders. The following categories, identified by the *DSM-5* (APA, 2013), are distinguished by the predominant features of the maladaptive response.

Adjustment Disorder with Depressed Mood

This category is the most commonly diagnosed adjustment disorder. The clinical presentation is one of predominant mood disturbance, although less pronounced than that of major depressive disorder (MDD). The symptoms, such as depressed mood, tearfulness, and feelings of hopelessness, exceed what is an expected or normative response to an identified stressor.

Adjustment Disorder with Anxiety

This category denotes a maladaptive response to a stressor in which the predominant manifestation is anxiety. For example, the symptoms may reveal nervousness, worry, and jitteriness. The clinician must differentiate this diagnosis from those of anxiety disorders.

Adjustment Disorder with Mixed Anxiety and Depressed Mood

The predominant features of this category include disturbances in mood (depression, feelings of hopelessness and sadness) and manifestations of anxiety (nervousness, worry, jitteriness) that are more intense than what would be expected or considered to be a normative response to an identified stressor.

Adjustment Disorder with Disturbance of Conduct

This category is characterized by conduct in which there is violation of the rights of others or of major age-appropriate societal norms and rules. Examples include truancy, vandalism, reckless driving, fighting, and defaulting on legal responsibilities. Differential diagnosis must be made from conduct disorder or antisocial personality disorder.

Adjustment Disorder with Mixed Disturbance of Emotions and Conduct

The predominant features of this category include emotional disturbances (e.g., anxiety or depression) as well as disturbances of conduct in which there is violation of the rights of others or of major age-appropriate societal norms and rules (e.g., truancy, vandalism, fighting).

Adjustment Disorder Unspecified

This subtype is used when the maladaptive reaction is not consistent with any of the other categories. The individual may have physical complaints, withdraw from relationships, or exhibit impaired work or academic performance but without significant disturbance in emotions or conduct.

■ PREDISPOSING FACTORS TO TRAUMA- AND STRESSOR-RELATED DISORDERS

PTSD and ASD

1. **Biological Theory**

Studies have suggested an endogenous opioid peptide response may assist in the maintenance of chronic PTSD. The hypothesis supports a type of "addiction to the trauma," which is explained in the following manner.

Opioids, including endogenous opioid peptides, have the following psychoactive properties:

- Tranquilizing action
- Reduction of rage/aggression

- Reduction of paranoia
- Reduction of feelings of inadequacy
- Antidepressant action

These studies suggest that physiological arousal initiated by re-exposure to trauma-like situations enhances production of endogenous opioid peptides and results in increased feelings of comfort and control. When the stressor terminates, the individual may experience opioid withdrawal, the symptoms of which bear strong resemblance to those of PTSD.

2. Psychosocial Theory

One psychosocial model that has become widely accepted seeks to explain why certain persons exposed to massive trauma develop trauma-related disorders and others do not. Variables include characteristics that relate to: (1) the traumatic experience; (2) the individual; and (3) the recovery environment.

> *The Traumatic Experience.* Specific characteristics relating to the trauma have been identified as crucial elements in the determination of an individual's long-term response to stress. They include:

- Severity and duration of the stressor
- Extent of anticipatory preparation for the event
- Exposure to death
- Numbers affected by life threat
- Amount of control over recurrence
- Location where the trauma was experienced (e.g., familiar surroundings, at home, in a foreign country)

> *The Individual.* Variables that are considered important in determining an individual's response to trauma include:

- Degree of ego strength
- Effectiveness of coping resources
- Presence of preexisting psychopathology
- Outcomes of previous experiences with stress/trauma
- Behavioral tendencies (temperament)
- Current psychosocial developmental stage
- Demographic factors (e.g., age, socioeconomic status, education)

> *The Recovery Environment.* It has been suggested that the quality of the environment in which the individual attempts to work through the traumatic experience is correlated with the outcome. Environmental variables include:

- Availability of social supports
- The cohesiveness and protectiveness of family and friends
- The attitudes of society regarding the experience
- Cultural and subcultural influences

In research with Vietnam veterans, it was shown that the best predictors of PTSD were the severity of the stressor and the degree of psychosocial isolation in the recovery environment.

3. Cognitive Theory

Most individuals hold positive beliefs of the world as a source of benevolence and joy and of the self as worthy and in control of his or her life. An individual is vulnerable to trauma-related disorders when his or her fundamental beliefs about the self and the world are invalidated by a trauma that cannot be comprehended and a sense of helplessness and hopelessness prevail.

Adjustment Disorder

1. Biological Theory

Chronic disorders, such as neurocognitive or intellectual developmental disorders, are thought to impair the ability of an individual to adapt to stress, causing increased vulnerability to adjustment disorder. Sadock and Sadock (2007) suggest that genetic factors also may influence individual risks for maladaptive response to stress.

2. Psychosocial Theories

Some proponents of psychoanalytic theory view adjustment disorder as a maladaptive response to stress that is caused by early childhood trauma, increased dependency, and retarded ego development. Other psychoanalysts put considerable weight on the constitutional factor, or birth characteristics that contribute to the manner in which individuals respond to stress. In many instances, adjustment disorder is precipitated by a specific meaningful stressor having found a point of vulnerability in an individual of otherwise adequate ego strength.

Some studies relate a predisposition to adjustment disorder to factors such as developmental stage, timing of the stressor, and available support systems. When a stressor occurs and the individual does not have the developmental maturity, available support systems, or adequate coping strategies to adapt, normal functioning is disrupted, resulting in psychological or somatic symptoms. The disorder also may be related to a dysfunctional grieving process. The individual may remain in the denial or anger stage, with inadequate defense mechanisms to complete the grieving process.

3. Stress-Adaptation Model

This model considers the type of stressor the individual experiences, the situational context in which it occurs, and intrapersonal factors in the predisposition to adjustment disorder. It has been found that continuous stressors (those to which an individual is exposed over an extended period of time) are more commonly cited than sudden-shock stressors (those that occur without warning) as precipitants to maladaptive functioning.

The situational context in which the stressor occurs may include factors such as personal and general economic conditions; occupational and recreational opportunities; the availability of social supports, such as family, friends, and neighbors; and the availability of cultural or religious support groups. Intrapersonal factors that have been implicated in the predisposition to adjustment disorder include birth temperament, learned social skills and coping strategies, the presence of psychiatric illness, degree of flexibility, and level of intelligence.

■ SYMPTOMATOLOGY (SUBJECTIVE AND OBJECTIVE DATA)

PTSD and ASD

1. Re-experiencing the traumatic event
2. Sustained high level of anxiety or arousal
3. A general numbing of responsiveness
4. Intrusive recollections
5. Nightmares of the event
6. Inability to remember certain aspects of the trauma
7. Depression
8. Survivor's guilt
9. Substance abuse
10. Anger and aggressive behavior
11. Relationship problems
12. Panic attacks

Adjustment Disorder

1. Depressed mood
2. Tearfulness
3. Hopelessness
4. Nervousness
5. Worry
6. Restlessness
7. Ambivalence
8. Anger, expressed inappropriately
9. Increased dependency
10. Violation of the rights of others
11. Violation of societal norms and rules, such as truancy, vandalism, reckless driving, fighting
12. Inability to function occupationally or academically
13. Manipulative behavior
14. Social isolation
15. Physical complaints, such as headache, backache, other aches and pains, fatigue

Common Nursing Diagnoses and Interventions

(Interventions are applicable to various health-care settings, such as inpatient and partial hospitalization, community outpatient clinic, home health, and private practice.)

■ POST-TRAUMA SYNDROME

Definition: *Sustained maladaptive response to a traumatic, overwhelming event* (NANDA International [NANDA-I], 2012, p. 335)

Possible Etiologies ("related to")

Being held prisoner of war
Criminal victimization
Disasters; epidemics
Physical or psychological abuse
Serious accidents
Serious threat to or injury of loved ones or self
Sudden destruction of one's home or community
Torture
Tragic occurrence involving multiple deaths
War
Witnessing mutilation or violent death

Defining Characteristics ("evidenced by")

[Physical injuries related to trauma]
Avoidance
Repression
Difficulty concentrating
Grieving; guilt
Intrusive thoughts
Neurosensory irritability
Palpitations
Anger and/or rage; aggression
Intrusive dreams; nightmares; flashbacks
Panic attacks; fear
Gastric irritability
Psychogenic amnesia
Substance abuse

Goals/Objectives

Short-term Goals

1. Client will begin a healthy grief resolution, initiating the process of psychological healing (within time frame specific to individual).
2. Client will demonstrate ability to deal with emotional reactions in an individually appropriate manner.

Long-term Goal

The client will integrate the traumatic experience into his or her persona, renew significant relationships, and establish meaningful goals for the future.

Interventions With *Selected Rationales*

1. Assign the same staff as often as possible. Use a nonthreatening, matter-of-fact but friendly approach. Respect the client's wishes regarding interaction with individuals of opposite gender at this time (especially important if the trauma was rape). Be consistent and keep all promises, and convey an attitude of unconditional acceptance. *A posttrauma client may be suspicious of others in his or her environment. These interventions serve to facilitate a trusting relationship.*

2. Stay with the client during periods of flashbacks and nightmares. Offer reassurance of safety and security and that these symptoms are not uncommon following a trauma of the magnitude he or she has experienced. *The presence of a trusted individual may help to calm fears for personal safety and reassure the anxious client that he or she is not "going crazy."*

3. Obtain an accurate history from significant others about the trauma and the client's specific response. *Various types of traumas elicit different responses in clients. For example, human-engendered traumas often generate a greater degree of humiliation and guilt in victims than trauma associated with natural disasters.*

4. Encourage the client to talk about the trauma at his or her own pace. Provide a nonthreatening, private environment, and include a significant other if the client wishes. Acknowledge and validate the client's feelings as they are expressed. *This debriefing process is the first step in the progression toward resolution.*

5. Discuss coping strategies used in response to the trauma, as well as those used during stressful situations in the past. Determine those that have been most helpful, and discuss alternative strategies for the future. Include available support systems, including religious and cultural influences. Identify maladaptive coping strategies, such as substance use or psychosomatic responses, and practice more adaptive coping strategies for possible future posttrauma responses. *Resolution of the posttrauma response is largely dependent on the effectiveness of the coping strategies employed.*

6. Assist the individual to try to comprehend the trauma if possible. Discuss feelings of vulnerability and the individual's "place" in the world following the trauma. *Posttrauma response is largely a function of the shattering of basic beliefs the survivor holds about self and world. Assimilation of the event into one's persona requires that some degree of meaning associated with the event be incorporated into the basic beliefs, which will affect how the individual eventually comes to reappraise self and world (Epstein, 1991).*

■ COMPLICATED GRIEVING

Definition: *A disorder that occurs after the death of a significant other [or any other loss of significance to the individual], in which the experience of distress accompanying bereavement fails to follow normative expectations and manifests in functional impairment* (NANDA-I, 2012, p. 365)

Possible Etiologies ("related to")

[Having experienced a trauma outside the range of usual human experience]
[Survivor's guilt]
[Real or perceived loss of any concept of value to the individual]
[Bereavement overload (cumulative grief from multiple unresolved losses)]
[Thwarted grieving response to a loss]
[Absence of anticipatory grieving]
[Feelings of guilt generated by ambivalent relationship with lost concept]

Defining Characteristics ("evidenced by")

[Verbal expression of distress at loss]
[Idealization of lost concept]
[Denial of loss]
[Excessive anger, expressed inappropriately]
[Developmental regression]
[Altered activities of daily living]
[Diminished sense of control]
[Persistent anxiety]
Depression
Self-blame
Traumatic distress

Goals/Objectives

Short-term Goals

1. By end of 1 week, client will express anger toward loss of valuable entity.
2. By end of 1 week, the client who has experienced a trauma will verbalize feelings (guilt, anger, self-blame, hopelessness) associated with the trauma.

Long-term Goal

Client will demonstrate progress in dealing with stages of grief and will verbalize a sense of optimism and hope for the future.

Interventions With *Selected Rationales*

1. Acknowledge feelings of guilt or self-blame that client may express. Guilt at having survived a trauma in which others died is

common. *The client needs to discuss these feelings and recognize that he or she is not responsible for what happened but must take responsibility for own recovery.*

2. Assess stage of grief in which the client is fixed. Discuss normalcy of feelings and behaviors related to stages of grief. *Knowledge of grief stage is necessary for accurate intervention. Guilt may be generated if client believes it is unacceptable to have these feelings. Knowing they are normal can provide a sense of relief.*

3. Assess impact of the trauma on client's ability to resume regular activities of daily living. Consider employment, marital relationship, and sleep patterns. *Following a trauma, individuals are at high risk for physical injury because of disruption in ability to concentrate and solve problems and because of lack of sufficient sleep. Isolation and avoidance behaviors may interfere with interpersonal relatedness.*

4. Assess for self-destructive ideas and behavior. *The trauma may result in feelings of hopelessness and worthlessness, leading to high risk for suicide.*

5. Assess for maladaptive coping strategies, such as substance abuse. *These behaviors interfere with and delay the recovery process.*

6. Identify available community resources from which the individual may seek assistance if problems with complicated grieving persist. Support groups for victims of various types of traumas exist within most communities. *The presence of support systems in the recovery environment has been identified as a major predictor in the successful recovery from trauma.*

7. Help client solve problems as he or she attempts to determine methods for more adaptive coping with the experienced loss. Provide positive feedback for strategies identified and decisions made. *Positive reinforcement enhances self-esteem and encourages repetition of desirable behaviors.*

8. Encourage the client to reach out for spiritual support during this time in whatever form is desirable to him or her. Assess spiritual needs of client, and assist as necessary in the fulfillment of those needs. *Spiritual support can enhance successful adaptation to painful life experiences for some individuals.*

■ RISK FOR SELF-DIRECTED OR OTHER-DIRECTED VIOLENCE

Definition: *At risk for behaviors in which an individual demonstrates that he/she can be physically, emotionally, and/or sexually harmful either to self or to others* (NANDA-I, 2012, p. 447–448)

Risk Factors ("related to")

[Negative role modeling]
[Dysfunctional family system]
[Low self-esteem]
[Unresolved grief]
[Psychic overload]
[Extended exposure to stressful situation]
[Lack of support systems]
[Biological factors, such as organic changes in the brain]
Body language (e.g., rigid posture, clenching of fists and jaw, hyperactivity, pacing, breathlessness, threatening stances)
[History or threats of violence toward self or others or of destruction to the property of others]
Impulsivity
Suicidal ideation, plan, available means
[Anger; rage]
[Increasing anxiety level]
[Depressed mood]

Goals/Objectives

Short-term Goals

1. Client will seek out staff member when hostile or suicidal feelings occur.
2. Client will verbalize adaptive coping strategies for use when hostile or suicidal feelings occur.

Long-term Goals

1. Client will demonstrate adaptive coping strategies for use when hostile or suicidal feelings occur.
2. Client will not harm self or others.

Interventions With *Selected Rationales*

1. Observe client's behavior frequently. Do this through routine activities and interactions; avoid appearing watchful and suspicious. Close observation is required so that intervention can occur if required to ensure client's (and others') safety.
2. Observe for suicidal behaviors: verbal statements, such as "I'm going to kill myself" and "Very soon my mother won't have to worry herself about me any longer," and nonverbal behaviors, such as giving away cherished items and mood swings. *Clients who are contemplating suicide often give clues regarding their potential behavior. The clues may be very subtle and require keen assessment skills by the nurse.*
3. Determine suicidal intent and available means. Ask direct questions, such as "Do you plan to kill yourself?" and "How do you plan to do it?" *The risk of suicide is greatly increased if the*

client has developed a plan and particularly if means exist for the client to execute the plan.

4. Obtain verbal or written contract from client agreeing not to harm self and to seek out staff in the event that suicidal ideation occurs. *Discussion of suicidal feelings with a trusted individual provides some relief to the client. A contract gets the subject out in the open and places some of the responsibility for his or her safety with the client. An attitude of acceptance of the client as a worthwhile individual is conveyed.*

5. Help client recognize when anger occurs and to accept those feelings as his or her own. Have client keep an "anger notebook," in which feelings of anger experienced during a 24-hour period are recorded. Information regarding source of anger, behavioral response, and client's perception of the situation should also be noted. Discuss entries with client and suggest alternative behavioral responses for those identified as maladaptive.

6. Act as a role model for appropriate expression of angry feelings and give positive reinforcement to client for attempting to conform. *It is vital that the client express angry feelings, because suicide and other self-destructive behaviors are often viewed as the result of anger turned inward on the self.*

7. Remove all dangerous objects from client's environment (e.g., sharp items, belts, ties, straps, breakable items, smoking materials). *Client safety is a nursing priority.*

8. Try to redirect violent behavior by means of physical outlets for the client's anxiety (e.g., punching bag, jogging). *Physical exercise is a safe and effective way of relieving pent-up tension.*

9. Be available to stay with client as anxiety level and tensions begin to rise. *Presence of a trusted individual provides a feeling of security and may help to prevent rapid escalation of anxiety.*

10. Staff should maintain and convey a calm attitude to client. *Anxiety is contagious and can be transmitted from staff members to client.*

11. Have sufficient staff available to indicate a show of strength to client if necessary. *This conveys to the client evidence of control over the situation and provides some physical security for staff.*

12. Administer tranquilizing medications as ordered by physician or obtain an order if necessary. Monitor client response for effectiveness of the medication and for adverse side effects. *Short-term use of tranquilizing medications such as anxiolytics or antipsychotics can induce a calming effect on the client and may prevent aggressive behaviors.*

13. Use of mechanical restraints or isolation room may be required if less restrictive interventions are unsuccessful. Follow policy and procedure prescribed by the institution in executing

this intervention. The Joint Commission (formerly the Joint Commission on Accreditation of Healthcare Organizations [JCAHO]) requires that an in-person evaluation by a physician or other licensed independent practitioner (LIP) be conducted within 1 hour of the initiation of the restraint or seclusion (The Joint Commission, 2010). The physician or LIP must reissue a new order for restraints every 4 hours for adults and every 1 to 2 hours for children and adolescents.

14. The Joint Commission requires that the client in restraints be observed at least every 15 minutes to ensure that circulation to extremities is not compromised (check temperature, color, pulses); to assist the client with needs related to nutrition, hydration, and elimination; and to position client so that comfort is facilitated and aspiration is prevented. Continuous one-to-one monitoring may be necessary for the client who is highly agitated or for whom there is a high risk of self- or accidental injury. *Client safety is a nursing priority.*

15. As agitation decreases, assess client's readiness for restraint removal or reduction. Remove one restraint at a time, while assessing client's response. *This minimizes risk of injury to the client and staff.*

Outcome Criteria

1. Anxiety is maintained at a level at which client feels no need for aggression.
2. Client denies any ideas of self-destruction.
3. Client demonstrates use of adaptive coping strategies when feelings of hostility or suicide occur.
4. Client verbalizes community support systems from which assistance may be requested when personal coping strategies are not successful.

▓ ANXIETY (MODERATE TO SEVERE)

Definition: *Vague uneasy feeling of discomfort or dread accompanied by an autonomic response (the source often nonspecific or unknown to the individual); a feeling of apprehension caused by anticipation of danger. It is an alerting signal that warns of impending danger and enables the individual to take measures to deal with threat.* (NANDA-I, 2012, p. 344)

Possible Etiologies ("related to")

Situational and maturational crises
[Low self-esteem]
[Complicated grieving]
[Feelings of powerlessness and lack of control in life situation]

[Having experienced a trauma outside the range of usual human experience]

Defining Characteristics ("evidenced by")

Increased tension
[Increased helplessness]
Overexcited
Apprehensive; fearful
Restlessness
Poor eye contact
Feelings of inadequacy
Insomnia
Focus on the self
Increased cardiac and respiratory rates
Diminished ability to problem solve and learn
Scanning; hypervigilance

Goals/Objectives

Short-term Goal

Client will demonstrate use of relaxation techniques to maintain anxiety at manageable level within 7 days.

Long-term Goal

By time of discharge from treatment, client will be able to recognize events that precipitate anxiety and intervene to prevent disabling behaviors.

Interventions With *Selected Rationales*

1. Be available to stay with client. Remain calm and provide assurance of safety. *Client safety and security is a nursing priority.*
2. Help client identify situation that precipitated onset of anxiety symptoms. *Client may be unaware that emotional issues are related to symptoms of anxiety. Recognition may be the first step in elimination of this maladaptive response.*
3. Review client's methods of coping with similar situations in the past. Discuss ways in which client may assume control over these situations. *In seeking to create change, it would be helpful for client to identify past responses and to determine whether they were successful and if they could be employed again. A measure of control reduces feelings of powerlessness in a situation, ultimately decreasing anxiety. Client strengths should be identified and used to his or her advantage.*
4. Provide quiet environment. Reduce stimuli: low lighting, few people. *Anxiety level may be decreased in calm atmosphere with few stimuli.*
5. Administer antianxiety medications as ordered by physician, or obtain order if necessary. Monitor client's response for effectiveness

of the medication as well as for adverse side effects. ***Short-term use of antianxiety medications (e.g., lorazepam, chlordiazepoxide, alprazolam) provide relief from the immobilizing effects of anxiety and facilitate client's cooperation with therapy***.

6. Discuss with client signs of increasing anxiety and ways of intervening to maintain the anxiety at a manageable level (e.g., exercise, walking, jogging, relaxation techniques). ***Anxiety and tension can be reduced safely and with benefit to the client through physical activities***.

Outcome Criteria

1. Client is able to verbalize events that precipitate anxiety and to demonstrate techniques for its reduction.
2. Client is able to verbalize ways in which he or she may gain more control of the environment and thereby reduce feelings of powerlessness.

■ INEFFECTIVE COPING

Definition: *Inability to form a valid appraisal of the stressors, inadequate choices of practiced responses, and/or inability to use available resources* (NANDA-I, 2012, p. 348)

Possible Etiologies ("related to")

Situational crises
Maturational crises
[Inadequate support systems]
[Low self-esteem]
[Unresolved grief]
[Inadequate coping strategies]

Defining Characteristics ("evidenced by")

Inability to meet role expectations
[Alteration in societal participation]
Inadequate problem solving
[Increased dependency]
[Manipulation of others in the environment for purposes of fulfilling own desires]
[Refusal to follow rules]

Goals/Objectives

Short-term Goal

By the end of 1 week, client will comply with rules of therapy and refrain from manipulating others to fulfill own desires.

Long-term Goal

By time of discharge from treatment, client will identify, develop, and use socially acceptable coping skills.

Interventions With *Selected Rationales*

1. Discuss with client the rules of therapy and consequences of noncompliance. Carry out the consequences matter-of-factly if rules are broken. *Negative consequences may work to decrease manipulative behaviors.*

2. Do not debate, argue, rationalize, or bargain with the client regarding limit setting on manipulative behaviors. *Ignoring these attempts may work to decrease manipulative behaviors. Consistency among all staff members is essential if this intervention is to be successful.*

3. Encourage discussion of angry feelings. Help client identify the true object of the hostility. Provide physical outlets for healthy release of the hostile feelings (e.g., punching bags, pounding boards). *Verbalization of feelings with a trusted individual may help client work through unresolved issues. Physical exercise provides a safe and effective means of releasing pent-up tension.*

4. Take care not to reinforce dependent behaviors. Encourage client to perform as independently as possible, and provide positive feedback. *Independent accomplishment and positive reinforcement enhance self-esteem and encourage repetition of desirable behaviors.*

5. Help client recognize some aspects of his or her life over which a measure of control is maintained. *Recognition of personal control, however minimal, diminishes the feeling of powerlessness and decreases the need for manipulation of others.*

6. Identify the stressor that precipitated the maladaptive coping. If a major life change has occurred, encourage client to express fears and feelings associated with the change. Assist client through the problem-solving process:
   a. Identify possible alternatives that indicate positive adaptation.
   b. Discuss benefits and consequences of each alternative.
   c. Select the most appropriate alternative.
   d. Implement the alternative.
   e. Evaluate the effectiveness of the alternative.
   f. Recognize areas of limitation, and make modifications. Request assistance with this process, if needed.

7. Provide positive reinforcement for application of adaptive coping skills and evidence of successful adjustment. *Positive reinforcement enhances self-esteem and encourages repetition of desirable behaviors.*

Outcome Criteria

1. Client is able to verbalize alternative, socially acceptable, and lifestyle-appropriate coping skills he or she plans to use in response to stress.

2. Client is able to solve problems and fulfill activities of daily living independently.
3. Client does not manipulate others for own gratification.

▨ RISK-PRONE HEALTH BEHAVIOR*

Definition: *Impaired ability to modify lifestyle/behaviors in a manner that improves health status* (NANDA-I, 2012, p. 155)

Possible Etiologies ("related to")

[Low self-esteem]
[Intense emotional state]
[Negative attitudes toward health behavior]
[Absence of intent to change behavior]
Multiple stressors
[Absence of social support for changed beliefs and practices]
[Disability or health status change requiring change in lifestyle]
[Lack of motivation to change behaviors]

Defining Characteristics ("evidenced by")

Minimizes health status change
Failure to achieve optimal sense of control
Failure to take actions that prevent health problems
Demonstrates nonacceptance of health status change

Goals/Objectives

Short-term Goals

1. Client will discuss with primary nurse the kinds of lifestyle changes that will occur because of the change in health status.
2. With the help of primary nurse, client will formulate a plan of action for incorporating those changes into his or her lifestyle.
3. Client will demonstrate movement toward independence, considering change in health status.

Long-term Goal

Client will demonstrate competence to function independently to his or her optimal ability, considering change in health status, by time of discharge from treatment.

Interventions With *Selected Rationales*

1. Encourage client to talk about lifestyle prior to the change in health status. Discuss coping mechanisms that were used at

---

*According to the NANDA-I definition, this diagnosis is appropriate for the person with adjustment disorder only if the precipitating stressor is a change in health status.

stressful times in the past. *It is important to identify the client's strengths so that they may be used to facilitate adaptation to the change or loss that has occurred.*

2. Encourage client to discuss the change or loss and particularly to express anger associated with it. *Some individuals may not realize that anger is a normal stage in the grieving process. If it is not released in an appropriate manner, it may be turned inward on the self, leading to pathological depression.*

3. Encourage client to express fears associated with the change or loss, or alteration in lifestyle that the change or loss has created. *Change often creates a feeling of disequilibrium and the individual may respond with fears that are irrational or unfounded. He or she may benefit from feedback that corrects misperceptions about how life will be with the change in health status.*

4. Provide assistance with activities of daily living (ADLs) as required, but encourage independence to the limit that client's ability will allow. Give positive feedback for activities accomplished independently. *Independent accomplishments and positive feedback enhance self-esteem and encourage repetition of desired behaviors. Successes also provide hope that adaptive functioning is possible and decrease feelings of powerlessness.*

5. Help client with decision making regarding incorporation of change or loss into lifestyle. Identify problems that the change or loss is likely to create. Discuss alternative solutions, weighing potential benefits and consequences of each alternative. Support client's decision in the selection of an alternative. *The great amount of anxiety that usually accompanies a major lifestyle change often interferes with an individual's ability to solve problems and to make appropriate decisions. Client may need assistance with this process in an effort to progress toward successful adaptation.*

6. Use role-playing of potential stressful situations that might occur in relation to the health status change. *Role-playing decreases anxiety and provides a feeling of security by providing client with a plan of action for responding in an appropriate manner when a stressful situation occurs.*

7. Ensure that client and family are fully knowledgeable regarding the physiology of the change in health status and its necessity for optimal wellness. Encourage them to ask questions, and provide printed material explaining the change to which they may refer following discharge. *Increased knowledge enhances successful adaptation.*

8. Help client identify resources within the community from which he or she may seek assistance in adapting to the change in health status. Examples include self-help or support groups and public health nurse, counselor, or social worker. Encourage

client to keep follow-up appointments with physician, or to call physician's office prior to follow-up date if problems or concerns arise.

Outcome Criteria

1. Client is able to perform ADLs independently.
2. Client is able to make independent decisions regarding lifestyle considering change in health status.
3. Client is able to express hope for the future with consideration of change in health status.

■ RELOCATION STRESS SYNDROME*

Definition: *Physiological and/or psychosocial disturbance following transfer from one environment to another* (NANDA-I, 2012, p. 338).

Possible Etiologies ("related to")

Move from one environment to another
[Losses involved with decision to move]
Feelings of powerlessness
Lack of adequate support system
[Little or no preparation for the impending move]
Impaired psychosocial health [status]
Decreased [physical] health status

Defining Characteristics ("evidenced by")

Anxiety
Depression
Loneliness
Reports unwillingness to move
Sleep pattern disturbance
Increased physical symptoms
Dependency
Insecurity
Withdrawal
Anger; fear

Goals/Objectives

Short-term Goal

Client will verbalize at least one positive aspect regarding relocation to new environment within (realistic time period).

*This diagnosis would be appropriate for the individual with adjustment disorder if the precipitating stressor was relocation to a new environment.

Long-term Goal

Client will demonstrate positive adaptation to new environment, as evidenced by involvement in activities, expression of satisfaction with new acquaintances, and elimination of previously evident physical and psychological symptoms associated with the relocation (time dimension to be determined individually).

Interventions With *Selected Rationales*

1. Encourage the individual to discuss feelings (concerns, fears, anger) regarding relocation. *Exploration of feelings with a trusted individual may help the individual perceive the situation more realistically and come to terms with the inevitable change.*

2. Encourage the individual to discuss how the change will affect his or her life. Ensure that the individual is involved in decision making and problem solving regarding the move. *Taking responsibility for making choices regarding the relocation will increase feelings of control and decrease feelings of powerlessness.*

3. Help the individual identify positive aspects about the move. *Anxiety associated with the opposed relocation may interfere with the individual's ability to recognize anything positive about it. Assistance may be required.*

4. Help the individual identify resources within the new community from which assistance with various types of services may be obtained. *Because of anxiety and depression, the individual may not be able to identify these resources alone. Assistance with problem solving may be required.*

5. Identify groups within the community that specialize in helping individuals adapt to relocation. Examples include Newcomers Club, Welcome Wagon Club, senior citizens groups, school and church organizations. *These groups offer support from individuals who may have encountered similar experiences. Adaptation may be enhanced by the reassurance, encouragement, and support of peers who exhibit positive adaptation to relocation stress.*

6. Refer the individual or family for professional counseling if deemed necessary. *An individual who is experiencing complicated grieving over loss of previous residence may require therapy to achieve resolution of the problem. It may be that other unresolved issues are interfering with successful adaptation to the relocation.*

Outcome Criteria

1. The individual no longer exhibits signs of anxiety, depression, or somatic symptoms.
2. The individual verbalizes satisfaction with the new environment.

3. The individual willingly participates in social and vocational activities within his or her new environment.

@ INTERNET REFERENCES

- Additional information about trauma- and stressor-related disorders may be located at the following Web sites:
  - a. www.mentalhealth.com/rx/p23-aj01.html
  - b. www.psyweb.com/Mdisord/jsp/adjd.jsp
  - c. http://emedicine.medscape.com/article/292759-overview
  - d. www.athealth.com/Consumer/disorders/Adjustment.html
  - e. www.nlm.nih.gov/medlineplus/ency/article/000932.htm
  - f. www.mayoclinic.com/health/adjustment-disorders/DS00584
  - g. www.ptsd.va.gov/
  - h. www.nimh.nih.gov/health/topics/post-traumatic-stress-disorder-ptsd/index.shtml
  - i. http://www.ptsd.va.gov/public/pages/acute-stress-disorder.asp

CHAPTER 10

Somatic Symptom and Related Disorders

■ BACKGROUND ASSESSMENT DATA

Somatic symptom disorders are characterized by physical symptoms suggesting medical disease but without demonstrable organic pathology or known pathophysiological mechanism to account for them. They are classified as mental disorders because pathophysiological processes are not demonstrable or understandable by existing laboratory procedures, and there is either evidence or strong presumption that psychological factors are the major cause of the symptoms. It is now well documented that a large proportion of clients in general medical outpatient clinics and private medical offices do not have organic disease requiring medical treatment. It is likely that many of these clients have somatic symptom disorders, but they do not perceive themselves as having a psychiatric problem and thus do not seek treatment from psychiatrists. The American Psychiatric Association (APA, 2013) *Diagnostic and Statistical Manual of Mental Disorders, Fifth Edition (DSM-5)* identifies the following categories of somatic symptom disorders.

Somatic Symptom Disorder

Somatic symptom disorder is a syndrome of multiple somatic symptoms that cannot be explained medically and are associated with psychosocial distress and long-term seeking of assistance from health-care professionals. Symptoms may be vague, dramatized, or exaggerated in their presentation, and an excessive amount of time and energy is devoted to worry and concern about the symptoms. Individuals with somatic symptom disorder are so totally convinced that their symptoms are related to organic pathology that they adamantly reject and are often irritated by any implication that stress or psychosocial factors play any role in their condition. The disorder is chronic, with symptoms beginning before age 30. Anxiety and depression are frequently manifested, and suicidal threats and attempts are not uncommon.

The disorder usually runs a fluctuating course, with periods of remission and exacerbation. Clients often receive medical care from several physicians, sometimes concurrently, leading to the possibility of dangerous combinations of treatments. They have a tendency to seek relief through overmedicating with prescribed analgesics or antianxiety agents. Drug abuse and dependence are common complications of somatic symptom disorder.

Illness Anxiety Disorder

Illness anxiety disorder may be defined as an unrealistic or inaccurate interpretation of physical symptoms or sensations, leading to preoccupation and fear of having a serious disease. The fear becomes disabling and persists despite appropriate reassurance that no organic pathology can be detected. Symptoms may be minimal or absent, but the individual is highly anxious about and suspicious of the presence of an undiagnosed, serious medical illness (APA, 2013).

Individuals with illness anxiety disorder are extremely conscious of bodily sensations and changes and may become convinced that a rapid heart rate indicates they have heart disease or that a small sore is skin cancer. They are profoundly preoccupied with their bodies and are totally aware of even the slightest change in feeling or sensation. Their response to these small changes, however, is usually unrealistic and exaggerated.

Some individuals with illness anxiety disorder have a long history of "doctor shopping" and are convinced that they are not receiving the proper care. Others avoid seeking medical assistance because to do so would increase their anxiety to intolerable levels. Depression is common, and obsessive-compulsive traits frequently accompany the disorder. Preoccupation with the fear of serious disease may interfere with social or occupational functioning. Some individuals are able to function appropriately on the job, however, while limiting their physical complaints to nonwork time.

Individuals with illness anxiety disorder are so apprehensive and fearful that they become alarmed at the slightest intimation of serious illness. Even reading about a disease or hearing that someone they know has been diagnosed with an illness precipitates alarm on their part.

Conversion Disorder (Functional Neurological Symptom Disorder)

Conversion disorder is a loss of or change in body function that cannot be explained by any known medical disorder or pathophysiological mechanism. There is most likely a psychological component involved in the initiation, exacerbation, or perpetuation of the symptom, although it may or may not be obvious or identifiable.

Conversion symptoms affect voluntary motor or sensory functioning suggestive of neurological disease. Examples include paralysis, aphonia (inability to produce voice), seizures, coordination disturbance, difficulty swallowing, urinary retention, akinesia, blindness, deafness, double vision, anosmia (inability to perceive smell), loss of pain sensation, and hallucinations. Pseudocyesis (false pregnancy) is a conversion symptom and may represent a strong desire to be pregnant.

Previous criteria in the *DSM-IV-TR* (APA, 2000) stated that the precipitation of conversion symptoms must be explained by psychological factors. This criterion has been removed in the *DSM-5*, which states, "The potential etiological relevance of stress or trauma may be suggested by a close temporal relationship. However, although assessment for stress and trauma is important, the diagnosis should not be withheld if none is found" (APA, 2013, pp. 319-320). It is likely that multiple causes play a role in the etiology. Most symptoms of conversion disorder resolve within a few weeks.

Psychological Factors Affecting Other Medical Conditions

Psychological factors may play a role in virtually any medical condition. In this disorder, it is evident that psychological or behavioral factors have been implicated in the development, exacerbation, or delayed recovery from a medical condition. Historically, mind and body have been viewed as two distinct entities, each subject to different laws of causality. Indeed, in many instances—particularly in highly specialized areas of medicine—the biological and psychological components of disease remain separate. However, medical research shows that a change is occurring. Research associated with biological functioning is being expanded to include the psychological and social determinants of health and disease. This psychobiological approach to illness reflects a more holistic perspective and one that promotes concern for helping clients achieve optimal functioning.

Factitious Disorder

Factitious disorders involve conscious, intentional feigning of physical or psychological symptoms (Black & Andreasen, 2011). Individuals with factitious disorder pretend to be ill in order to receive emotional care and support commonly associated with the role of "patient." Even though the behaviors are deliberate and intentional, there may be an associated compulsive element that diminishes personal control. Individuals may aggravate existing symptoms, induce new ones, or even inflict painful injuries on themselves (Sadock & Sadock, 2007). The disorder may also be identified as *Munchausen syndrome*, and symptoms may be psychological, physical, or a combination of both.

The disorder may be imposed on oneself, or on another person (previously called *Factitious Disorder by Proxy*). In the latter case, physical symptoms are intentionally imposed on a person under the care of the perpetrator. Diagnosis of factitious disorder can be very difficult, as individuals become very inventive in their quest to produce symptoms. Examples include self-inflicted wounds, injection or insertion of contaminated substances, manipulating a thermometer to feign a fever, urinary tract manipulation, and surreptitious use of medications (Black & Andreasen, 2011, p. 236).

■ PREDISPOSING FACTORS TO SOMATIC SYMPTOM DISORDERS

1. **Physiological**
   a. *Genetic.* Studies have shown an increased incidence of somatic symptom disorder, conversion disorder, and illness anxiety disorder in first-degree relatives, implying a possible inheritable predisposition (Sadock & Sadock, 2007; Soares & Grossman, 2012; Yutzy & Parish, 2008).
   b. *Biochemical.* Decreased levels of serotonin and endorphins may play a role in the etiology of somatic symptom disorder, predominantly pain. Serotonin is probably the main neurotransmitter involved in inhibiting the firing of afferent pain fibers (Parcell, 2008). The deficiency of endorphins seems to correlate with an increase of incoming sensory (pain) stimuli (Wootton, 2008).
   c. *Neuroanatomical.* Brain dysfunction has been proposed by some researchers as a factor in factitious disorders (Sadock & Sadock, 2007). The hypothesis is that impairment in information processing contributes to the aberrant behaviors associated with the disorder. However, no genetic patterns have been identified, nor have specific electroencephalographic (EEG) abnormalities been noted in clients with factitious disorder.

2. **Psychosocial**
   a. *Psychodynamic Theory.* Some psychodynamic theorists view illness anxiety disorder as an ego defense mechanism. They suggest that physical complaints are the expression of low self-esteem and feelings of worthlessness and that the individual believes it is easier to feel something is wrong with the body than to feel something is wrong with the self. Another psychodynamic view of illness anxiety disorder (as well as somatic symptom disorder, predominantly pain) is related to a defense against guilt. The individual views the self as "bad," based on real or imagined past misconduct, and views physical suffering as the deserved punishment required for atonement. This view has also been related to individuals with factitious disorders.

   The psychodynamic theory of conversion disorder proposes that emotions associated with a traumatic event that the individual cannot express because of moral or ethical unacceptability are "converted" into physical symptoms.

The unacceptable emotions are repressed and converted to a somatic hysterical symptom that is symbolic in some way of the original emotional trauma.

Some reports suggest that individuals with factitious disorders were victims of child abuse or neglect. Frequent childhood hospitalizations provided a reprieve from the traumatic home situation and a loving and caring environment that was absent in the child's family. This theory proposes that the individual with factitious disorder is attempting to recapture the only positive support he or she may have known by seeking out the environment in which it was received as a child. Regarding factitious disorder imposed on another, Sadock and Sadock (2007) have stated, "One apparent purpose of the behavior is for the caretaker to indirectly assume the sick role; another is to be relieved of the caretaking role by having the child hospitalized" (p. 661).

b. *Family Dynamics.* Some families have difficulty expressing emotions openly and resolving conflicts verbally. When this occurs, the child may become ill, and a shift in focus is made from the open conflict to the child's illness, leaving unresolved the underlying issues that the family cannot confront openly. Thus, somatization by the child brings some stability to the family, as harmony replaces discord and the child's welfare becomes the common concern. The child in turn receives positive reinforcement for the illness. This shift in focus from family discord to concern for the child is sometimes called *tertiary gain.*

c. *Learning Theory.* Somatic complaints are often reinforced when the sick role relieves the individual from the need to deal with a stressful situation, whether it be within society or within the family. The sick person learns that he or she may avoid stressful obligations, may postpone unwelcome challenges, and is excused from troublesome duties (primary gain); becomes the prominent focus of attention because of the illness (secondary gain); or relieves conflict within the family as concern is shifted to the ill person and away from the real issue (tertiary gain). These types of positive reinforcements virtually guarantee repetition of the response.

d. *Past Experience with Physical Illness.* Past experience with serious or life-threatening physical illness, either personal or that of close family members, can predispose an individual to illness anxiety disorder. Once an individual has experienced a threat to biological integrity, he or she may develop a fear of recurrence. The fear of recurring illness generates an exaggerated response to minor physical changes, leading to excessive anxiety and health concerns.

■ SYMPTOMATOLOGY (SUBJECTIVE AND OBJECTIVE DATA)

1. Any physical symptom for which there is no organic basis but for which evidence exists for the implication of psychological factors.
2. Depressed mood is common.
3. Loss or alteration in physical functioning, with no organic basis. Examples include the following:
   a. Blindness or tunnel vision
   b. Paralysis
   c. Anosmia (inability to smell)
   d. Aphonia (inability to speak)
   e. Seizures
   f. Coordination disturbances
   g. Pseudocyesis (false pregnancy)
   h. Akinesia or dyskinesia
   i. Anesthesia or paresthesia
4. "Doctor shopping."
5. Excessive use of analgesics.
6. Requests for surgery.
7. Assumption of an invalid role.
8. Impairment in social or occupational functioning because of preoccupation with physical complaints.
9. Psychosexual dysfunction (impotence, dyspareunia [painful coitus], sexual indifference).
10. Excessive dysmenorrhea.
11. Excessive anxiety and fear of having a serious illness.
12. Objective evidence that a general medical condition has been precipitated by or is being perpetuated by psychological or behavioral circumstances.
13. Conscious, intentional feigning of physical or psychological symptoms (may be imposed on the self or on another person).

Common Nursing Diagnoses and Interventions

(Interventions are applicable to various health-care settings, such as inpatient and partial hospitalization, community outpatient clinic, home health, and private practice.)

▓ INEFFECTIVE COPING

Definition: *Inability to form a valid appraisal of the stressors, inadequate choices of practiced responses, and/or inability to use available resources* (NANDA International [NANDA-I], 2012, p. 348)

Possible Etiologies ("related to")

[Severe level of anxiety, repressed]
[Low self-esteem]

[Unmet dependency needs]
[History of self or loved one having experienced a serious illness or disease]
[Regression to, or fixation in, an earlier level of development]
[Retarded ego development]
[Inadequate coping skills]
[Possible child abuse or neglect]

Defining Characteristics ("evidenced by")

[Numerous physical complaints verbalized, in the absence of any pathophysiological evidence]
[Total focus on the self and physical symptoms]
[History of doctor shopping]
[Demanding behaviors]
[Refuses to attend therapeutic activities]
[Does not correlate physical symptoms with psychological problems]
[Feigning of physical or psychological symptoms to gain attention]
Inability to meet basic needs
Inability to meet role expectations
Inadequate problem solving
Sleep pattern disturbance

Goals/Objectives

Short-term Goal

Within (specified time), client will verbalize understanding of correlation between physical symptoms and psychological problems.

Long-term Goal

By time of discharge from treatment, client will demonstrate ability to cope with stress by means other than preoccupation with physical symptoms.

Interventions With *Selected Rationales*

1. Monitor physician's ongoing assessments, laboratory reports, and other data to maintain assurance that possibility of organic pathology is clearly ruled out. Review findings with the client. *Accurate medical assessment is vital for the provision of adequate and appropriate care. Honest explanation may help the client understand the psychological implications.*

2. Recognize and accept that the physical complaint is indeed real to the individual, even though no organic etiology can be identified. *Denial of the client's feelings is nontherapeutic and interferes with establishment of a trusting relationship.*

3. Provide pain medication as prescribed by the physician. *Client comfort and safety are nursing priorities.*

4. Identify gains that the physical symptoms are providing for the client: increased dependency, attention, and distraction from other problems. *Identification of underlying motivation is important in assisting the client with problem resolution.*

5. Initially, fulfill client's most urgent dependency needs. *Failure to do this may cause client to become extremely anxious, with an increase in maladaptive behaviors.*

6. Gradually withdraw attention to physical symptoms. Minimize time given in response to physical complaints. *Lack of positive response will discourage repetition of maladaptive behaviors.*

7. Explain to client that any new physical complaints will be referred to the physician, and give no further attention to them. Follow up on physician's assessment of the complaint. *The possibility of organic pathology must always be considered. Failure to do so could jeopardize client's safety.*

8. Encourage client to verbalize fears and anxieties. Explain that attention will be withdrawn if rumination about physical complaints begins. Follow through. *Without consistency of limit setting, change will not occur.*

9. Help the client recognize that physical symptoms occur because of or are exacerbated by specific stressors. Discuss alternative coping strategies that the client may use in response to stress (e.g., relaxation exercises, physical activities, assertiveness skills). The client may need help with problem solving.

10. Give positive reinforcement for adaptive coping strategies. *Positive reinforcement encourages repetition of desired behaviors.*

11. Have the client keep a diary of appearance, duration, and intensity of physical symptoms. A separate record of situations that the client finds especially stressful should also be kept. *Comparison of these records may provide objective data from which to observe the relationship between physical symptoms and stress.*

12. Help client identify ways to achieve recognition from others without resorting to physical symptoms. *Positive recognition from others enhances self-esteem and minimizes the need for attention through maladaptive behaviors.*

13. Discuss how interpersonal relationships are affected by client's narcissistic behavior. Explain how this behavior alienates others. *Client may not realize how he or she is perceived by others.*

14. Provide instruction in relaxation techniques and assertiveness skills. *These approaches decrease anxiety and increase self-esteem, which facilitate adaptive responses to stressful situations.*

Outcome Criteria

1. Client is able to demonstrate techniques that may be used in response to stress to prevent the occurrence or exacerbation of physical symptoms.
2. Client verbalizes an understanding of the relationship between emotional problems and physical symptoms.

■ DISTURBED SENSORY PERCEPTION

Definition: *Change in the amount or patterning of incoming stimuli [either internally or externally initiated] accompanied by a diminished, exaggerated, distorted, or impaired response to such stimuli* (Note: This diagnosis has been retired by NANDA-I but is retained in this text because of its appropriateness in describing these specific behaviors.)

Possible Etiologies ("related to")

[Severe level of anxiety, repressed]
[Low self-esteem]
[Unmet dependency needs]
[Regression to or fixation in an earlier level of development]
[Retarded ego development]
[Inadequate coping skills]
Psychological stress [narrowed perceptual fields caused by anxiety]

Defining Characteristics ("evidenced by")

[Loss or alteration in physical functioning suggesting a physical disorder (often neurological in nature), but for which organic pathology is not evident. Common alterations include paralysis, anosmia, aphonia, deafness, blindness]

Goals/Objectives

Short-term Goal

The client will verbalize understanding of emotional problems as a contributing factor to the alteration in physical functioning (within time limit appropriate for specific individual).

Long-term Goal

The client will demonstrate recovery of lost or altered function.

Interventions With *Selected Rationales*

1. Monitor the physician's ongoing assessments, laboratory reports, and other data to maintain assurance that possibility of organic pathology is clearly ruled out. *Failure to do so may jeopardize client's safety.*

2. Identify primary or secondary gains that the physical symptom is providing for the client (e.g., increased dependency, attention, protection from experiencing a stressful event). *These are considered to be etiological factors and may be used to assist in problem resolution.*

3. Fulfill client's needs related to activities of daily living (ADLs) with which the physical symptom is interfering. *Client comfort and safety are nursing priorities.*

4. Do not focus on the disability, and encourage the client to be as independent as possible. Intervene only when the client requires assistance. *Positive reinforcement would encourage continual use of the maladaptive response for secondary gains, such as dependency.*

5. Maintain a nonjudgmental attitude when providing assistance with self-care activities to the client. The physical symptom is not within the client's conscious control and is very real to him or her.

6. Encourage the client to participate in therapeutic activities to the best of his or her ability. Do not allow client to use the disability as a manipulative tool. Withdraw attention if client continues to focus on physical limitation. Reinforce reality as required, but ensure maintenance of a nonthreatening environment.

7. Encourage client to verbalize fears and anxieties. Help client to recognize that the physical symptom appears at a time of extreme stress and is a mechanism used for coping. *Client may be unaware of the relationship between physical symptom and emotional stress.*

8. Help the client identify coping mechanisms that he or she could use when faced with stressful situations rather than retreating from reality with a physical disability.

9. Explain assertiveness techniques and practice use of same through role-playing. *Use of assertiveness techniques enhances self-esteem and minimizes anxiety in interpersonal relationships.*

10. Help the client identify a satisfactory support system within the community from which he or she may seek assistance as needed to cope with overwhelming stress.

Outcome Criteria

1. Client is no longer experiencing symptoms of altered physical functioning.

2. Client verbalizes an understanding of the relationship between extreme psychological stress and loss of physical functioning.

3. Client is able to verbalize adaptive ways of coping with stress and identify community support systems to which he or she may go for help.

■ DEFICIENT KNOWLEDGE (PSYCHOLOGICAL FACTORS AFFECTING MEDICAL CONDITION)

Definition: *Absence or deficiency of cognitive information related to a specific topic* (NANDA-I, 2012, p. 271)

Possible Etiologies ("related to")

Lack of interest in learning
[Severe level of anxiety]
[Low self-esteem]
[Regression to earlier level of development]
Cognitive limitation
Information misinterpretation

Defining Characteristics ("evidenced by")

[Denial of emotional problems]
[Statements such as, "I don't know why the doctor put me on the psychiatric unit. I have a physical problem."]
[Evidence of a general medical condition that is being precipitated by psychological or behavioral circumstances]
[History of numerous exacerbations of physical illness]
[Noncompliance with psychiatric treatment]
Inappropriate or exaggerated behaviors (e.g., hysterical, hostile, agitated, apathetic)

Goals/Objectives

Short-term Goal

Client will cooperate with plan for teaching provided by primary nurse.

Long-term Goal

By time of discharge from treatment, client will be able to verbalize psychological factors affecting his or her medical condition.

Interventions With *Selected Rationales*

1. Assess client's level of knowledge regarding effects of psychological problems on the body. *An adequate database is necessary for the development of an effective teaching plan.*
2. Assess client's level of anxiety and readiness to learn. *Learning does not occur beyond the moderate level of anxiety.*
3. Discuss physical examinations and laboratory tests that have been conducted. Explain purpose and results of each. *Fear of the unknown may contribute to elevated level of anxiety. The client has the right to know about and accept or refuse any medical treatment.*

4. Explore client's feelings and fears. Go slowly. These feelings may have been suppressed or repressed for so long that their disclosure may be very painful. Be supportive. *Expression of feelings in a nonthreatening environment and with a trusting individual may encourage the individual to confront unresolved issues.*

5. Have the client keep a diary of appearance, duration, and intensity of physical symptoms. A separate record of situations that the client finds especially stressful should also be kept. *Comparison of these records may provide objective data from which to observe the relationship between physical symptoms and stress.*

6. Help client identify needs that are being met through the sick role. Together, formulate more adaptive means for fulfilling these needs. Practice by role-playing. *Repetition through practice serves to reduce discomfort in the actual situation.*

7. Provide instruction in assertiveness techniques, especially the ability to recognize the differences among passive, assertive, and aggressive behaviors, and the importance of respecting the human rights of others while protecting one's own basic human rights. *These skills will preserve client's self-esteem while also improving his or her ability to form satisfactory interpersonal relationships.*

8. Discuss adaptive methods of stress management such as relaxation techniques, physical exercise, meditation, breathing exercises, and autogenics. *Use of these adaptive techniques may decrease appearance or exacerbation of physical symptoms in response to stress.*

Outcome Criteria

1. Client verbalizes an understanding of the relationship between psychological stress and exacerbation (or perpetuation) of physical illness.

2. Client demonstrates the ability to use adaptive coping strategies in the management of stress.

■ FEAR (OF HAVING A SERIOUS ILLNESS)

Definition: *Response to perceived threat that is consciously recognized as a danger* (NANDA-I, 2012, p. 361)

Possible Etiologies ("related to")

[Past experience with life-threatening illness, either personal or that of close family members]

Defining Characteristics ("evidenced by")

[Preoccupation with and unrealistic interpretation of bodily signs and sensations]

[Excessive anxiety over health concerns]

Goals/Objectives

Short-term Goal

Client will verbalize that fears associated with bodily sensations are irrational (within time limit deemed appropriate for specific individual).

Long-term Goal

Client interprets bodily sensations correctly.

Interventions With *Selected Rationales*

1. Monitor the physician's ongoing assessments and laboratory reports. *Organic pathology must be clearly ruled out.*
2. Refer all new physical complaints to the physician. *To ignore all physical complaints could place the client's safety in jeopardy.*
3. Assess what function the client's illness is fulfilling for him or her (e.g., unfulfilled needs for dependency, nurturing, caring, attention, or control). *This information may provide insight into reasons for maladaptive behavior and provide direction for planning client care.*
4. Identify times during which the preoccupation with physical symptoms is worse. Determine the extent of correlation of physical complaints with times of increased anxiety. *The client may be unaware of the psychosocial implications of the physical complaints. Knowledge of the relationship is the first step in the process for creating change.*
5. Convey empathy. Let the client know that you understand how a specific symptom may conjure up fears of previous life-threatening illness. *Unconditional acceptance and empathy promote a therapeutic nurse-client relationship.*
6. Initially allow the client a limited amount of time (e.g., 10 minutes each hour) to discuss physical symptoms. *Because this has been his or her primary method of coping for so long, complete prohibition of this activity would likely raise the client's anxiety level significantly, further exacerbating the behavior.*
7. Help the client determine what techniques may be most useful for him or her to implement when fear and anxiety are exacerbated (e.g., relaxation techniques; mental imagery; thought-stopping techniques; physical exercise). *All of these techniques are effective in reducing anxiety and may assist the client in*

the transition from focusing on fear of physical illness to the discussion of honest feelings.

8. Gradually increase the limit on amount of time spent each hour in discussing physical symptoms. If the client violates the limits, withdraw attention. *Lack of positive reinforcement may help to extinguish the maladaptive behavior.*

9. Encourage the client to discuss feelings associated with fear of serious illness. *Verbalization of feelings in a nonthreatening environment facilitates expression and resolution of disturbing emotional issues. When the client can express feelings directly, there is less need to express them through physical symptoms.*

10. Role-play the client's plan for dealing with the fear the next time it assumes control and before anxiety becomes disabling. *Anxiety and fears are minimized when the client has achieved a degree of comfort through practicing a plan for dealing with stressful situations in the future.*

@ INTERNET REFERENCES

- Additional information about somatic symptom disorders may be located at the following Web sites:
  a. www.psyweb.com/Mdisord/somatd.html
  b. http://my.clevelandclinic.org/disorders/hypochondriasis/hic_hypochondriasis.aspx
  c. http://emedicine.medscape.com/article/805361-overview
  d. http://emedicine.medscape.com/article/291304-overview

Movie Connections

Bandits (Illness anxiety disorder) • *Hanna and Her Sisters* (Illness anxiety disorder) • *Send Me No Flowers* (Illness anxiety disorder)

CHAPTER **11**

Dissociative Disorders

■ BACKGROUND ASSESSMENT DATA

Dissociative disorders are defined by a disturbance of or alteration in the usually integrated functions of consciousness, memory, and identity (Black & Andreasen, 2011). During periods of intolerable stress, the individual blocks off part of his or her life from consciousness. The stressful emotion becomes a separate entity, as the individual "splits" from it and mentally drifts into a fantasy state. The following categories are defined in the *Diagnostic and Statistical Manual of Mental Disorders, Fifth Edition (DSM-5)* (American Psychiatric Association [APA], 2013):

1. **Dissociative Amnesia.** An inability to recall important personal information, usually of a traumatic or stressful nature. The extent of the disturbance is too great to be explained by ordinary forgetfulness. Types of impairment in recall include the following:
   a. *Localized Amnesia:* Inability to recall all incidents associated with a traumatic event. It may be broader than just a single event, however, such as being unable to remember months or years of child abuse (APA, 2013).
   b. *Selective Amnesia:* Inability to recall only certain incidents associated with a traumatic event for a specific period following the event.
   c. *Generalized Amnesia:* Inability to recall all events encompassing one's entire life, including one's identity.
   A specific subtype of dissociative amnesia is *with dissociative fugue.* Dissociative fugue is characterized by a sudden, unexpected travel away from customary place of daily activities or by bewildered wandering, with the inability to recall some or all of one's past. An individual in a fugue state may not be able to recall personal identity and sometimes assumes a new identity (Black & Andreasen, 2011).

2. **Dissociative Identity Disorder (DID).** The existence within the individual of two or more distinct personalities, each of which is dominant at a particular time. The original personality usually is not aware (at least initially) of the existence of subpersonalities. When there are more than two subpersonalities, however, they are usually aware of each other. Transition from

one personality to another is usually sudden and often associated with psychosocial stress. The course tends to be more chronic than in the other dissociative disorders. This disorder was previously called *multiple personality disorder.*

3. **Depersonalization-Derealization Disorder.** Characterized by a temporary change in the quality of self-awareness, which often takes the form of feelings of unreality, changes in body image, feelings of detachment from the environment, or a sense of observing oneself from outside the body. *Depersonalization* (a disturbance in the perception of oneself) is differentiated from *derealization*, which describes an alteration in the perception of the external environment. Both of these phenomena also occur in a variety of psychiatric illnesses such as schizophrenia, depression, anxiety states, and neurocognitive disorders.

■ PREDISPOSING FACTORS TO DISSOCIATIVE DISORDERS

1. **Physiological**
   a. *Genetics.* Regarding DID, Maldonado and Spiegel (2008) report on twin studies with monozygotic and dizygotic pairs in which the results suggested "common genetic factors underlying pathological and nonpathological dissociative capacity" (p. 685). Further research is required to determine if there is a true genetic influence associated with the etiology of DID.
   b. *Neurobiological.* Some clinicians have suggested a possible correlation between neurological alterations and dissociative disorders. Although available information is inadequate, it is possible that dissociative amnesia may be related to neurophysiological dysfunction. Areas of the brain that have been associated with memory include the hippocampus, amygdala, fornix, mammillary bodies, thalamus, and frontal cortex. Some studies have suggested a possible link between DID and certain neurological conditions, such as temporal lobe epilepsy and severe migraine headaches. Electroencephalographic abnormalities have been observed in some clients with DID.
2. **Psychosocial**
   a. *Psychodynamic Theory.* Freud (1962) believed that dissociative behaviors occurred when individuals repressed distressing mental contents from conscious awareness. He believed that the unconscious was a dynamic entity in which repressed mental contents were stored and unavailable to conscious recall. Current psychodynamic explanations of dissociation are based on Freud's concepts. The repression

of mental contents is perceived as a coping mechanism for protecting the client from emotional pain that has arisen from either disturbing external circumstances or anxiety-provoking internal urges and feelings (Maldonado & Spiegel, 2008). In the case of depersonalization and de-realization, the pain and anxiety are expressed as feelings of unreality or detachment from the environment of the painful situation.

b. *Psychological Trauma.* A growing body of evidence points to the etiology of DID as a set of traumatic experiences that overwhelms the individual's capacity to cope by any means other than dissociation. These experiences usually take the form of severe physical, sexual, and/or psychological abuse by a parent or significant other in the child's life. The most widely accepted explanation for DID is that it begins as a survival strategy that serves to help children cope with the horrifying sexual, physical, or psychological abuse. In this traumatic environment, the child uses dissociation to become a passive victim of the cruel and unwanted experience. He or she creates a new being who is able to endure the overwhelming pain of the cruel reality, while the primary self can then escape awareness of the pain. Each new personality has as its nucleus a means of responding without anxiety and distress to various painful or dangerous stimuli.

■ SYMPTOMATOLOGY (SUBJECTIVE AND OBJECTIVE DATA)

1. Impairment in recall.
   a. Inability to remember specific incidents.
   b. Inability to recall any of one's past life, including one's identity.
2. Sudden travel away from familiar surroundings; assumption of new identity with inability to recall past.
3. Assumption of additional identities within the personality; behavior involves transition from one identity to another as a method of dealing with stressful situations.
4. Feeling of unreality; detachment from a stressful situation—may be accompanied by light-headedness, depression, obsessive rumination, somatic concerns, anxiety, fear of going insane, and a disturbance in the subjective sense of time (APA, 2013).

Common Nursing Diagnoses and Interventions

(Interventions are applicable to various health-care settings, such as inpatient and partial hospitalization, community outpatient clinic, home health, and private practice.)

■ INEFFECTIVE COPING

Definition: *Inability to form a valid appraisal of the stressors, inadequate choices of practiced responses, and/or inability to use available resources* (NANDA International [NANDA-I], 2012, p. 348)

Possible Etiologies ("related to")

[Severe level of anxiety, repressed]
[Childhood trauma]
[Childhood abuse]
[Low self-esteem]
[Unmet dependency needs]
[Regression to or fixation in an earlier level of development]
[Inadequate coping skills]

Defining Characteristics ("evidenced by")

[Dissociating self from painful situation by experiencing:
    Memory loss (partial or complete)
    Sudden travel away from home with inability to recall previous
        identity
    The presence of more than one personality within the individual
    Detachment from reality]
Inadequate problem solving
Inability to meet role expectations
[Inappropriate use of defense mechanisms]

Goals/Objectives

Short-term Goals

1. Client will verbalize understanding that he or she is employing dissociative behaviors in times of psychosocial stress.
2. Client will verbalize more adaptive ways of coping in stressful situations than resorting to dissociation.

Long-term Goal

Client will demonstrate ability to cope with stress (employing means other than dissociation).

Interventions With *Selected Rationales*

1. Reassure client of safety and security by your presence. Dissociative behaviors may be frightening to the client. *Presence of a trusted individual provides feeling of security and assurance of freedom from harm.*
2. Identify stressor that precipitated severe anxiety. *This information is necessary to the development of an effective plan of client care and problem resolution.*

3. Explore feelings that client experienced in response to the stressor. Help client understand that the disequilibrium felt is acceptable—indeed, even expected—in times of severe stress. *Client's self-esteem is preserved by the knowledge that others may experience these behaviors in similar circumstances.*

4. As anxiety level decreases (and memory returns), use exploration and an accepting, nonthreatening environment to encourage client to identify repressed traumatic experiences that contribute to chronic anxiety.

5. Have client identify methods of coping with stress in the past and determine whether the response was adaptive or maladaptive. *In times of extreme anxiety, client is unable to evaluate appropriateness of response. This information is necessary for client to develop a plan of action for the future.*

6. Help client define more adaptive coping strategies. Make suggestions of alternatives that might be tried. Examine benefits and consequences of each alternative. Assist client in the selection of those that are most appropriate for him or her. *Depending on current level of anxiety, client may require assistance with problem solving and decision making.*

7. Provide positive reinforcement for client's attempts to change. *Positive reinforcement enhances self-esteem and encourages repetition of desired behaviors.*

8. Identify community resources to which the individual may go for support if past maladaptive coping patterns return.

Outcome Criteria

1. Client is able to demonstrate techniques that may be used in response to stress to prevent dissociation.
2. Client verbalizes an understanding of the relationship between severe anxiety and the dissociative response.

■ IMPAIRED MEMORY

Definition: *Inability to remember or recall bits of information or behavioral skills* (NANDA-I, 2012, p. 273)

Possible Etiologies ("related to")

[Severe level of anxiety, repressed]
[Childhood trauma]
[Childhood abuse]
[Threat to physical integrity]
[Threat to self-concept]

Defining Characteristics ("evidenced by")

[Memory loss—inability to recall selected events related to a stressful situation]
[Memory loss—inability to recall events associated with entire life]
[Memory loss—inability to recall own identity]

Goals/Objectives

Short-term Goal

Client will verbalize understanding that loss of memory is related to a stressful situation and begin discussing stressful situation with nurse or therapist.

Long-term Goal

Client will recover deficits in memory and develop more adaptive coping mechanisms to deal with stressful situations.

Interventions With *Selected Rationales*

1. Obtain as much information as possible about client from family and significant others, if possible. Consider likes, dislikes, important people, activities, music, and pets. *A comprehensive baseline assessment is important for the development of an effective plan of care.*
2. Do not flood client with data regarding his or her past life. *Individuals who are exposed to painful information from which the amnesia is providing protection may decompensate even further into a psychotic state.*
3. Instead, expose the client to stimuli that represent pleasant experiences from the past, such as smells associated with enjoyable activities, beloved pets, and music known to have been pleasurable to client.
4. As memory begins to return, engage the client in activities that may provide additional stimulation. *Recall often occurs during activities that simulate life experiences.*
5. Encourage the client to discuss situations that have been especially stressful and to explore the feelings associated with those times. *Verbalization of feelings in a nonthreatening environment may help the client come to terms with unresolved issues that may be contributing to the dissociative process.*
6. Identify specific conflicts that remain unresolved, and help the client to identify possible solutions. *Unless these underlying conflicts are resolved, any improvement in coping behaviors must be viewed as only temporary.*
7. Provide instruction regarding more adaptive ways to respond to anxiety *so that dissociative behaviors are no longer needed.*

8. Provide positive feedback for decisions made. Respect the client's right to make those decisions independently, and refrain from attempting to influence him or her toward those that may seem more logical. *Independent choice provides a feeling of control, decreases feelings of powerlessness, and increases self-esteem.*

Outcome Criteria

1. Client has recovered lost memories for events of past life.
2. Client is able to demonstrate adaptive coping strategies that may be used in response to severe anxiety to avert amnestic behaviors.

■ DISTURBED PERSONAL IDENTITY

Definition: *Inability to maintain an integrated and complete perception of self* (NANDA-I, 2012, p. 282)

Possible Etiologies ("related to")

[Severe level of anxiety, repressed]
[Childhood trauma]
[Childhood abuse]
[Threat to physical integrity]
[Threat to self-concept]

Defining Characteristics ("evidenced by")

[Presence of more than one personality within the individual]

Goals/Objectives

Short-term Goals

1. Client will verbalize understanding of the existence of multiple personalities within the self.
2. Client will be able to recognize stressful situations that precipitate transition from one personality to another.

Long-term Goals

1. Client will verbalize understanding of the need for existence of each personality and the role each plays for the individual.
2. Client will enter into and cooperate with long term therapy, with the ultimate goal being integration into one personality.

Interventions With *Selected Rationales*

1. The nurse must develop a trusting relationship with the original personality and with each of the subpersonalities. *Trust is the basis of a therapeutic relationship. Each of the personalities*

views itself as a separate entity and must initially be treated as such.

2. Help the client understand the existence of the subpersonalities. *Client may be unaware of this dissociative response to stressful situations.*

3. Help client identify the need each subpersonality serves in the personal identity of the individual. *Knowledge of the needs each personality fulfills is the first step in the integration process and the client's ability to face unresolved issues without dissociation.*

4. Help the client identify stressful situations that precipitate the transition from one personality to another. Carefully observe and record these transitions. *This knowledge is required to assist the client in responding more adaptively and to eliminate the need for transition to another personality.*

5. Use nursing interventions necessary to deal with maladaptive behaviors associated with individual subpersonalities. For example, if one personality is suicidal, precautions must be taken to guard against client's self-harm. If another personality has a tendency toward physical hostility, precautions must be taken for the protection of others. *Safety of the client and others is a nursing priority.*

CLINICAL PEARL It may be possible to seek assistance from one of the personalities. For example, a strong-willed personality may help to control the behaviors of a "suicidal" personality.

---

6. Help subpersonalities to understand that their "being" will not be destroyed, but integrated into a unified identity within the individual. *Because subpersonalities function as separate entities, the idea of total elimination generates fear and defensiveness.*

7. Provide support during disclosure of painful experiences and reassurance when the client becomes discouraged with lengthy treatment.

Outcome Criteria

1. Client recognizes the existence of more than one personality.
2. Client is able to verbalize the purpose these personalities serve.
3. Client verbalizes the intention of seeking long-term outpatient psychotherapy.

■ DISTURBED SENSORY PERCEPTION (Visual/Kinesthetic)

Definition: *Change in the amount or patterning of incoming stimuli [either internally or externally initiated] accompanied by a diminished, exaggerated, distorted, or impaired response to such stimuli* (NANDA-I, 2012, p. 490) (***Note:*** This nursing diagnosis has been retired by NANDA. It is retained in this text because of its appropriateness to the specific behaviors described.)

Possible Etiologies ("related to")

[Severe level of anxiety, repressed]
[Childhood trauma]
[Childhood abuse]
[Threat to physical integrity]
[Threat to self-concept]

Defining Characteristics ("evidenced by")

[Alteration in the perception or experience of the self]
[Loss of one's own sense of reality]
[Loss of the sense of reality of the external world]

Goals/Objectives

Short-term Goal

Client will verbalize adaptive ways of coping with stress.

Long-term Goal

By time of discharge from treatment, client will demonstrate the ability to perceive stimuli correctly and maintain a sense of reality during stressful situations.

Interventions With *Selected Rationales*

1. Provide support and encouragement during times of depersonalization. The client manifesting these symptoms may express fear and anxiety. They do not understand the response and may express a fear of "going insane." *Support and encouragement from a trusted individual provide a feeling of security when fears and anxieties are manifested.*
2. Explain the depersonalization behaviors and the purpose they usually serve for the client. *This knowledge may help to minimize fears and anxieties associated with their occurrence.*
3. Explain the relationship between severe anxiety and depersonalization behaviors. *The client may be unaware that the occurrence of depersonalization behaviors is related to severe anxiety.*

4. Help client relate these behaviors to times of severe psychological stress that he or she has experienced personally. ***Knowledge of this relationship is the first step in the process of behavioral change.***

5. Explore past experiences and possibly repressed painful situations such as trauma or abuse. ***It is thought that traumatic experiences predispose individuals to dissociative disorders.***

6. Discuss these painful experiences with the client and encourage him or her to deal with the feelings associated with these situations. Work to resolve the conflicts these repressed feelings have nurtured. ***Conflict resolution will serve to decrease the need for the dissociative response to anxiety.***

7. Discuss ways the client may more adaptively respond to stress, and use role-play to practice using these new methods. ***Having practiced through role-play helps to prepare the client to face stressful situations by using these new behaviors when they occur in real life.***

Outcome Criteria

1. Client perceives stressful situations correctly and is able to maintain a sense of reality.

2. Client demonstrates use of adaptive strategies for coping with stress.

@ INTERNET REFERENCES

- Additional information about dissociative disorders may be located at the following Web sites:
  a. www.nami.org/helpline/dissoc.htm
  b. www.isst-d.org
  c. www.mental-health-matters.com/disorders
  d. http://emedicine.medscape.com/article/294508-overview

Movie Connections

Dead Again (Amnesia) • *Mirage* (Amnesia) • *Suddenly Last Summer* (Amnesia) • *The Three Lives of Karen* (Dissociative fugue) • *Sybil* (DID) • *The Three Faces of Eve* (DID) • *Identity* (DID)

CHAPTER **12**

Sexual Disorders and Gender Dysphoria

■ BACKGROUND ASSESSMENT DATA

The *Diagnostic and Statistical Manual of Mental Disorders, Fifth Edition (DSM-5)* (American Psychiatric Association [APA], 2013) identifies three categories of disorders associated with sexuality: paraphilic disorders, sexual dysfunctions, and gender dysphoria. The term *paraphilia* is used to identify repetitive or preferred sexual fantasies or behaviors that involve: (1) nonhuman objects; (2) suffering or humiliation of oneself or one's partner; or (3) nonconsenting persons (Black & Andreasen, 2011). In a *paraphilic disorder*, these sexual fantasies or behaviors are recurrent over a period of at least 6 months and cause the individual clinically significant distress or impairment in social, occupational, or other important areas of functioning (APA, 2013). *Sexual dysfunction disorders* can be described as an impairment or disturbance in any of the phases of the sexual response cycle. These include disorders of desire, arousal, orgasm, and disorders that relate to the experience of genital pain during intercourse. *Gender dysphoria* refers to the "distress that may accompany the incongruence between one's experienced or expressed gender and one's assigned gender" (APA, 2013, p. 451).

■ PARAPHILIC DISORDERS

Paraphilic disorders are characterized by recurrent and intense sexual arousal of at least 6 months' duration involving any of the following:

1. The preference for use of a nonhuman object.
2. Repetitive sexual activity with humans involving real or simulated suffering or humiliation.
3. Repetitive sexual activity with nonconsenting partners.

The individual has acted on these sexual urges, or the urges or fantasies cause clinically significant distress or impairment in social, occupational, or other important areas of functioning (APA, 2013).

Types of paraphilic disorders include the following:

1. **Exhibitionistic Disorder.** The major symptoms include recurrent, intense sexual urges, behaviors, or sexually arousing fantasies, of at least 6 months' duration, involving the exposure of one's genitals to an unsuspecting stranger (APA, 2013). Masturbation may occur during the exhibitionism. Most individuals with exhibitionistic disorder are men, and the behavior is generally established in adolescence.

2. **Fetishistic Disorder.** Fetishistic disorder involves recurrent, intense sexual urges, behaviors, or sexually arousing fantasies, of at least 6 months' duration, involving the use of nonliving objects, a specific nongenital body part, or a combination of both (APA, 2013). Commonly, the sexual focus is on objects intimately associated with the human body (e.g., shoes, gloves, stockings) or on a nongenital body part (e.g., feet, hair). The fetish object is generally used during masturbation or incorporated into sexual activity with another person to produce sexual excitation.

3. **Frotteuristic Disorder.** This disorder is defined as the recurrent preoccupation with intense sexual urges or fantasies, of at least 6 months' duration, involving touching or rubbing against a nonconsenting person (APA, 2013). Sexual excitement is derived from the actual touching or rubbing, not from the coercive nature of the act. The disorder is significantly more common in men than in women.

4. **Pedophilic Disorder.** The *DSM-5* describes the essential feature of pedophilic disorder as recurrent sexual urges, behaviors, or sexually arousing fantasies, of at least 6 months' duration, involving sexual activity with a prepubescent child. The age of the molester is 16 years or older, and he or she is at least 5 years older than the child. This category of paraphilic disorder is the most common of sexual assaults.

5. **Sexual Masochism Disorder.** The identifying feature of this disorder is recurrent, intense sexual urges, behaviors, or sexually arousing fantasies, of at least 6 months' duration, involving the act of being humiliated, beaten, bound, or otherwise made to suffer (APA, 2013). These masochistic activities may be fantasized, solitary, or with a partner. Examples include becoming sexually aroused by self-inflicted pain, or by being restrained, raped, or beaten by a sexual partner.

6. **Sexual Sadism Disorder.** The essential feature of sexual sadism disorder is identified as recurrent, intense, sexual urges, behaviors, or sexually arousing fantasies, of at least 6 months' duration, of acts involving the psychological or physical suffering of another person (APA, 2013). The sadistic activities may be fantasized or acted on with a nonconsenting partner.

In all instances, sexual excitation occurs in response to the suffering of the victim. Examples include rape, beating, torture, or even killing.

7. **Voyeuristic Disorder.** This disorder is identified by recurrent, intense sexual urges, behaviors, or sexually arousing fantasies, of at least 6 months' duration, involving the act of observing an unsuspecting person who is naked, in the process of disrobing, or engaging in sexual activity (APA, 2013). Sexual excitement is achieved through the act of looking, and no contact with the person is attempted. Masturbation usually accompanies the "window peeping" but may occur later as the individual fantasizes about the voyeuristic act.

8. **Transvestic Disorder.** This disorder involves recurrent and intense sexual arousal (as manifested by fantasies, urges, or behaviors of at least 6 months duration) from dressing in the clothes of the opposite gender. The individual is commonly a heterosexual man who keeps a collection of women's clothing that he intermittently uses to dress in when alone. The sexual arousal may be produced by an accompanying fantasy of the individual as a woman with female genitalia or merely by the view of himself fully clothed as a woman without attention to the genitalia. The disorder causes marked distress to the individual, or interferes with social, occupational, or other important areas of functioning.

Predisposing Factors to Paraphilic Disorders

1. **Physiological**
   a. ***Biological.*** Various studies have implicated several organic factors in the etiology of paraphilic disorder. Destruction of parts of the limbic system in animals has been shown to cause hypersexual behavior (Becker & Johnson, 2008). Temporal lobe diseases, such as psychomotor seizures or temporal lobe tumors, have been implicated in some individuals with paraphilias. Abnormal levels of androgens also may contribute to inappropriate sexual arousal. The majority of studies involved violent sex offenders, and the results cannot accurately be generalized.

2. **Psychosocial**
   a. ***Psychoanalytic Theory.*** The psychoanalytic approach defines a paraphilic as one who has failed the normal developmental process toward heterosexual adjustment (Sadock & Sadock, 2007). This occurs when the individual fails to resolve the oedipal crisis and either identifies with the parent of the opposite gender or selects an inappropriate object for libido cathexis. This creates intense anxiety, which leads the individual to seek sexual gratification in ways that provide a "safe substitution" for the parent (Becker & Johnson, 2008).

b. ***Behavioral Theory.*** The behavioral model hypothesizes that whether or not an individual engages in paraphilic behavior depends on the type of reinforcement he or she receives following the behavior. The initial act may be committed for various reasons. Some examples include recalling memories of experiences from an individual's early life (especially the first shared sexual experience), modeling behavior of others who have carried out paraphilic acts, mimicking sexual behavior depicted in the media, and recalling past trauma such as one's own molestation (Sadock & Sadock, 2007). Once the initial act has been committed, the individual with paraphilic disorder consciously evaluates the behavior and decides whether to repeat it. A fear of punishment or perceived harm or injury to the victim, or a lack of pleasure derived from the experience, may extinguish the behavior. However, when negative consequences do not occur, when the act itself is highly pleasurable, or when the person with the paraphilic disorder immediately escapes and thereby avoids seeing any negative consequences experienced by the victim, the activity is more likely to be repeated.

Symptomatology (Subjective and Objective Data)

1. Exposure of one's genitals to a stranger.
2. Sexual arousal in the presence of nonliving objects.
3. Touching and rubbing one's genitals against a nonconsenting person.
4. Sexual attraction to or activity with a prepubescent child.
5. Sexual arousal from being humiliated, beaten, bound, or otherwise made to suffer (through fantasy, self-infliction, or by a sexual partner).
6. Sexual arousal by inflicting psychological or physical suffering on another individual (either consenting or nonconsenting).
7. Sexual arousal from dressing in the clothes of the opposite gender.
8. Sexual arousal from observing unsuspecting people either naked or engaged in sexual activity.
9. Masturbation often accompanies the activities described when they are performed solitarily.
10. The individual is markedly distressed by these activities.

■ SEXUAL DYSFUNCTIONS

Sexual dysfunctions may occur in any phase of the sexual response cycle. Types of sexual dysfunctions include the following:

1. **Sexual Interest/Arousal Disorders**
   a. ***Female Sexual Interest/Arousal Disorder.*** This disorder is characterized by a reduced or absent interest or pleasure in

sexual activity (APA, 2013). The individual typically does not initiate sexual activity and is commonly unreceptive to partner's attempts to initiate. There is an absence of sexual thoughts or fantasies and absent or reduced arousal in response to sexual or erotic cues. The condition has persisted for at least 6 months and causes the individual significant distress.

b. ***Male Hypoactive Sexual Desire Disorder.*** This disorder is defined by the *DSM-5* as a persistent or recurrent deficiency or absence of sexual fantasies and desire for sexual activity. In making the judgment of deficiency or absence, the clinician considers factors that affect sexual functioning, such as age and circumstances of the person's life (APA, 2013). The condition has persisted for at least 6 months and causes the individual significant distress.

c. ***Erectile Disorder.*** Erectile disorder is characterized by marked difficulty in obtaining or maintaining an erection during sexual activity or a decrease in erectile rigidity that interferes with sexual activity (APA, 2013). The problem has persisted for at least 6 months and causes the individual significant distress. *Primary erectile disorder* refers to cases in which the man has never been able to have intercourse; *secondary erectile disorder* refers to cases in which the man has difficulty getting or maintaining an erection but has been able to have vaginal or anal intercourse at least once.

2. **Orgasmic Disorders**

a. ***Female Orgasmic Disorder.*** Female orgasmic disorder is defined by the *DSM-5* as a marked delay in, infrequency of, or absence of orgasm during sexual activity (APA, 2013). It may also be characterized by a reduced intensity of orgasmic sensation. The condition, which is sometimes referred to as **anorgasmia**, has lasted at least 6 months and causes the individual significant distress. Women who can achieve orgasm through noncoital clitoral stimulation but are not able to experience it during coitus in the absence of manual clitoral stimulation are not necessarily categorized as anorgasmic. A woman is considered to have *primary orgasmic disorder* when she has never experienced orgasm by any kind of stimulation. *Secondary orgasmic disorder* exists if the woman has experienced at least one orgasm, regardless of the means of stimulation, but no longer does so.

b. ***Delayed Ejaculation.*** Delayed ejaculation is characterized by marked delay in ejaculation or marked infrequency or absence of ejaculation during partnered sexual activity (APA, 2013). The condition has lasted for at least 6 months and causes the individual significant distress. With this disorder, the man is unable to ejaculate, even though he has a firm erection and has had more than adequate stimulation. The severity of the problem may range from only occasional problems ejaculating (*secondary disorder*) to a history of never having experienced an orgasm (*primary disorder*). In the most common version, the man cannot ejaculate during coitus but may be able to ejaculate as a result of other types of stimulation.

  c. ***Premature (Early) Ejaculation.*** The *DSM-5* describes premature (early) ejaculation as persistent or recurrent ejaculation occurring within one minute of beginning partnered sexual activity and before the person wishes it (APA, 2013). The condition has lasted at least 6 months and causes the individual significant distress. The diagnosis should take into account factors that affect the duration of the excitement phase, such as the person's age, the uniqueness of the sexual partner, and frequency of sexual activity (Sadock & Sadock, 2007). Premature (early) ejaculation is the most common sexual disorder for which men seek treatment. It is particularly common among young men who have a very high sex drive and have not yet learned to control ejaculation.

3. **Sexual Pain Disorders**
  a. ***Genito-Pelvic Pain/Penetration Disorder.*** With this disorder, the individual experiences considerable difficulty with vaginal intercourse and attempts at penetration. Pain is felt in the vagina, around the vaginal entrance and clitoris, or deep in the pelvis. There is fear and anxiety associated with anticipation of pain or vaginal penetration. A tensing and tightening of the pelvic floor muscles occurs during attempted vaginal penetration (APA, 2013). The condition may be *lifelong* (present since the individual became sexually active) or *acquired* (began after a period of relatively normal sexual function). It has persisted for at least 6 months and causes the individual clinically significant distress.

4. **Substance/Medication-Induced Sexual Dysfunction**
  a. With these disorders, the sexual dysfunction developed after substance intoxication or withdrawal or after exposure to a medication (APA, 2013). The dysfunction may involve pain, impaired desire, impaired arousal, or impaired orgasm. Some substances/medications that can interfere with sexual functioning include alcohol, amphetamines, cocaine, opioids, sedatives, hypnotics, anxiolytics, antidepressants, antipsychotics, antihypertensives, and others.

Predisposing Factors to Sexual Dysfunctions

1. **Physiological**
  a. ***Sexual Interest/Arousal Disorders.*** In men, these disorders have been linked to low levels of serum testosterone and to

elevated levels of serum prolactin. Evidence also exists that suggests a relationship between serum testosterone and increased female libido. Various medications, such as antihypertensives, antipsychotics, antidepressants, anxiolytics, and anticonvulsants, as well as chronic use of drugs such as alcohol and cocaine, have also been implicated in sexual desire disorders. Problems with sexual arousal may occur in response to decreased estrogen levels in postmenopausal women. Medications such as antihistamines and cholinergic blockers may produce similar results. Erectile dysfunction in men may be attributed to arteriosclerosis, diabetes, temporal lobe epilepsy, multiple sclerosis, some medications (e.g, antihypertensives, antidepressants, anxiolytics), spinal cord injury, pelvic surgery, and chronic use of alcohol.

b. ***Orgasmic Disorders.*** In women these may be attributed to some medical conditions (hypothyroidism, diabetes, and depression), and certain medications (antihypertensives, antidepressants). Medical conditions that may interfere with male orgasm include genitourinary surgery (e.g., prostatectomy), Parkinson's disease, and diabetes. Various medications have also been implicated, including antihypertensives, antidepressants, and antipsychotics. Transient cases of the disorder may occur with excessive alcohol intake. Although early ejaculation is commonly caused by psychological factors, general medical conditions or substance use may also be contributing influences. Particularly in cases of secondary dysfunction, in which a man at one time had ejaculatory control but later lost it, physical factors may be involved. Examples include a local infection such as prostatitis or a degenerative neural disorder such as multiple sclerosis.

c. ***Sexual Pain Disorders.*** In women, sexual pain disorders may be caused by intact hymen, episiotomy scar, vaginal or urinary tract infection, ligament injuries, endometriosis, or ovarian cysts or tumors. Painful intercourse in men may be attributed to penile infections, phimosis, urinary tract infections, or prostate problems.

2. **Psychosocial**

a. ***Sexual Interest/Arousal Disorders.*** Phillips (2000) has identified a number of individual and relationship factors that may contribute to hypoactive sexual desire disorder. Individual causes include religious orthodoxy; sexual identity conflicts; past sexual abuse; financial, family, or job problems; depression; and concerns related to aging (e.g., changes in physical appearance). Among the relationship causes are interpersonal conflicts; current physical, verbal, or sexual abuse; extramarital affairs; and desire or practices different from partner. Arousal disorders in the female may be attributed to doubts, fears, guilt, anxiety, shame, conflict, embarrassment, tension, disgust, resentment, grief, anger toward the partner, and puritanical or moralistic upbringing. A history of sexual abuse may also be an important etiologic factor (Leiblum, 1999). The etiology of male erectile disorder may be related to chronic stress, anxiety, or depression. Early developmental factors that promote feelings of inadequacy and a sense of being unloving or unlovable may also result in impotence. Difficulties in the relationship may also be a contributing factor.

b. ***Orgasmic Disorders.*** A number of factors have been implicated in the etiology of female orgasm disorders. They include fear of becoming pregnant, hostility toward men, negative cultural conditioning, childhood exposure to rigid religious orthodoxy, and traumatic sexual experiences during childhood or adolescence. Orgasm disorders in men may be related to a rigid, puritanical background in which sex was perceived as sinful and the genitals as dirty; or interpersonal difficulties, such as ambivalence about commitment, fear of pregnancy, or unexpressed hostility may be implicated. Premature (early) ejaculation may be related to a lack of physical awareness on the part of a sexually inexperienced man. The ability to control ejaculation occurs as a gradual maturing process with a sexual partner in which foreplay becomes more give-and-take "pleasuring," rather than strictly goal-oriented. The man becomes aware of the sensations and learns to delay the point of ejaculatory inevitability. Relationship problems such as a stressful marriage, negative cultural conditioning, anxiety over intimacy, and lack of comfort in the sexual relationship may also contribute to this disorder.

c. ***Sexual Pain Disorders.*** Penetration disorders may occur after having experienced painful intercourse for any organic reason, after which involuntary constriction of the vagina occurs in anticipation and fear of recurring pain. The diagnosis does not apply if the etiology is determined to be due to another medical condition. A variety of psychosocial factors have been implicated, including negative childhood conditioning of sex as dirty, sinful, and shameful; early childhood sexual trauma; homosexual orientation; traumatic experience with an early pelvic examination; pregnancy phobia; sexually transmitted disease phobia; or cancer phobia (Dreyfus, 2012; King, 2011; Leiblum, 1999; Phillips, 2000; Sadock & Sadock, 2007).

Symptomatology (Subjective and Objective Data)

1. Absence of sexual fantasies and desire for sexual activity.
2. Discrepancy between partners' levels of desire for sexual activity.

3. Inability to produce adequate lubrication for sexual activity.
4. Absence of a subjective sense of sexual excitement during sexual activity.
5. Failure to attain or maintain penile erection until completion of sexual activity.
6. Inability to achieve orgasm (in men, to ejaculate) following a period of sexual excitement judged adequate in intensity and duration to produce such a response.
7. Ejaculation occurs with minimal sexual stimulation or before, on, or shortly after penetration and before the individual wishes it.
8. Genital pain occurring before, during, or after sexual intercourse.
9. Fear or anxiety in anticipation of vaginal penetration, with tensing or tightening of the pelvic floor muscles.

Common Nursing Diagnoses and Interventions for Paraphilic Disorders And Sexual Dysfunctions

(Interventions are applicable to various health-care settings, such as inpatient and partial hospitalization, community outpatient clinic, home health, and private practice.)

■ SEXUAL DYSFUNCTION

Definition: *The state in which an individual experiences a change in sexual function during the sexual response phases of desire, excitation, and/or orgasm, which is viewed as unsatisfying, unrewarding, or inadequate* (NANDA International [NANDA-I], 2012, p. 323)

Possible Etiologies ("related to")

Ineffectual or absent role models
Physical [or sexual] abuse
Psychosocial abuse
Values conflict
Lack of privacy
Lack of significant other
Altered body structure or function (pregnancy, recent childbirth, drugs, surgery, anomalies, disease process, trauma, radiation)
Misinformation or deficient knowledge
[Depression]
[Pregnancy phobia]
[Sexually transmitted disease phobia]
[Cancer phobia]
[Previous painful experience]
[Severe anxiety]
[Relationship difficulties]

Defining Characteristics ("evidenced by")

Verbalization of problem:

- [Absence of desire for sexual activity
- Absence of lubrication or subjective sense of sexual excitement during sexual activity
- Failure to attain or maintain penile erection during sexual activity
- Inability to achieve orgasm or ejaculation
- Premature ejaculation
- Genital pain during intercourse
- Constriction of the vagina that prevents penile penetration]

Inability to achieve desired satisfaction

Goals/Objectives

Short-term Goals

1. Client will identify stressors that may contribute to loss of sexual function within 1 week.

or

2. Client will discuss pathophysiology of disease process that contributes to sexual dysfunction within 1 week.

For client with permanent dysfunction due to disease process:

3. Client will verbalize willingness to seek professional assistance from a sex therapist in order to learn alternative ways of achieving sexual satisfaction with partner by (time is individually determined).

Long-term Goal

Client will resume sexual activity at level satisfactory to self and partner by (time is individually determined).

Interventions With *Selected Rationales*

1. Assess client's sexual history and previous level of satisfaction in his or her sexual relationship. *This establishes a database from which to work and provides a foundation for goal setting.*
2. Assess the client's perception of the problem. *The client's idea of what constitutes a problem may differ from the nurse. It is the client's perception on which the goals of care must be established.*
3. Help the client determine time dimension associated with the onset of the problem and discuss what was happening in his or her life situation at that time. *Stress in all areas of life can affect sexual functioning. Client may be unaware of correlation between stress and sexual dysfunction.*
4. Assess the client's mood and level of energy. *Depression and fatigue decrease desire and enthusiasm for participation in sexual activity.*

5. Review medication regimen; observe for side effects. *Many medications can affect sexual functioning. Evaluation of the drug and the individual's response is important to ascertain whether the drug may be contributing to the problem.*
6. Encourage the client to discuss the disease process that may be contributing to sexual dysfunction. Ensure that the client is aware that alternative methods of achieving sexual satisfaction exist and can be learned through sex counseling if he or she and the partner desire to do so. *Client may be unaware that satisfactory changes can be made in his or her sex life. He or she may also be unaware of the availability of sex counseling.*
7. Provide information regarding sexuality and sexual functioning. *Increasing knowledge and correcting misconceptions can decrease feelings of powerlessness and anxiety and facilitate problem resolution.*
8. Make a referral for additional counseling or sex therapy, if required. Client may even request that an initial appointment be made for him or her. *Complex problems are likely to require assistance from an individual who is specially trained to treat problems related to sexuality. Client and partner may be somewhat embarrassed to seek this kind of assistance. Support from a trusted nurse can provide the impetus for them to pursue the help they need.*

Outcome Criteria

1. Client is able to correlate physical or psychosocial factors that interfere with sexual functioning.
2. Client is able to communicate with partner about their sexual relationship without discomfort.
3. Client and partner verbalize willingness and desire to seek assistance from a professional sex therapist.

or

4. Client verbalizes resumption of sexual activity at level satisfactory to self and partner.

■ INEFFECTIVE SEXUALITY PATTERN

Definition: *Expressions of concern regarding own sexuality* (NANDA-I, 2012, p. 325)

Possible Etiologies ("related to")

Lack of significant other
Ineffective or absent role models
[Illness-related alterations in usual sexuality patterns]
Conflicts with sexual orientation or variant preferences

[Unresolved Oedipal conflict]
[Delayed sexual adjustment]

Defining Characteristics ("evidenced by")

Reports difficulties, limitations, or changes in sexual behaviors or activities
[Expressed dissatisfaction with sexual behaviors]
[Reports that sexual arousal can only be achieved through variant practices, such as pedophilia, fetishism, masochism, sadism, frotteurism, exhibitionism, voyeurism]
[Desires to experience satisfying sexual relationship with another individual without need for arousal through variant practices]

Goals/Objectives

(Time elements to be determined by individual situation.)

Short-term Goals

1. Client will verbalize aspects about sexuality that he or she would like to change.
2. Client and partner will communicate with each other ways in which each believes their sexual relationship could be improved.

Long-term Goals

1. Client will express satisfaction with own sexuality pattern.
2. Client and partner will express satisfaction with sexual relationship.

Interventions With *Selected Rationales*

1. Take sexual history, noting client's expression of areas of dissatisfaction with his or her sexual pattern. *Knowledge of what client perceives as the problem is essential for providing the type of assistance he or she may need.*
2. Assess areas of stress in the client's life and examine the relationship with his or her sexual partner. *Variant sexual behaviors are often associated with added stress in the client's life. The relationship with his or her partner may deteriorate as individual eventually gains sexual satisfaction only from variant practices.*
3. Note cultural, social, ethnic, racial, and religious factors that may contribute to conflicts regarding variant sexual practices. *The client may be unaware of the influence these factors exert in creating feelings of discomfort, shame, and guilt regarding sexual attitudes and behavior.*
4. Be accepting and nonjudgmental. *Sexuality is a very personal and sensitive subject. The client is more likely to share this information if he or she does not fear being judged by the nurse.*

5. Assist the therapist in a plan of behavior modification to help the client who desires to decrease variant sexual behaviors. *Individuals with paraphilic disorders are treated by specialists who have experience in modifying variant sexual behaviors. Nurses can intervene by providing assistance with implementation of the plan for behavior modification.*

6. If altered sexuality patterns are related to illness or medical treatment, provide information to the client and partner regarding the correlation between the illness and the sexual alteration. Explain possible modifications in usual sexual patterns that client and partner may try in an effort to achieve a satisfying sexual experience in spite of the limitation. *The client and his or her partner may be unaware of alternate possibilities for achieving sexual satisfaction, or anxiety associated with the limitation may interfere with rational problem solving.*

7. Explain to client that sexuality is a normal human response and does not relate exclusively to the sex organs or sexual behavior. Sexuality involves complex interrelationships among one's self-concept, body image, personal history, family and cultural influences; and all interactions with others. *If client feels "abnormal" or very unlike everyone else, the self-concept is likely to be very low—he or she may even feel worthless. To increase the client's feelings of self-worth and desire to change behavior, help him or her to understand that even though the behavior is variant, feelings and motivations are common.*

Outcome Criteria

1. Client is able to verbalize fears about abnormality and inappropriateness of sexual behaviors.
2. Client expresses desire to change variant sexual behavior and cooperates with plan of behavior modification.
3. Client and partner verbalize modifications in sexual activities in response to limitations imposed by illness or medical treatment.
4. Client expresses satisfaction with own sexuality pattern or satisfying sexual relationship with another.

■ GENDER DYSPHORIA

Gender *identity* is the sense of knowing to which gender one belongs—that is, the awareness of one's masculinity or femininity. Gender *dysphoria* is the "distress that accompanies the incongruence between one's experienced and expressed gender and one's assigned or natal gender" (APA, 2013, p. 822). The *DSM-5* (APA, 2013) identifies two categories of gender dysphoria: gender dysphoria in children and gender dysphoria in adolescents and adults.

Intervention with adolescents and adults with gender dysphoria is difficult. Adolescents rarely have the desire or motivation to alter their cross-gender roles, and disruptive behaviors are not uncommon. Some adults seek therapy to learn how to cope with their altered sexual identity, whereas others have direct and immediate request for hormonal therapy and surgical sex reassignment. Treatment of the adult with gender dysphoria is a complex process. The true transgendered individual intensely desires to have the genitalia and physical appearance of the assigned gender changed to conform to his or her gender identity. This change requires a great deal more than surgical alteration of physical features. In most cases, the individual must undergo extensive psychological testing and counseling, as well as live in the role of the desired gender for up to 2 years before surgery.

Treatment of children with gender dysphoria may be initiated when the behaviors cause significant distress and when the client desires it. Several controversial issues exist relative to treatment of these children. One type of treatment suggests that they should be encouraged to become satisfied with their assigned gender. Behavior modification therapy serves to help the child embrace the games and activities of his or her assigned gender and promotes development of friendships with same gender peers. A somewhat effeminate boy will not be forced to become an aggressive and competitive type nor will a "tomboy" be expected to turn into a "girly-girl." The goal is acceptance of a culturally-appropriate self-image without mental health concerns from discomfort associated with the assigned gender.

Another treatment model suggests that children who have problems with gender identity are dysphoric only because of their image within the culture. In this view, children should be accepted as they see themselves—different from their assigned gender—and supported in their efforts to live as the gender in which they feel most comfortable. Some professionals are recommending pubertal delay for adolescents aged 12 to 16 years who have suffered with extreme lifelong gender dysphoria, and who have supportive parents that encourage the child to pursue a desired change in gender (Gibson & Catlin, 2010). A gonadotropin-releasing hormone agonist is administered, which suppresses pubertal changes. The treatment is reversible if the adolescent decides later not to pursue the gender change. When the medication is withdrawn, external sexual development proceeds, and the individual has avoided permanent surgical intervention. If he or she decides as an adult to advance to the surgical intervention, the proponents of the hormonal treatment suggest that initiating pubertal delay at an early age will "most certainly result in high percentages of individuals who will more easily pass into the opposite gender role than when treatment commenced well after the development of secondary sexual characteristics" (Delemarre-van de Waal & Cohen-Kettenis, 2006). The type of treatment one chooses for gender dysphoria (if any) is very individual and a matter of personal choice. However, issues associated with mental health concerns, such as depression, anxiety, social isolation, anger, self-esteem, and parental conflict, must be addressed, even if the client elects not to proceed with the behavior modification approach.

Predisposing Factors Associated with Gender Dysphoria

1. **Physiological**
   a. *Genetics.* Studies of genetics and physiological alterations have been conducted in an attempt to determine whether or not a biological predisposition to problems with gender identity exists. The research has dealt largely with the study of abnormal levels of sex hormones. To date, no clear evidence has been demonstrated.
2. **Psychosocial**
   a. *Family Dynamics.* It appears that family dynamics may play an influential role in the etiology of gender disorders. Sadock and Sadock (2007) state, "Children develop a gender identity consonant with their sex of rearing (also known as *assigned sex*)." Gender roles are culturally determined, and parents encourage masculine or feminine behaviors in their children. Although "temperament" may play a role with certain behavioral characteristics being present at birth, mothers usually foster a child's pride in their gender. Sadock and Sadock (2007) state:

   The father's role is also important in the early years, and his presence normally helps the separation-individuation process. Without a father, mother and child may remain overly close. For a girl, the father is normally the prototype of future love objects; for a boy, the father is a model for male identification" (p. 719).

   In a 2003 study, Zucker and associates found a high rate of psychopathology and family dysfunction in children with gender dysphoria. Maternal depression and bipolar disorder was frequently demonstrated, whereas fathers often exhibited depression and substance use disorders. The authors recommended that parental conflicts and psychopathology must be given careful consideration as an aspect in childhood gender dysphoria.
   b. *Psychoanalytic Theory.* This theory suggests that gender identity problems begin during the struggle of the Oedipal/Electra conflict. Problems may reflect both real family events and those created in the child's imagination. These conflicts, whether real or imagined, interfere with the child's loving of the opposite-gender parent and identifying with the same-gender parent, and ultimately with normal gender identity.

Symptomatology (Subjective and Objective Data)

In children or adolescents:
1. Repeatedly stating intense desire to be of the opposite gender.
2. Insistence that one is of the opposite gender.

3. Preference in males for crossdressing or simulating female attire.
4. Insistence by females on wearing only stereotypical masculine clothing.
5. Fantasies of being of the opposite gender.
6. Strong desire to participate only in the stereotypical games and pastimes of the opposite gender.
7. Strong preference for playmates (peers) of the opposite gender.

In adults:
1. A stated desire to be of the opposite gender.
2. Frequently passing as the opposite gender.
3. Desire to live or be treated as the opposite gender. Stated conviction that one has the typical feelings and reactions of the opposite gender.
5. Persistent discomfort with or sense of inappropriateness in the assigned gender role.
6. Request for opposite gender hormones or surgery to alter sexual characteristics.

Common Nursing Diagnoses and Interventions for Gender Dysphoria

(Interventions are applicable to various health-care settings, such as inpatient and partial hospitalization, community outpatient clinic, home health, and private practice.)

NOTE: Because adults and adolescents rarely have the desire or motivation to modify their gender identity, nursing interventions in this section are focused on working with gender dysphoria in children. Becker and Johnson (2008) state, "It is important to note that not all children with gender identity disorder become adults with gender identity disorder" (p. 733).

▓ DISTURBED PERSONAL IDENTITY

Definition: *Inability to maintain an integrated and complete perception of self* (NANDA-I, 2012, p. 282)

Possible Etiologies ("related to")

[Parenting patterns that encourage culturally unacceptable behaviors for assigned gender]
[Unresolved Oedipal/Electra conflict]

Defining Characteristics ("evidenced by")

[Statements of desire to be opposite gender]
[Statements that one is the opposite gender]
[Cross-dressing, or passing as the opposite gender]
[Strong preference for playmates (peers) of the opposite gender]

[Stated desire to be treated as the opposite gender]
[Statements of having feelings and reactions of the opposite gender]

Goals/Objectives

Short-term Goals

1. Client will verbalize knowledge of behaviors that are appropriate and culturally acceptable for assigned gender.
2. Client will verbalize desire for congruence between personal feelings and behavior and assigned gender.

Long-term Goals

1. Client will demonstrate behaviors that are appropriate and culturally acceptable for assigned gender.
2. Client will express personal satisfaction and feelings of being comfortable in assigned gender.

Interventions With *Selected Rationales*

1. Spend time with the client and show positive regard. ***Trust and unconditional acceptance are essential to the establishment of a therapeutic nurse-client relationship.***
2. Be aware of own feelings and attitudes toward this client and his or her behavior. ***Attitudes influence behavior. The nurse must not allow negative attitudes to interfere with the effectiveness of interventions.***
3. Allow the client to describe his or her perception of the problem. ***It is important to know how the client perceives the problem before attempting to correct misperceptions.***
4. Discuss with the client the types of behaviors that are more culturally acceptable. Practice these behaviors through role-playing or with play therapy strategies (e.g., male and female dolls). Positive reinforcement or social attention may be given for use of appropriate behaviors. No response is given for stereotypical opposite-gender behaviors.

> **CLINICAL PEARL** The objective in working for behavioral change in a child who has gender dysphoria is to enhance culturally appropriate same-gender behaviors but not necessarily to extinguish all coexisting opposite-gender behaviors.

5. Behavioral change is attempted with the child's best interests in mind—that is, to help him or her with cultural and societal integration, while maintaining individuality. ***To preserve self-esteem and enhance self-worth, the child must know that he or she is accepted unconditionally as a unique and worthwhile individual.***

Outcome Criteria

1. Client demonstrates behaviors that are culturally appropriate for assigned gender.
2. Client verbalizes and demonstrates self-satisfaction with assigned gender role.
3. Client demonstrates development of a close relationship with the parent of the same gender.

■ IMPAIRED SOCIAL INTERACTION

Definition: *Insufficient or excessive quantity or ineffective quality of social exchange* (NANDA-I, 2012, p. 320)

Possible Etiologies ("related to")

[Socially and culturally unacceptable behavior]
[Negative role modeling]
[Low self-esteem]

Defining Characteristics ("evidenced by")

Discomfort in social situations
Inability to receive or communicate a satisfying sense of belonging, caring, interest, or shared history
Use of unsuccessful social interaction behaviors
Dysfunctional interaction with others

Goals/Objectives

Short-term Goal

Client will verbalize possible reasons for ineffective interactions with others.

Long-term Goal

Client will interact with others using culturally acceptable behaviors.

Interventions With *Selected Rationales*

1. Once client feels comfortable with the new behaviors in role playing or one-to-one nurse-client interactions, the new behaviors may be tried in group situations. If possible, remain with the client during initial interactions with others. ***Presence of a trusted individual provides security for the client in a new situation. It also provides the potential for feedback to the client about his or her behavior.***
2. Observe client behaviors and the responses he or she elicits from others. Give social attention (e.g., smile, nod) to desired

behaviors. Follow up these "practice" sessions with one-to-one processing of the interaction. Give positive reinforcement for efforts. *Positive reinforcement encourages repetition of desirable behaviors. One-to-one processing provides time for discussing the appropriateness of specific behaviors and why they should or should not be repeated.*

3. Offer support if client is feeling hurt from peer ridicule. Discuss in a matter-of-fact manner the behaviors that elicited the ridicule. Offer no personal reaction to the behavior. *Personal reaction from the nurse would be considered judgmental. Validation of the client's feelings is important, yet it is also important that the client understand why his or her behavior was the subject of ridicule and how to avoid it in the future.*

4. The goal is to create a trusting, nonthreatening atmosphere for the client in an attempt to change behavior and improve social interactions. Long-term studies have not yet revealed the significance of therapy with these children for psychosexual relationship development in adolescence or adulthood. One variable that must be considered is the evidence of psychopathology within the families of many of these children.

Outcome Criteria

1. Client interacts appropriately with others demonstrating culturally acceptable behaviors.
2. Client verbalizes and demonstrates comfort in assigned gender role in interactions with others.

■ LOW SELF-ESTEEM

Definition: *Negative self-evaluating/feelings about self or self-capabilities* (NANDA-I, 2012, p. 285-287)

Possible Etiologies ("related to")

[Rejection by peers]
Lack of approval and/or affection
Repeated negative reinforcement
[Lack of personal satisfaction with assigned gender]

Defining Characteristics ("evidenced by")

[Inability to form close, personal relationships]
[Negative view of self]
[Expressions of worthlessness]
[Social isolation]
[Hypersensitivity to slight or criticism]
Reports feelings of shame or guilt

Self-negating verbalizations

Lack of eye contact

Goals/Objectives

Short-term Goal

Client will verbalize positive statements about self, including past accomplishments and future prospects.

Long-term Goal

Client will verbalize and demonstrate behaviors that indicate self-satisfaction with assigned gender, ability to interact with others, and a sense of self as a worthwhile person.

Interventions With *Selected Rationales*

1. *To enhance the child's self-esteem:*
   a. Encourage the child to engage in activities in which he or she is likely to achieve success.
   b. Help the child to focus on aspects of his or her life for which positive feelings exist. Discourage rumination about situations that are perceived as failures or over which the client has no control. Give positive feedback for these behaviors.
2. Help the client identify behaviors or aspects of life he or she would like to change. If realistic, assist the child in problem-solving ways to bring about the change. *Having some control over his or her life may decrease feelings of powerlessness and increase feelings of self-worth and self-satisfaction.*
3. Offer to be available for support to the child when he or she is feeling rejected by peers. *Having an available support person who does not judge the child's behavior and who provides unconditional acceptance assists the child to progress toward acceptance of self as a worthwhile person.*

Outcome Criteria

1. Client verbalizes positive perception of self.
2. Client verbalizes self-satisfaction about accomplishments and demonstrates behaviors that reflect self-worth.

@ INTERNET REFERENCES

- Additional information about sexual disorders and gender dysphoria may be located at the following Web sites:
   a. www.sexualhealth.com
   b. www.priory.com/sex.htm
   c. http://emedicine.medscape.com/article/293890-overview
   d. http://emedicine.medscape.com/article/291419-overview

Movie Connections

Mystic River (Pedophilic disorder) • *Blue Velvet* (Sexual masochism disorder) • *Looking for Mr. Goodbar* (Sadism/masochism disorders) • *Normal* (Transvestic disorder) • *Transamerica* (Gender dysphoria)

CHAPTER 13

Eating Disorders

■ BACKGROUND ASSESSMENT DATA

The *Diagnostic and Statistical Manual of Mental Disorders, Fifth Edition (DSM-5)* (American Psychiatric Association [APA], 2013) states that eating disorders are characterized by "a persistent disturbance of eating or eating-related behavior that results in the altered consumption or absorption of food and that significantly impairs physical health or psychosocial functioning" (p. 329). Three such disorders that are described in the *DSM-5* include anorexia nervosa, bulimia nervosa, and binge-eating disorder. Obesity is not classified as a psychiatric disorder per se; however, because of the strong emotional factors associated with it, it is suggested that obesity may be considered within the category of *Psychological Factors Affecting Medical Condition*. Obesity is also considered as a factor associated with binge-eating disorder.

Anorexia Nervosa

Defined

Anorexia nervosa is a clinical syndrome in which the person has a morbid fear of obesity. It is characterized by the individual's gross distortion of body image, preoccupation with food, and refusal to eat. The disorder occurs predominantly in females 12 to 30 years of age. Without intervention, death from starvation can occur.

Symptomatology (Subjective and Objective Data)

1. Morbid fear of obesity. Preoccupied with body size. Reports "feeling fat" even when in an emaciated condition.
2. Refusal to eat. Reports "not being hungry," although it is thought that the actual feelings of hunger do not cease until late in the disorder.
3. Preoccupation with food. Thinks and talks about food at great length. Prepares enormous amounts of food for friends and family members but refuses to eat any of it. Amenorrhea is common, often appearing even before noticeable weight loss has occurred.
5. Delayed psychosexual development.
6. Compulsive behavior, such as excessive hand washing, may be present.

7. Extensive exercising is common.
8. Feelings of depression and anxiety often accompany this disorder.
9. May engage in the binge-and-purge syndrome from time to time (see following section on Bulimia Nervosa).

Bulimia Nervosa

Defined

Bulimia nervosa is an eating disorder (commonly called "the binge-and-purge syndrome") characterized by extreme overeating, followed by self-induced vomiting and abuse of laxatives and diuretics. The disorder occurs predominantly in females and begins in adolescence or early adult life.

Symptomatology (Subjective and Objective Data)

1. Binges are usually solitary and secret, and the individual may consume thousands of calories in one episode.
2. After the binge has begun, there is often a feeling of loss of control or inability to stop eating.
3. Following the binge, the individual engages in inappropriate compensatory measures to avoid gaining weight (e.g., self-induced vomiting; excessive use of laxatives, diuretics, or enemas; fasting; and extreme exercising).
4. Eating binges may be viewed as pleasurable but are followed by intense self-criticism and depressed mood.
5. Individuals with bulimia are usually within normal weight range—some a few pounds underweight, some a few pounds overweight.
6. Obsession with body image and appearance is a predominant feature of this disorder. Individuals with bulimia display undue concern with sexual attractiveness and how they will appear to others.
7. Binges usually alternate with periods of normal eating and fasting.
8. Excessive vomiting may lead to problems with dehydration and electrolyte imbalance.
9. Gastric acid in the vomitus may contribute to the erosion of tooth enamel.

Predisposing Factors to Anorexia Nervosa and Bulimia Nervosa

1. **Physiological**
   a. *Genetics*. A hereditary predisposition to eating disorders has been hypothesized on the basis of family histories and an apparent association with other disorders for which the likelihood of genetic influences exist. Anorexia nervosa is more common among sisters and mothers of those with the disorder than among the general population. Several studies have reported a higher than expected frequency of mood

and substance use disorders among first-degree biological relatives of individuals with eating disorders (Puri & Treasaden, 2011).

b. *Neuroendocrine Abnormalities.* Some speculation has occurred regarding a primary hypothalamic dysfunction in anorexia nervosa. Studies consistent with this theory have revealed elevated cerebrospinal fluid cortisol levels and a possible impairment of dopaminergic regulation in individuals with anorexia (Halmi, 2008). Additional evidence in the etiological implication of hypothalamic dysfunction is gathered from the fact that many people with anorexia nervosa experience amenorrhea before the onset of starvation and significant weight loss.

c. *Neurochemical Influences.* Neurochemical influences in bulimia nervosa may be associated with the neurotransmitters serotonin and norepinephrine. This hypothesis has been supported by the positive response these individuals have shown to therapy with the selective serotonin reuptake inhibitors (SSRIs). Some studies have found high levels of endogenous opioids in the spinal fluid of clients with anorexia nervosa, promoting the speculation that these chemicals may contribute to denial of hunger (Sadock & Sadock, 2007). Some of these individuals have been shown to gain weight when given naloxone, an opioid antagonist.

2. **Psychosocial**

a. *Psychodynamic Theory.* The psychodynamic theory suggests that behaviors associated with eating disorders reflect a developmental arrest in the very early years of childhood caused by disturbances in mother-infant interactions. The tasks of trust, autonomy, and separation-individuation go unfulfilled, and the individual remains in the dependent position. Ego development is delayed. The problem is compounded when the mother responds to the child's physical and emotional needs with food. Manifestations include a disturbance in body identity and a distortion in body image. When events occur that threaten the vulnerable ego, feelings of lack of control over one's body (self) emerge. Behaviors associated with food and eating provide feelings of control over one's life.

b. *Family Dynamics.* This theory proposes that the issue of control becomes the overriding factor in the family of the individual with an eating disorder. These families often consist of a passive father, a domineering mother, and an overly dependent child. A high value is placed on perfectionism in this family, and the child feels he or she must satisfy these standards. Parental criticism promotes an increase in obsessive and perfectionistic behavior on the part of the child, who continues to seek love, approval, and recognition. The child eventually begins to feel helpless and ambivalent toward the parents. In adolescence, these distorted eating patterns may represent a rebellion against the parents, viewed by the child as a means of gaining and remaining in control. The symptoms are often triggered by a stressor that the adolescent perceives as a loss of control in some aspect of his or her life.

Obesity

Defined

The following formula is used to determine the degree of obesity in an individual:

$$\text{Body mass index (BMI)} = \frac{\text{weight (kg)}}{\text{height (m)}^2}$$

The BMI range for normal weight is 20 to 24.9. Studies by the National Center for Health Statistics indicate that *overweight* is defined as a BMI of 25.0 to 29.9 (based on U.S Dietary Guidelines for Americans). Based on criteria of the World Health Organization, *obesity* is defined as a BMI of 30.0 or greater. These guidelines, which were released by the National Heart, Lung, and Blood Institute in July 1998, markedly increased the number of Americans considered to be overweight. The average American woman has a BMI of 26, and fashion models typically have BMIs of 18 (Priesnitz, 2005). Anorexia nervosa is characterized by a BMI of 17.5 or lower (Black & Andreasen, 2011).

Binge-Eating Disorder

Binge-eating disorder is characterized by recurrent episodes of binge eating; that is, eating in a discrete period of time an excessive amount of food and feeling a sense that the episode of eating is beyond the individual's control. The eating usually takes place in isolation, and the individual feels disgusted with himself or herself, depressed, or very guilty afterward (APA, 2013). Binge-eating disorder differs from bulimia nervosa in that the individual does not engage in compensatory behaviors (e.g., self-induced vomiting, laxatives, diuretics) following the binge to rid the body of the excess calories. Therefore, obesity becomes a factor in the disorder.

Obesity is known to contribute to a number of health problems, including hyperlipidemia, diabetes mellitus, osteoarthritis, and increased workload on the heart and lungs.

Predisposing Factors to Obesity

1. **Physiological**
   a. *Genetics.* Genetics have been implicated in the development of obesity in that 80% of offspring of two obese parents are

obese (Halmi, 2008). This hypothesis has also been supported by studies of twins reared by normal and overweight parents.

b. *Physical.* Overeating and/or obesity have also been associated with lesions in the appetite and satiety centers of the hypothalamus, hypothyroidism, decreased insulin production in diabetes mellitus, and increased cortisone production in Cushing's disease.

c. *Lifestyle.* On a more basic level, obesity can be viewed as the ingestion of a greater number of calories than are expended. Weight gain occurs when caloric intake exceeds caloric output in terms of basal metabolism and physical activity. Many overweight individuals lead sedentary lifestyles, making it very difficult to burn off calories.

2. **Psychosocial**

a. *Psychoanalytic Theory.* This theory suggests that obesity is the result of unresolved dependency needs, with the individual being fixed in the oral stage of psychosexual development. The symptoms of obesity are viewed as depressive equivalents, attempts to regain "lost" or frustrated nurturance and caring. Depression and binge eating are strongly linked: As many as half of individuals with binge-eating disorder have a history of depression (Jaret, 2010). Depression may be a cause of binge eating when food provides comfort for the despondent mood. Binge-eating disorder can also lead to depression, with respect to the feelings of disgust and despair that occur following episodes of binging.

Common Nursing Diagnoses and Interventions (For Anorexia Nervosa and Bulimia Nervosa)

(Interventions are applicable to various health-care settings, such as inpatient and partial hospitalization, community outpatient clinic, home health, and private practice.)

■ IMBALANCED NUTRITION: LESS THAN BODY REQUIREMENTS

Definition: *Intake of nutrients insufficient to meet metabolic needs* (NANDA International [NANDA-I], 2012, p. 174)

Possible Etiologies ("related to")

[Refusal to eat]

[Ingestion of large amounts of food, followed by self-induced vomiting]

[Abuse of laxatives, diuretics, and/or diet pills]

[Physical exertion in excess of energy produced through caloric intake]

Defining Characteristics ("evidenced by")

[Loss of 15% of expected body weight (anorexia nervosa)]
Pale mucous membranes
Poor muscle tone
Excessive loss of hair [or increased growth of hair on body (lanugo)]
[Amenorrhea]
[Poor skin turgor]
[Electrolyte imbalances]
[Hypothermia]
[Bradycardia]
[Hypotension]
[Cardiac irregularities]
[Edema]

Goals/Objectives

Short-term Goal

Client will gain _____ pounds per week (amount to be established by client, nurse, and dietitian).

Long-term Goal

By discharge from treatment, client will exhibit no signs or symptoms of malnutrition.

Interventions With *Selected Rationales*

1. If client is unable or unwilling to maintain adequate oral intake, physician may order a liquid diet to be administered via nasogastric tube. Nursing care of the individual receiving tube feedings should be administered according to established hospital procedures. *The client's physical safety is a nursing priority, and without adequate nutrition, a life-threatening situation exists.*

For oral diet:

2. In collaboration with dietitian, determine number of calories required to provide adequate nutrition and realistic (according to body structure and height) weight gain. *Adequate calories are required to affect a weight gain of 2-3 pounds per week.*

3. Explain to client details of behavior modification program as outlined by physician. Explain benefits of compliance with prandial routine and consequences for noncompliance. *Behavior modification bases privileges granted or restricted directly on weight gain and loss. Focus is placed on emotional issues, rather than food and eating specifically.*

4. Sit with client during mealtimes for support and to observe amount ingested. A limit (usually 30 minutes) should be imposed on time allotted for meals. *Without a time limit, meals*

can become lengthy, drawn-out sessions, providing client with attention based on food and eating.

5. Client should be observed for at least 1 hour following meals. *This time may be used by client to discard food stashed from tray or to engage in self-induced vomiting.*

6. Client may need to be accompanied to bathroom *if self-induced vomiting is suspected.*

7. Strict documentation of intake and output. *This information is required to promote client safety and plan nursing care.*

8. Weigh client daily immediately on arising and following first voiding. Always use same scale, if possible. *Client care, privileges, and restrictions will be based on accurate daily weights.*

9. If weight loss occurs, enforce restrictions. *Restrictions and limits must be established and carried out consistently to avoid power struggles and to encourage client compliance with therapy.*

10. Do not discuss food or eating with client, once protocol has been established. However, do offer support and positive reinforcement for obvious improvements in eating behaviors. *Discussing food with client provides positive feedback for maladaptive behaviors.*

11. Client must understand that if, because of poor oral intake, nutritional status deteriorates, tube feedings will be initiated *to ensure client's safety.* Staff must be consistent and firm with this action, using a matter-of-fact, nonpunitive approach regarding the tube insertion and subsequent feedings.

12. As nutritional status improves and eating habits are established, begin to explore with client the feelings associated with his or her extreme fear of gaining weight. *Emotional issues must be resolved if maladaptive responses are to be eliminated.*

Outcome Criteria

1. Client has achieved and maintained at least 85% of expected body weight.
2. Vital signs, blood pressure, and laboratory serum studies are within normal limits.
3. Client verbalizes importance of adequate nutrition.

■ DEFICIENT FLUID VOLUME

Definition: *Decreased intravascular, interstitial, and/or intracellular fluid; this refers to dehydration, water loss alone without change in sodium* (NANDA-I, 2012, p. 186)

Possible Etiologies ("related to")

[Decreased fluid intake]
[Abnormal fluid loss caused by self-induced vomiting]

[Excessive use of laxatives or enemas]
[Excessive use of diuretics]
[Electrolyte or acid-base imbalance brought about by malnourished condition or self-induced vomiting]

Defining Characteristics ("evidenced by")

Decreased urine output
Increased urine concentration
Elevated hematocrit
Decreased blood pressure
Increased pulse rate
Increased body temperature
Dry skin
Decreased skin turgor
Weakness
Change in mental status
Dry mucous membranes

Goals/Objectives

Short-term Goal

Client will drink 125 mL of fluid each hour during waking hours.

Long-term Goal

By discharge from treatment, client will exhibit no signs or symptoms of dehydration (as evidenced by quantity of urinary output sufficient to individual client; normal specific gravity; vital signs within normal limits; moist, pink mucous membranes; good skin turgor; and immediate capillary refill).

Interventions With *Selected Rationales*

1. Keep strict record of intake and output. Teach client the importance of daily fluid intake of 2000 to 3000 mL. *This information is required to promote client safety and plan nursing care.*
2. Weigh client daily immediately on arising and following first voiding. Always use same scale, if possible. *An accurate daily weight is needed to plan nursing care for the client.*
3. Assess and document the condition of skin turgor and any changes in skin integrity. *Condition of the skin provides valuable data regarding client hydration.*
4. Discourage client from bathing every day if skin is very dry. *Hot water and soap are drying to the skin.*
5. Monitor laboratory serum values, and notify physician of significant alterations. *Laboratory data provide an objective measure for evaluating adequate hydration.*
6. Client should be observed for at least 1 hour following meals and may need to be accompanied to the bathroom if

self-induced vomiting is suspected. *Vomiting causes active loss of body fluids and can precipitate fluid volume deficit.*

7. Assess and document moistness and color of oral mucous membranes. *Dry, pale mucous membranes may be indicative of malnutrition or dehydration.*

8. Encourage frequent oral care *to moisten mucous membranes, reducing discomfort from dry mouth, and to decrease bacterial count, minimizing risk of tissue infection.*

9. Help the client identify true feelings and fears that contribute to maladaptive eating behaviors. *Emotional issues must be resolved if maladaptive behaviors are to be eliminated.*

Outcome Criteria

1. Client's vital signs, blood pressure, and laboratory serum studies are within normal limits.

2. No abnormalities of skin turgor and dryness of skin and oral mucous membranes are evident.

3. Client verbalizes knowledge regarding consequences of fluid loss due to self-induced vomiting and importance of adequate fluid intake.

■ INEFFECTIVE DENIAL

Definition: *Conscious or unconscious attempt to disavow the knowledge or meaning of an event to reduce anxiety and/or fear, leading to the detriment of health* (NANDA-I, 2012, p. 358)

Possible Etiologies ("related to")

[Delayed ego development]
[Unfulfilled tasks of trust and autonomy]
[Dysfunctional family system]
[Unmet dependency needs]
[Feelings of helplessness and lack of control in life situation]
[Possible chemical imbalance caused by malfunction of hypothalamus]
[Unrealistic perceptions]

Defining Characteristics ("evidenced by")

[Preoccupation with extreme fear of obesity, and distortion of own body image]
[Refusal to eat]
[Obsessed with talking about food]
[Compulsive behavior (e.g., excessive hand washing)]
[Excessive overeating, followed by self-induced vomiting and/or abuse of laxatives and diuretics]
[Poor self-esteem]
[Chronic fatigue]

[Chronic anxiety]
[Chronic depression]
Does not perceive personal relevance of symptoms
Does not perceive personal relevance of danger
Minimizes symptoms
Unable to admit impact of disease on life pattern

Goals/Objectives

Short-term Goal

The client will verbalize understanding of the correlation between emotional issues and maladaptive eating behaviors (within time deemed appropriate for individual client).

Long-term Goal

By time of discharge from treatment, the client will demonstrate the ability to discontinue use of maladaptive eating behaviors and to cope with emotional issues in a more adaptive manner.

Interventions With *Selected Rationales*

1. Establish a trusting relationship with client by being honest, accepting, and available and by keeping all promises. Convey unconditional positive regard. *The therapeutic nurse-client relationship is built on trust.*
2. Acknowledge client's anger at feelings of loss of control brought about by the established eating regimen associated with the program of behavior modification. *Anger is a normal human response, and should be expressed in an appropriate manner. Feelings that are not expressed remain unresolved and add an additional component to an already serious situation.*
3. When nutritional status has improved, begin to explore with client the feelings associated with his or her extreme fear of gaining weight. *Emotional issues must be resolved if maladaptive behaviors are to be eliminated.*
4. Avoid arguing or bargaining with the client who is resistant to treatment. State matter-of-factly which behaviors are unacceptable and how privileges will be restricted for noncompliance. *It is essential that all staff members are consistent with this intervention if positive change is to occur.*
5. Explore family dynamics. Help client to identify his or her role contributions and their appropriateness within the family system. Assist client to identify specific concerns within the family structure and ways to help relieve those concerns. Also, discuss importance of client's separation of self as individual within the family system and of identifying independent emotions and accepting them as his or her own. *Client must recognize how maladaptive eating behaviors are related to*

emotional problems—often issues of control within the family structure.

6. Explore with client ways in which he or she may feel in control within the environment, without resorting to maladaptive eating behaviors. *When client feels control over major life issues, the need to gain control through maladaptive eating behaviors will diminish.*

Outcome Criteria

1. Client verbalizes understanding of the correlation between emotional issues and maladaptive eating behaviors.
2. Client demonstrates the use of adaptive coping strategies unrelated to eating behaviors.

■ ANXIETY (Moderate to Severe)

Definition: *Vague uneasy feeling of discomfort or dread accompanied by an autonomic response (the source often nonspecific or unknown to the individual); a feeling of apprehension caused by anticipation of danger. It is alerting signal that warns of impending danger and enables the individual to take measures to deal with threat* (NANDA-I, 2012, p. 344)

Possible Etiologies ("related to")

Situational and maturational crises
[Unmet dependency needs]
[Low self-esteem]
[Dysfunctional family system]
[Feelings of helplessness and lack of control in life situation]
[Unfulfilled tasks of trust and autonomy]

Defining Characteristics ("evidenced by")

Increased tension
Increased helplessness
Overexcited
Apprehensive; fearful
Restlessness
Poor eye contact
[Increased difficulty taking oral nourishment]
[Inability to learn]

Goals/Objectives

Short-term Goal

Client will demonstrate use of relaxation techniques to maintain anxiety at manageable level within 7 days.

Long-term Goal

By time of discharge from treatment, client will be able to recognize events that precipitate anxiety and intervene to prevent disabling behaviors.

Interventions With *Selected Rationales*

1. Be available to stay with client. Remain calm and provide reassurance of safety. *Client safety and security is a nursing priority.*
2. Help client identify the situation that precipitated onset of anxiety symptoms. *Client may be unaware that emotional issues are related to symptoms of anxiety. Recognition may be the first step in elimination of this maladaptive response.*
3. Review client's methods of coping with similar situations in the past. *In seeking to create change, it is helpful for client to identify past responses and determine whether they were successful and whether they could be employed again. Client strengths should be identified and used to his or her advantage.*
4. Provide quiet environment. Reduce stimuli: low lighting, few people. *Anxiety level may be decreased in calm atmosphere with few stimuli.*
5. Administer antianxiety medications, as ordered by physician. Monitor for effectiveness of medication as well as for adverse side effects. *Short-term use of antianxiety medications (e.g., lorazepam, chlordiazepoxide, alprazolam) provides relief from the immobilizing effects of anxiety, and facilitates client's cooperation with therapy.*
6. Teach client to recognize signs of increasing anxiety and ways to intervene for maintaining the anxiety at a manageable level (e.g., exercise, walking, jogging, relaxation techniques). *Anxiety and tension can be reduced safely and with benefit to the client through physical activities and relaxation techniques.*

Outcome Criteria

1. Client is able to verbalize events that precipitate anxiety and demonstrate techniques for its reduction.
2. Client is able to verbalize ways in which he or she may gain more control of the environment and thereby reduce feelings of helplessness.

■ DISTURBED BODY IMAGE/LOW SELF-ESTEEM

Definition: Disturbed body image is defined as *confusion in mental picture of one's physical self* (NANDA-I, 2012, p. 291). Low self-esteem is defined as *negative self-evaluating/feelings about self or self-capabilities* (p. 285–287).

Possible Etiologies ("related to")

[Lack of positive feedback]
[Perceived failures]
[Unrealistic expectations (on the part of self and others)]
[Delayed ego development]
[Unmet dependency needs]
[Threat to security caused by dysfunctional family dynamics]
[Morbid fear of obesity]
[Perceived loss of control in some aspect of life]

Defining Characteristics ("evidenced by")

[Distorted body image, views self as fat, even in the presence of normal body weight or severe emaciation]
[Denial that problem with low body weight exists]
[Difficulty accepting positive reinforcement]
[Not taking responsibility for self-care (self-neglect)]
[Nonparticipation in therapy]
[Self-destructive behavior (self-induced vomiting; abuse of laxatives or diuretics; refusal to eat)]
Lack of eye contact
[Depressed mood and self-deprecating thoughts following episode of binging and purging]
[Preoccupation with appearance and how others perceive them]

Goals/Objectives

Short-term Goal

Client will verbally acknowledge misperception of body image as "fat" within specified time (depending on severity and chronicity of condition).

Long-term Goal

Client will demonstrate an increase in self-esteem as manifested by verbalizing positive aspects of self and exhibiting less preoccupation with own appearance as a more realistic body image is developed by time of discharge from therapy.

Interventions With *Selected Rationales*

1. Help client reexamine negative perceptions of self and recognize positive attributes. ***Client's own identification of strengths and positive attributes can increase sense of self-worth.***
2. Offer positive reinforcement for independently made decisions influencing client's life. ***Positive reinforcement enhances self-esteem and may encourage client to continue functioning more independently.***

3. Offer positive reinforcement when honest feelings related to autonomy and dependence issues remain separated from maladaptive eating behaviors.

4. Help client develop a realistic perception of body image and relationship with food. Compare specific measurement of the client's body with the client's perceived calculations. There may be a large discrepancy between the actual body size and the client's perception of his or her body size. *The client needs to recognize that his or her perception of body image is unhealthy and that maintaining control through maladaptive eating behaviors is dangerous—even life-threatening.*

5. Promote feelings of control within the environment through participation and independent decision making. Through positive feedback, help the client learn to accept self as is, including weaknesses as well as strengths. *Client must come to understand that he or she is a capable, autonomous individual who can perform outside the family unit and who is not expected to be perfect. Control of his or her life must be achieved in other ways besides dieting and weight loss.*

6. Help client realize that perfection is unrealistic, and explore this need with him or her. *As client begins to feel better about self and identifies positive self-attributes, and develops the ability to accept certain personal inadequacies, the need for unrealistic achievements should diminish.*

7. Help client claim ownership of angry feelings and recognize that expressing them is acceptable if done so in an appropriate manner. Be an effective role model. *Unexpressed anger is often turned inward on the self, resulting in depreciation of self-esteem.*

Outcome Criteria

1. Client is able to verbalize positive aspects about self.
2. Client expresses interest in welfare of others and less preoccupation with own appearance.
3. Client verbalizes that image of body as "fat" was misperception and demonstrates ability to take control of own life without resorting to maladaptive eating behaviors.

Common Nursing Diagnoses and Interventions (for Obesity)

(Interventions are applicable to various health-care settings, such as inpatient and partial hospitalization, community outpatient clinic, home health, and private practice.)

■ IMBALANCED NUTRITION: MORE THAN BODY REQUIREMENTS

Definition: *Intake of nutrients that exceeds metabolic needs* (NANDA-I, 2012, p. 175)

Possible Etiologies ("related to")

[Compulsive eating]
Excessive intake in relation to metabolic needs
[Sedentary lifestyle]
[Genetics]
[Unmet dependency needs—fixation in oral developmental stage]

Defining Characteristics ("evidenced by")

Weight 20% over ideal for height and frame
[Body mass index of 30 or more]

Goals/Objectives

Short-term Goal

Client will verbalize understanding of what must be done to lose
   weight.

Long-term Goal

Client will demonstrate change in eating patterns resulting in a
   steady weight loss.

Interventions With *Selected Rationales*

1. Encourage the client to keep a diary of food intake. *A food
   diary provides the opportunity for the client to gain a realistic
   picture of the amount of food ingested and provides data on
   which to base the dietary program.*
2. Discuss feelings and emotions associated with eating. *This
   helps to identify when client is eating to satisfy an emotional
   need rather than a physiological one.*
3. With input from the client, formulate an eating plan that includes food from the required food groups with emphasis on
   low-fat intake. It is helpful to keep the plan as similar to the
   client's usual eating pattern as possible. *Diet must eliminate
   calories while maintaining adequate nutrition. Client is more
   likely to stay on the eating plan if he or she is able to participate in its creation and if it deviates as little as possible from
   usual types of foods.*
4. Identify realistic increment goals for weekly weight loss. *Reasonable weight loss (1 to 2 pounds per week) results in more
   lasting effects. Excessive, rapid weight loss may result in fatigue and irritability and may ultimately lead to failure in
   meeting goals for weight loss. Motivation is more easily sustained by meeting "stair-step" goals.*
5. Plan a progressive exercise program tailored to individual goals
   and choice. *Exercise may enhance weight loss by burning calories and reducing appetite, increasing energy, toning muscles,
   and enhancing a sense of well-being and accomplishment.
   Walking is an excellent choice for overweight individuals.*

6. Discuss the probability of reaching plateaus when weight remains stable for extended periods. *Client should know that this is likely to happen as changes in metabolism occur. Plateaus cause frustration, and client may need additional support during these times to remain on the weight-loss program.*

7. Provide instruction about medications to assist with weight loss if ordered by the physician. *Appetite-suppressant drugs (e.g., lorcaserin; phentermine) and others that have weight loss as a side effect (e.g., fluoxetine; topiramate) may be helpful to someone who is severely overweight. Drugs should be used for this purpose for only a short period while the individual attempts to adjust to the new pattern of eating.*

Outcome Criteria

1. Client has established a healthy pattern of eating for weight control with weight loss progressing toward a desired goal.
2. Client verbalizes plans for future maintenance of weight control.

■ DISTURBED BODY IMAGE/LOW SELF-ESTEEM

Definition: Disturbed body image is defined as *confusion in mental picture of one's physical self* (NANDA-I, 2012, p. 291). Low self-esteem is defined as *negative self-evaluating/feelings about self or self-capabilities* (p. 285–287).

Possible Etiologies ("related to")

[Dissatisfaction with appearance]
[Unmet dependency needs]
[Lack of adequate nurturing by maternal figure]

Defining Characteristics ("evidenced by")

Negative feelings about body (e.g., feelings of helplessness, hopelessness, or powerlessness)
[Verbalization of desire to lose weight]
[Failure to take responsibility for self-care (self-neglect)]
Lack of eye contact
[Expressions of low self-worth]

Goals/Objectives

Short-term Goal

Client will begin to accept self based on self-attributes rather than on appearance.

Long-term Goal

Client will pursue loss of weight as desired.

Interventions With *Selected Rationales*

1. Assess client's feelings and attitudes about being obese. *Obesity and compulsive eating behaviors may have deep-rooted psychological implications, such as compensation for lack of love and nurturing or a defense against intimacy.*

2. Ensure that the client has privacy during self-care activities. *The obese individual may be sensitive or self-conscious about his or her body.*

3. Have client recall coping patterns related to food in family of origin, and explore how these may affect current situation. *Parents are role models for their children. Maladaptive eating behaviors are learned within the family system and are supported through positive reinforcement. Food may be substituted by the parent for affection and love, and eating is associated with a feeling of satisfaction, becoming the primary defense.*

4. Determine client's motivation for weight loss and set goals. *The individual may harbor repressed feelings of hostility, which may be expressed inward on the self. Because of a poor self-concept, the person often has difficulty with relationships. When the motivation is to lose weight for someone else, successful weight loss is less likely to occur.*

5. Help the client identify positive self-attributes. Focus on strengths and past accomplishments unrelated to physical appearance. *It is important that self-esteem not be tied solely to size of the body. The client needs to recognize that obesity need not interfere with positive feelings regarding self-concept and self-worth.*

6. Refer client to a support or therapy group. *Support groups can provide companionship, increase motivation, decrease loneliness and social ostracism, and give practical solutions to common problems. Group therapy can be helpful in dealing with underlying psychological concerns.*

Outcome Criteria

1. Client verbalizes self-attributes not associated with physical appearance.
2. Client attends regular support group for social interaction and for assistance with weight management.

@ INTERNET REFERENCES

- Additional information about anorexia nervosa, bulimia nervosa, and BED may be located at the following Web sites:
  a. www.anad.org
  b. http://healthyminds.org
  c. www.nationaleatingdisorders.org
  d. www.mentalhealth.com/dis/p20-et01.html

   e. www.mentalhealth.com/dis/p20-et02.html
   f. www.nimh.nih.gov/health/publications/eating-disorders/
      complete-index.shtml
   g. www.nlm.nih.gov/medlineplus/eatingdisorders.html
   h. www.mayoclinic.com/health/binge-eating-disorder/DS00608
   i. www.bedaonline.com
   j. http://psychcentral.com/disorders/eating_disorders
- Additional information about obesity may be located at the following Web sites:
   a. www.shapeup.org
   b. www.obesity.org
   c. www.nlm.nih.gov/medlineplus/obesity.html
   d. www.asbp.org
   e. http://win.niddk.nih.gov/publications/binge.htm

Movie Connections

The Best Little Girl in the World (Anorexia nervosa) • *Kate's Secret* (Bulimia nervosa) • *For the Love of Nancy* (Anorexia nervosa) • *Super Size Me* (Obesity)

CHAPTER **14**

Personality Disorders

■ BACKGROUND ASSESSMENT DATA

The *Diagnostic and Statistical Manual of Mental Disorders, Fifth Edition (DSM-5)* (American Psychiatric Association [APA], 2013) defines *personality disorder* as "an enduring pattern of inner experience and behavior that deviates markedly from the expectations of the individual's culture, is pervasive and inflexible, has an onset in adolescence or early adulthood, is stable over time, and leads to distress or impairment" (p. 645).

The *DSM-5* groups the personality disorders into three clusters. These clusters, and the disorders classified under each, are described as follows:

1. **Cluster A:** Behaviors described as odd or eccentric
   a. Paranoid personality disorder
   b. Schizoid personality disorder
   c. Schizotypal personality disorder
2. **Cluster B:** Behaviors described as dramatic, emotional, or erratic
   a. Antisocial personality disorder
   b. Borderline personality disorder
   c. Histrionic personality disorder
   d. Narcissistic personality disorder
3. **Cluster C:** Behaviors described as anxious or fearful
   a. Avoidant personality disorder
   b. Dependent personality disorder
   c. Obsessive-compulsive personality disorder

A description of these personality disorders is presented in the following sections.

1. **Cluster A**
   a. *Paranoid Personality Disorder.* The essential feature is a pervasive and unwarranted suspiciousness and mistrust of people. There is a general expectation of being exploited or harmed by others in some way. Symptoms include guardedness in relationships with others, pathological jealousy, hypersensitivity, inability to relax, unemotionality, and lack of a sense of humor. These individuals are very critical of others but have much difficulty accepting criticism themselves.

b. ***Schizoid Personality Disorder.*** This disorder is characterized by an inability to form close, personal relationships. Symptoms include social isolation; absence of warm, tender feelings for others; indifference to praise, criticism, or the feelings of others; and flat, dull affect (appears cold and aloof).

c. ***Schizotypal Personality Disorder.*** This disorder is characterized by peculiarities of ideation, appearance, and behavior and by deficits in interpersonal relatedness that are not severe enough to meet the criteria for schizophrenia. Symptoms include magical thinking; ideas of reference; social isolation; illusions; odd speech patterns; aloof, cold, suspicious behavior; and undue social anxiety.

2. **Cluster B**

a. ***Antisocial Personality Disorder.*** This disorder is characterized by a pattern of socially irresponsible, exploitative, and guiltless behavior, as evidenced by the tendency to fail to conform to the law, to sustain consistent employment, to exploit and manipulate others for personal gain, to deceive, and to fail to develop stable relationships. The individual must be at least 18 years of age and have a history of conduct disorder before the age of 15. (Symptoms of this disorder are identified later in this chapter, along with predisposing factors and nursing care.)

b. ***Borderline Personality Disorder.*** The features of this disorder are described as marked instability in interpersonal relationships, mood, and self-image. The instability is significant to the extent that the individual seems to hover on the border between neurosis and psychosis. (Symptoms of this disorder are identified later in this chapter, along with predisposing factors and nursing care.)

c. ***Histrionic Personality Disorder.*** The essential feature of this disorder is described by the *DSM-5* as a "pervasive pattern of excessive emotionality and attention-seeking behavior" (APA, 2013, p. 667). Symptoms include exaggerated expression of emotions, incessant drawing of attention to oneself, overreaction to minor events, constantly seeking approval from others, egocentricity, vain and demanding behavior, extreme concern with physical appearance, and inappropriately sexually seductive appearance or behavior.

d. ***Narcissistic Personality Disorder.*** This disorder is characterized by a grandiose sense of self-importance; preoccupation with fantasies of success, power, brilliance, beauty, or ideal love; a constant need for admiration and attention; exploitation of others for fulfillment of own desires; lack of empathy; response to criticism or failure with indifference or humiliation and rage; and preoccupation with feelings of envy.

3. **Cluster C**
   a. ***Avoidant Personality Disorder.*** This disorder is characterized by social withdrawal brought about by extreme sensitivity to rejection. Symptoms include unwillingness to enter into relationships unless given unusually strong guarantees of uncritical acceptance; low self-esteem; and social withdrawal in spite of a desire for affection and acceptance. Depression and anxiety are common. Social phobia may be a complication of this disorder.
   b. ***Dependent Personality Disorder.*** Individuals with this disorder passively allow others to assume responsibility for major areas of life because of their inability to function independently. They lack self-confidence, are unable to make decisions, perceive themselves as helpless and stupid, possess fear of being alone or abandoned, and seek constant reassurance and approval from others.
   c. ***Obsessive-Compulsive Personality Disorder.*** This disorder is characterized by a pervasive pattern of perfectionism and inflexibility. Interpersonal relationships have a formal and serious quality, and others often perceive these individuals as stilted or "stiff." Other symptoms include difficulty expressing tender feelings, insistence that others submit to his or her way of doing things, excessive devotion to work and productivity to the exclusion of pleasure, indecisiveness, perfectionism, preoccupation with details, depressed mood, and being judgmental of self and others.

Many of the behaviors associated with the various personality disorders may be manifested by clients with virtually every psychiatric diagnosis, as well as by those individuals described as "healthy." It is only when personality traits or styles repetitively interfere with an individual's ability to function within age-appropriate cultural and developmental expectations, disrupt interpersonal relationships, and distort a person's pattern of perception and thinking about the environment that a diagnosis of personality disorder is assigned.

Individuals with personality disorders may be encountered in all types of treatment settings. They are not often treated in acute care settings, but because of the instability of the borderline client, hospitalization is necessary from time to time. The individual with antisocial personality disorder also may be hospitalized as an alternative to imprisonment when a legal determination is made that psychiatric intervention may be helpful. Because of these reasons, suggestions for inpatient care of individuals with these disorders are included in this chapter; however, these interventions may be used in other types of treatment settings as well. Undoubtedly, these clients represent the ultimate challenge for the psychiatric nurse.

■ BORDERLINE PERSONALITY DISORDER
Defined

This personality disorder is characterized by instability of affect, behavior, object relationships, and self-image. The term "borderline" came into being because these clients' emotionally unstable behavior seems to fall *on the border* between neurotic and psychotic. Transient psychotic symptoms appear during periods of extreme stress. The disorder is more commonly diagnosed in women than in men.

Predisposing Factors to Borderline Personality Disorder

1. **Physiological**
   a. ***Biochemical.*** Cummings and Mega (2003) have suggested a possible serotonergic defect in clients with borderline personality disorder. In positron emission tomography using α-[11C] methyl-L-tryptophan (α-[11C]-MTrp), which reflects serotonergic synthesis capability, clients with borderline personality demonstrated significantly decreased α-[11C]-MTrp in medial frontal, superior temporal, and striatal regions of the brain. Cummings and Mega (2003) state:

   > These functional imaging studies support a medial and orbitofrontal abnormality that may promote the impulsive aggression demonstrated by patients with the borderline personality disorder (p. 230).

   b. ***Genetic.*** The decrease in serotonin may also have genetic implications for borderline personality disorder. Sadock and Sadock (2007) report that depression is common in the family backgrounds of clients with borderline personality disorder. They state:

   > These patients have more relatives with mood disorders than do control groups, and persons with borderline personality disorder often have mood disorder as well (p. 791).

2. **Psychosocial**
   a. ***Childhood Trauma.*** Studies have shown that many individuals with borderline personality disorder were reared in families with chaotic environments. Lubit (2013) states, "Risk factors [for borderline personality disorder] include family environments characterized by trauma, neglect, and/or separation; exposure to sexual and physical abuse; and serious parental psychopathology such as substance abuse and antisocial personality disorder." Seventy percent of borderline personality disorder clients report a history of physical and/or sexual abuse (Gunderson, 2011). In some instances, this disorder has been likened to posttraumatic

stress disorder in response to childhood trauma and abuse. Oldham and associates (2006) state:

> Even when full criteria for comorbid PTSD are not present, patients with borderline personality disorder may experience PTSD-like symptoms. For example, symptoms such as intrusion, avoidance, and hyperarousal may emerge during psychotherapy. Awareness of the trauma-related nature of these symptoms can facilitate both psychotherapeutic and pharmacological efforts in symptom relief (p. 1267).

b. ***Theory of Object Relations.*** This theory suggests that the basis for borderline personality lies in the ways the child relates to the mother and does not separate from her. Mahler and associates (1975) define this process in a series of phases described as follows:

- **Phase 1 (Birth to 1 month), Autistic Phase.** Most of the infant's time is spent in a half-waking, half-sleeping state. The main goal is fulfillment of needs for survival and comfort.
- **Phase 2 (1 to 5 months), Symbiotic Phase.** A type of psychic fusion of mother and child. The child views the self as an extension of the parenting figure, although there is a developing awareness of external sources of need fulfillment.
- **Phase 3 (5 to 10 months), Differentiation Phase.** The child is beginning to recognize that there is separateness between the self and the parenting figure.
- **Phase 4 (10 to 16 months), Practicing Phase.** This phase is characterized by increased locomotor functioning and the ability to explore the environment independently. A sense of separateness of the self is increased.
- **Phase 5 (16 to 24 months), Rapprochement Phase.** Awareness of separateness of the self becomes acute. This is frightening to the child, who wants to regain some lost closeness but not return to symbiosis. The child wants the mother there as needed for "emotional refueling" and to maintain feelings of security.
- **Phase 6 (24 to 36 months), On the Way to Object Constancy Phase.** In this phase, the child completes the individuation process and learns to relate to objects in an effective, constant manner. A sense of separateness is established, and the child is able to internalize a sustained image of the loved object or person when out of sight. Separation anxiety is resolved.

The theory of object relations suggests that the individual with borderline personality is fixed in the rapprochement phase of development. This fixation occurs when the mother begins to feel threatened by the increasing autonomy of her child and so withdraws her emotional support during those times *or* she may instead reward clinging, dependent behaviors. In this way, the child comes to believe that:

"To grow up and be independent = a 'bad' child."
"To stay immature and dependent = a 'good' child."
"Mom withholds nurturing from 'bad' child."

Consequently, the child develops a deep fear of abandonment that persists into adulthood. In addition, because object constancy is never achieved, the child continues to view objects (people) as parts—either good or bad. This is called splitting, the primary defense mechanism of borderline personality.

Symptomatology (Subjective and Objective Data)

Individuals with borderline personality always seem to be in a state of crisis. Their affect is one of extreme intensity and their behavior reflects frequent changeability. These changes can occur within days, hours, or even minutes. Often these individuals exhibit a single, dominant affective tone, such as depression, which may give way periodically to anxious agitation or inappropriate outbursts of anger.

Common symptoms include the following:

1. **Chronic depression.** Depression is so common in clients with this disorder that before the inclusion of borderline personality disorder in the *DSM*, many of these clients were diagnosed as depressed. Depression occurs in response to feelings of abandonment by the mother in early childhood. It also may occur as a result of biochemical alterations or as a complicated grieving process in response to childhood trauma (see *Predisposing Factors*). Underlying the depression is a sense of rage that is sporadically turned inward on the self and externally on the environment. Seldom is the individual aware of the true source of these feelings until well into long-term therapy.

2. **Inability to be alone.** Because of this chronic fear of abandonment, clients with borderline personality disorder have little tolerance for being alone. They prefer a frantic search for companionship, no matter how unsatisfactory, to sitting with feelings of loneliness, emptiness, and boredom (Sadock & Sadock, 2007).

3. **Clinging and distancing.** The client with borderline personality disorder commonly exhibits a pattern of interaction with others that is characterized by clinging and distancing behaviors. When clients are clinging to another individual, they may exhibit helpless, dependent, or even childlike behaviors. They overidealize a single individual with whom they want to spend

all their time, with whom they express a frequent need to talk, or from whom they seek constant reassurance. Acting-out behaviors, even self-mutilation, may result when they cannot be with this chosen individual. Distancing behaviors are characterized by hostility, anger, and devaluation of others, arising from a feeling of discomfort with closeness. Distancing behaviors also occur in response to separations, confrontations, or attempts to limit certain behaviors. Devaluation of others is manifested by discrediting or undermining their strengths and personal significance.

4. **Splitting.** Splitting is a primitive ego defense mechanism that is common in people with borderline personality disorder. It arises from their lack of achievement of object constancy and is manifested by an inability to integrate and accept both positive and negative feelings. In their view, people—including themselves—and life situations are either all good or all bad.

5. **Manipulation.** In their efforts to prevent the separation they so desperately fear, clients with this disorder become masters of manipulation. Virtually any behavior becomes an acceptable means of achieving the desired result: relief from separation anxiety. Playing one individual against another is a common ploy to allay these fears of abandonment.

6. **Self-destructive behaviors.** Repetitive, self-mutilative behaviors, such as cutting, scratching, and burning, are classic manifestations of borderline personality disorder. Although these acts can be fatal, most commonly they are manipulative gestures designed to elicit a rescue response from significant others. Suicide attempts are not uncommon and often result from feelings of abandonment following separation from a significant other.

7. **Impulsivity.** Individuals with borderline personality disorder have poor impulse control based on primary process functioning. Impulsive behaviors associated with borderline personality disorder include substance abuse, gambling, promiscuity, reckless driving, and binging and purging (APA, 2013). Many times these acting-out behaviors occur in response to real or perceived feelings of abandonment.

8. **Feelings of unreality.** Transient episodes of extreme stress can precipitate periods of dissociation in the individual with borderline personality disorder.

9. **Rage reactions.** Difficulty controlling anger.

Common Nursing Diagnoses and Interventions

(Interventions are applicable to various health-care settings, such as inpatient and partial hospitalization, community outpatient clinic, home health, and private practice.)

■ RISK FOR SELF-MUTILATION/RISK FOR SELF-DIRECTED OR OTHER-DIRECTED VIOLENCE

Definition: Risk for self-mutilation is defined as *at risk for deliberate self-injurious behavior causing tissue damage with the intent of causing non-fatal injury to attain relief of tension* (NANDA International [NANDA-I], 2012, p. 451). Risk for self- or other-directed violence is defined as *at risk for behaviors in which an individual demonstrates that he or she can be physically, emotionally, and/or sexually harmful to self or others* (NANDA-I, 2012, p. 447, 448).

Risk Factors ("related to")

[Extreme fears of abandonment]
[Feelings of unreality]
[Depressed mood]
[Use of suicidal gestures for manipulation of others]
[Unmet dependency needs]
[Unresolved grief]
[Rage reactions]
[Physically self-damaging acts (cutting, burning, drug overdose, etc.)]
Body language (e.g., rigid posture, clenching of fists and jaw, hyperactivity, pacing, breathlessness, threatening stances)
History or threats of violence toward self or others or of destruction to the property of others
Impulsivity
Suicidal ideation, plan, available means
History of suicide attempts
Low self-esteem
Irresistible urge to [injure] self
[Childhood abuse]

Goals/Objectives

Short-term Goals

1. Client will seek out staff member if feelings of harming self or others emerge.
2. Client will not harm self or others.

Long-term Goal

Client will not harm self or others.

Interventions With *Selected Rationales*

1. Observe client's behavior frequently. Do this through routine activities and interactions; avoid appearing watchful and suspicious. *Close observation is required so that intervention can occur if required to ensure client's (and others') safety.*

2. Secure a verbal contract from client that he or she will seek out a staff member when the urge for self-mutilation is experienced. *Discussing feelings of self-harm with a trusted individual provides some relief to the client. A contract gets the subject out in the open and places some of the responsibility for his or her safety with the client. An attitude of acceptance of the client as a worthwhile individual is conveyed.*

3. If self-mutilation occurs, care for the client's wounds in a matter-of-fact manner. Do not give positive reinforcement to this behavior by offering sympathy or additional attention. *Lack of attention to the maladaptive behavior may decrease repetition of its use.*

4. Encourage the client to talk about feelings he or she was having just before this behavior occurred. *To problem-solve the situation with the client, knowledge of the precipitating factors is important.*

5. Act as a role model for appropriate expression of angry feelings, and give positive reinforcement to the client when attempts to conform are made. *It is vital that the client expresses angry feelings, because suicide and other self-destructive behaviors are often viewed as a result of anger turned inward on the self.*

6. Remove all dangerous objects from the client's environment *so that he or she may not purposefully or inadvertently use them to inflict harm to self or others. Client safety is a nursing priority.*

7. Try to redirect violent behavior with physical outlets for the client's anxiety (e.g., punching bag, jogging). *Physical exercise is a safe and effective way of relieving pent-up tension.*

8. Have sufficient staff available to indicate a show of strength to the client if necessary. *This conveys to the client evidence of control over the situation and provides some physical security for staff.*

9. Administer tranquilizing medications as ordered by the physician or obtain an order if necessary. Monitor the client for effectiveness of the medication and for the appearance of adverse side effects. *Tranquilizing medications such as anxiolytics or antipsychotics may have a calming effect on the client and may prevent aggressive behaviors.*

10. If the client is not calmed by "talking down" or by medication, use of mechanical restraints may be necessary. The avenue of the "least restrictive alternative" must be selected when planning interventions for a violent client. Restraints should be used only as a last resort, after all other interventions have been unsuccessful, and the client is clearly at risk of harm to self or others.

11. If restraint is deemed necessary, ensure that sufficient staff is available to assist. Follow protocol established by the institution.

The Joint Commission requires that an in-person evaluation by a physician or other licensed independent practitioner (LIP) be conducted within 1 hour of the initiation of the restraint or seclusion (The Joint Commission, 2010). The physician or LIP must reissue a new order for restraints every 4 hours for adults and every 1 to 2 hours for children and adolescents.

12. The Joint Commission requires that the client in restraints be observed at least every 15 minutes to ensure that circulation to extremities is not compromised (check temperature, color, pulses); to assist the client with needs related to nutrition, hydration, and elimination; and to position the client so that comfort is facilitated and aspiration is prevented. Some institutions may require continuous one-to-one monitoring of restrained clients, particularly those who are highly agitated, and for whom there is a high risk of self- or accidental injury.

13. As agitation decreases, assess the client's readiness for restraint removal or reduction. Remove one restraint at a time while assessing the client's response. *This minimizes the risk of injury to client and staff.*

14. If warranted by high acuity of the situation, staff may need to be assigned on a one-to-one basis. *Because of their extreme fear of abandonment, clients with borderline personality disorder should not be left alone at a stressful time as it may cause an acute rise in anxiety and agitation levels.*

Outcome Criteria

1. Client has not harmed self or others.
2. Anxiety is maintained at a level in which client feels no need for aggression.
3. Client denies any ideas of self-harm.
4. Client verbalizes community support systems from which assistance may be requested when personal coping strategies are unsuccessful.

■ ANXIETY (SEVERE TO PANIC)

Definition: *Vague uneasy feeling of discomfort or dread accompanied by an autonomic response (the source often nonspecific or unknown to the individual); a feeling of apprehension caused by anticipation of danger. It is an alerting signal that warns of impending danger and enables the individual to take measures to deal with threat* (NANDA-I, 2012, p. 344)

Possible Etiologies ("related to")

Threat to self-concept
Unmet needs
[Extreme fear of abandonment]

Unconscious conflicts [associated with fixation in earlier level of development]

Defining Characteristics ("evidenced by")

[Transient psychotic symptoms in response to severe stress, manifested by disorganized thinking, confusion, altered communication patterns, disorientation, misinterpretation of the environment]

[Excessive use of projection (attributing own thoughts and feelings to others)]

[Depersonalization (feelings of unreality)]

[Derealization (a feeling that the environment is unreal)]

[Acts of self-mutilation in an effort to find relief from feelings of unreality]

Goals/Objectives

Short-term Goal

Client will demonstrate use of relaxation techniques to maintain anxiety at manageable level.

Long-term Goal

Client will be able to recognize events that precipitate anxiety and intervene to prevent disabling behaviors.

Interventions With *Selected Rationales*

1. Symptoms of depersonalization often occur at the panic level of anxiety. Clients with borderline personality disorder often resort to cutting or other self-mutilating acts in an effort to relieve the anxiety. Being able to feel pain or see blood is a reassurance of existence to the person. If injury occurs, care for the wounds in a matter-of-fact manner without providing reinforcement for this behavior. *Lack of reinforcement may discourage repetition of the maladaptive behavior.*

2. During periods of panic anxiety, stay with the client and provide reassurance of safety and security. Orient client to the reality of the situation. *Client comfort and safety are nursing priorities.*

3. Administer tranquilizing medications as ordered by physician, or obtain order if necessary. Monitor client for effectiveness of the medication as well as for adverse side effects. *Antianxiety medications (e.g., lorazepam, chlordiazepoxide, alprazolam) provide relief from the immobilizing effects of anxiety and facilitate client's cooperation with therapy.*

4. Correct misinterpretations of the environment as expressed by client. *Confronting misinterpretations honestly, with a caring and accepting attitude, provides a therapeutic orientation to reality and preserves the client's feelings of dignity and self-worth.*

5. Encourage the client to talk about true feelings. Help him or her recognize ownership of these feelings rather than projecting them onto others in the environment. *Exploration of feelings with a trusted individual may help the client perceive the situation more realistically and come to terms with unresolved issues.*

6. Help the client work toward achievement of object constancy. Client may feel totally abandoned when nurse or therapist leaves at shift change or at end of therapy session. There may even be feelings that the therapist ceases to exist. Leaving a signed note or card with the client for reassurance may help. It is extremely important for more than one nurse to develop a therapeutic relationship with the borderline client. It is also necessary that staff maintain open communication and consistency in the provision of care for these individuals. *Individuals with borderline personality disorder have a tendency to cling to one staff member, if allowed, transferring their maladaptive dependency to that individual. This dependency can be avoided if the client is able to establish therapeutic relationships with two or more staff members who encourage independent self-care activities.*

Outcome Criteria

1. Client is able to verbalize events that precipitate anxiety and demonstrate techniques for its reduction.
2. Client manifests no symptoms of depersonalization.
3. Client interprets the environment realistically.

■ COMPLICATED GRIEVING

Definition: *A disorder that occurs after the death of a significant other [or any other loss of significance to the individual], in which the experience of distress accompanying bereavement fails to follow normative expectations and manifests in functional impairment* (NANDA-I, 2012, p. 365)

Possible Etiologies ("related to")

[Maternal deprivation during rapprochement phase of development (internalized as a loss, with fixation in the anger stage of the grieving process)]

[Loss of self-esteem as a result of childhood trauma]

Defining Characteristics ("evidenced by")

Persistent emotional distress

[Anger]

[Internalized rage]

Depression

[Labile affect]

[Extreme fear of being alone (fear of abandonment)]

[Acting-out behaviors, such as sexual promiscuity, suicidal gestures, temper tantrums, substance abuse]

[Difficulty expressing feelings]

[Altered activities of daily living]

[Reliving of past experiences with little or no reduction of intensity of the grief]

[Feelings of inadequacy; dependency]

Goals/Objectives

Short-term Goal

Client will discuss with nurse or therapist maladaptive patterns of expressing anger.

Long-term Goal

Client will be able to identify the true source of angry feelings, accept ownership of these feelings, and express them in a socially acceptable manner, in an effort to satisfactorily progress through the grieving process.

Interventions With *Selected Rationales*

1. Convey an accepting attitude—one that creates a nonthreatening environment for the client to express feelings. Be honest and keep all promises. *An accepting attitude conveys to the client that you believe he or she is a worthwhile person. Trust is enhanced.*

2. Identify the function that anger, frustration, and rage serve for the client. Allow the client to express these feelings within reason. *Verbalization of feelings in a nonthreatening environment may help the client come to terms with unresolved issues.*

3. Encourage the client to discharge pent-up anger through participation in large motor activities (e.g., brisk walks, jogging, physical exercises, volleyball, punching bag, exercise bike). *Physical exercise provides a safe and effective method for discharging pent-up tension.*

4. Explore with client the true source of the anger. This is painful therapy that often leads to regression as the client deals with the feelings of early abandonment or abuse. It seems that sometimes the client must "get worse before he or she can get better." *Reconciliation of the feelings associated with this stage is necessary before progression through the grieving process can continue.*

5. As anger is displaced onto the nurse or therapist, caution must be taken to guard against the negative effects of countertransference. *These are very difficult clients who have the capacity*

for eliciting a whole array of negative feelings from the therapist. The existence of negative feelings by the nurse or therapist must be acknowledged, but they must not be allowed to interfere with the therapeutic process.

6. Explain the behaviors associated with the normal grieving process. Help the client to recognize his or her position in this process. *Knowledge of the acceptability of the feelings associated with normal grieving may help to relieve some of the guilt that these responses generate.*

7. Help the client understand appropriate ways of expressing anger. Give positive reinforcement for behaviors used to express anger appropriately. Act as a role model. *Positive reinforcement enhances self-esteem and encourages repetition of desirable behaviors. It is appropriate to let the client know when he or she has done something that has generated angry feelings in you. Role modeling ways to express anger in an appropriate manner is a powerful learning tool.*

8. Set limits on acting-out behaviors and explain consequences of violation of those limits. Be supportive, yet consistent and firm, in caring for this client. *Client lacks sufficient self-control to limit maladaptive behaviors so assistance is required from staff. Without consistency on the part of all staff members working with this client, a positive outcome will not be achieved.*

Outcome Criteria

1. Client is able to verbalize how anger and acting-out behaviors are associated with maladaptive grieving.
2. Client is able to discuss the original source of the anger and demonstrates socially acceptable ways of expressing the emotion.

■ IMPAIRED SOCIAL INTERACTION

Definition: *Insufficient or excessive quantity or ineffective quality of social exchange* (NANDA-I, 2012, p. 320)

Possible Etiologies ("related to")

[Fixation in rapprochement phase of development]
[Extreme fears of abandonment and engulfment]
[Lack of personal identity]

Defining Characteristics ("evidenced by")

[Alternating clinging and distancing behaviors]
[Inability to form satisfactory intimate relationship with another person]

Use of unsuccessful social interaction behaviors
[Use of primitive dissociation (splitting) in their relationships
(viewing others as all good or all bad)]
[Manipulative behaviors]

Goals/Objectives

Short-term Goal

Client will discuss with nurse or therapist behaviors that impede
the development of satisfactory interpersonal relationships.

Long-term Goal

By time of discharge from treatment, client will interact appropriately with others in the therapy setting in both social and
therapeutic activities (evidencing a discontinuation of splitting
and clinging and distancing behaviors).

Interventions With *Selected Rationales*

1. Encourage the client to examine these behaviors (to recognize
   that they are occurring). *Client may be unaware of splitting
   or of clinging and distancing pattern of interaction with
   others. Recognition must take place before change can occur.*
2. Help the client understand that you will be available, without
   reinforcing dependent behaviors. *Knowledge of your availability
   may provide needed security for the client.*
3. Give positive reinforcement for independent behaviors. *Positive reinforcement enhances self-esteem and encourages repetition of desirable behaviors.*
4. Rotate staff who work with the client in order to avoid the
   client's developing dependence on particular staff members.
   *Client must learn to relate to more than one staff member in
   an effort to decrease use of splitting and to diminish fears of
   abandonment.*

> **CLINICAL PEARL** Recognize when client is playing one staff member against an-
> other. Remember that splitting is the primary defense mechanism of these individuals, and
> the impressions they have of others as either "good" or "bad" are a manifestation of this
> defense. Do not listen as client tries to degrade other staff members. Suggest that client
> discuss the problem directly with staff person involved.

5. With the client, explore feelings that relate to fears of abandonment and engulfment. Help client understand that clinging
   and distancing behaviors are engendered by these fears. *Exploration of feelings with a trusted individual may help client
   come to terms with unresolved issues.*
6. Help the client understand how these behaviors interfere with
   satisfactory relationships. *Client may be unaware of how others
   perceive these behaviors and why they are not acceptable.*

7. Assist the client to work toward achievement of object constancy. Be available, without promoting dependency. *This may help client resolve fears of abandonment and develop the ability to establish satisfactory intimate relationships.*

Outcome Criteria

1. Client is able to interact with others in both social and therapeutic activities in a socially acceptable manner.
2. Client does not use splitting or clinging and distancing behaviors in relationships and is able to relate the use of these behaviors to failure of past relationships.

■ DISTURBED PERSONAL IDENTITY

Definition: *Inability to maintain an integrated and complete perception of self* (NANDA-I, 2012, p. 282)

Possible Etiologies ("related to")

[Failure to complete tasks of separation/individuation stage of development]
[Underdeveloped ego]
[Unmet dependency needs]
[Absence of or rejection by parental gender-role model]

Defining Characteristics ("evidenced by")

[Excessive use of projection]
[Vague self-image]
[Unable to tolerate being alone]
[Feelings of depersonalization and derealization]
[Self-mutilation (cutting, burning) to validate existence of self]
Gender confusion
Feelings of emptiness
Uncertainties about goals and values

Goals/Objectives

Short-term Goal

Client will describe characteristics that make him or her a unique individual.

Long-term Goal

Client will be able to distinguish own thoughts, feelings, behaviors, and image from those of others as the initial step in the development of a healthy personal identity.

Interventions With *Selected Rationales*

1. Help the client recognize the reality of his or her separateness. Do not attempt to translate his or her thoughts and feelings into words. ***Because of the blurred ego boundaries, the client may believe you can read his or her mind.*** For this reason, caution should be taken in the use of empathetic understanding. For example, avoid statements such as "I know how you must feel about that."

2. Help the client recognize separateness from nurse by clarifying which behaviors and feelings belong to whom. If deemed appropriate, allow the client to touch your hand or arm. ***Touch and physical presence provide reality for the client and serve to strengthen weak ego boundaries.***

3. Encourage the client to discuss thoughts and feelings. Help the client recognize ownership of these feelings rather than projecting them onto others in the environment. ***Verbalization of feelings in a nonthreatening environment may help the client come to terms with unresolved issues.***

4. Confront statements that project the client's feelings onto others. Ask the client to validate that others possess those feelings. The expression of *reasonable doubt* as a therapeutic technique may be helpful ("I find that hard to believe").

5. If the problem is with gender identity, ask the client to describe his or her perception of appropriate male and female behaviors. Provide information about role behaviors and sex education, if necessary. Convey acceptance of the person regardless of preferred identity. ***Client may require clarification of distorted ideas or misinformation. An attitude of acceptance reinforces the client's feelings of self-worth.***

6. Always call the client by his or her name. If the client experiences feelings of depersonalization or derealization, orientation to the environment and correction of misperceptions may be helpful. ***These interventions help to preserve the client's feelings of dignity and self-worth.***

7. Help the client understand that there are more adaptive ways of validating his or her existence than self-mutilation. Contract with the client to seek out a staff member when these feelings occur. ***A contract gets the subject out in the open and places some of the responsibility for his or her safety with the client. Client safety is a nursing priority.***

8. Work with the client to clarify values. Discuss beliefs, attitudes, and feelings underlying his or her behaviors. Help the client to identify those values that have been (or are intended to be) incorporated as his or her own. Care must be taken by the nurse to avoid imposing his or her own value system on the client.

Because of an underdeveloped ego and fixation in an early developmental level, the client may not have established his or her own value system. In order to accomplish this, ownership of beliefs and attitudes must be identified and clarified.

9. Use of photographs of the client may help to establish or clarify ego boundaries. *Photographs may help to increase the client's awareness of self as separate from others.*

10. Alleviate anxiety by providing assurance to the client that he or she will not be left alone. *Early childhood traumas may predispose clients with borderline personality disorder to extreme fears of abandonment.*

11. Use of touch is sometimes therapeutic in identity confirmation. Before this technique is used, however, assess cultural influences and degree of trust. *Touch and physical presence provide reality for the client and serve to strengthen weak ego boundaries.*

Outcome Criteria

1. Client is able to distinguish between own thoughts and feelings and those of others.
2. Client claims ownership of those thoughts and feelings and does not use projection in relationships with others.
3. Client has clarified own feelings regarding sexual identity.

■ CHRONIC LOW SELF-ESTEEM

Definition: *Long-standing negative self-evaluating/feelings about self or self-capabilities* (NANDA-I, 2012, p. 285)

Possible Etiologies ("related to")

[Lack of positive feedback]
[Unmet dependency needs]
[Retarded ego development]
[Repeated negative feedback, resulting in diminished self-worth]
[Dysfunctional family system]
[Fixation in earlier level of development]
[Childhood trauma]

Defining Characteristics ("evidenced by")

[Difficulty accepting positive reinforcement]
[Self-destructive behavior]
[Frequent use of derogatory and critical remarks against the self]
Lack of eye contact
[Manipulation of one staff member against another in an attempt to gain special privileges]

[Inability to form close, personal relationships]
[Inability to tolerate being alone]
[Degradation of others in an attempt to increase own feelings of self-worth]
Hesitant to try new things or situations [because of fear of failure]
Excessively seeks reassurance

Goals/Objectives

Short-term Goals

1. Client will discuss fear of failure with nurse or therapist.
2. Client will verbalize things he or she likes about self.

Long-term Goals

1. Client will exhibit increased feelings of self-worth as evidenced by verbal expression of positive aspects about self, past accomplishments, and future prospects.
2. Client will exhibit increased feelings of self-worth by setting realistic goals and trying to reach them, thereby demonstrating a decrease in fear of failure.

Interventions With *Selected Rationales*

1. Ensure that goals are realistic. It is important for the client to achieve something, so plan for activities in which success is likely. *Success increases self-esteem.*
2. Convey unconditional positive regard for the client. Promote understanding of your acceptance of him or her as a worthwhile human being. *Acceptance by others increases feelings of self-worth.*
3. Set limits on manipulative behavior. Identify the consequences for violation of those limits. Minimize negative feedback to the client. Enforce the limits and impose the consequences for violations in a matter-of-fact manner. Consistency among all staff members is essential. *Negative feedback can be extremely threatening to a person with low self-esteem and possibly aggravate the problem. Consequences should convey unacceptability of the* behavior *but not the* person.
4. Encourage independence in the performance of personal responsibilities, as well as in decision making related to the client's self-care. Offer recognition and praise for accomplishments. *Positive reinforcement enhances self-esteem and encourages repetition of desirable behaviors.*
5. Help the client increase level of self-awareness through critical examination of feelings, attitudes, and behaviors. *Self-exploration in the presence of a trusted individual may help the client come to terms with unresolved issues.*
6. Help the client identify positive self-attributes as well as those aspects of the self he or she finds undesirable. Discuss ways to

effect change in these areas. *Individuals with low self-esteem often have difficulty recognizing their positive attributes. They may also lack problem-solving ability and require assistance to formulate a plan for implementing the desired changes.*

7. Discuss the client's future. Assist the client in the establishment of short-term and long-term goals. What are his or her strengths? How can he or she best use those strengths to achieve those goals? Encourage the client to perform at a level realistic to his or her ability. Offer positive reinforcement for decisions made.

Outcome Criteria

1. Client verbalizes positive aspects about self.
2. Client demonstrates the ability to make independent decisions regarding management of own self-care.
3. Client expresses some optimism and hope for the future.
4. Client sets realistic goals for self and demonstrates willingness to reach them.

■ ANTISOCIAL PERSONALITY DISORDER

Defined

Antisocial personality disorder is characterized by a pattern of antisocial behavior that began before the age of 15. These behaviors violate the rights of others, and individuals with this disorder display no evidence of guilt feelings at having done so. There is often a long history of involvement with law-enforcement agencies. Substance abuse is not uncommon. The disorder is more frequently diagnosed in men than in women. Individuals with antisocial personalities are often labeled *sociopathic* or *psychopathic* in the lay literature.

Predisposing Factors to Antisocial Personality Disorder

1. **Physiological**
   a. **Genetic.** The *DSM-5* reports that antisocial personality is more common among first-degree biological relatives of those with the disorder than among the general population (APA, 2013). Twin and adoptive studies have implicated the role of genetics in antisocial personality disorder (Skodol & Gunderson, 2008). These studies of families of individuals with antisocial personality show higher numbers of relatives with antisocial personality or alcoholism than are found in the general population. Additional studies have shown that children of parents with antisocial behavior are more likely to be diagnosed as antisocial personality, even when they are separated at birth from their biological parents and reared by individuals without the disorder.

b. ***Temperament.*** Characteristics associated with temperament in the newborn may be significant in the predisposition to antisocial personality. Parents who bring their children with behavior disorders to clinics often report that the child displayed temper tantrums from infancy and would become furious when awaiting a bottle or a diaper change. As these children mature, they commonly develop a bullying attitude toward other children. Parents report that they are undaunted by punishment and generally quite unmanageable. They are daring and foolhardy in their willingness to chance physical harm and, they seem unaffected by pain.

2. **Psychosocial**

a. ***Theories of Family Dynamics.*** Antisocial personality disorder frequently arises from a chaotic home environment. Parental deprivation during the first 5 years of life appears to be a critical predisposing factor in the development of antisocial personality disorder. Separation due to parental delinquency appears to be more highly correlated with the disorder than is parental loss from other causes. The presence or intermittent appearance of inconsistent impulsive parents, not the loss of a consistent parent, is environmentally *most* damaging.

Studies have shown that individuals with antisocial personality disorder often have been severely physically abused in childhood. The abuse contributes to the development of antisocial behavior in several ways. First, it provides a model for behavior. Second, it may result in injury to the child's central nervous system, thereby impairing the child's ability to function appropriately. Finally, it engenders rage in the victimized child, which is then displaced onto others in the environment.

Disordered family functioning has been implicated as an important factor in determining whether or not an individual develops antisocial personality (Hill, 2003; Ramsland, 2013; Skodol & Gunderson, 2008). The following circumstances may be influential in the predisposition to the disorder:

a) Absence of parental discipline.
b) Extreme poverty.
c) Removal from the home.
d) Growing up without parental figures of both genders.
e) Erratic and inconsistent methods of discipline.
f) Being "rescued" each time they are in trouble (never having to suffer the consequences of their own behavior).
g) Maternal deprivation.

Symptomatology (Subjective and Objective Data)

1. Extremely low self-esteem (abuses other people in an attempt to validate his or her own superiority).
2. Inability to sustain satisfactory job performance.
3. Inability to function as a responsible parent.
4. Failure to follow social and legal norms; repeated performance of antisocial acts that are grounds for arrest (whether arrested or not).
5. Inability to develop satisfactory, enduring, intimate relationship with a sexual partner.
6. Aggressive behaviors; repeated physical fights; spouse or child abuse.
7. Extreme impulsivity.
8. Repeated lying for personal benefit.
9. Reckless driving; driving while intoxicated.
10. Inability to learn from punishment.
11. Lack of guilt or remorse felt in response to exploitation of others.
12. Difficulty with interpersonal relationships.
13. Social extroversion; stimulation through interaction with and abuse of others.
14. Repeated failure to honor financial obligations.

Common Nursing Diagnoses and Interventions

(Interventions are applicable to various health-care settings, such as inpatient and partial hospitalization, community outpatient clinic, home health, and private practice.)

■ RISK FOR OTHER-DIRECTED VIOLENCE

Definition: *At risk for behaviors in which an individual demonstrates that he or she can be physically, emotionally, and/or sexually harmful to others* (NANDA-I, 2012, p. 447)

Risk Factors ("related to")

[Rage reactions]
History of witnessing family violence
Neurological impairment (e.g., positive EEG)
[Suspiciousness of others]
[Interruption of client's attempt to fulfill own desires]
[Inability to tolerate frustration]
[Learned behavior within client's subculture]
[Vulnerable self-esteem]
Body language (e.g., rigid posture, clenching of fists and jaw, hyperactivity, pacing, breathlessness, threatening stances)

[History or threats of violence toward self or others or of destruction to the property of others]

Impulsivity

Availability of weapon(s)

[Substance abuse or withdrawal]

[Provocative behavior: Argumentative, dissatisfied, overreactive, hypersensitive]

History of childhood abuse

Goals/Objectives

Short-term Goals

1. Client will discuss angry feelings and situations that precipitate hostility.
2. Client will not harm others.

Long-term Goal

Client will not harm others.

Interventions With Selected Rationales

1. Convey an accepting attitude toward this client. Feelings of rejection are undoubtedly familiar to him or her. Work on development of trust. Be honest, keep all promises, and convey the message to the client that it is not *him* or *her*, but the *behavior* that is unacceptable. *An attitude of acceptance promotes feelings of self-worth. Trust is the basis of a therapeutic relationship.*
2. Maintain a low level of stimuli in the client's environment (low lighting, few people, simple decor, low noise level). *A stimulating environment may increase agitation and promote aggressive behavior.*
3. Observe the client's behavior frequently. Do this through routine activities and interactions; avoid appearing watchful and suspicious. *Close observation is required so that intervention can occur if needed to ensure the client's (and others') safety.*
4. Remove all dangerous objects from client's environment so that he or she may not purposefully or inadvertently use them to inflict harm to self or others. *Client safety is a nursing priority.*
5. Help the client identify the true object of his or her hostility (e.g., "You seem to be upset with . . ."). *Because of weak ego development, client may be misusing the defense mechanism of displacement. Helping him or her recognize this in a nonthreatening manner may help reveal unresolved issues so that they may be confronted.*
6. Encourage client to gradually verbalize hostile feelings. *Verbalization of feelings in a nonthreatening environment may help client come to terms with unresolved issues.*

7. Explore with the client alternative ways of handling frustration (e.g., large motor skills that channel hostile energy into socially acceptable behavior). *Physically demanding activities help to relieve pent-up tension.*

8. Staff should maintain and convey a calm attitude toward the client. *Anxiety is contagious and can be transferred from staff to client. A calm attitude provides the client with a feeling of safety and security.*

9. Have sufficient staff available to present a show of strength to the client if necessary. *This conveys to the client evidence of control over the situation and provides some physical security for staff.*

10. Administer tranquilizing medications as ordered by the physician or obtain an order if necessary. Monitor the client for effectiveness of the medication as well as for appearance of adverse side effects. *Antianxiety agents (e.g., lorazepam, chlordiazepoxide, oxazepam) produce a calming effect and may help to allay hostile behaviors.* (NOTE: Medications are often not prescribed for clients with antisocial personality disorder because of these individuals' strong susceptibility to addictions.)

11. If the client is not calmed by "talking down" or by medication, use of mechanical restraints may be necessary. The avenue of the "least restrictive alternative" must be selected when planning interventions for a violent client. Restraints should be used only as a last resort, after all other interventions have been unsuccessful, and the client is clearly at risk of harm to self or others.

12. If restraint is deemed necessary, ensure that sufficient staff is available to assist. Follow protocol established by the institution. The Joint Commission requires that an in-person evaluation by a physician or other licensed independent practitioner (LIP) be conducted within 1 hour of the initiation of the restraint or seclusion (The Joint Commission, 2010). The physician or LIP must reissue a new order for restraints every 4 hours for adults and every 1 to 2 hours for children and adolescents.

13. The Joint Commission requires that the client in restraints be observed at least every 15 minutes to ensure that circulation to extremities is not compromised (check temperature, color, pulses); to assist the client with needs related to nutrition, hydration, and elimination; and to position the client so that comfort is facilitated and aspiration is prevented. Some institutions may require continuous one-to-one monitoring of restrained clients, particularly those who are highly agitated, and for whom there is a high risk of self- or accidental injury.

14. As agitation decreases, assess the client's readiness for restraint removal or reduction. Remove one restraint at a time while

assessing the client's response. ***This minimizes the risk of injury to client and staff.***

Outcome Criteria

1. Client is able to rechannel hostility into socially acceptable behaviors.
2. Client is able to discuss angry feelings and verbalize ways to tolerate frustration appropriately.

▨ DEFENSIVE COPING

Definition: *Repeated projection of falsely positive self-evaluation based on a self-protective pattern that defends against underlying perceived threats to positive self-regard* (NANDA-I, 2012, p. 346)

Possible Etiologies ("related to")

[Inadequate support systems]
[Inadequate coping method]
[Underdeveloped ego]
[Underdeveloped superego]
[Dysfunctional family system]
[Negative role modeling]
[Absent, erratic, or inconsistent methods of discipline]
[Extreme poverty]

Defining Characteristics ("evidenced by")

[Disregard for societal norms and laws]
[Absence of guilt feelings]
[Inability to delay gratification]
Denial of obvious problems
Grandiosity
Hostile laughter
Projection of blame and responsibility
Ridicule of others
Superior attitude toward others

Goals/Objectives

Short-term Goals

1. Within 24 hours after admission, client will verbalize understanding of treatment setting rules and regulations and the consequences for violation of them.
2. Client will verbalize personal responsibility for difficulties experienced in interpersonal relationships within (time period reasonable for client).

Long-term Goals

1. By the time of discharge from treatment, the client will be able to cope more adaptively by delaying gratification of own desires and following rules and regulations of the treatment setting.

2. By the time of discharge from treatment, the client will demonstrate ability to interact with others without becoming defensive, rationalizing behaviors, or expressing grandiose ideas.

Interventions With *Selected Rationales*

1. From the onset, client should be made aware of which behaviors are acceptable and which are not. Explain consequences of violation of the limits. Consequences must involve something of value to the client. All staff must be consistent in enforcing these limits. Consequences should be administered in a matter-of-fact manner immediately following the infraction. *Because client cannot (or will not) impose own limits on maladaptive behaviors, these behaviors must be delineated and enforced by staff. Undesirable consequences may help to decrease repetition of these behaviors.*

2. Do not attempt to coax or convince client to do the "right thing." Do not use the words "You should (or shouldn't) . . ."; instead, use "You will be expected to . . . ." The ideal would be for this client to eventually internalize societal norms, beginning with this step-by-step, "either/or" approach on the unit (*either* you do [don't do] this, *or* this will occur). *Explanations must be concise, concrete, and clear, with little or no capacity for misinterpretation.*

3. Provide positive feedback or reward for acceptable behaviors. *Positive reinforcement enhances self-esteem and encourages repetition of desirable behaviors.*

4. *In an attempt to assist the client to delay gratification*, begin to increase the length of time requirement for acceptable behavior in order to achieve the reward. For example, 2 hours of acceptable behavior may be exchanged for a phone call; 4 hours of acceptable behavior for 2 hours of television; 1 day of acceptable behavior for a recreational therapy bowling activity; 5 days of acceptable behavior for a weekend pass.

5. A milieu unit provides an appropriate environment for the client with antisocial personality. *The democratic approach, with specific rules and regulations, community meetings, and group therapy sessions emulates the type of societal situation in which the client must learn to live. Feedback from peers is often more effective than confrontation from an authority figure. The client learns to follow the rules of the group as a positive step in the progression toward internalizing the rules of society.*

6. Help the client gain insight into his or her own behavior. Often, these individuals rationalize to such an extent that they

deny that their behavior is inappropriate. (For example, thinking may be reflected in statements such as, "The owner of this store has so much money, he'll never miss the little bit I take. He has everything, and I have nothing. It's not fair! I deserve to have some of what he has."). *Client must come to understand that certain behaviors will not be tolerated within the society and that severe consequences will be imposed on those individuals who refuse to comply. Client must want to become a productive member of society before he or she can be helped.*

7. Talk about past behaviors with client. Discuss which behaviors are acceptable by societal norms and which are not. Help the client identify ways in which he or she has exploited others. Encourage the client to explore how he or she would feel if the circumstances were reversed. *An attempt may be made to enlighten the client to the sensitivity of others by promoting self-awareness in an effort to help the client gain insight into his or her own behavior.*

8. Throughout the relationship with the client, maintain attitude of "It is not *you*, but your *behavior*, that is unacceptable." *An attitude of acceptance promotes feelings of dignity and self-worth.*

Outcome Criteria

1. Client follows rules and regulations of the milieu environment.
2. Client is able to verbalize which of his or her behaviors are not acceptable.
3. Client shows regard for the rights of others by delaying gratification of own desires when appropriate.

■ CHRONIC LOW SELF-ESTEEM

Definition: *Long-standing negative self-evaluating/feelings about self or self-capabilities* (NANDA-I, 2012, p. 285)

Possible Etiologies ("related to")

[Lack of positive feedback]
[Unmet dependency needs]
[Retarded ego development]
[Repeated negative feedback, resulting in diminished self-worth]
[Dysfunctional family system]
[Absent, erratic, or inconsistent parental discipline]
[Extreme poverty]
[History of childhood abuse]

Defining Characteristics ("evidenced by")

[Denial of problems obvious to others]

[Projection of blame or responsibility for problems]
[Grandiosity]
[Aggressive behavior]
[Frequent use of derogatory and critical remarks against others]
[Manipulation of others to fulfill own desires]
[Inability to form close, personal relationships]

Goals/Objectives

Short-term Goal

Client will verbalize an understanding that derogatory and critical remarks against others reflect feelings of self-contempt.

Long-term Goal

Client will experience an increase in self-esteem, as evidenced by verbalizations of positive aspects of self and the lack of manipulative behaviors toward others.

Interventions With *Selected Rationales*

1. Ensure that goals are realistic. It is important for client to achieve something, so plan for activities in which success is likely. *Success increases self-esteem.*
2. Identify ways in which client is manipulating others. Set limits on manipulative behavior. *Because client is unable (or unwilling) to limit own maladaptive behaviors, assistance is required from staff.*
3. Explain the consequences of manipulative behavior. All staff must be consistent and follow through with consequences in a matter-of-fact manner. *From the onset, client must be aware of the consequences of his or her maladaptive behaviors. Without consistency of follow-through from all staff, a positive outcome cannot be achieved.*
4. Encourage the client to talk about his or her behavior, the limits, and consequences for violation of those limits. *Discussion of feelings regarding these circumstances may help the client achieve some insight into his or her situation.*
5. Discuss how manipulative behavior interferes with formation of close, personal relationships. *Client may be unaware of others' perception of him or her and of why these behaviors are not acceptable to others.*
6. Help the client identify more adaptive interpersonal strategies. Provide positive feedback for nonmanipulative behaviors. *Client may require assistance with solving problems. Positive reinforcement enhances self-esteem and encourages repetition of desirable behaviors.*
7. Encourage the client to confront the fear of failure by attending therapy activities and undertaking new tasks. Offer recognition of successful endeavors.

8. Help the client identify positive aspects of the self and develop ways to change the characteristics that are socially unacceptable. *Individuals with low self-esteem often have difficulty recognizing their positive attributes. They may also lack problem-solving ability and require assistance to formulate a plan for implementing the desired changes.*

9. Minimize negative feedback to client. Enforce limit setting in a matter-of-fact manner, imposing previously established consequences for violations. *Negative feedback can be extremely threatening to a person with low self-esteem, possibly aggravating the problem. Consequences should convey unacceptability of the behavior but not the person.*

10. Encourage independence in the performance of personal responsibilities and in decision making related to own self-care. Offer recognition and praise for accomplishments. *Positive reinforcement enhances self-esteem and encourages repetition of desirable behaviors.*

11. Help the client increase level of self-awareness through critical examination of feelings, attitudes, and behaviors. Help the client understand that it is perfectly acceptable for attitudes and behaviors to differ from those of others, as long as they do not become intrusive. *As the client becomes more aware and accepting of himself or herself, the need for judging the behavior of others will diminish.*

12. Teach the client assertiveness techniques, especially the ability to recognize the differences among passive, assertive, and aggressive behaviors and the importance of respecting the human rights of others while protecting one's own basic human rights. *These techniques increase self-esteem while enhancing the ability to form satisfactory interpersonal relationships.*

Outcome Criteria

1. Client verbalizes positive aspects about self.
2. Client does not manipulate others in an attempt to increase feelings of self-worth.
3. Client considers the rights of others in interpersonal interactions.

▨ IMPAIRED SOCIAL INTERACTION

Definition: *Insufficient or excessive quantity or ineffective quality of social exchange* (NANDA-I, 2012, p. 320)

Possible Etiologies ("related to")

Self-concept disturbance

[Unmet dependency needs]
[Retarded ego development]
[Retarded superego development]
[Negative role modeling]
Knowledge deficit about ways to enhance mutuality

Defining Characteristics ("evidenced by")

Discomfort in social situations

Inability to receive or communicate a satisfying sense of social engagement (e.g., belonging, caring, interest, shared history)

Use of unsuccessful social interaction behaviors

Dysfunctional interaction with others

[Exploitation of others for the fulfillment of own desires]

[Inability to develop satisfactory, enduring, intimate relationship with a sexual partner]

[Physical and verbal hostility toward others when fulfillment of own desires is thwarted]

Goals/Objectives

Short-term Goal

Client will develop satisfactory relationship (no evidence of manipulation or exploitation) with nurse or therapist within 1 week.

Long-term Goal

Client will interact appropriately with others, demonstrating concern for the needs of others as well as for his or her own needs, by time of discharge from treatment.

Interventions With *Selected Rationales*

1. Develop therapeutic rapport with client. Establish trust by always being honest; keep all promises; convey acceptance of person, separate from unacceptable behaviors ("It is not *you*, but your *behavior*, that is unacceptable."). *An attitude of acceptance promotes feelings of self-worth. Trust is the basis of a therapeutic relationship.*

2. Offer to remain with client during initial interactions with others. *Presence of a trusted individual increases feelings of security during uncomfortable situations.*

3. Provide constructive criticism and positive reinforcement for efforts. *Positive feedback enhances self-esteem and encourages repetition of desirable behaviors.*

4. Confront client as soon as possible when interactions with others are manipulative or exploitative. Establish consequences for unacceptable behavior, and always follow through. *Because of the strong id influence on client's behavior, he or she should receive immediate feedback when behavior is unacceptable. Consistency in enforcing the consequences is essential if*

positive outcomes are to be achieved. Inconsistency creates confusion and encourages testing of limits.

5. Act as a role model for client through appropriate interactions with him or her and with others. *Role modeling is a powerful and effective form of learning.*

6. Provide group situations for client. *It is through these group interactions with positive and negative feedback from his or her peers, that client will learn socially acceptable behavior.*

Outcome Criteria

1. Client willingly and appropriately participates in group activities.

2. Client has satisfactorily established and maintained one interpersonal relationship with nurse or therapist, without evidence of manipulation or exploitation.

3. Client demonstrates ability to interact appropriately with others, showing respect for self and others.

4. Client is able to verbalize reasons for inability to form close interpersonal relationships with others in the past.

■ DEFICIENT KNOWLEDGE (SELF-CARE ACTIVITIES TO ACHIEVE AND MAINTAIN OPTIMAL WELLNESS)

Definition: *Absence or deficiency of cognitive information related to a specific topic* (NANDA-I, 2012, p. 271)

Possible Etiologies ("related to")

Lack of interest in learning
[Low self-esteem]
[Denial of need for information]
[Denial of risks involved with maladaptive lifestyle]
Unfamiliarity with information sources

Defining Characteristics ("evidenced by")

[History of substance abuse]
[Statement of lack of knowledge]
[Statement of misconception]
[Request for information]
[Demonstrated lack of knowledge regarding basic health practices]
[Reported or observed inability to take the responsibility for meeting basic health practices in any or all functional pattern areas]
[History of lack of health-seeking behavior]
Inappropriate or exaggerated behaviors (e.g., hysterical, hostile, agitated, apathetic)

Goals/Objectives

Short-term Goal

Client will verbalize understanding of knowledge required to fulfill basic health needs following implementation of teaching plan.

Long-term Goal

Client will be able to demonstrate skills learned for fulfillment of basic health needs by time of discharge from therapy.

Interventions With *Selected Rationales*

1. Assess the client's level of knowledge regarding positive self-care practices. *An adequate database is necessary for the development of an effective teaching plan.*
2. Assess the client's level of anxiety and readiness to learn. *Learning does not occur beyond the moderate level of anxiety.*
3. Determine the method of learning most appropriate for the client (e.g., discussion, question and answer, use of audio or visual aids, oral, written). Be sure to consider level of education and development. *Teaching will be ineffective if presented at a level or by a method inappropriate to the client's ability to learn.*
4. Develop a teaching plan, including measurable objectives for the learner. Provide information regarding healthful strategies for activities of daily living as well as about harmful effects of substance abuse on the body. Include suggestions for community resources to assist client when adaptability is impaired. *Client needs this information to promote effective health maintenance.*
5. Include significant others in the learning activity, if possible. *Input from individuals who are directly involved in the potential change increases the likelihood of a positive outcome.*
6. Implement the teaching plan at a time that facilitates and in a place that is conducive to optimal learning (e.g., in the evening when family members visit; in an empty, quiet classroom or group therapy room). *Learning is enhanced by an environment with few distractions.*
7. Begin with simple concepts and progress to the more complex. *Retention is increased if introductory material is easy to understand.*
8. Provide activities for the client and significant others in which to actively participate during the learning exercise. *Active participation increases retention.*
9. Ask client and significant others to demonstrate knowledge gained by verbalizing information regarding positive self-care practices. *Verbalization of knowledge gained is a measurable method of evaluating the teaching experience.*

10. Provide positive feedback for participation, as well as for accurate demonstration of knowledge gained. ***Positive feedback enhances self-esteem and encourages repetition of desirable behaviors.***

Outcome Criteria

1. Client is able to verbalize information regarding positive self-care practices.
2. Client is able to verbalize available community resources for obtaining knowledge about and help with deficits related to health care.

@ INTERNET REFERENCES

- Additional information about personality disorders may be located at the following Web sites:
  a. http://www.mentalhealth.com/dis/p20-pe01.html
  b. http://www.mentalhealth.com/dis/p20-pe02.html
  c. http://www.mentalhealth.com/dis/p20-pe03.html
  d. http://www.mentalhealth.com/dis/p20-pe04.html
  e. http://www.mentalhealth.com/dis/p20-pe05.html
  f. http://www.mentalhealth.com/dis/p20-pe06.html
  g. http://www.mentalhealth.com/dis/p20-pe07.html
  h. http://www.mentalhealth.com/dis/p20-pe08.html
  i. http://www.mentalhealth.com/dis/p20-pe09.html
  j. http://www.mentalhealth.com/dis/p20-pe10.html
  k. http://www.mentalhealth.com/p13.html#Per
  l. http://www.ncbi.nlm.nih.gov/pubmedhealth/PMH0001935
  m. http://www.mayoclinic.com/health/personality-disorders/DS00562

Movie Connections

Taxi Driver (Schizoid personality) • *One Flew Over the Cuckoo's Nest* (Antisocial) • *The Boston Strangler* (Antisocial) • *Just Cause* (Antisocial) • *The Dream Team* (Antisocial) • *Goodfellas* (Antisocial) • *Fatal Attraction* (Borderline) • *Play Misty for Me* (Borderline) • *Girl, Interrupted* (Borderline) • *Gone With the Wind* (Histrionic) • *Wall Street* (Narcissistic) • *The Odd Couple* (Obsessive-compulsive) • *As Good As It Gets* (Obsessive-compulsive)

SPECIAL TOPICS IN PSYCHIATRIC/MENTAL HEALTH NURSING

CHAPTER 15

Problems Related to Abuse or Neglect

■ BACKGROUND ASSESSMENT DATA

Categories of Abuse and Neglect

Physical Abuse of a Child

Physical abuse of a child includes "any nonaccidental physical injury (ranging from minor bruises to severe fractures or death) as a result of punching, beating, kicking, biting, shaking, throwing, stabbing, choking, hitting (with a hand, stick, strap, or other object), burning, or any other method that is inflicted by a parent, caregiver, or other individual who has responsibility for the child" (American Psychiatric Association [APA], 2013, p. 717). The most obvious way to detect it is by outward physical signs. However, behavioral indicators may also be evident.

Sexual Abuse of a Child

This category is defined as "employment, use, persuasion, inducement, enticement, or coercion of any child to engage in, or assist any other person to engage in, any sexually explicit conduct or any simulation of such conduct for the purpose of producing any visual depiction of such conduct; or the rape, and in cases of caretaker or interfamilial relationships, statutory rape, molestation, prostitution, or other form of sexual exploitation of children, or incest with children" (CWIG, 2013). **Incest** is the occurrence of sexual contacts or interaction between, or sexual exploitation of, close relatives, or between participants who are related to each other by a kinship bond that is regarded as a prohibition to sexual relations (e.g., caretakers, stepparents, stepsiblings) (Sadock & Sadock, 2007).

Neglect of a Child

Physical neglect of a child includes refusal of or delay in seeking health care, abandonment, expulsion from the home or refusal to allow a runaway to return home, and inadequate supervision. *Emotional neglect* refers to a chronic failure by the parent or caretaker to provide the child with the hope, love, and support necessary for the development of a sound, healthy personality.

Physical Abuse of an Adult

Physical abuse of an adult may be defined as behavior used with the intent to cause harm and to establish power and control over another person. It may include slaps, punches, biting, hair pulling, choking, kicking, stabbing or shooting, or forcible restraint.

Sexual Abuse of an Adult

Sexual abuse of an adult may be defined as the expression of power and dominance by means of sexual violence, most commonly by men over women, although men may also be victims of sexual assault. Sexual assault is identified by the use of force and executed against the person's will.

Predisposing Factors (that Contribute to Patterns of Abuse)

1. **Physiological**
   a. *Neurophysiological Influences.* Various components of the neurological system in both humans and animals have been implicated in both the facilitation and inhibition of aggressive impulses. Areas of the brain that may be involved include the temporal lobe, the limbic system, and the amygdaloid nucleus (Tardiff, 2003).
   b. *Biochemical Influences.* Studies show that various neurotransmitters—in particular norepinephrine, dopamine, and serotonin—may play a role in the facilitation and inhibition of aggressive impulses (Hollander, Berlin, & Stein, 2008).
   c. *Genetic Influences.* Some studies have implicated heredity as a component in the predisposition to aggressive behavior. Both direct genetic links and the genetic karyotype XYY have been investigated as possibilities. Evidence remains inconclusive.
   d. *Disorders of the Brain.* Various disorders of the brain, including tumors, trauma, and certain diseases (e.g., encephalitis

and epilepsy), have been implicated in the predisposition to aggressive behavior.

2. **Psychosocial**

   a. *Psychodynamic Theory.* The psychodynamic theorists imply that unmet needs for satisfaction and security result in an underdeveloped ego and a weak superego. It is thought that when frustration occurs, aggression and violence supply this individual with a dose of power and prestige that boosts the self-image and validates significance to his or her life that is lacking. The immature ego cannot prevent dominant id behaviors from occurring, and the weak superego is unable to produce feelings of guilt.

   b. *Learning Theory.* This theory postulates that aggressive and violent behaviors are learned from prestigious and influential role models. Individuals who were abused as children or whose parents disciplined with physical punishment are more likely to behave in a violent manner as adults (Hornor, 2005).

   c. *Societal Influences.* Social scientists believe that aggressive behavior is primarily a product of one's culture and social structure. Societal influences may contribute to violence when individuals believe that their needs and desires cannot be met through conventional means, and they resort to delinquent behaviors in an effort to obtain desired ends.

Symptomatology (Subjective and Objective Data)

1. Signs of physical abuse may include the following:
   a. Bruises over various areas of the body. They may present with different colors of bluish-purple to yellowish-green (indicating various stages of healing).
   b. Bite marks, skin welts, burns.
   c. Fractures, scars, serious internal injuries, brain damage.
   d. Lacerations, abrasions, or unusual bleeding.
   e. Bald spots indicative of severe hair pulling.
   f. In a child, regressive behaviors (such as thumb-sucking and enuresis) are common.
   g. Extreme anxiety and mistrust of others.
2. Signs of neglect of a child may include the following:
   a. Soiled clothing that does not fit and may be inappropriate for the weather.
   b. Poor hygiene.
   c. Always hungry, with possible signs of malnutrition (e.g., emaciated with swollen belly).
   d. Listless and tired much of the time.
   e. Unattended medical problems.
   f. Social isolation; unsatisfactory peer relationships.
   g. Poor school performance and attendance record.

3. Signs of sexual abuse of a child include the following:
   a. Frequent urinary infections.
   b. Difficulty or pain in walking or sitting.
   c. Rashes or itching in the genital area; scratching the area a great deal or fidgeting when seated.
   d. Frequent vomiting.
   e. Seductive behavior; compulsive masturbation; precocious sex play.
   f. Excessive anxiety and mistrust of others.
   g. Sexually abusing another child.
4. Signs of sexual abuse of an adult include the following (Burgess, 2010):
   a. Contusions and abrasions about various parts of the body.
   b. Headaches, fatigue, sleep-pattern disturbances.
   c. Stomach pains, nausea, and vomiting.
   d. Vaginal discharge and itching, burning on urination, rectal bleeding and pain.
   e. Rage, humiliation, embarrassment, desire for revenge, self-blame.
   f. Fear of physical violence and death.

Common Nursing Diagnoses and Interventions

(Interventions are applicable to various health-care settings, such as inpatient and partial hospitalization, community outpatient clinic, home health, and private practice.)

■ RAPE-TRAUMA SYNDROME

Definition: *Sustained maladaptive response to a forced, violent sexual penetration against the victim's will and consent* (NANDA International [NANDA-I], 2012, p. 337)

Possible Etiologies ("related to")

[Having been the victim of sexual violence executed with the use of force and against one's personal will and consent]

Defining Characteristics ("evidenced by")

Disorganization
Change in relationships
Confusion
Physical trauma (e.g., bruising, tissue irritation)
Suicide attempts
Denial; guilt
Paranoia; humiliation, embarrassment
Aggression; muscle tension and/or spasms
Mood swings

Dependence
Powerlessness; helplessness
Nightmares and sleep disturbances
Sexual dysfunction
Revenge; phobias
Loss of self-esteem
Impaired decision making
Substance abuse; depression
Anger; anxiety; agitation
Shame; shock; fear

Goals/Objectives

Short-term Goal

The client's physical wounds will heal without complication.

Long-term Goal

The client will begin a healthy grief resolution, initiating the process of physical and psychological healing (time to be individually determined).

Interventions With *Selected Rationales*

1. It is important to communicate the following to the individual who has been sexually assaulted:
   a. You are safe here.
   b. I'm sorry that it happened.
   c. I'm glad that you survived.
   d. It's not your fault. No one deserves to be treated this way.
   e. You did the best that you could.
   The woman who has been sexually assaulted fears for her life and must be reassured of her safety. She may also be overwhelmed with self-doubt and self-blame, and these statements instill trust and validate self-worth.
2. Explain every assessment procedure that will be conducted and why it is being conducted. Ensure that data collection is conducted in a caring, nonjudgmental manner *to decrease fear and anxiety and increase trust.*
3. Ensure that the client has adequate privacy for all immediate postcrisis interventions. Try to have as few people as possible providing the immediate care or collecting immediate evidence. *The posttrauma client is extremely vulnerable. Additional people in the environment increase this feeling of vulnerability and serve to escalate anxiety.*
4. Encourage the client to give an account of the assault. Listen, but do not probe. *Nonjudgmental listening provides an avenue for catharsis that the client needs to begin healing. A detailed account may be required for legal follow-up, and a caring nurse, as client advocate, may help to lessen the trauma of evidence collection.*

5. Discuss with the client whom to call for support or assistance. Provide information about referrals for aftercare. *Because of severe anxiety and fear, client may need assistance from others during this immediate postcrisis period. Provide referral information in writing for later reference (e.g., psychotherapist, mental health clinic, community advocacy group).*

Outcome Criteria

1. Client is no longer experiencing panic anxiety.
2. Client demonstrates a degree of trust in the primary nurse.
3. Client has received immediate attention to physical injuries.
4. Client has initiated behaviors consistent with the grief response.

■ POWERLESSNESS

Definition: *The lived experience of lack of control over a situation, including a perception that one's actions do not significantly affect an outcome* (NANDA-I, 2012, p. 370)

Possible Etiologies ("related to")

[Lifestyle of helplessness]
[Low self-esteem]
[Living with, or in a long-term relationship with, an individual who victimizes by inflicting physical pain or injury with the intent to cause harm, and continues to do so over a long period of time]
[Lack of support network of caring others]
[Lack of financial independence]

Defining Characteristics ("evidenced by")

Reports lack of control [over situation or outcome]
[Reluctance to express true feelings]
[Passivity]
[Verbalizations of abuse]
[Lacerations over areas of body]
[Fear for personal and children's safety]
[Verbalizations of no way to get out of relationship]

Goals/Objectives

Short-term Goal

Client will recognize and verbalize choices that are available, thereby perceiving some control over life situation (time dimension to be individually determined).

Long-term Goal

Client will exhibit control over life situation by making decision about what to do regarding living with cycle of abuse (time dimension to be individually determined).

Interventions With *Selected Rationales*

1. In collaboration with physician, ensure that all physical wounds, fractures, and burns receive immediate attention. Take photographs if the victim will permit. *Client safety is a nursing priority. Photographs may be called in as evidence if charges are filed.*

2. Take the client to a private area to do the interview. *If the client is accompanied by the person who did the battering, he or she is not likely to be truthful about the injuries.*

3. If she has come alone or with her children, assure her of her safety. (Author's note: *Female gender is used here because most intimate partner violence [IPV] is directed by men toward women, although it is understood that men are also victims of IPV.)* Encourage her to discuss the battering incident. Ask questions about whether this has happened before, whether the abuser takes drugs, whether the woman has a safe place to go, and whether she is interested in pressing charges. *Some women will attempt to keep secret how their injuries occurred in an effort to protect the partner or because they are fearful that the partner will kill them if they tell.*

4. Ensure that "rescue" efforts are not attempted by the nurse. Offer support, but remember that the final decision must be made by the client. *Making her own decision will give the client a sense of control over her life situation. Imposing judgments and giving advice are nontherapeutic.*

5. Stress to the victim the importance of safety. She must be made aware of the variety of resources that are available to her. These may include crisis hotlines, community groups for women who have been abused, shelters, counseling services, and information regarding the victim's rights in the civil and criminal justice system. Following a discussion of these available resources, the woman may choose for herself. If her decision is to return to the marriage and home, this choice also must be respected. *Knowledge of available choices can serve to decrease the victim's sense of powerlessness, but true empowerment comes only when she chooses to use that knowledge for her own benefit.*

Outcome Criteria

1. Client has received immediate attention to physical injuries.
2. Client verbalizes assurance of her immediate safety.
3. Client discusses life situation with primary nurse.

4. Client is able to verbalize choices available to her from which she may receive assistance.

■ RISK FOR DELAYED DEVELOPMENT

Definition: *At risk for delay of 25% or more in one or more of the areas of social or self-regulatory behavior, or in cognitive, language, gross or fine motor skills* (NANDA-I, 2012, p. 485)

Risk Factors ("related to")

[The infliction by caretakers of physical or sexual abuse, usually occurring over an extended period of time]
[Ignoring the child's basic physiological needs]
[Indifference to the child]
[Ignoring the child's presence]
[Ignoring the child's social, educational, recreational, and developmental needs]

Goals/Objectives

Short-term Goal

Client will develop a trusting relationship with the nurse and report how evident injuries were sustained (time dimension to be individually determined).

Long-term Goal

Client will demonstrate behaviors consistent with age-appropriate growth and development.

Interventions With *Selected Rationales*

1. Perform complete physical assessment of the child. Take particular note of bruises (in various stages of healing), lacerations, and client complaints of pain in specific areas. Do not overlook or discount the possibility of sexual abuse. Assess for nonverbal signs of abuse: aggressive conduct, excessive fears, extreme hyperactivity, apathy, withdrawal, age-inappropriate behaviors. *An accurate and thorough physical assessment is required in order to provide appropriate care for the client.*
2. Conduct an in-depth interview with the parent or adult who accompanies the child. Consider: If the injury is being reported as an accident, is the explanation reasonable? Is the injury consistent with the explanation? Is the injury consistent with the child's developmental capabilities? *Fear of imprisonment or loss of child custody may place the abusive parent on the defensive. Discrepancies may be evident in the description of the incident, and lying to cover up involvement*

is a common defense that may be detectable in an in-depth interview.

3. Use games or play therapy to gain the child's trust. Use these techniques to assist in describing his or her side of the story. *Establishing a trusting relationship with an abused child is extremely difficult. The child may not even want to be touched. These types of play activities can provide a nonthreatening environment that may enhance the child's attempt to discuss these painful issues.*

4. Determine whether the nature of the injuries warrants reporting to authorities. Specific state statutes must enter into the decision of whether to report suspected child abuse. Individual state statues regarding what constitutes child abuse and neglect may be found at www.childwelfare.gov/systemwide/laws_policies/state. *A report is commonly made if there is reason to suspect that a child has been injured as a result of physical, mental, emotional, or sexual abuse. "Reason to suspect" exists when there is evidence of a discrepancy or inconsistency in explaining a child's injury. Most states require that the following individuals report cases of suspected child abuse: all health-care workers, all mental health therapists, teachers, childcare providers, firefighters, emergency medical personnel, and law enforcement personnel. Reports are made to the Department of Health and Human Services or a law enforcement agency.*

Outcome Criteria

1. Client has received immediate attention to physical injuries.
2. Client demonstrates trust in the primary nurse by discussing abuse through the use of play therapy.
3. Client is demonstrating a decrease in regressive behaviors.

@ INTERNET REFERENCES

- Additional information related to child abuse may be located at the following Web sites:
  a. www.childwelfare.gov
  b. http://endabuse.org/
  c. www.child-abuse.com
  d. www.nlm.nih.gov/medlineplus/childabuse.html
- Additional information related to Sexual Assault may be located at the following Web sites:
  a. www.vaw.umn.edu/
  b. www.nlm.nih.gov/medlineplus/rape.html

- Additional information related to Intimate Partner Violence may be located at the following Web sites:
  a. www.thehotline.org
  b. www.nursingworld.org/MainMenuCategories/ANA Marketplace/ANAPeriodicals/OJIN/TableofContents/ Volume72002/No1Jan2002/DomesticViolenceChallenge .html
  c. www.cdc.gov/ViolencePrevention/intimatepartnerviolence/ index.html
  d. www.nursingworld.org/MainMenuCategories/ANA Marketplace/ANAPeriodicals/OJIN/TableofContents/ Volume72002/No1Jan2002/IntimatePartnerViolence.html

---

Movie Connections

The Burning Bed (Domestic violence) • *Life With Billy* (Domestic violence) • *Two Story House* (Child abuse) • *The Prince of Tides* (Domestic violence) • *Radio Flyer* (Child abuse) • *Flowers in the Attic* (Child abuse) • *A Case of Rape* (Sexual assault) • *The Accused* (Sexual assault)

CHAPTER 16

Premenstrual Dysphoric Disorder

■ BACKGROUND ASSESSMENT DATA

Defined

The essential features of premenstrual dysphoric disorder (PMDD) are identified by the *Diagnostic and Statistical Manual of Mental Disorders, Fifth Edition* (DSM-5, American Psychiatric Association [APA], 2013) as "the expression of mood lability, irritability, dysphoria, and anxiety symptoms that occur repeatedly during the premenstrual phase of the cycle and remit around the onset of menses or shortly thereafter" (p. 172). The symptoms are sufficiently severe to cause marked impairment in social, occupational, and other important areas of functioning, and have occurred during most of the menstrual cycles during the past year.

Predisposing Factors to PMDD

1. **Physiological**
   a. *Biochemical.* An imbalance of the hormones estrogen and progesterone has been implicated in the predisposition to PMDD. It is postulated that excess estrogen or a high estrogen-to-progesterone ratio during the luteal phase causes water retention and that this hormonal imbalance has other effects as well, resulting in the symptoms associated with premenstrual syndrome.
   b. *Nutritional.* A number of nutritional alterations have been implicated in the etiology of PMDD, although the exact role is unsubstantiated. Deficiencies in the B vitamins, calcium, magnesium, manganese, vitamin E, and linolenic acid have been suggested. Glucose tolerance fluctuations, abnormal fatty acid metabolism, and sensitivity to caffeine and alcohol may also play a role in contributing to the symptoms associated with this disorder.

Symptomatology (Subjective and Objective Data)

The following symptoms have been associated with PMDD (APA, 2013; Sadock & Sadock, 2007):

1. Feelings of depression and hopelessness
2. Increased anxiety and restlessness
3. Mood swings
4. Anger and irritability
5. Decreased interest in usual activities
6. Difficulty concentrating
7. Anergia; increased fatigability
8. Appetite changes (e.g., food cravings)
9. Changes in sleep patterns (e.g., hypersomnia or insomnia)
10. Somatic complaints (e.g., breast tenderness, headaches, edema)

Other subjective symptoms that have been reported include:

11. Cramps
12. Alcohol intolerance
13. Acne
14. Cystitis
15. Oliguria
16. Altered sexual drive
17. Forgetfulness
18. Suicidal ideations or attempts

Common Nursing Diagnoses And Interventions

(Interventions are applicable to various health-care settings, such as in-patient and partial hospitalization, community outpatient clinic, home health, and private practice.)

■ ACUTE PAIN

Definition: *Unpleasant sensory and emotional experience arising from actual or potential tissue damage or described in terms of such damage (International Association for the Study of Pain); sudden or slow onset of any intensity from mild to severe with an anticipated or predictable end and a duration of less than 6 months (NANDA International [NANDA-I], 2012, p. 478)*

Possible Etiologies ("related to")

[Imbalance in estrogen and progesterone levels]
[Possible nutritional alterations, including the following:
   Vitamin B deficiencies
   Glucose tolerance fluctuations
   Abnormal fatty acid metabolism, which may contribute to alterations in prostaglandin synthesis
   Magnesium deficiency

Vitamin E deficiency
Caffeine sensitivity
Alcohol intolerance]
[Fluid retention]

Defining Characteristics ("evidenced by")

[Subjective communication of:
Headache
Backache
Joint or muscle pain
A sensation of "bloating"
Abdominal cramping
Breast tenderness and swelling]
Facial mask [of pain]
Sleep disturbance
Self-focus
Changes in appetite [and eating]

Goals/Objectives

Short-term Goal

Client cooperates with efforts to manage symptoms of PMDD and minimize feelings of discomfort.

Long-term Goal

Client verbalizes relief from discomfort associated with symptoms of PMDD.

Interventions With *Selected Rationales*

1. Assess and record location, duration, and intensity of pain. *Background assessment data are necessary to formulate an accurate plan of care for the client.*
2. Provide nursing comfort measures with a matter-of-fact approach that does not give positive reinforcement to the pain behavior (e.g., backrub, warm bath, heating pad). Give additional attention at times when client is not focusing on physical symptoms. *These measures may serve to provide some temporary relief from pain. Absence of secondary gains in the form of positive reinforcement may discourage client's use of the pain as an attention-seeking behavior.*
3. Encourage the client to get adequate rest and sleep and avoid stressful activity during the premenstrual period. *Fatigue exaggerates symptoms associated with PMDD. Stress elicits heightened symptoms of anxiety, which may contribute to exacerbation of symptoms and altered perception of pain.*
4. Assist the client with activities that distract from focus on self and pain. Demonstrate techniques such as visual or auditory

distractions, guided imagery, breathing exercises, massage, application of heat or cold, and relaxation techniques that may provide symptomatic relief. *These techniques may help to maintain anxiety at a manageable level and prevent the discomfort from becoming disabling.*

5. *In an effort to correct the possible nutritional alterations that may be contributing to PMDD,* the following guidelines may be suggested:

   a. Reduce intake of fats in the diet, particularly saturated fats.

   b. Limit intake of dairy products to two servings a day (excessive dairy products block the absorption of magnesium).

   c. Increase intake of complex carbohydrates (vegetables, legumes, cereals, and whole grains) and *cis*-linoleic acid-containing foods (e.g., safflower oil).

   d. Decrease refined and simple sugars. (Excess sugar is thought to cause nervous tension, palpitations, headache, dizziness, drowsiness, and excretion of magnesium in the urine.)

   e. Decrease salt intake to no more than 2300 mg per day but not less than 500 mg per day. (Salt restriction prevents edema; too little salt stimulates norepinephrine and causes sleep disturbances.)

   f. Limit intake of caffeine (coffee, tea, colas, and chocolate) and alcohol (one to two drinks a week). Caffeine increases breast tenderness and pain. Alcohol can cause reactive hypoglycemia and fluid retention.

   g. Because some women crave junk food during the premenstrual period, it is important that they take a multiple vitamin or mineral tablet daily to ensure that adequate nutrients are consumed.

6. Administer medications as prescribed. Monitor client response for effectiveness of the medication, as well as for appearance of adverse side effects. *When other measures are insufficient to bring about relief,* physician may prescribe symptomatic drug therapy. Provide client with information about the medication to be administered. *Client has the right to know about the treatment she is receiving.* Some medications commonly used for symptomatic treatment of PMDD are presented in Table 16-1 (following page). Some women have experienced relief from the symptoms of PMDD with herbal medications. Some of these are listed in Table 16-2.

Outcome Criteria

1. Client demonstrates ability to manage premenstrual symptoms with minimal discomfort.

2. Client verbalizes relief of painful symptoms.

TABLE 16–1 Medications for Symptomatic Relief of PMDD

Medication	Indication
Fluoxetine (Sarafem), sertraline (Zoloft), paroxetine (Paxil)	These medications have been approved by the FDA for treatment of PMDD.
Hydrochlorothiazide (Ezide, HydroDiuril), furosemide (Lasix)	Diuretics may provide relief from edema when diet and sodium restriction are not sufficient.
Ibuprofen (Advil, Motrin), naproxen (Naprosyn, Aleve)	Nonsteroidal anti-inflammatory agents may provide relief from joint, muscle, and lower abdominal pain related to increased prostaglandins.
Propranolol (Inderal), verapamil (Isoptin)	β-Blockers and calcium channel blockers are often given for prophylactic treatment of migraine headaches.
Sumatriptan (Imitrex), naratriptan (Amerge), rizatriptan (Maxalt), zolmitriptan (Zomig), frovatriptan (Frova), almotriptan (Axert), eletriptan (Relpax)	These serotonin 5-HT$_1$ receptor agonists are highly effective in the treatment of acute migraine attack.
Bromocriptine (Parlodel)	This drug may be prescribed to relieve breast pain and other symptoms of PMDD that may be caused by elevated prolactin.

TABLE 16–2 Herbal Medications Used to Treat Symptoms of PMDD

Herbal	Precautions/Adverse Effects	Contraindications
Black cohosh (Cimicifuga racemosa)	May potentiate the effects of antihypertensive medications. Some individuals may experience nausea or headache.	Pregnancy
Bugleweed (Lycopus virginicus)	No side effects known. Should not be taken concomitantly with thyroid preparations.	Thyroid disease

TABLE 16–2	Herbal Medications Used to Treat Symptoms of PMDD—cont'd	
Herbal	**Precautions/Adverse Effects**	**Contraindications**
Chaste tree (*Vitex agnus-castus*)	Occasional rashes may occur. Should not be taken concomitantly with dopamine-receptor antagonists.	Pregnancy and lactation
Evening primrose (*Oenothera biennis*)	May lower the seizure threshold. Should not be taken concomitantly with other drugs that lower the seizure threshold.	
Potentilla (*Potentilla anserine*)	May cause stomach irritation.	
Shepherd's purse (*Capsella bursa-pastoris*)	No side effects known.	Pregnancy
Valerian (*Valeriana officinalis*)	With long-term use: headache, restless states, sleeplessness, mydriasis, disorders of cardiac function. Should not be taken concomitantly with CNS depressants.	Pregnancy and lactation

Source: *PDR for herbal medicines* (4th ed.). (2007). Montvale, NJ: Thomson Healthcare Inc.; Presser, A.M. (2000). *Pharmacist's guide to medicinal herbs*. Petaluma, CA: Smart Publications.

▓ INEFFECTIVE COPING

Definition: *Inability to form a valid appraisal of the stressors, inadequate choices of practiced responses, and/or inability to use available resources* (NANDA-I, 2012, p. 348)

Possible Etiologies ("related to")

[Imbalance in estrogen and progesterone levels]
[Possible nutritional alterations, including the following:
    Vitamin B deficiencies
    Glucose tolerance fluctuations
    Abnormal fatty acid metabolism, which may contribute to alterations in prostaglandin synthesis
    Magnesium deficiency

Vitamin E deficiency
Caffeine sensitivity
Alcohol intolerance]

Defining Characteristics ("evidenced by")

[Mood swings]
[Marked anger or irritability]
[Increased anxiety and restlessness]
[Feelings of depression and hopelessness]
[Decreased interest in usual activities]
[Anergia; easy fatigability]
[Difficulty concentrating; forgetfulness]
[Changes in appetite]
[Hypersomnia or insomnia]
[Altered sexual drive]
[Suicidal ideations or attempts]
Inadequate problem solving
Inability to meet role expectations

Goals/Objectives

Short-term Goals

1. Client will seek out support person if thoughts of suicide emerge.
2. Client will verbalize ways to express anger in an appropriate manner and maintain anxiety at a manageable level.

Long-term Goals

1. Client will not harm self while experiencing symptoms associated with PMDD.
2. Client will demonstrate adaptive coping strategies to use in an effort to minimize disabling behaviors during the premenstrual and perimenstrual periods.

Interventions With *Selected Rationales*

1. Assess client's potential for suicide. Has she expressed feelings of not wanting to live? Does she have a plan? A means? *Depression is the most prevalent disorder that precedes suicide. The risk of suicide is greatly increased if the client has developed a plan and particularly if means exist for the client to execute the plan.*
2. Formulate a short-term verbal contract with the client that she will not harm herself during specific period of time. When that contract expires, make another, and so forth. *Discussion of suicidal feelings with a trusted individual provides a degree of relief to the client. A contract gets the subject out in the open and places some of the responsibility for the client's safety with the client. An attitude*

of acceptance of the client as a worthwhile individual is conveyed.

3. Secure a promise from client that she will seek out a staff member if thoughts of suicide emerge. *Suicidal clients are often very ambivalent about their feelings. Discussion of feelings with a trusted individual may provide assistance before the client experiences a crisis situation.*

4. Encourage the client to express angry feelings within appropriate limits. Provide a safe method of hostility release. Help the client to identify the source of anger, if possible. Work on adaptive coping skills for use outside the health-care system. *Depression and suicidal behaviors are sometimes viewed as anger turned inward on the self. If this anger can be verbalized in a nonthreatening environment, the client may be able to resolve these feelings, regardless of the discomfort involved.*

5. Encourage the client to discharge pent-up anger through participation in large motor activities (e.g., brisk walks, jogging, physical exercises, volleyball, punching bag, exercise bike). *Physical exercise provides a safe and effective method for discharging pent-up tension.*

6. Help the client identify stressors that precipitate anxiety and irritability and develop new methods of coping with these situations (e.g., stress reduction techniques, relaxation, and visualization skills). *Knowing stress factors and ways of handling them reduces anxiety and allows client to feel a greater measure of control over the situation.*

7. Identify the extent of feelings and situations when loss of control occurs. Assist with problem solving to identify behaviors for protection of self and others (e.g., call support person, remove self from situation). *Recognition of potential for harm to self or others and development of a plan enables the client to take effective actions to meet safety needs.*

8. Encourage the client to reduce or shift workload and social activities during the premenstrual period as part of a total stress management program. *Stress may play a role in the exacerbation of symptoms.*

9. At each visit, evaluate symptoms. Discuss those that may be most troublesome and continue to persist well after initiation of therapy. *If traditional measures are inadequate, pharmacological intervention may be required to enhance coping abilities. For example, antidepressants may be administered for depression that remains unresolved after other symptoms have been relieved.*

10. Encourage participation in a support group, psychotherapy, marital counseling, or other type of therapy as deemed necessary. *Professional assistance may be required to help the client and family members learn effective coping strategies and support lifestyle changes that may be needed.*

Outcome Criteria

1. Client participates willingly in treatment regimen and initiates necessary lifestyle changes.
2. Client demonstrates adaptive coping strategies to deal with episodes of depression and anxiety.
3. Client verbalizes that she has no suicidal thoughts or intentions.

@ INTERNET REFERENCES

Additional information related to premenstrual dysphoric disorder may be located at the following Web sites:

a. www.aafp.org/afp/1998/0701/p183.html
b. www.drdonnica.com/display.asp?article=1086
c. www.usdoctor.com/pms.htm
d. www.healthyplace.com/depression/pmdd/pmdd-premenstrual-dysphoric-disorder-symptoms-treatment/
e. http://hcp.obgyn.net/home

CHAPTER 17

Homelessness

■ BACKGROUND ASSESSMENT DATA

It is difficult to determine how many individuals are homeless in the United States. Estimates have been made at somewhere between 250,000 and 4 million.

Who Are the Homeless?

1. **Age.** Studies have produced a variety of statistics related to age of the homeless: 39% are younger than 18 years of age; individuals between the ages of 25 and 34 comprise 25%; and 6% are ages 55 to 64.
2. **Gender.** More men than women are homeless. Statistics suggest that 62% of homeless individuals are male and 38% are female (Substance Abuse and Mental Health Services Administration [SAMHSA], 2011).
3. **Families.** Families with children are among the fastest growing segments of the homeless population. They make up 33% of the homeless population, but research indicates that this number is higher in rural areas, where families, single mothers, and children account for the largest group of homeless people.
4. **Ethnicity.** The homeless population is estimated to be 37% African-American; 41% Caucasian; 10% Hispanic; 5% of other single races; and 7% of multiple races (SAMHSA, 2011). The ethnic makeup of homeless populations varies according to geographic location.

Mental Illness and Homelessness

A U.S. Conference of Mayors (USCM, 2012) survey revealed that approximately 30% of the homeless population suffers from some form of mental illness. Schizophrenia is frequently described as the most common diagnosis. Other prevalent disorders include bipolar disorder, substance addiction, depression, personality disorders, and neurocognitive disorders.

Predisposing Factors to Homelessness Among the Mentally Ill

1. **Deinstitutionalization.** Deinstitutionalization is frequently implicated as a contributing factor to homelessness among persons with mental illness. Deinstitutionalization began out of

expressed concern by mental health professionals and others who described the "deplorable conditions" under which mentally ill individuals were housed. Some individuals believed that institutionalization deprived the mentally ill of their civil rights. Not the least of the motivating factors for deinstitutionalization was the financial burden these clients placed on state governments.

2. **Poverty.** Cuts in various government entitlement programs have depleted the allotments available for individuals with severe and persistent mental illness living in the community. The job market is prohibitive for individuals whose behavior is incomprehensible or even frightening to many. The stigma and discrimination associated with mental illness may be diminishing slowly, but it is highly visible to those who suffer from its effects.

3. **A Scarcity of Affordable Housing.** The National Coalition for the Homeless (NCH, 2009) states:

   > A lack of affordable housing and the limited scale of housing assistance programs have contributed to the current housing crisis and to homelessness. The lack of affordable housing has led to high rent burdens (rents which absorb a high proportion of income), overcrowding, and substandard housing. These phenomena, in turn, have not only forced many people to become homeless; they have put a large and growing number of people at risk of becoming homeless. Recently, [a rise in the percentage of housing] foreclosures has increased the number of people who experience homelessness.

   In addition, the number of single-room-occupancy (SRO) hotels has diminished drastically. These SRO hotels provided a means of relatively inexpensive housing, and although some people believe that these facilities nurtured isolation, they provided adequate shelter from the elements for their occupants. So many individuals currently frequent the shelters of our cities that there is concern that the shelters are becoming miniinstitutions for people with serious mental illness.

4. **Lack of Affordable Health Care.** For families barely able to scrape together enough money to pay for day-to-day living, a catastrophic illness can create the level of poverty that starts the downward spiral to homelessness.

5. **Domestic Violence.** The NCH (2009) reports that domestic violence is a primary cause of homelessness, with approximately 63% of homeless women having experienced domestic violence in their adult lives. Battered women are often forced to choose between an abusive relationship and homelessness.

6. **Addiction Disorders.** For individuals with alcohol or drug addictions, in the absence of appropriate treatment, the chances increase for being forced into life on the street. The following have been cited as obstacles to addiction treatment for homeless persons: lack of health insurance, lack of documentation,

waiting lists, scheduling difficulties, daily contact requirements, lack of transportation, ineffective treatment methods, lack of supportive services, and cultural insensitivity.

Symptomatology (Commonly Associated With Homelessness)

1. Mobility and migration (the penchant for frequent movement to various geographic locations)
2. Substance abuse
3. Nutritional deficiencies
4. Difficulty with thermoregulation
5. Increased incidence of tuberculosis
6. Increased incidence of sexually transmitted diseases
7. Increased incidence of gastrointestinal (GI) and respiratory disorders
8. Among homeless children (compared with control samples), increased incidence of:
   a. Ear infections
   b. GI and respiratory disorders
   c. Infestational ailments
   d. Developmental delays
   e. Psychological problems

Common Nursing Diagnoses and Interventions

(Interventions are applicable to various health-care settings, such as inpatient and partial hospitalization, community health clinic, "street clinic," and homeless shelters.)

▓ INEFFECTIVE HEALTH MAINTENANCE

Definition: *Inability to identify, manage and/or seek out help to maintain health* (NANDA International [NANDA-I], 2012, p. 157)

Possible Etiologies ("related to")

Perceptual/cognitive impairment
Deficient communication skills
Unachieved developmental tasks
Insufficient resources (e.g., equipment, finances)
Inability to make appropriate judgments
Ineffective individual coping

Defining Characteristics ("evidenced by")

History of lack of health-seeking behavior
Impairment of personal support systems
Demonstrated lack of knowledge about basic health practices

Demonstrated lack of adaptive behaviors to environmental changes
Inability to take responsibility for meeting basic health practices

Goals/Objectives

Short-term Goal

Client will seek and receive assistance with current health matters.

Long-term Goals

1. Client will assume responsibility for own health care needs within level of ability.
2. Client will adopt lifestyle changes that support individual health care needs.

Interventions With *Selected Rationales*

1. The triage nurse in the emergency department, street clinic, or shelter will begin the biopsychosocial assessment of the homeless client. *An adequate assessment is required to ensure appropriate nursing care is provided.*
2. Assess developmental level of functioning and ability to communicate. Use language that the client can comprehend. *This information is essential to ensure that client achieves an accurate understanding of information presented and that the nurse correctly interprets what the client is attempting to convey.*
3. Assess the client's use of substances, including use of tobacco. Discuss eating and sleeping habits. *These actions may be contributing to current health problems.*
4. Assess sexual practices, *to determine level of personal risk.*
5. Assess oral hygiene practices, *to determine specific self-care needs.*
6. Assess the client's ability to make decisions. *Client may need assistance in determining the type of care that is required, how to determine the most appropriate time to seek that care, and where to go to receive it.*
7. It is important to ask the following basic questions of the homeless client:
   a. Do you understand what your problem is?
   b. How will you get your prescriptions filled?
   c. Where are you going when you leave here, or where will you sleep tonight?
   Answers to these questions at admission will initiate discharge planning for the client.
8. Teach the client the basics of self-care (e.g., proper hygiene, facts about nutrition). *The client must have this type of knowledge if he or she is to become more self-sufficient.*
9. Teach the client about safe-sex practices *in an effort to avoid sexually transmitted diseases.*

10. Identify immediate problems and assist with crisis intervention. *Emergency departments, "storefront" clinics, or shelters may be the homeless client's only resource in a crisis situation.*

11. Tend to physical needs immediately. Ensure that the client has a thorough physical examination. *The client cannot deal with psychosocial issues until physical problems have been addressed.*

12. Assess mental health status. *Many homeless individuals have some form of mental illness.* Ensure that appropriate psychiatric care is provided. If possible, inquire about possible long-acting medication injections for the client. *The client may be less likely to discontinue the medication if he or she does not have to take pills every day.*

13. Refer the client to others who can provide assistance (e.g., case manager, social worker). *If the client is to be discharged to a shelter, a case manager or social worker may be the best link between the client and the health-care system to ensure that he or she obtains appropriate follow-up care.*

Outcome Criteria

1. Client verbalizes understanding of information presented regarding optimal health maintenance.
2. Client is able to verbalize signs and symptoms that should be reported to a health care professional.
3. Client verbalizes knowledge of available resources from which he or she may seek assistance as required.

■ POWERLESSNESS

Definition: *The lived experience of lack of control over a situation, including a perception that one's actions do not significantly affect an outcome* (NANDA-I, 2012, p. 370)

Possible Etiologies ("related to")

[Lifestyle of helplessness]
[Homelessness]

Defining Characteristics ("evidenced by")

Reports lack of control (e.g., over self-care, situation, outcome)
[Apathy]
[Inadequate coping patterns]

Goals/Objectives

Short-term Goal

Client will identify areas over which he or she has control.

Long-term Goal

Client will make decisions that reflect control over present situation and future outcome.

Interventions With *Selected Rationales*

1. Provide opportunities for the client to make choices about his or her present situation. *Providing client with choices will increase his or her feeling of control.*
2. Avoid arguing or using logic with the client who feels powerless. *Client will not believe it can make a difference.*
3. Accept expressions of feelings, including anger and hopelessness. *An attitude of acceptance enhances feelings of trust and self-worth.*
4. Help the client identify personal strengths and establish realistic life goals. *Unrealistic goals set the client up for failure and reinforce feelings of powerlessness.*
5. Help the client identify areas of life situation that he or she can control. *Client's emotional condition interferes with his or her ability to solve problems. Assistance is required to accurately perceive the benefits and consequences of available alternatives.*
6. Help the client identify areas of life situation that are not within his or her ability to control. Encourage verbalization of feelings related to this inability *in an effort to deal with unresolved issues and accept what cannot be changed.*
7. Encourage the client to seek out a support group or shelter resources. *Social isolation promotes feelings of powerlessness and hopelessness.*

Outcome Criteria

1. Client verbalizes choices made in a plan to maintain control over his or her life situation.
2. Client verbalizes honest feelings about life situations over which he or she has no control.
3. Client is able to verbalize a system for problem solving as required to maintain hope for the future.

@ INTERNET REFERENCES

Additional information related to homelessness may be located at the following Web sites:

a. www.nationalhomeless.org
b. www.endhomelessness.org
c. http://portal.hud.gov/portal/page/portal/HUD/topics/homelessness
d. www.hhs.gov/homeless

e. http://homeless.samhsa.gov/Default.aspx
f. http://www.americanbar.org/groups/public_services/homelessness_poverty.html

Movie Connections

The Soloist • *The Grapes of Wrath* • *Generosity* • *The Redemption*

CHAPTER 18

Psychiatric Home Nursing Care

■ BACKGROUND ASSESSMENT DATA

Dramatic changes in the health-care delivery system and skyrocketing costs have created a need to find a way to provide quality, cost-effective care to psychiatric clients. Home care has become one of the fastest growing areas in the health-care system and is now recognized by many reimbursement agencies as a preferred method of community-based service. Just what is home health care? The American Nurses Association (ANA, 2008) contributes the following definition:

> Home health nursing is nursing practice applied to patients of all ages in the patients' residences, which may include private homes, assisted living, or personal care facilities. Patients and their families and other caregivers are the focus of home health nursing practice. The goal of care is to maintain or improve the quality of life for patients and the families and other caregivers, or to support patients in their transition to end of life (p. 3).

The psychiatric home-care nurse must have knowledge and skills to meet both the physical and psychosocial needs of the homebound client. Serving health-care consumers in their home environment charges the nurse with the responsibility of providing holistic care.

Predisposing Factors

An increase in psychiatric home care may be associated with the following factors:
1. Earlier hospital discharges
2. Increased demand for home care as an alternative to institutional care
3. Broader third-party payment coverage
4. Greater physician acceptance of home care
5. The increasing need to contain health-care costs and the growth of managed care

Psychiatric home nursing care is provided through private home health agencies; private hospitals; public hospitals; government institutions, such as the Veterans Administration; and community mental health centers. Most often, home care is viewed as follow-up care to inpatient, partial, or outpatient hospitalization. The majority of home health care is paid for by Medicare. Other sources include Medicaid, private insurance, self-pay, and others. An acute psychiatric diagnosis is not enough to qualify for the service. The client must show that he or she is unable to leave the home without considerable difficulty or the assistance of another person. The plan of treatment and subsequent charting must explain why the client's psychiatric disorder keeps him or her at home and justify the need for home services. Home care must be prescribed by a physician.

Although Medicare and Medicaid are the largest reimbursement providers, a growing number of health maintenance organizations (HMOs) and preferred provider organizations (PPOs) are recognizing the cost effectiveness of psychiatric home nursing care and are including it as part of their benefit packages. Most managed care agencies require that treatment, or even a specific number of visits, be preauthorized for psychiatric home nursing care. The plan of treatment and subsequent charting must explain why the client's psychiatric disorder keeps him or her at home and justify the need for services.

Symptomatology (Subjective and Objective Data)

Homebound psychiatric clients most often have a diagnosis of depressive disorder, neurocognitive disorder, anxiety disorder, bipolar disorder, or schizophrenia. Psychiatric nurses also provide consultation for clients with primary medical disorders. Many elderly clients are homebound because of medical conditions that impair mobility and necessitate home care. Psychiatric nurses may provide the following types of home nursing care:

- To clients with primary psychiatric diagnoses, the symptoms of which are immobilizing, and the client and family require assistance with management of the symptoms
- To clients who are homebound for medical conditions but have a psychiatric condition for which they have been receiving (and continue to need ongoing) treatment
- To clients who are homebound with medical conditions and who may develop serious psychiatric symptoms in response to their medical illness

Table 18-1 identifies some of the conditions for which a psychiatric nursing home-care consultation may be sought.

The following components should be included in the comprehensive assessment of the homebound client:

1. Client's perception of the problem and need for assistance
2. Information regarding client's strengths and personal habits
3. Health history, review of systems, and vital signs

TABLE 18–1	**Conditions that Warrant Psychiatric Nursing Consultation**

- When a client has a new psychiatric diagnosis
- When a new psychotropic medication has been added to the regimen
- When the client's mental status exacerbates or causes deterioration in his or her medical condition
- When the client is suspected of abusing alcohol or drugs
- When a client is expressing suicidal ideation
- When a client is noncompliant with psychotropic medication
- When a client develops a fundamental change in mood or a thought disorder
- When a client is immobilized by severe depression or anxiety

Source: Adapted from Schroeder, 2013.

4. Any recent changes (physical, psychosocial, environmental)
5. Availability of support systems
6. Current medication regimen (including client's understanding about the medications and reason for taking)
7. Nutritional and elimination assessment
8. Activities of daily living (ADLs) assessment
9. Substance use assessment
10. Neurological assessment
11. Mental status examination (see Appendices K and M)

Other important assessments include information about acute or chronic medical conditions, patterns of sleep and rest, solitude and social interaction, use of leisure time, education and work history, issues related to religion or spirituality, and adequacy of the home environment.

Nursing Diagnoses and Interventions Common to Psychiatric Homebound Clients

■ INEFFECTIVE SELF-HEALTH MANAGEMENT

Definition: *Pattern of regulating and integrating into daily living a therapeutic regime for treatment of illness and its sequelae that is unsatisfactory for meeting specific health goals* (NANDA-I, 2012, p. 161)

Possible Etiologies ("related to")

Perceived barriers
Social support deficit
Powerlessness
Perceived benefits
[Mistrust of regimen and/or health-care personnel]

Deficient knowledge
Complexity of therapeutic regimen

Defining Characteristics ("evidenced by")

Ineffective choices in daily living for meeting health goals
Failure to include treatment regimens in daily living
Failure to take action to reduce risk factors
Reports difficulty with prescribed regimens
Reports desire to manage the illness

Goals/Objectives

Short-term Goals

1. Client will verbalize understanding of barriers to self-health management.
2. Client will participate in problem-solving efforts toward adequate self-health management.

Long-term Goal

Client will incorporate changes in lifestyle necessary to maintain effective self-health management.

Interventions With *Selected Rationales*

1. Assess the client's knowledge of condition and treatment needs. ***Client may lack full comprehension of need for treatment regimen.***
2. Identify the client's perception of treatment regimen. ***Client may be mistrustful of treatment regimen or of health-care system in general.***
3. ***Promote a trusting relationship with the client*** by being honest, encouraging client to participate in decision making, and conveying genuine positive regard.
4. Assist the client in recognizing strengths and past successes. ***Recognition of strengths and past successes increases self-esteem and indicates to client that he or she can be successful in managing therapeutic regimen.***
5. Provide positive reinforcement for efforts. ***Positive reinforcement increases self-esteem and encourages repetition of desirable behaviors.***
6. Emphasize importance of need for treatment and/or medication. ***Client must understand that the consequence of lack of follow-through is possible decompensation.***
7. ***In an effort to incorporate lifestyle changes and promote wellness,*** help the client develop plans for managing therapeutic regimen, such as attending support groups, integration in social and family systems, and seeking financial assistance.

Outcome Criteria

1. Client verbalizes understanding of information presented regarding management of therapeutic regimen.
2. Client demonstrates desire and ability to perform strategies necessary to maintain adequate management of therapeutic regimen.
3. Client verbalizes knowledge of available resources from which he or she may seek assistance as required.

■ RISK-PRONE HEALTH BEHAVIOR

Definition: *Impaired ability to modify lifestyle/behaviors in a manner that improves health status* (NANDA-I, 2012, p. 155)

Possible Etiologies ("related to")

Inadequate comprehension
Inadequate social support
Low self-efficacy
Low socioeconomic status
Multiple stressors
Negative attitude toward health care
[Intense emotional state]

Defining Characteristics ("evidenced by")

Demonstrates nonacceptance of health status change
Failure to achieve optimal sense of control
Failure to take action that prevents health problems
Minimizes health status change

Goals/Objectives

Short-term Goals

1. Client will discuss with home health nurse the kinds of lifestyle changes that will occur because of the change in health status.
2. With the help of home health nurse, client will formulate a plan of action for incorporating those changes into his or her lifestyle.
3. Client will demonstrate movement toward independence, considering change in health status.

Long-term Goal

Client will demonstrate competence to function independently to his or her optimal ability, considering change in health status, by time of discharge from home health care.

Interventions With *Selected Rationales*

1. Encourage the client to talk about lifestyle prior to the change in health status. Discuss coping mechanisms that were used at stressful times in the past. *It is important to identify the client's strengths so that they may be used to facilitate adaptation to the change or loss that has occurred.*

2. Encourage the client to discuss the change or loss and particularly to express anger associated with it. *Some individuals may not realize that anger is a normal stage in the grieving process. If it is not released in an appropriate manner, it may be turned inward on the self, leading to pathological depression.*

3. Encourage the client to express fears associated with the change or loss or alteration in lifestyle that the change or loss has created. *Change often creates a feeling of disequilibrium and the individual may respond with fears that are irrational or unfounded. He or she may benefit from feedback that corrects misperceptions about how life will be with the change in health status.*

4. Provide assistance with ADLs as required, but encourage independence to the limit that the client's ability will allow. Give positive feedback for activities accomplished independently. *Independent accomplishments and positive feedback enhance self-esteem and encourage repetition of desired behaviors. Successes also provide hope that adaptive functioning is possible and decrease feelings of powerlessness.*

5. Help the client with decision making regarding incorporation of the change or loss into his or her lifestyle. Identify problems that the change or loss is likely to create. Discuss alternative solutions, weighing potential benefits and consequences of each alternative. Support the client's decision in the selection of an alternative. *The great amount of anxiety that usually accompanies a major lifestyle change often interferes with an individual's ability to solve problems and to make appropriate decisions. Client may need assistance with this process in an effort to progress toward successful adaptation.*

6. Use role playing *to decrease anxiety* as the client anticipates stressful situations that might occur in relation to the health status change. *Role playing decreases anxiety and provides a feeling of security by arming the client with a plan of action with which to respond in an appropriate manner when a stressful situation occurs.*

7. Ensure that the client and family are fully knowledgeable regarding the physiology of the change in health status and its necessity for optimal wellness. Encourage them to ask questions, and provide printed material explaining the change to which they may refer following discharge.

8. Help the client identify resources within the community from which he or she may seek assistance in adapting to the change in

health status. Examples include self-help or support groups, counselor, or social worker. Encourage the client to keep follow-up appointments with the physician or to call the physician's office prior to follow-up date if problems or concerns arise.

Outcome Criteria

1. Client is able to perform ADLs independently.
2. Client is able to make independent decisions regarding lifestyle considering the change in health status.
3. Client is able to express hope for the future with consideration of change in health status.

■ SOCIAL ISOLATION

Definition: *Aloneness experienced by the individual and perceived as imposed by others and as a negative or threatening state* (NANDA-I, 2012, p. 480)

Possible Etiologies ("related to")

Alterations in mental status
Inability to engage in satisfying personal relationships
Unaccepted social values
Unaccepted social behavior
Inadequate personal resources
Immature interests
Alterations in physical appearance
Altered state of wellness

Defining Characteristics ("evidenced by")

Reports feelings of aloneness imposed by others
Reports feelings of rejection
Developmentally inappropriate interests
Inability to meet expectations of others
Insecurity in public
Absence of supportive significant other(s)
Projects hostility
Withdrawn; uncommunicative
Seeks to be alone
Preoccupation with own thoughts
Sad, dull affect

Goals/Objectives

Short-term Goal
Client will verbalize willingness to be involved with others.

Long-term Goal

Client will participate in interactions with others at level of ability or desire.

Interventions With *Selected Rationales*

1. Convey an accepting attitude by making regular visits. *An accepting attitude increases feelings of self-worth and facilitates trust.*
2. Show unconditional positive regard. *This conveys your belief in the client as a worthwhile human being.*
3. Be honest and keep all promises. *Honesty and dependability promote a trusting relationship.*
4. Be cautious with touch until trust has been established. *A suspicious client may perceive touch as a threatening gesture.*
5. Be with the client to offer support during activities that may be frightening or difficult for him or her. *The presence of a trusted individual provides emotional security for the client.*
6. Take walks with the client. Help him or her perform simple tasks around the house. *Increased activity enhances both physical and mental status.*
7. Assess lifelong patterns of relationships. *Basic personality characteristics will not change. Most individuals keep the same style of relationship development that they had in the past.*
8. Help the client identify present relationships that are satisfying and activities that he or she considers interesting. *Only the client knows what he or she truly likes, and these personal preferences will facilitate success in reversing social isolation.*
9. Consider the feasibility of a pet. *There are many documented studies of the benefits of companion animals.*

Outcome Criteria

1. Client demonstrates willingness and desire to socialize with others.
2. Client independently pursues social activities with others.

■ RISK FOR CAREGIVER ROLE STRAIN

Definition: *At risk for caregiver vulnerability for felt difficulty in performing the family caregiver role (NANDA-I, 2012, p. 301)*

Risk Factors

Caregiver not developmentally ready for caregiver role
Inadequate physical environment for providing care (e.g., housing, transportation, community services, equipment)
Unpredictable illness course or instability in the care receiver's health

Psychological or cognitive problems in care receiver
Presence of abuse or violence
Past history of poor relationship between caregiver and care receiver
Marginal caregiver's coping patterns
Lack of respite and recreation for caregiver
Substance abuse or codependency
Caregiver's competing role commitments
Illness severity of the care receiver
Duration of caregiving required
Family/caregiver isolation

Goals/Objectives

Short-term Goal

Caregivers will verbalize understanding of ways to facilitate the caregiver role.

Long-term Goal

Caregivers will demonstrate effective problem-solving skills and develop adaptive coping mechanisms to regain equilibrium.

Interventions With *Selected Rationales*

1. Assess caregivers' abilities to anticipate and fulfill client's unmet needs. Provide information to assist caregivers with this responsibility. Ensure that caregivers encourage client to be as independent as possible. *Caregivers may be unaware of what the client can realistically accomplish. They may be unaware of the nature of the illness.*
2. Ensure that caregivers are aware of available community support systems from which they can seek assistance when required. Examples include respite care services, day treatment centers, and adult day-care centers. *Caregivers require relief from the pressures and strain of providing 24-hour care for their loved one. Studies have shown that abuse arises out of caregiving situations that place overwhelming stress on the caregivers.*
3. Encourage caregivers to express feelings, particularly anger. *Release of these emotions can serve to prevent psychopathology, such as depression or psychophysiological disorders, from occurring.*
4. Encourage participation in support groups composed of members with similar life situations. Provide information about support groups that may be helpful:
   a. National Alliance on Mental Illness—(800) 950-NAMI
   b. American Association on Intellectual and Developmental Disabilities—(202) 387-1968
   c. Alzheimer's Association—(800) 272-3900

Hearing others who are experiencing the same problems discuss ways in which they have coped may help the caregiver adopt more adaptive strategies. Individuals who are experiencing similar life situations provide empathy and support for each other.

Outcome Criteria

1. Caregivers are able to solve problems effectively regarding care of the client.
2. Caregivers demonstrate adaptive coping strategies for dealing with stress of the caregiver role.
3. Caregivers openly express feelings.
4. Caregivers express desire to join a support group of other caregivers.

@ INTERNET REFERENCES

Additional information related to psychiatric home nursing care may be located at the following Web sites:

a. www.cms.gov
b. www.nahc.org
c. www.aahomecare.org

CHAPTER 19

Forensic Nursing

■ BACKGROUND ASSESSMENT DATA

The International Association of Forensic Nurses (IAFN) and the American Nurses Association (ANA) (2009) have defined forensic nursing as "the practice of nursing globally when health and legal systems intersect" (ANA, 2009, p. 3).

Bellfield and Catalano (2012) offer the following:

> Forensic nursing is an emerging field that forms an alliance between nursing, law enforcement, and the forensic sciences. The term *forensic* means anything belonging to, or pertaining to, the law. Forensic nurses provide a continuum of care to victims and their families beginning in the emergency room or crime scene and leading to participation in the criminal investigation and the courts of law (p. 450).

Constantino, Crane, and Young (2013) state:

> Forensic nursing is defined as the application of forensic science, biopsychosocial knowledge, and clinical nursing skills in the scientific investigation, collection, preservation, analysis, and examination of evidence (p. vii).

Areas of forensic nursing include:
1. Clinical Forensic Nursing
2. The Sexual Assault Nurse Examiner (SANE)
3. Forensic Mental Health Nursing
4. Forensic Correctional Nursing
5. Legal Nurse Consultant
6. Forensic Nurse Death Investigator
7. Nurses in General Practice

Clinical Forensic Nursing in Trauma Care

Assessment

Forensic nurse examiners (FNEs) are included as valuable members of trauma units in many emergency departments. They are specifically trained to perform sexual assault examinations, conduct formal assessments for abuse and neglect, and provide other services such as forensic photography, wound identification, evidence collection, and expert testimony (Dougherty, 2011). All traumatic injuries in which liability is suspected are considered within the scope of forensic nursing. Reports to legal agencies are required to ensure follow-up investigation; however, the protection of clients' rights remains a nursing priority.

Several areas of assessment in which the clinical forensic nurse specialist in trauma care may become involved include:

1. **Preservation of Evidence.** Evidence from both crime-related and self-inflicted traumas must be safeguarded in a manner consistent with the investigation. Evidence such as clothing, bullets, blood stains, hairs, fibers and small pieces of material such as fragments of metal, glass, paint, and wood should be saved and documented in all medical accident instances that have legal implications.

2. **Investigation of Wound Characteristics.** Wounds that the nurse must be able to identify include:
   a. *Sharp-Force Injuries:* Sharp force injuries including stab wounds and other wounds resulting from penetration with a sharp object.
   b. *Blunt-Force Injuries:* Includes cuts and bruises resulting from the impact of a blunt object against the body.
   c. *Dicing Injuries:* Multiple, minute cuts and abrasions caused by contact with shattered glass (e.g., often occur in motor vehicle accidents).
   d. *Patterned Injuries:* Specific injuries that reflect the pattern of the weapon used to inflict the injury.
   e. *Bite-Mark Injuries:* A type of patterned injury inflicted by human or animal.
   f. *Defense Wounds:* Injuries that reflect the victim's attempt to defend him- or herself from attack.
   g. *Hesitation Wounds:* Usually superficial, sharp-force wounds; often found perpendicular to the lower part of the body and may reflect self-inflicted wounds.
   h. *Fast-Force Injuries:* Usually gunshot wounds; may reflect various patterns of injury.

3. **Deaths in the Emergency Department.** When deaths occur in the emergency department as a result of abuse or accident, evidence must be retained, the death must be reported to legal authorities, and an investigation is conducted. It is therefore essential that the nurse carefully document the appearance, condition, and behavior of the victim upon arrival at the hospital. The information gathered from the client and family (or others accompanying the client) may serve to facilitate the postmortem investigation and may be used during criminal justice proceedings.

The critical factor is to be able to determine if the cause of death is natural or unnatural. *Natural* deaths occur because of disease pathology of the internal organs or the degenerative aging process (Lynch & Koehler, 2011). In the emergency department, most deaths are sudden and unexpected. Those that are considered natural most commonly involve the cardiovascular, respiratory, and central nervous systems. Deaths that are considered *unnatural* include those from trauma, from self-inflicted acts, or from injuries inflicted by another. Legal authorities must be notified of all deaths related to unnatural circumstances.

Common Nursing Diagnoses and Interventions
(For Forensic Nursing in Trauma Care)

■ POST-TRAUMA SYNDROME/RAPE-TRAUMA SYNDROME

Definition: Post-trauma syndrome is defined as *sustained maladaptive response to a traumatic, overwhelming event* (NANDA International, [NANDA-I], 2012, p. 335). Rape-trauma syndrome is defined as *sustained maladaptive response to a forced, violent sexual penetration against the victim's will and consent* (NANDA-I, 2012, p. 337).

Possible Etiologies ("related to")

Physical and/or psychosocial abuse
Tragic occurrence involving multiple deaths
Sudden destruction of one's home or community
Epidemics
Disasters
Serious accidents (e.g., industrial, motor vehicle)
Witnessing mutilation, violent death, [or other horrors]
Serious threat or injury to self or loved ones
Rape

Defining Characteristics ("evidenced by")

[Physical injuries related to trauma]
Avoidance
Repression
Difficulty concentrating
Grieving; guilt
Intrusive thoughts
Neurosensory irritability
Palpitations
Anger and/or rage; aggression
Intrusive dreams; nightmares; flashbacks
Panic attacks; fear
Gastric irritability
Psychogenic amnesia
Substance abuse

Goals/Objectives

Short-term Goals

1. The client's physical wounds will heal without complication.
2. The client will begin a healthy grief resolution, initiating the process of psychological healing.

Long-term Goal

The client will demonstrate ability to deal with emotional reactions in an individually appropriate manner.

Interventions With *Selected Rationales*

1. It is important to communicate the following to the victim of sexual assault:
   a. You are safe here.
   b. I'm sorry that it happened.
   c. I am very glad you survived.
   d. It is not your fault. No one deserves to be treated this way.
   e. You did the best that you could.
   The woman who has been sexually assaulted fears for her life and must be reassured of her safety. She may also be overwhelmed with self-doubt and self-blame, and these statements instill trust and validate self-worth.

2. Explain every assessment procedure that will be conducted and why it is being conducted. Ensure that data collection is conducted in a caring, nonjudgmental manner *to decrease fear and anxiety and increase trust.*

3. Ledray (2009) suggests the following five essential components of a forensic examination of the sexual assault survivor in the emergency department:
   a. *Treatment and documentation injuries.* Samples of blood, semen, hair, and fingernail scrapings should be sealed in paper—not plastic—bags *to prevent the possible growth of mildew from accumulation of moisture inside the plastic container and the subsequent contamination of the evidence.*
   b. *Maintaining the proper chain of evidence.* Samples must be properly labeled, sealed, and refrigerated when necessary and kept under observation or properly locked until rendered to the proper legal authority *in order to ensure the proper chain of evidence and freshness of the samples.*
   c. *Treatment and evaluation of sexually transmitted diseases (STDs).* If conducted within 72 hours of the attack, several tests and interventions are available for prophylactic treatment of certain STDs.
   d. *Pregnancy risk evaluation and prevention.* Prophylactic regimens, such as the postcoital progestin-only contraceptive (Plan B One-Step; Next Choice), significantly reduce the

risk of pregnancy, especially when administered within the first 24 hours. The effectiveness decreases as the time between the assault and the first dose increases.

  e. *Crisis intervention and arrangements for follow-up counseling.* **Because a survivor is often too ashamed or fearful to seek follow-up counseling,** it may be important for the nurse to obtain the individual's permission to allow a counselor to call her to make a follow-up appointment.

4. In the case of other types of trauma (e.g., gunshot victims; automobile/pedestrian hit-and-run victims), ***ensure that any possible evidence is not lost.*** Clothing that is removed from a victim should not be shaken, and each separate item of clothing should be placed carefully in a paper bag, which should be sealed, dated, timed, and signed.

5. Ensure that the client has adequate privacy for all immediate postcrisis interventions. Try to have as few people as possible providing the immediate care or collecting immediate evidence. ***The posttrauma client is extremely vulnerable. Additional people in the environment may increase this feeling of vulnerability and escalate anxiety.***

6. Encourage the client to give an account of the trauma/assault. Listen, but do not probe. ***Nonjudgmental listening provides an opportunity for catharsis that the client needs to begin healing. A detailed account may be required for legal follow-up, and a caring nurse, as client advocate, may help to lessen the trauma of evidence collection.***

7. Discuss with the client whom to call for support or assistance. Provide information about referrals for aftercare. ***Because of severe anxiety and fear, the client may need assistance from others during this immediate postcrisis period. Provide referral information in writing for later reference (e.g., psychotherapist, mental health clinic, community advocacy group).***

8. In the event of a sudden and unexpected death in the trauma care setting, the clinical forensic nurse may be called upon to present information associated with an anatomical donation request to the survivors. ***The clinical forensic nurse specialist is an expert in legal issues and has the knowledge and sensitivity to provide coordination between the medical examiner and families who are grieving the loss of loved ones.***

Outcome Criteria

1. The client is no longer experiencing panic anxiety.
2. The client demonstrates a degree of trust in the primary nurse.
3. The client has received immediate attention to physical injuries.
4. The client has initiated behaviors consistent with the grief response.
5. Necessary evidence has been collected and preserved in order to proceed appropriately within the legal system.

Forensic Mental Health Nursing in Correctional Facilities

Assessment

It was believed that deinstitutionalization increased the freedom of mentally ill individuals in accordance with the principle of "least restrictive alternative." However, because of inadequate community-based services, many of these individuals drift into poverty and homelessness, increasing their vulnerability to criminalization. Because the bizarre behavior of mentally ill individuals living on the street is sometimes offensive to community standards, law enforcement officials have the authority to protect the welfare of the public, as well as the safety of the individual, by initiating emergency hospitalization. However, legal criteria for commitment are so stringent in most cases, that arrest becomes an easier way of getting the mentally ill person off the street if a criminal statute has been violated. According to the Bureau of Justice, more than half of all prison and jail inmates have some form of mental health problem (James & Glaze, 2006). Some of these individuals are incarcerated as a result of the increasingly popular "guilty but mentally ill" verdict. With this verdict, individuals are deemed mentally ill, yet are held criminally responsible for their actions. The individual is incarcerated and receives special treatment, if needed, but it is no different from that available for and needed by any prisoner.

Psychiatric diagnoses commonly identified at the time of incarceration include schizophrenia, bipolar disorder, major depression, personality disorders, and substance use disorders, and many have dual diagnoses. Common psychiatric behaviors include hallucinations, suspiciousness, thought disorders, anger/agitation, and impulsivity. Denial of problems is a common behavior among this population. Use of substances and nonadherence to medication regimen are common obstacles to rehabilitation. Substance abuse has been shown to have a strong correlation with recidivism among the prison population. Many individuals report that they were under the influence of substances at the time of their criminal actions. Detoxification frequency occurs in jails and prisons, and some inmates have died from the withdrawal syndrome because of inadequate treatment during this process.

Common Nursing Diagnoses and Interventions
(For Forensic Nursing in Correctional Facilities)

■ DEFENSIVE COPING

Definition: *Repeated projection of falsely positive self-evaluation based on a self-protective pattern that defends against underlying perceived threats to positive self-regard* (NANDA-I, 2012, p. 346)

Possible Etiologies ("related to")

Low level of self-confidence
[Retarded ego development]
[Underdeveloped superego]
[Negative role models]
[Lack of positive feedback]
[Absent, erratic, or inconsistent methods of discipline]
[Dysfunctional family system]

Defining Characteristics ("evidenced by")

Denial of obvious problems or weaknesses
Projection of blame or responsibility
Rationalization of failures
Hypersensitivity to criticism
Grandiosity
Superior attitude toward others
Difficulty establishing or maintaining relationships
Hostile laughter or ridicule of others
Difficulty in perception of reality testing
Lack of follow-through or participation in treatment or therapy

Goals/Objectives

Short-term Goal

Client will verbalize personal responsibility for own actions, successes, and failures.

Long-term Goal

Client will demonstrate ability to interact with others and adapt to lifestyle goals without becoming defensive, rationalizing behaviors, or expressing grandiose ideas.

Interventions With *Selected Rationales*

1. Recognize and support basic ego strengths. *Focusing on positive aspects of the personality may help to improve self-concept.*
2. Encourage the client to recognize and verbalize feelings of inadequacy and need for acceptance from others and how these feelings provoke defensive behaviors, such as blaming others for own behaviors. *Recognition of the problem is the first step in the change process toward resolution.*
3. Provide immediate, matter-of-fact, nonthreatening feedback for unacceptable behaviors. *Client may lack knowledge about how he or she is being perceived by others. Direct the behavior in a nonthreatening manner to a more acceptable behavior.*
4. Help the client identify situations that provoke defensiveness and practice more appropriate responses through role playing.

Role playing provides confidence to deal with difficult situations when they actually occur.

5. Provide immediate positive feedback for acceptable behaviors. *Positive feedback enhances self-esteem and encourages repetition of desirable behaviors.*

6. Help the client set realistic, concrete goals and determine appropriate actions to meet those goals. *Success increases self-esteem.*

7. Evaluate with the client the effectiveness of the new behaviors and discuss any modifications for improvement. *Because of limited problem-solving ability, assistance may be required to reassess and develop new strategies, in the event that certain of the new coping methods prove ineffective.*

8. Use confrontation judiciously *to help client begin to identify defense mechanisms (e.g., denial and projection) that are hindering development of satisfying relationships and adaptive behaviors.*

Outcome Criteria

1. Client verbalizes and accepts responsibility for own behavior.
2. Client verbalizes correlation between feelings of inadequacy and the need to defend the ego through rationalization and grandiosity.
3. Client does not ridicule or criticize others.
4. Client interacts with others in group situations without taking a defensive stance.

■ COMPLICATED GRIEVING

Definition: *A disorder that occurs after the death of a significant other [or any other loss of significance to the individual], in which the experience of distress accompanying bereavement fails to follow normative expectations and manifests in functional impairment* (NANDA-I, 2012, p. 365)

Possible Etiologies ("related to")

[Loss of freedom]

Defining Characteristics ("evidenced by")

[Anger]
[Internalized rage]
Depression
[Labile affect]
[Suicidal ideation]
[Difficulty expressing feelings]
[Altered activities of daily living]
[Prolonged difficulty coping]

Goals/Objectives

Short-term Goal

Client will verbalize feelings of grief related to loss of freedom.

Long-term Goal

Client will progress satisfactorily through the grieving process.

Interventions With *Selected Rationales*

1. Convey an accepting attitude—one that creates a nonthreatening environment for the client to express feelings. Be honest and keep all promises. *An accepting attitude conveys to the client that you believe he or she is a worthwhile person. Trust is enhanced.*

2. Identify the function that anger, frustration, and rage serve for the client. Allow the client to express these feelings within reason. *Verbalization of feelings in a nonthreatening environment may help the client come to terms with unresolved grief.*

3. Encourage the client to discharge pent-up anger through participation in large motor activities (e.g., physical exercises, volleyball, punching bag). *Physical exercise provides a safe and effective method for discharging pent-up tension.*

4. Anger may be displaced onto the nurse or therapist, and caution must be taken to guard against the negative effects of countertransference. These are very difficult clients who have the capacity for eliciting a whole array of negative feelings from the therapist. These feelings must be acknowledged but not allowed to interfere with the therapeutic process.

5. Explain the behaviors associated with the normal grieving process. Help the client to recognize his or her position in this process. *This knowledge about normal grieving may help facilitate the client's progression toward resolution of grief.*

6. Help the client understand appropriate ways to express anger. Give positive reinforcement for behaviors used to express anger appropriately. Act as a role model. *Positive reinforcement enhances self-esteem and encourages repetition of desirable behaviors. It is appropriate to let the client know when he or she has done something that has generated angry feelings in you. Role modeling ways to express anger in an appropriate manner is a powerful learning tool.*

7. Set limits on acting-out behaviors and explain consequences of violation of those limits. Be supportive, yet consistent and firm in working with this client. *Client lacks sufficient self-control to limit maladaptive behaviors; therefore, assistance is required from staff. Without consistency on the part of all staff members working with the client, a positive outcome will not be achieved.*

8. Provide a safe and protective environment for the client against risk of self-directed violence. ***Depression is the emotion that most commonly precedes suicidal attempts.***

Outcome Criteria

1. Client is able to verbalize ways in which anger and acting-out behaviors are associated with maladaptive grieving.
2. Client expresses anger and hostility outwardly in a safe and acceptable manner.
3. Client has not harmed self or others.

■ RISK FOR INJURY

Definition: *At risk for injury as a result of [internal or external] environmental conditions interacting with the individual's adaptive and defensive resources* (NANDA-I, 2012, p. 430)

Risk Factors ("related to")

[Substance use/detoxification at time of incarceration, exhibiting any of the following:
  Substance intoxication
  Substance withdrawal
  Disorientation
  Seizures
  Hallucinations
  Psychomotor agitation
  Unstable vital signs
  Delirium
  Flashbacks
  Panic level of anxiety]

Goals/Objectives

Short-term Goal
Client's condition will stabilize within 72 hours.

Long-term Goal
Client will not experience physical injury.

Interventions With *Selected Rationales*

1. Assess the client's level of disorientation to determine specific requirements for safety. ***Knowledge of the client's level of functioning is necessary to formulate an appropriate plan of care.***
2. Obtain a drug history, if possible, to determine:
   a. Type of substance(s) used.

   b. Time of last ingestion and amount consumed.
   c. Duration and frequency of consumption.
   d. Amount consumed on a daily basis.
3. Obtain a urine sample for laboratory analysis of substance content. *Subjective history often is not accurate. Knowledge regarding substance ingestion is important for accurate assessment of client condition.*
4. Place the client in a quiet room, if possible. *Excessive stimuli increase client agitation.*
5. Institute necessary safety precautions. *Client safety is a nursing priority.*
   a. Observe client behaviors frequently; assign staff on a one-to-one basis if condition warrants it; accompany and assist the client when ambulating; use a wheelchair for transporting long distances.
   b. Be sure that side rails are up when the client is in bed.
   c. Pad headboard and side rails of bed with thick towels to protect client in case of a seizure.
   d. Use mechanical restraints as necessary to protect the client if excessive hyperactivity accompanies the disorientation.
6. Ensure that smoking materials and other potentially harmful objects are stored outside the client's access. *Client may harm self or others in disoriented, confused state.*
7. Monitor vital signs every 15 minutes initially and less frequently as acute symptoms subside. *Vital signs provide the most reliable information regarding the client's condition and need for medication during the acute detoxification period.*
8. Follow medication regimen, as ordered by the physician. Common medical interventions for detoxification from substances include the following:
   a. **Alcohol.** Benzodiazepines are the most widely used group of drugs for substitution therapy in alcohol withdrawal. The approach to treatment is to start with relatively high doses and reduce the dosage by 20% to 25% each day until withdrawal is complete. In clients with liver disease, accumulation of the longer-acting agents, such as chlordiazepoxide (Librium), may be problematic, and the use of the shorter-acting benzodiazepine, oxazepam (Serax), is more appropriate. Some physicians may order anticonvulsant medication to be used prophylactically; however, this is not a universal intervention. Multivitamin therapy, in combination with daily thiamine (either orally or by injection), is common protocol.
   b. **Opioids.** Narcotic antagonists, such as naloxone (Narcan), naltrexone (ReVia), or nalmefene (Revex), are administered for opioid intoxication. Withdrawal is managed with rest and nutritional therapy. Substitution therapy may be instituted

with methadone (Dolophine) to decrease withdrawal symptoms. In October 2002, the FDA approved two forms of the drug buprenorphine for treating opiate dependence. Buprenorphine is less powerful than methadone but is considered to be somewhat safer and causes fewer side effects, making it especially attractive for clients who are mildly or moderately addicted.

c. **Depressants.** Substitution therapy may be instituted to decrease withdrawal symptoms using a long-acting barbiturate, such as phenobarbital (Luminal). Some physicians prescribe oxazepam (Serax) as needed for objective symptoms, gradually decreasing the dosage until the drug is discontinued. Long-acting benzodiazepines are commonly used for substitution therapy when the abused substance is a nonbarbiturate CNS depressant.

d. **Stimulants.** Treatment of stimulant intoxication is geared toward stabilization of vital signs. Intravenous antihypertensives may be used, along with intravenous diazepam (Valium) to control seizures. Minor tranquilizers, such as chlordiazepoxide, may be administered orally for the first few days while the client is "crashing." Treatment is aimed at reducing drug craving and managing severe depression. Suicide precautions may be required. Therapy with antidepressant medication is not uncommon.

e. **Hallucinogens and Cannabinoids.** Medications are normally not prescribed for withdrawal from these substances. However, in the event of overdose or the occurrence of adverse reactions (e.g., anxiety or panic), benzodiazepines (e.g., diazepam or chlordiazepoxide) may be given as needed to decrease agitation. Should psychotic reactions occur, they may be treated with antipsychotics.

Outcome Criteria

1. Client is no longer exhibiting any signs or symptoms of substance intoxication or withdrawal.
2. Client shows no evidence of physical injury obtained during substance intoxication or withdrawal.

@ INTERNET REFERENCES

Additional information related to forensic nursing may be found at the following Web sites:
a. www.forensiceducation.com/
b. www.forensicnurse.org/
c. www.amrn.com/
d. http://nursing.advanceweb.com/Editorial/Content/Editorial.aspx?CC=40302
e. http://onlinelibrary.wiley.com/journal/10.1111/(ISSN)1939-3938

CHAPTER 20

Complementary Therapies

■ INTRODUCTION

The connection between mind and body, and the influence of each on the other, is well recognized by all clinicians and particularly by psychiatrists. Conventional medicine as it is currently practiced in the United States is based solely on scientific methodology. Conventional, science-based medicine, also known as *allopathic* medicine, is the type of medicine historically taught in U.S. medical schools.

The term *alternative medicine* has come to be recognized as practices that differ from the usual traditional practices in the treatment of disease. "Alternative" refers to an intervention that is used *instead of* conventional treatment. "Complementary therapy" is an intervention that is different from, but used *in conjunction with*, traditional or conventional medical treatment. In the United States, approximately 38% of adults and 12% of children use some form of complementary or alternative therapy (Nahin, Barnes, Stussman, & Bloom, 2009). When prayer specifically for health reasons is included in the definition of complementary and alternative medicine, the numbers are even higher. Approximately $34 billion a year is spent on these types of therapies in the United States.

In 1991, an Office of Alternative Medicine (OAM) was established by the National Institutes of Health (NIH) to study nontraditional therapies and to evaluate their usefulness and their effectiveness. Since that time, the name has been changed to the National Center for Complementary and Alternative Medicine (NCCAM or CAM). The mission statement of the CAM states:

> NCCAM's mission is to explore complementary and alternative healing practices in the context of rigorous science, train CAM researchers, and disseminate authoritative information to the public and professionals (NCCAM, 2008, p. 4).

Some health insurance companies and health maintenance organizations (HMOs) appear to be bowing to public pressure by including alternative providers in their networks of providers for treatments such as acupuncture and massage therapy. Chiropractic care has been covered by some third-party payers for many years. Individuals who seek alternative therapy, however, are often reimbursed at lower rates than those who choose conventional practitioners.

Client education is an important part of complementary care. Positive lifestyle changes are encouraged, and practitioners serve as educators as well as treatment specialists. Complementary medicine is viewed as *holistic* health care, which deals not only with the physical perspective, but also the emotional and spiritual components of the individual. Interest in holistic health care is increasing worldwide. A large number of U.S. medical schools—among them Harvard, Yale, Johns Hopkins, and Georgetown universities—now offer coursework in holistic methods (Neddermeyer, 2006). The American Medical Association (AMA, 2010), in its Policy #H-480-973, "encourages its members to become better informed regarding the practices and techniques of alternative or unconventional medicine."

■ TYPES OF COMPLEMENTARY THERAPIES

Herbal Medicine

The use of plants to heal is probably as old as humankind. Virtually every culture in the world has relied on herbs and plants to treat illness. Clay tablets from about 4000 B.C. reveal that the Sumerians had apothecaries for dispensing medicinal herbs. At the root of Chinese medicine is the *Pen Tsao*, a Chinese text written around 3000 B.C., which contained hundreds of herbal remedies. When the Pilgrims came to America in the 1600s, they brought with them a variety of herbs to be established and used for medicinal purposes. The new settlers soon discovered that the Native Americans also had their own varieties of plants that they used for healing.

Many people are seeking a return to herbal remedies because they perceive these remedies as being less potent than prescription drugs and as being free of adverse side effects. However, because the Food and Drug Administration (FDA) classifies herbal remedies as dietary supplements or food additives, their labels cannot indicate medicinal uses. They are not subject to FDA approval, and they lack uniform standards of quality control.

Several organizations have been established to attempt regulation and control of the herbal industry. They include the Council for Responsible Nutrition, the American Herbal Association, and the American Botanical Council. The Commission E of the German Federal Health Agency is the group responsible for researching and regulating the safety and efficacy of herbs and plant medicines in Germany. All of the Commission E monographs of herbal medicines have been translated into English and compiled into one text (Blumenthal, 1998).

Until more extensive testing has been completed on humans and animals, the use of herbal medicines must be approached with caution and responsibility. *The notion that something being "natural" means it is therefore completely safe is a myth.* In fact, some of the plants from which prescription drugs are derived are highly toxic in their natural state. Also, because of lack of regulation and standardization, ingredients may be adulterated. Their method of manufacture also may alter potency. For example, dried herbs lose potency rapidly because of exposure to air. In addition, it is often safer to use preparations that contain only one herb. There is a greater likelihood of unwanted side effects with combined herbal preparations.

Table 20-1 lists information about common herbal remedies, with possible implications for psychiatric/mental health nursing. Botanical names, medicinal uses, and safety profiles are included.

TABLE 20–1	Herbal Remedies	
Common Name (Botanical Name)	**Medicinal Uses/ Possible Action**	**Safety Profile**
Black cohosh (*Cimicifuga racemosa*)	May provide relief of menstrual cramps; improved mood; calming effect. Extracts from the roots are thought to have action similar to estrogen.	Generally considered safe in low doses. Occasionally causes GI discomfort. Toxic in large doses, causing dizziness, nausea, headaches, stiffness, and trembling. Should not take with heart problems, concurrently with antihypertensives, or during pregnancy.
Cascara sagrada (*Rhamnus purshiana*)	Relief of constipation	Generally recognized as safe; sold as over-the-counter drug in the United States. Should not be used during pregnancy. Contraindicated in bowel obstruction or inflammation.
Chamomile (*Matricaria chamomilla*)	As a tea, is effective as a mild sedative in the relief of insomnia. May also aid digestion, relieve menstrual cramps, and settle upset stomach.	Generally recognized as safe when consumed in reasonable amounts.
Echinacea (*Echinacea angustifolia* and *Echinacea purpurea*)	Stimulates the immune system; may have value in fighting infections and easing the symptoms of colds and flu.	Considered safe in reasonable doses. Observe for side effects or allergic reaction.

TABLE 20–1 Herbal Remedies—cont'd

Common Name (Botanical Name)	Medicinal Uses/ Possible Action	Safety Profile
Fennel *(Foeniculum vulgare or Foeniculum officinale)*	Used to ease stomachaches and to aid digestion. Taken in a tea or in extracts to stimulate the appetites of people with anorexia (1–2 tsp. seeds steeped in boiling water for making tea).	Generally recognized as safe when consumed in reasonable amounts.
Feverfew *(Tanacetum parthenium)*	Prophylaxis and treatment of migraine headaches. Effective in either the fresh leaf or freeze-dried forms (2–3 fresh leaves [or equivalent] per day).	A small percentage of individuals may experience the adverse effect of temporary mouth ulcers. Considered safe in reasonable doses.
Ginger *(Zingiber officinale)*	Ginger tea to ease stomachaches and to aid digestion. Two powdered gingerroot capsules have shown to be effective in preventing motion sickness.	Generally recognized as safe in designated therapeutic doses.
Ginkgo *(Ginkgo biloba)*	Used to treat senility, short-term memory loss, and peripheral insufficiency. Has been shown to dilate blood vessels. Usual dosage is 120–240 mg/day.	Safety has been established with recommended dosages. Possible side effects include headache, GI problems, and dizziness. Contraindicated in pregnancy and lactation and in patients with bleeding disorder. Possible compound effect with concomitant use of aspirin or anticoagulants.
Ginseng *(Panax ginseng)*	The ancient Chinese saw this herb as one that increased wisdom and longevity. Current studies support a possible positive effect on the cardiovascular system. Action not known.	Generally considered safe. Side effects may include headache, insomnia, anxiety, skin rashes, diarrhea. Avoid concomitant use with anticoagulants.

(Continued)

TABLE 20–1	Herbal Remedies—cont'd	
Common Name (Botanical Name)	**Medicinal Uses/ Possible Action**	**Safety Profile**
Hops *(Humulus lupulus)*	Used in cases of nervousness, mild anxiety, and insomnia. Also may relieve the cramping associated with diarrhea. May be taken as a tea, in extracts, or capsules.	Generally recognized as safe when consumed in recommended dosages.
Kava-Kava *(Piper methylsticum)*	Used to reduce anxiety while promoting mental acuity. Dosage: 150–300 mg bid.	Scaly skin rash may occur when taken at high dosage for long periods. Motor reflexes and judgment when driving may be reduced while taking the herb. Concurrent use with CNS depressants may produce additive tranquilizing effects. Reports of potential for liver damage. Investigations continue. Should not be taken for longer than 3 months without a doctor's supervision.
Passion flower *(Passiflora incarnata)*	Used in tea, capsules, or extracts to treat nervousness and insomnia. Depresses the central nervous system to produce a mild sedative effect.	Generally recognized as safe in recommended doses.
Peppermint *(Mentha piperita)*	Used as a tea to relieve upset stomachs and headaches and as a mild sedative. Pour boiling water over 1 tbsp. dried leaves and steep to make a tea. Oil of peppermint is also used for inflammation of the mouth, pharynx, and bronchus.	Considered to be safe when consumed in designated therapeutic dosages.

TABLE 20–1	Herbal Remedies—cont'd	
Common Name (Botanical Name)	**Medicinal Uses/ Possible Action**	**Safety Profile**
Psyllium (*Plantago ovata*)	Psyllium seeds are a popular bulk laxative commonly used for chronic constipation. Also found to be useful in the treatment of hypercholesterolemia.	Approved as an over-the-counter drug in the United States.
Skullcap (*Scutellaria lateriflora*)	Used as a sedative for mild anxiety and nervousness.	Considered safe in reasonable amounts.
St. John's Wort (*Hypericum perforatum*)	Used in the treatment of mild to moderate depression. May block reuptake of serotonin/norepinephrine and have a mild MAO inhibiting effect. Effective dose: 900 mg/day. May also have antiviral, antibacterial, and anti-inflammatory properties.	Generally recognized as safe when taken at recommended dosages. Side effects include mild GI irritation that is lessened with food; photosensitivity when taken in high dosages over long periods. Should not be taken with other psychoactive medications.
Valerian (*Valeriana officinals*)	Used to treat nervousness and insomnia. Produces restful sleep without morning "hangover." The root may be used to make a tea, or capsules are available in a variety of dosages. Mechanism of action is similar to benzodiazepines, but without addicting properties. Daily dosage range: 100–1000 mg.	Generally recognized as safe when taken at recommended dosages. Side effects may include mild headache or upset stomach. Taking doses higher than recommended may result in severe headache, nausea, morning grogginess, blurry vision. Should not be taken concurrently with CNS depressants or during pregnancy.

Sources: Adapted from Holt and Kouzi (2002); PDR for Herbal Medicines (2007); Pranthikanti (2007), Sadock and Sadock (2007); Trivieri and Anderson (2002), and Ulbricht, 2011.

Acupressure and Acupuncture

Acupressure and acupuncture are healing techniques based on the ancient philosophies of traditional Chinese medicine dating back to 3000 B.C. The main concept behind Chinese medicine is that healing energy (*qi*) flows through the body along specific pathways called *meridians*. It is believed that these meridians of *qi* connect various parts of the body in a way similar to the way in which lines on a road map link various locations. The pathways link a conglomerate of points, called *acupoints*. Therefore, it is possible to treat a part of the body distant to another because they are linked by a meridian. Trivieri and Anderson (2002) state, "The proper flow of *qi* along energy channels (meridians) within the body is crucial to a person's health and vitality" (p. 435).

In acupressure, the fingers, thumbs, palms, or elbows are used to apply pressure to the acupoints. This pressure is thought to dissolve any obstructions in the flow of healing energy and to restore the body to a healthier functioning. In acupuncture, hair-thin, sterile, disposable, stainless-steel needles are inserted into acupoints to dissolve the obstructions along the meridians. The needles may be left in place for a specified length of time, they may be rotated, or a mild electric current may be applied. An occasional tingling or numbness is experienced, but little to no pain is associated with the treatment (NCCAM, 2012a).

The Western medical philosophy regarding acupressure and acupuncture is that they stimulate the body's own painkilling chemicals—the morphine-like substances known as *endorphins*. The treatment has been found to be effective in the treatment of asthma, dysmenorrhea, cervical pain, insomnia, anxiety, depression, substance abuse, stroke rehabilitation, nausea of pregnancy, postoperative and chemotherapy-induced nausea and vomiting, tennis elbow, fibromyalgia, low back pain, carpal tunnel syndrome and many other conditions (Council of Acupuncture and Oriental Medicine Associations [CAOMA], 2013; NCCAM, 2012a; Sadock & Sadock, 2007). Some studies suggest that acupuncture may aid in the treatment of cocaine dependence and chronic daily headaches (Avants et al, 2000; Coeytaux et al, 2005).

Acupuncture is gaining wide acceptance is the United States by both patients and physicians. This treatment can be administered at the same time other techniques are being used, such as conventional Western techniques, although it is essential that all health-care providers have knowledge of all treatments being received. Acupuncture should be administered by a physician or an acupuncturist who is licensed by the state in which the service is provided. Typical training for licensed acupuncturists, doctors of oriental medicine, and acupuncture physicians is a 3- or 4-year program of 2500 to 3500 hours.

Diet and Nutrition

The value of nutrition in the healing process has long been underrated. Lutz and Przytulski (2011) state:

> Good nutrition is essential for good health and important for physical growth and development, good body composition, and mental development. A person's nutritional state can protect him from or predispose him toward chronic disease. Only recently has it been discovered that nutrition influences our genetic code. Medical treatment for many diseases includes diet therapy. Nutrition is thus both a preventive and a therapeutic science (p. 5).

Individuals select the foods they eat based on a number of factors, not the least of which is enjoyment. Eating must serve social and cultural, as well as nutritional, needs. The U.S. Departments of Agriculture (USDA) and Health and Human Services (USDHHS) have collaborated on a set of guidelines to help individuals understand what types of foods to eat and the healthy lifestyle they need to pursue in order to promote health and prevent disease. Following is a list of key recommendations from these guidelines (USDA/USDHHS, 2010):

1. Balancing Calories to Manage Weight
   - Prevent and/or reduce overweight and obesity through improved eating and physical activity behaviors.
   - Control total calorie intake to manage body weight. For people who are overweight or obese, this will mean consuming fewer calories from foods and beverages.
   - Increase physical activity and reduce time spent in sedentary behaviors.
   - Maintain appropriate calorie balance during each stage of life—childhood, adolescence, adulthood, pregnancy and breastfeeding, and older age.
2. Foods and Food Components to Reduce
   - Reduce daily sodium intake to less than 2300 milligrams (mg) and further reduce intake to 1500 mg among persons who are 51 and older and those of any age who are African American or have hypertension, diabetes, or chronic kidney disease. The 1500 mg recommendation applies to about half of the U.S. population, including children and the majority of adults.
   - Consume less than 10% of calories from saturated fatty acids by replacing them with monounsaturated and polyunsaturated fatty acids.
   - Consume less than 300 mg per day of dietary cholesterol.
   - Keep *trans*-fatty acid consumption as low as possible by limiting foods that contain synthetic sources of *trans*-fats, such as partially hydrogenated oils, and by limiting other solid fats.

- Reduce the intake of calories from solid fats and added sugars.
- Limit the consumption of foods that contain refined grains, especially refined grain foods that contain solid fats, added sugars, and sodium.
- If alcohol is consumed, it should be consumed in moderation—up to one drink per day for women and two drinks per day for men—and only by adults of legal drinking age.

One drink is defined as:

- 12 ounces of regular beer (150 calories)
- 5 ounces of wine (100 calories)
- 1.5 ounces of 80-proof distilled spirits (100 calories)

Alcohol should be avoided by individuals who are unable to restrict their intake; women who are pregnant, may become pregnant, or are breastfeeding; and individuals who are taking medications that may interact with alcohol or who have specific medical conditions.

3. Foods and Nutrients to Increase

   Individuals should meet the following recommendations as part of a healthy eating pattern while staying within their calorie needs:

   - Increase vegetable and fruit intake.
   - Eat a variety of vegetables, especially dark-green, red, and orange vegetables and beans and peas.
   - Consume at least half of all grains as whole grains. Increase whole-grain intake by replacing refined grains with whole grains.
   - Increase intake of fat-free or low-fat milk and milk products, such as milk, yogurt, cheese, or fortified soy beverages.
   - Choose a variety of protein foods, which include seafood, lean meat and poultry, eggs, beans and peas, soy products, and unsalted nuts and seeds.
   - Increase the amount and variety of seafood consumed by choosing seafood in place of some meat and poultry.
   - Replace protein foods that are higher in solid fats with choices that are lower in solid fats and calories and/or are sources of oils.
   - Use oils to replace solid fats when possible.
   - Choose foods that provide more potassium, dietary fiber, calcium, and vitamin D, which are nutrients of concern in American diets. These foods include vegetables, fruits, whole grains, and milk and milk products.
   - Meet recommended intakes within energy needs by adopting a balanced eating pattern, such as the USDA Food Guide (Table 20-2). Table 20-3 provides a summary of information about essential vitamins and minerals.

4. Building Healthy Eating Patterns

   - Select an eating pattern that meets nutrient needs over time at an appropriate calorie level.
   - Account for all foods and beverages consumed and assess how they fit within a total healthy eating pattern.
   - Follow food safety recommendations when preparing and eating foods to reduce the risk of food-borne illnesses.

TABLE 20–2	Sample USDA Food Guide at the 2000-Calorie Level	
Food Groups and Subgroups	**USDA Food Guide Daily Amount**	**Examples/ Equivalent Amounts**
Fruit Group	2 cups (4 servings)	½ cup equivalent is: • ½ cup fresh, frozen, or canned fruit • 1 medium fruit • ¼ cup dried fruit • ½ cup fruit juice
Vegetable Group	2.5 cups (5 servings) • Dark green vegetables: 3 cups/week • Orange vegetables: 2 cups/week • Legumes (dry beans/peas): 3 cups/week • Starchy vegetables: 3 cups/week • Other vegetables: 6.5 cups/week	½ cup equivalent is: • ½ cup cut-up raw or cooked vegetable • 1 cup raw leafy vegetable • ½ cup vegetable juice
Grain Group	6 ounce-equivalents • Whole grains: 3 ounce-equivalents • Other grains: 3 ounce-equivalents	1 ounce-equivalent is: • 1 slice bread • 1 cup dry cereal • ½ cup cooked rice, pasta, cereal
Meat and Beans Group	5.5 ounce-equivalents	1 ounce-equivalent is: • 1 oz. cooked lean meat, poultry, or fish • 1 egg • ¼ cup cooked dry beans or tofu • 1 tbsp. peanut butter • ½ oz. nuts or seeds
Milk Group	3 cups	1 cup equivalent is: • 1 cup low fat/fat-free milk • 1 cup low fat/fat-free yogurt • 1½ oz. low-fat or fat-free natural cheese • 2 oz. low-fat or fat-free processed cheese
Oils	24 grams (6 tsp.)	1 tsp. equivalent is: • 1 tbsp. low-fat mayo

(Continued)

TABLE 20–2	Sample USDA Food Guide at the 2000-Calorie Level—cont'd	
Food Groups and Subgroups	**USDA Food Guide Daily Amount**	**Examples/ Equivalent Amounts**
		• 2 tbsp. light salad dressing
		• 1 tsp. vegetable oil
		• 1 tsp. soft margarine with zero *trans*-fat
Discretionary Calorie Allowance	267 calories Example of distribution: • Solid fats, 18 grams (e.g., saturated & *trans*-fats) • Added sugars, 8 tsp. (e.g., sweetened cereals)	1 added sugar equivalent is: • ½ oz. jelly beans • 8 oz. lemonade Examples of solid fats: • Fat in whole milk or ice cream • Fatty meats Essential oils (above) are not considered part of the discretionary calories

Source: *Dietary Guidelines for Americans 2010.* Washington, DC: USDA/ USDHHS, 2010.

Chiropractic Medicine

Chiropractic medicine is probably the most widely used form of alternative healing in the United States. It was developed in the late 1800s by a self-taught healer named David Palmer. It was later reorganized and expanded by his son Joshua, a trained practitioner. Palmer's objective was to find a cure for disease and illness that did not use drugs, but instead relied on more natural methods of healing (Trivieri & Anderson, 2002). Palmer's theory behind chiropractic medicine was that energy flows from the brain to all parts of the body through the spinal cord and spinal nerves. When vertebrae of the spinal column become displaced, they may press on a nerve and interfere with the normal nerve transmission. Palmer named the displacement of these vertebrae *subluxation*, and he alleged that the way to restore normal function was to manipulate the vertebrae back into their normal positions. These manipulations are called *adjustments*.

Adjustments are usually performed by hand, although some chiropractors have special treatment tables equipped to facilitate these manipulations. Other processes used to facilitate the outcome of the spinal adjustment by providing muscle relaxation include massage tables, application of heat or cold, and ultrasound treatments.

(*Text continued on page 366*)

TABLE 20-3 Essential Vitamins and Minerals

Vitamin/ Mineral	Function	DRI (UL)*	Food Sources	Comments
Vitamin A	Prevention of night blindness; calcification of growing bones; resistance to infection	Men: 900 mcg (3000 mcg) Women: 700 mcg (3000 mcg)	Liver, butter, cheese, whole milk, egg yolk, fish, green leafy vegetables, carrots, pumpkin, sweet potatoes	May be of benefit in prevention of cancer, because of its antioxidant properties which are associated with control of free radicals that damage DNA and cell membranes.[†]
Vitamin D	Promotes absorption of calcium and phosphorus in the small intestine; prevention of rickets	Men and women: 15 mcg (100 mcg) Men and women >70 years of age: 20 mcg (100 mcg)	Fortified milk and dairy products, egg yolk, fish liver oils, liver, oysters; formed in the skin by exposure to sunlight	Without vitamin D, very little dietary calcium can be absorbed.
Vitamin E	An antioxidant that prevents cell membrane destruction	Men and women: 15 mg (1000 mg)	Vegetable oils, wheat germ, whole grain or fortified cereals, green leafy vegetables, nuts	As an antioxidant, may have implications in the prevention of Alzheimer's Disease, heart disease, breast cancer.[†]
Vitamin K	Synthesis of prothrombin and other clotting factors; normal blood coagulation	Men: 120 mcg (ND)*** Women: 90 mcg (ND)***	Green vegetables (collards, spinach, lettuce, kale, broccoli, Brussels sprouts,	Individuals on anticoagulant therapy should monitor vitamin K intake.

(Continued)

TABLE 20-3	Essential Vitamins and Minerals—cont'd			
Vitamin/ Mineral	Function	DRI (UL)*	Food Sources	Comments
			cabbage), plant oils, and margarine	
Vitamin C	Formation of collagen in connective tissues; a powerful antioxidant; facilitates iron absorption; aids in the release of epinephrine from the adrenal glands during stress	Men: 90 mg (2000 mg) Women: 75 mg (2000 mg)	Citrus fruits, tomatoes, potatoes, green leafy vegetables, strawberries	As an antioxidant, may have implications in the prevention of cancer, cataracts, heart disease. It may stimulate the immune system to fight various types of infection.†
Vitamin B₁ (thiamine)	Essential for normal functioning of nervous tissue; coenzyme in carbohydrate metabolism	Men: 1.2 mg (ND)*** Women: 1.1 mg (ND)***	Whole grains, legumes, nuts, egg yolk, meat, green leafy vegetables	Large doses may improve mental performance in people with Alzheimer's disease.
Vitamin B₂ (riboflavin)	Coenzyme in the metabolism of protein and carbohydrate for energy	Men: 1.3 mg (ND)*** Women: 1.1 mg (ND)***	Meat, dairy products, whole or enriched grains, legumes, nuts	May help in the prevention of cataracts; high dose therapy may be effective in migraine prophylaxis (Schoenen et al, 1998).
Vitamin B₃ (niacin)	Coenzyme in the metabolism of protein	Men: 16 mg (35 mg) Women: 14 mg (35 mg)	Milk, eggs, meats, legumes, whole grain	High doses of niacin have been successful in decreasing

	and carbohydrates for energy		and enriched cereals, nuts	levels of cholesterol in some individuals.
Vitamin B$_6$ (pyridoxine)	Coenzyme in the synthesis and catabolism of amino acids; essential for metabolism of tryptophan to niacin	Men and women: 1.3 mg (100 mg) After age 50: Men: 1.7 mg Women: 1.5 mg	Meat, fish, grains, legumes, bananas, nuts, white and sweet potatoes	May decrease depression in some individuals by increasing levels of serotonin; deficiencies may contribute to memory problems; also used in the treatment of migraines and premenstrual discomfort.
Vitamin B$_{12}$	Necessary in the formation of DNA and the production of red blood cells; associated with folic acid metabolism	Men and women: 2.4 mcg (ND)***	Found in animal products (e.g., meats, eggs, dairy products)	Deficiency may contribute to memory problems. Vegetarians can get this vitamin from fortified foods. Intrinsic factor must be present in the stomach for absorption of vitamin B$_{12}$.
Folic acid (folate)	Necessary in the formation of DNA and the production of red blood cells	Men and women: 400 mcg (1,000 mcg) Pregnant women: 600 mcg	Meat; green leafy vegetables; beans; peas; fortified cereals, breads, rice, and pasta	Important in women of childbearing age to prevent fetal neural tube defects; may contribute to prevention of heart disease and colon cancer.
Calcium	Necessary in the formation of bones and teeth; neuron and muscle	Men and women: 1,000 mg (2500 mg) After age 50:	Dairy products, kale, broccoli, spinach, sardines, oysters, salmon	Calcium has been associated with preventing headaches, muscle cramps, osteoporosis,

(Continued)

TABLE 20-3	Essential Vitamins and Minerals—cont'd			
Vitamin/ Mineral	**Function**	**DRI (UL)***	**Food Sources**	**Comments**
	functioning; blood clotting	Men and women: 1200 mg		and premenstrual problems. Requires vitamin D for absorption.
Phosphorus	Necessary in the formation of bones and teeth; a component of DNA, RNA, ADP, and ATP; helps control acid-base balance in the blood	Men and women: 700 mg (4000 mg)	Milk, cheese, fish, meat, yogurt, ice cream, peas, eggs	
Magnesium	Protein synthesis and carbohydrate metabolism; muscular relaxation following contraction; bone formation	Men: 420 mg (350 mg)** Women: 320 mg (350 mg)**	Green vegetables, legumes, seafood, milk, nuts, meat	May aid in prevention of asthmatic attacks and migraine headaches. Deficiencies may contribute to insomnia, premenstrual problems.
Iron	Synthesis of hemoglobin and myoglobin; cellular oxidation	Men: 8 mg (45 mg) Women: (45 mg) Childbearing age: 18 mg Over 50: 8 mg Pregnant: 27 mg Breastfeeding: 9 mg	Meat, fish, poultry, eggs, nuts, dark green leafy vegetables, dried fruit, enriched pasta and bread	Iron deficiencies can result in headaches and feeling chronically fatigued.

	Function	RDA (UL)	Food Sources	Comments
Iodine	Aids in the synthesis of T3 and T4	Men and women: 150 mcg (1100 mcg)	Iodized salt, seafood	Exerts strong controlling influence on overall body metabolism.
Selenium	Works with vitamin E to protect cellular compounds from oxidation	Men and women: 55 mcg (400 mcg)	Seafood, low-fat meats, dairy products, liver	As an antioxidant combined with vitamin E, may have some anticancer effect.† Deficiency has also been associated with depressed mood.
Zinc	Involved in synthesis of DNA and RNA; energy metabolism and protein synthesis; wound healing; increased immune functioning; necessary for normal smell and taste sensation.	Men: 11 mg (40 mg) Women: 8 mg (40 mg)	Meat, seafood, fortified cereals, poultry, eggs, milk	An important source for the prevention of infection and improvement in wound healing.

†The health benefits of antioxidants continue to be investigated.

*Dietary Reference Intakes (UL), the most recent set of dietary recommendations for adults established by the Food and Nutrition Board of the Institute of Medicine, © 2004. UL is the upper limit of intake considered to be safe for use by adults (includes total intake from food, water, and supplements). In addition to the UL, DRIs are composed of the Recommended Dietary Allowance (RDA, the amount considered sufficient to meet the requirements of 97% to 98% of all healthy individuals) and the Adequate Intake (AI, the amount considered sufficient where no RDA has been established).

**UL for magnesium applies only to intakes from dietary supplements, excluding intakes from food and water.

***ND, not determined.

Source: Adapted from National Academy of Sciences (2004).

The chiropractor takes a medical history and performs a clinical examination, which usually includes X-ray films of the spine. Today's chiropractors may practice "straight" therapy: that is, the only therapy provided is that of subluxation adjustments. *Mixer* is a term applied to a chiropractor who combines adjustments with adjunct therapies, such as exercise, heat treatments, or massage.

Individuals seek treatment from chiropractors for many types of ailments and illnesses; the most common is back pain. In addition, chiropractors treat clients with headaches, neck injuries, scoliosis, carpal tunnel syndrome, respiratory and gastrointestinal disorders, menstrual difficulties, allergies, sinusitis, and certain sports injuries (Trivieri & Anderson, 2002). Some chiropractors are employed by professional sports teams as their team physicians.

Chiropractors are licensed to practice in all 50 states and treatment costs are covered by government and most private insurance plans. They treat more than 20 million people in the United States annually (NCCAM, 2012b).

Therapeutic Touch and Massage
Therapeutic Touch

The technique of therapeutic touch was developed in the 1970s by Dolores Krieger, a nurse associated with the New York University School of Nursing. This therapy is based on the philosophy that the human body projects a field of energy around it. When this field of energy becomes blocked, pain or illness occurs. Practitioners of therapeutic touch use this technique to correct the blockages, thereby relieving the discomfort and improving health.

Based on the premise that the energy field extends beyond the surface of the body, the practitioner need not actually touch the client's skin. The therapist's hands are passed over the client's body, remaining 2 to 4 inches from the skin. The goal is to repattern the energy field by performing slow, rhythmic, sweeping hand motions over the entire body. Heat should be felt where the energy is blocked. The therapist "massages" the energy field in that area, smoothing it out, and thus correcting the obstruction. Therapeutic touch is thought to reduce pain and anxiety and promote relaxation and health maintenance. It has been useful in the treatment of chronic health conditions.

Massage

Massage is the technique of manipulating the muscles and soft tissues of the body. Chinese physicians prescribed massage for the treatment of disease more than 5000 years ago. The

Eastern style focuses on balancing the body's vital energy (*qi*) as it flows through pathways (meridians), as described earlier in the discussion of acupressure and acupuncture. The Western style of massage affects muscles, connective tissues (e.g., tendons and ligaments), and the cardiovascular system. Swedish massage, which is probably the best-known Western style, uses a variety of gliding and kneading strokes along with deep circular movements and vibrations to relax the muscles, improve circulation, and increase mobility (Trivieri & Anderson, 2002).

Massage has been shown to be beneficial in the following conditions: anxiety, chronic back and neck pain, arthritis, sciatica, migraine headaches, muscle spasms, insomnia, pain of labor and delivery, stress-related disorders, and whiplash. Massage is contraindicated in certain conditions, such as high blood pressure, acute infection, osteoporosis, phlebitis, skin conditions, and varicose veins. It also should not be performed over the site of a recent injury, bruise, or burn.

Massage therapists require specialized training in a program accredited by the American Massage Therapy Association and must pass the National Certification Examination for Therapeutic Massage and Bodywork.

Yoga

Yoga is thought to have developed in India some 5000 years ago and is attributed to an Indian physician and Sanskrit scholar named Patanjali. The objective of yoga is to integrate the physical, mental, and spiritual energies that enhance health and well-being (Trivieri & Anderson, 2002). Yoga has been found to be especially helpful in relieving stress and in improving overall physical and psychological wellness. Proper breathing is a major component of yoga. It is believed that yoga breathing—a deep, diaphragmatic breathing—increases oxygen to brain and body tissues, thereby easing stress and fatigue and boosting energy.

Another component of yoga is meditation. Individuals who practice the meditation and deep breathing associated with yoga find that they are able to achieve a profound feeling of relaxation. The most familiar type of yoga practiced in Western countries is hatha yoga. Hatha yoga uses body postures, along with the meditation and breathing exercises, to achieve a balanced, disciplined workout that releases muscle tension, tones the internal organs, and energizes the mind, body, and spirit, to allow natural healing to occur. The complete routine of poses is designed to work all parts of the body—stretching and toning muscles and keeping joints flexible. Studies have shown that yoga has provided beneficial effects to some individuals with back pain, stress, migraine, insomnia, high blood pressure, rapid heart rates, and limited mobility (Sadock & Sadock, 2007; Steinberg, 2002; Trivieri & Anderson, 2002).

Pet Therapy

The therapeutic value of pets is no longer just theory. Evidence has shown that animals can directly influence a person's mental and physical well-being. Many pet therapy programs have been established across the country, and the numbers are increasing regularly. Several studies have provided information about the positive results of human interaction with pets. Some of these include the following:

1. Petting a dog or cat has been shown to lower blood pressure. In one study, volunteers experienced a 7.1 mm Hg drop in systolic and an 8.1 mm Hg decrease in diastolic blood pressure when they talked to and petted their dogs, as opposed to reading aloud or resting quietly (Whitaker, 2000).

2. Bringing a pet into a nursing home or other institution for the elderly has been shown to enhance a client's mood and social interaction (Godenne, 2001). Another study revealed that animal-assisted therapy with nursing home residents significantly reduced loneliness for those in the study group (Banks & Banks, 2002).

3. One study of 96 patients who had been admitted to a coronary care unit for heart attack or angina revealed that in the year following hospitalization, the mortality rate among those who did not own pets was 22% higher than among pet owners (Whitaker, 2000).

4. Individuals with AIDS who have pets are less likely to suffer from depression than people with AIDS who don't own pets (Siegel et al, 1999).

5. Studies are ongoing at the Research Center for Human-Animal Interaction (ReCHAI), a part of the College of Veterinary Medicine at the University of Missouri, in its Veterans and Shelter Dogs Initiative. This program allows military veterans to participate in the training of shelter dogs to work as service dogs for veterans with PTSD (ReCHAI, 2008).

6. Animal-assisted therapy with patients in acute care centers has been shown to decrease anxiety, reduce blood pressure, lower stress hormone release, increase feelings of safety, and improve cooperation and participation in the patient's own recovery (Ernst, 2012).

7. The American Heart Association has recently released a statement based on a survey of research studies stating that "there is a substantial body of data that suggests that pet ownership is

associated with a reduction in CVD risk factors and increased survival in individuals with established CVD" (Levine et al., 2013, p. 7).

Some researchers believe that animals actually may retard the aging process among those who live alone. Loneliness often results in premature death, and having a pet mitigates the effects of loneliness and isolation.

Whitaker (2000) suggests:

> Though owning a pet doesn't make you immune to illness, pet owners are on the whole healthier than those who don't own pets. Study after study shows that people with pets have fewer minor health problems, require fewer visits to the doctor and less medication, and have fewer risk factors for heart disease, such as high blood pressure or cholesterol levels (p. 7).

It may never be known precisely why animals affect humans they way they do, but for those who have pets to love, the therapeutic benefits come as no surprise. Pets provide unconditional, nonjudgmental love and affection, which can be the perfect antidote for a depressed mood or a stressful situation. The role of animals in the human healing process still requires more research, but its validity is now widely accepted in both the medical and lay communities.

■ SUMMARY

Complementary therapies help the practitioner view the client in a holistic manner. Most complementary therapies consider the mind and body connection and strive to enhance the body's own natural healing powers. The Office of Alternative Medicine of the National Institutes of Health has established a list of alternative therapies to be used in practice and for investigative purposes. Approximately $34 billion a year is spent on alternative medical therapies in the United States.

This chapter examined herbal medicine, acupressure, acupuncture, diet and nutrition, chiropractic medicine, therapeutic touch, massage, yoga, and pet therapy. Nurses must be familiar with these therapies, as more and more clients seek out the healing properties of these complementary care strategies.

@ INTERNET REFERENCES

Additional information related to complementary therapies may be located at the following Web sites:

a. www.herbalgram.org
b. www.herbmed.org/
c. http://nutritiondata.self.com
d. www.nutrition.gov
e. www.chiropractic.org

f. www.pawssf.org
g. www.therapydogs.com
h. www.angelonaleash.org
i. www.holisticmed.com/www/acupuncture.html
j. www.americanyogaassociation.org

CHAPTER 21

Loss and Bereavement

■ BACKGROUND ASSESSMENT DATA

Loss is the experience of separation from something of personal importance. Loss is anything that is perceived as such by the individual. The separation from loved ones or the giving up of treasured possessions, for whatever reason; the experience of failure, either real or perceived; or life events that create change in a familiar pattern of existence—all can be experienced as loss, and all can trigger behaviors associated with the grieving process. Loss and bereavement are universal events encountered by all beings that experience emotions. Following are examples of some notable forms of loss:

1. A significant other (person or pet) through death, divorce, or separation for any reason.
2. Illness or debilitating conditions. Examples include (but are not limited to) diabetes, stroke, cancer, rheumatoid arthritis, multiple sclerosis, Alzheimer's disease, hearing or vision loss, and spinal cord or head injuries. Some of these conditions not only incur a loss of physical and/or emotional wellness but may also result in the loss of personal independence.
3. Developmental/maturational changes or situations, such as menopause, andropause, infertility, "empty nest" syndrome, aging, impotence, or hysterectomy.
4. A decrease in self-esteem due to inability to meet self-expectations or the expectations of others (even if these expectations are only perceived by the individual as unfulfilled). This includes a loss of potential hopes and dreams.
5. Personal possessions that symbolize familiarity and security in a person's life. Separation from these familiar and personally valued external objects represents a loss of material extensions of the self.

Some texts differentiate the terms *mourning* and *grief* by describing mourning as the psychological process (or stages) through which the individual passes on the way to successful adaptation to the loss of a valued object. Grief may be viewed as the subjective states that accompany mourning, or the emotional work involved in the mourning process. For purposes of this text, grief work and the process of mourning are collectively referred to as the *grief response*.

Theoretical Perspectives on Loss and Bereavement (Symptomatology)

Stages of Grief

Behavior patterns associated with the grief response include many individual variations. However, sufficient similarities have been observed to warrant characterization of grief as a syndrome that has a predictable course with an expected resolution. Early theorists, including Elisabeth Kübler-Ross (1969), John Bowlby (1961), and George Engel (1964), described behavioral stages through which individuals advance in their progression toward resolution. A number of variables influence one's progression through the grief process. Some individuals may reach acceptance, only to revert back to an earlier stage; some may never complete the sequence; and some may never progress beyond the initial stage.

A more contemporary grief specialist, J. William Worden (2009), offers a set of tasks that must be processed in order to complete the grief response. He suggests that it is possible for a person to accomplish some of these tasks and not others, resulting in an incomplete bereavement, and thus impairing further growth and development.

Elisabeth Kübler-Ross

These well-known stages of the grief process were identified by Kübler-Ross in her extensive work with dying patients. Behaviors associated with each of these stages can be observed in individuals experiencing the loss of any concept of personal value.

- **Stage I: Denial.** The individual does not acknowledge that the loss has occurred. He or she may say, "No, it can't be true!" or "It's just not possible." This stage may protect the individual against the psychological pain of reality.
- **Stage II: Anger.** This is the stage when reality sets in. Feelings associated with this stage include sadness, guilt, shame, helplessness, and hopelessness. Self-blame or blaming of others may lead to feelings of anger toward the self and others. The anxiety level may be elevated, and the individual may experience confusion and a decreased ability to function independently. He or she may be preoccupied with an idealized image of what has been lost. Numerous somatic complaints are common.
- **Stage III: Bargaining.** The individual attempts to strike a bargain with God for a second chance or for more time. The person acknowledges the loss, or impending loss, but holds out hope for additional alternatives, as evidenced by such statements as, "If only I could . . ." or "If only I had . . . ."
- **Stage IV: Depression.** The individual mourns for that which has been or will be lost. This is a very painful stage, during which the individual must confront feelings associated

with having lost someone or something of value (called *reactive* depression). An example might be the individual who is mourning a change in body image. Feelings associated with an impending loss (called *preparatory* depression) are also confronted. Examples include permanent lifestyle changes related to the altered body image or even an impending loss of life itself. Regression, withdrawal, and social isolation may be observed behaviors with this stage. Therapeutic intervention should be available, but not imposed, and with guidelines for implementation based on client readiness.

- **Stage V: Acceptance.** The individual has worked through the behaviors associated with the other stages and either accepts or is resigned to the loss. Anxiety decreases, and methods for coping with the loss have been established. The client is less preoccupied with what has been lost and increasingly interested in other aspects of the environment. If this is an impending death of self, the individual is ready to die. The person may become very quiet and withdrawn, seemingly devoid of feelings. These behaviors are an attempt to facilitate the passage by slowly disengaging from the environment.

John Bowlby

John Bowlby hypothesized four stages in the grief process. He implied that these behaviors can be observed in all individuals who have experienced the loss of something or someone of value, even in infants as young as 6 months of age.

- **Stage I: Numbness or Protest.** This stage is characterized by a feeling of shock and disbelief that the loss has occurred. Reality of the loss is not acknowledged.
- **Stage II: Disequilibrium.** During this stage, the individual has a profound urge to recover what has been lost. Behaviors associated with this stage include a preoccupation with the loss, intense weeping and expressions of anger toward the self and others, and feelings of ambivalence and guilt associated with the loss.
- **Stage III: Disorganization and Despair.** Feelings of despair occur in response to the realization that the loss has occurred. Activities of daily living become increasingly disorganized, and behavior is characterized by restlessness and aimlessness. Efforts to regain productive patterns of behavior are ineffective and the individual experiences fear, helplessness, and hopelessness. Somatic complaints are common. Perceptions of visualizing or being in the presence of that which has been lost may occur. Social isolation is common, and the individual may feel a great deal of loneliness.
- **Stage IV: Reorganization.** The individual accepts or becomes resigned to the loss. New goals and patterns of organization are established. The individual begins a reinvestment

in new relationships and indicates a readiness to move forward within the environment. Grief subsides and recedes into valued remembrances.

George Engel

- **Stage I: Shock and Disbelief.** The initial reaction to a loss is a stunned, numb feeling and refusal by the individual to acknowledge the reality of the loss. Engel states that this stage is an attempt by the individual to protect the self "against the effects of the overwhelming stress by raising the threshold against its recognition or against the painful feelings evoked thereby."

- **Stage II: Developing Awareness.** This stage begins within minutes to hours of the loss. Behaviors associated with this stage include excessive crying and regression to a state of helplessness and a childlike manner. Awareness of the loss creates feelings of emptiness, frustration, anguish, and despair. Anger may be directed toward the self or toward others in the environment who are held accountable for the loss.

- **Stage III: Restitution.** The various rituals associated with loss within a culture are performed. Examples include funerals, wakes, special attire, a gathering of friends and family, and religious practices customary to the spiritual beliefs of the bereaved. Participation in these rituals is thought to assist the individual to accept the reality of the loss and to facilitate the recovery process.

- **Stage IV: Resolution of the Loss.** This stage is characterized by a preoccupation with the loss. The concept of the loss is idealized, and the individual may even imitate admired qualities of the lost entity. Preoccupation with the loss gradually decreases over a year or more, and the individual eventually begins to reinvest feelings in others.

- **Stage V: Recovery.** Obsession with the loss has ended, and the individual is able to go on with his or her life.

J. William Worden

Worden views the bereaved person as active and self-determining rather than a passive participant in the grief process. He proposes that bereavement includes a set of tasks that must be reconciled in order to complete the grief process. Worden's four tasks of mourning include the following:

- **Task I: Accepting the Reality of the Loss.** When something of value is lost, it is common for individuals to refuse to believe that the loss has occurred. Behaviors include misidentifying individuals in the environment for their lost loved one, retaining possessions of the lost loved one as though he or she has not died, and removing all reminders of the lost loved one so as not to have to face the reality of the loss. Worden (2009) states:

Coming to an acceptance of the reality of the loss takes time since it involves not only an intellectual acceptance but also an emotional one.

The bereaved person may be intellectually aware of the finality of the loss long before the emotions allow full acceptance of the information as true (p. 42).

Belief and denial are intermittent when grappling with this task. It is thought that traditional rituals such as the funeral help some individuals move toward acceptance of the loss.

- **Task II: Processing the Pain of Grief.** Pain associated with a loss includes both physical pain and emotional pain. This pain must be acknowledged and worked through. To avoid or suppress it serves only to delay or prolong the grieving process. People accomplish this by refusing to allow themselves to think painful thoughts, by idealizing or avoiding reminders of the lost entity, and by using alcohol or drugs. The intensity of the pain and the manner in which it is experienced are different for all individuals. But the commonality is that it *must* be experienced. Failure to do so generally results in some form of depression that commonly requires therapy, which then focuses on working through the pain of grief that the individual failed to work through at the time of the loss. In this very difficult Task II, individuals must "allow themselves to process the pain—to feel it and to know that one day it will pass" (Worden, 2009, p. 45).
- **Task III: Adjusting to a World without the Lost Entity.** It usually takes a number of months for a bereaved person to realize what his or her world will be like without the lost entity. In the case of a lost loved one, how the environment changes will depend on the types of roles that person fulfilled in life. In the case of a changed lifestyle, the individual will be required to make adaptations to his or her environment in terms of the changes as they are presented in daily life. In addition, those individuals who had defined their identity through the lost entity will require an adjustment to their own sense of self. Worden (2009) states:

The coping strategy of redefining the loss in such a way that it can redound to the benefit of the survivor is often part of the successful completion of Task III" (p. 47).

If the bereaved person experiences failures in his or her attempt to adjust in an environment without the lost entity, feelings of low self-esteem may result. Regressed behaviors and feelings of helplessness and inadequacy are not uncommon. Worden (2009) states:

[Another] area of adjustment may be to one's sense of the world. Loss through death can challenge one's fundamental life values and philosophical beliefs—beliefs that are influenced by our families, peers, education, and religion as well as life experiences. The bereaved person searches for meaning in the loss and its attendant life changes in order to make sense of it and to regain some control of his or her life (pp. 48–49).

To be successful in Task III, bereaved individuals must develop new skills to cope and adapt to their new environment without the lost entity. Successful achievement of this task determines the outcome of the mourning process—that of continued growth or a state of arrested development.

- **Task IV: Finding an Enduring Connection With the Lost Entity in the Midst of Embarking on a New Life.** This task allows for the bereaved person to identify a special place for the lost entity. Individuals need not purge from their history or find a replacement for that which has been lost. Instead, there is a kind of continued presence of the lost entity that only becomes *relocated* in the life of the bereaved. Successful completion of Task IV involves letting go of past attachments and forming new ones. However, there is also the recognition that although the relationship between the bereaved and what has been lost is changed, it is nonetheless still a relationship. Worden (2009) suggests that one never loses memories of a significant relationship. He states:

> For many people Task IV is the most difficult one to accomplish. They get stuck at this point in their grieving and later realize that their life in some way stopped at the point the loss occurred (p. 52).

Worden (2009) relates the story of a teenaged girl who had a difficult time adjusting to the death of her father. After two years, when she began to finally fulfill some of the tasks associated with successful grieving, she wrote these words that express rather clearly what bereaved people in Task IV are struggling with: "There are other people to be loved, and it doesn't mean that I love Dad any less" (p. 52).

Length of the Grief Process

Stages of grief allow bereaved persons an orderly approach to the resolution of mourning. Each stage presents tasks that must be overcome through a painful experiential process. Engel (1964) stated that successful resolution of the grief response is thought to have occurred when a bereaved individual is able "to remember comfortably and realistically both the pleasures and disappointments of [what has been lost]." The duration of the grief process depends on the individual and can last for a number of years without being maladaptive. The acute phase of normal grieving usually lasts 6 to 8 weeks—longer in older adults—but complete resolution of the grief response may take much longer. Sadock and Sadock (2007) state:

> Ample evidence suggests that the bereavement process does not end within a prescribed interval; certain aspects persist indefinitely for many otherwise high-functioning, normal individuals. Common manifestations of protracted grief occur intermittently. Most grief does not fully

resolve or permanently disappear; rather grief becomes circumscribed and submerged only to reemerge in response to certain triggers (p. 64).

A number of factors influence the eventual outcome of the grief response. The grief response can be more difficult if:

- The bereaved person was strongly dependent on or perceived the lost entity as an important means of physical and/or emotional support.
- The relationship with the lost entity was highly ambivalent. A love-hate relationship may instill feelings of guilt that can interfere with the grief work.
- The individual has experienced a number of recent losses. Grief tends to be cumulative, and if previous losses have not been resolved, each succeeding grief response becomes more difficult.
- The loss is that of a young person. Grief over loss of a child is often more intense than it is over the loss of an elderly person.
- The state of the person's physical or psychological health is unstable at the time of the loss.
- The bereaved person perceives (whether real or imagined) some responsibility for the loss.

The grief response may be facilitated if:

- The individual has the support of significant others to assist him or her through the mourning process.
- The individual has the opportunity to prepare for the loss. Grief work is more intense when the loss is sudden and unexpected. The experience of *anticipatory grieving* is thought to facilitate the grief response that occurs at the time of the actual loss.

Worden (2009) states:

> There is a sense in which mourning can be finished, when people regain an interest in life, feel more hopeful, experience gratification again, and adapt to new roles. There is also a sense in which mourning is never finished. [People must understand] that mourning is a long-term process, and that the culmination [very likely] will not be to a pre-grief state (p. 77).

Anticipatory Grief

Anticipatory grieving is the experiencing of the feelings and emotions associated with the normal grief response before the loss actually occurs. One dissimilar aspect relates to the fact that conventional grief tends to diminish in intensity with the passage of time. Anticipatory grief can become more intense as the expected loss becomes imminent.

Although anticipatory grief is thought to facilitate the actual mourning process following the loss, there may be some problems. In the case of a dying person, difficulties can arise when the family members complete the process of anticipatory grief, and detachment from the dying person occurs prematurely. The person who is dying experiences feelings of loneliness and isolation as the psychological pain of imminent death is faced without family support. Another example of difficulty associated with premature completion of the grief response is one that can occur on the return of persons long absent and presumed dead (e.g., soldiers missing in action or prisoners of war). In this instance, resumption of the previous relationship may be difficult for the bereaved person.

Anticipatory grieving may serve as a defense for some individuals to ease the burden of loss when it actually occurs. It may prove to be less functional for others who, because of interpersonal, psychological, or sociocultural variables, are unable in advance of the actual loss to express the intense feelings that accompany the grief response.

Maladaptive Responses to Loss

When, then, is the grieving response considered to be maladaptive? Three types of pathological grief reactions have been described. These include delayed or inhibited grief, an exaggerated or distorted grief response, and chronic or prolonged grief.

Delayed or Inhibited Grief

Delayed or inhibited grief refers to the absence of evidence of grief when it ordinarily would be expected. Many times, cultural influences, such as the expectation to keep a "stiff upper lip," cause the delayed response.

Delayed or inhibited grief is potentially pathological because the person is simply not dealing with the reality of the loss. He or she remains fixed in the denial stage of the grief process, sometimes for many years. When this occurs, the grief response may be triggered, sometimes many years later, when the individual experiences a subsequent loss. Sometimes the grief process is triggered spontaneously or in response to a seemingly insignificant event. Overreaction to another person's loss may be one manifestation of delayed grief.

The recognition of delayed grief is critical because, depending on the profoundness of the loss, the failure of the mourning process may prevent assimilation of the loss and thereby delay a return to satisfying living. Delayed grieving most commonly occurs because of ambivalent feelings toward the lost entity, outside pressure to resume normal function, or perceived lack of internal and external resources to cope with a profound loss.

Distorted (Exaggerated) Grief Response

In the distorted grief reaction, all of the symptoms associated with normal grieving are exaggerated. Feelings of sadness, helplessness, hopelessness, powerlessness, anger, and guilt, as well as numerous somatic complaints, render the individual dysfunctional in terms of management of daily living. Murray, Zentner, and Yakimo (2009) describe an exaggerated grief reaction in the following way:

> An intensification of grief to the point that the person is overwhelmed, demonstrates prolonged maladaptive behavior, manifests excessive symptoms and extensive interruptions in healing, and does not progress to integration of the loss, finding meaning in the loss, and resolution of the mourning process (p. 706).

When the exaggerated reaction occurs, the individual remains fixed in the anger stage of the grief response. This anger may be directed toward others in the environment to whom the individual may be attributing the loss. However, many times the anger is turned inward on the self. When this occurs, depression is the result. Depressive mood disorder is a type of exaggerated grief reaction.

Chronic or Prolonged Grieving

Some authors have discussed a chronic or prolonged grief response as a type of maladaptive grief response. Care must be taken in making this determination because, as was stated previously, length of the grief response depends on the individual. An adaptive response may take years for some people. A prolonged process may be considered maladaptive when certain behaviors are exhibited. Prolonged grief may be a problem when behaviors such as maintaining personal possessions aimed at keeping a lost loved one alive (as though he or she will eventually reenter the life of the bereaved) or disabling behaviors that prevent the bereaved from adaptively performing activities of daily living are in evidence. Another example is of a widow who refused to participate in family gatherings following the death of her husband. For many years until her own death, she took a sandwich to the cemetery on holidays, sat on the tombstone, and ate her "holiday meal" with her husband. Other bereaved individuals have been known to set a place at the table for the deceased loved one long after the completed mourning process would have been expected.

Normal versus Maladaptive Grieving

Several authors have identified one crucial difference between normal and maladaptive grieving: the loss of self-esteem. Marked feelings of worthlessness are indicative of depression rather than uncomplicated bereavement. Corr and Corr (2013) state, "Normal grief reactions do not include the loss of self-esteem commonly found in most clinical depression" (p. 215). Pies (2013) affirmed:

> Unlike the person with [Major Depressive Disorder] MDD, most recently bereaved individuals are usually not preoccupied with feelings of worthlessness, hopelessness, or unremitting gloom; rather, self-esteem is usually preserved; the bereaved person can envision a "better day;" and positive thoughts and feelings are often interspersed with negative ones.

It is thought that this major difference between normal grieving and maladaptive grieving (the feeling of worthlessness or low self-esteem) ultimately precipitates depression, which can be a progressive process for some individuals.

Concepts of Death—Developmental Issues

Children

- **Birth to Age 2.** Infants are unable to recognize and understand death, but they can experience the feelings of loss and separation. Infants who are separated from their mothers may become quiet, lose weight, and sleep less. Children at this age will likely sense changes in the atmosphere of the home in which a death has occurred. They often react to the emotions of adults by becoming more irritable and crying more.
- **Ages 3 to 5.** Preschoolers and kindergartners have some understanding about death but often have difficulty distinguishing between fantasy and reality. They believe death is reversible, and their thoughts about death may include magical thinking. For example, they may believe that their thoughts or behaviors caused a person to become sick or to die.

Children of this age are capable of understanding at least some of what they see and hear from adult conversations or media reports. They become frightened if they feel a threat to themselves or to their loved ones. They are concerned with safety issues and require a great deal of personal reassurance that they will be protected. Regressive behaviors, such as loss of bladder or bowel control, thumb-sucking, and temper tantrums, are not uncommon. Changes in eating and sleeping patterns may also occur.

- **Ages 6 to 9.** Children at this age begin to understand the finality of death. They are able to understand a more detailed explanation of why or how the person died, although the concept of death is often associated with old age or with accidents. They may believe that death is contagious and avoid association with individuals who have experienced a loss by death. Death is often personified in the form of a "bogey man" or a monster—someone who takes people away or someone they can avoid if they try hard enough. It is difficult for them to perceive their own death. Normal grief reactions at this age include regressive and aggressive behaviors, withdrawal, school phobias, somatic symptoms, and clinging behaviors.
- **Ages 10 to 12.** Preadolescent children are able to understand that death is final and eventually affects everyone, including themselves. They are interested in the physical aspects of dying and the final disposition of the body. They may ask questions about how the death will affect them personally. Feelings of anger, guilt, and depression are common. Peer

relationships and school performance may be disrupted. There may be a preoccupation with the loss and a withdrawal into the self. They will require reassurance of their own safety and self-worth.

Adolescents

Adolescents are usually able to view death on an adult level. They understand death to be universal and inevitable; however, they have difficulty tolerating the intense feelings associated with the death of a loved one. They may or may not cry. They may withdraw into themselves or attempt to go about usual activities in an effort to avoid dealing with the pain of the loss. Some teens exhibit acting-out behaviors, such as aggression and defiance. It is often easier for adolescents to discuss their feelings with peers than with their parents or other adults. Some adolescents may show regressive behaviors whereas others react by trying to take care of their loved ones who are also grieving. In general, individuals of this age group have an attitude of immortality. Although they understand that their own death is inevitable, the concept is so far-reaching as to be imperceptible.

Adults

The adult's concept of death is influenced by cultural and religious backgrounds (Murray et al., 2009). Behaviors associated with grieving in the adult were discussed in the section on "Theoretical Perspectives on Loss and Bereavement."

Older Adults

Philosophers and poets have described late adulthood as the "season of loss." Jeffreys (2010) states:

> The grief of older people is unique because of the many nondeath losses that are a part of aging. These include physical changes, changes in family, occupational and social roles, relocation, and shifts in mental functioning (p. 18).

By the time individuals reach their 60s and 70s, they have experienced numerous losses, and mourning has become a life-long process. Those who are most successful at adapting to losses earlier in life will similarly cope better with the losses and grief inherent in aging. Unfortunately, with the aging process comes a convergence of losses, the timing of which makes it impossible for the aging individual to complete the grief process in response to one loss before another occurs. Because grief is cumulative, this can result in *bereavement overload*; the person is less able to adapt and reintegrate, and mental and physical health is jeopardized (Halstead, 2005). Bereavement overload has been implicated as a predisposing factor in the development of depressive disorder in older adults.

Depression is a common symptom in the grief response to significant losses. It is important to understand the difference between the depression of normal grieving and the disorder of clinical depression. Some of these differences are presented in Table 21-1.

TABLE 21-1	Normal Grief Reactions versus Symptoms of Clinical Depression	
Normal Grief	**Clinical Depression**
Self-esteem intact	Self-esteem is disturbed
May openly express anger	Usually does not directly express anger
Experiences a mixture of "good and bad days"	Persistent state of dysphoria
Able to experience moments of pleasure	Anhedonia is prevalent
Accepts comfort and support from others	Does not respond to social interaction and support from others
Maintains feeling of hope	Feelings of hopelessness prevail
May express guilt feelings over some aspect of the loss	Has generalized feelings of guilt
Relates feelings of depression to specific loss experienced	Does not relate feelings to a particular experience
May experience transient physical symptoms	Expresses chronic physical complaints

Sources: Corr and Corr (2013); Pies (2013); and Sadock and Sadock (2007).

Common Nursing Diagnoses and Interventions for the Individual Who Is Grieving

■ RISK FOR COMPLICATED GRIEVING

Definition: *At risk for a disorder that occurs after the death of a significant other [or any other loss of significance to the individual], in which the experience of distress accompanying bereavement fails to follow normative expectations and manifests in functional impairment* (NANDA International [NANDA-I], 2012, p. 367)

Risk Factors ("related to")

[Actual or perceived object loss (e.g., people, pets, possessions, job, status, home, ideals, parts and process of the body)]
[Denial of loss]
[Interference with life functioning]
[Reliving of past experiences with little or no reduction (diminishment) of intensity of the grief]
Lack of social support
Emotional instability

Goals/Objectives

Short-term Goals

1. Client will acknowledge awareness of the loss.
2. Client will express feelings about the loss.
3. Client will verbalize own position in the grief process.

Long-term Goal

Client will progress through the grief process in a healthful manner toward resolution.

Interventions With *Selected Rationales*

1. Assess client's stage in the grief process. *Accurate baseline data are required to provide appropriate assistance.*
2. Develop trust. Show empathy, concern, and unconditional positive regard. *Developing trust provides the basis for a therapeutic relationship.*
3. 🐾 Help the client actualize the loss by talking about it. "When did it happen? How did it happen?" and so forth. *Reviewing the events of the loss can help the client come to full awareness of the loss.*
4. Help the client identify and express feelings. *Until client can recognize and accept personal feelings regarding the loss, grief work cannot progress.* Some of the more problematic feelings include:
   a. *Anger.* The anger may be directed at the deceased, at God, displaced on others, or retroflected inward on the self. Encourage the client to examine this anger and validate the appropriateness of this feeling. *Many people will not admit to angry feelings, believing it is inappropriate and unjustified. Expression of this emotion is necessary to prevent fixation in this stage of grief.*
   b. *Guilt.* The client may feel that he or she did not do enough to prevent the loss. Help the client by reviewing the circumstances of the loss and the reality that it could not be prevented. *Feelings of guilt prolong resolution of the grief process.*
   c. *Anxiety and helplessness.* Help the client to recognize the way that life was managed before the loss. Help the client to put the feelings of helplessness into perspective by pointing out ways that he or she managed situations effectively without help from others. Role-play life events and assist with decision-making situations. *The client may have fears that he or she may not be able to carry on alone.*
5. Interpret normal behaviors associated with grieving and provide client with adequate time to grieve. *Understanding of the grief process will help prevent feelings of guilt generated by these responses. Individuals need adequate time to adjust to*

the loss and all its ramifications. This involves getting past birthdays and anniversaries of which the deceased was a part.

6. Provide continuing support. If this is not possible by the nurse, then offer referrals to support groups. Support groups of individuals going through the same experiences can be very helpful for the grieving individual. *The availability of emotional support systems facilitates the grief process.*

7. Identify pathological defenses that the client may be using (e.g., drug/alcohol use, somatic complaints, social isolation). Assist the client in understanding why these are not healthy defenses and how they delay the process of grieving. *The bereavement process is impaired by behaviors that mask the pain of the loss.*

8. Encourage the client to make an honest review of the relationship with the lost entity. Journal-keeping is a facilitative tool with this intervention. *Only when the client is able to see both positive and negative aspects related to the loss will the grieving process be complete.*

Outcome Criteria

1. Client is able to express feelings about the loss.
2. Client verbalizes stages of the grief process and behaviors associated with each.
3. Client acknowledges own position in the grief process and recognizes the appropriateness of the associated feelings and behaviors.

■ RISK FOR SPIRITUAL DISTRESS

Definition: *At risk for an impaired ability to experience and integrate meaning and purpose in life through connectedness with self, others, art, music, literature, nature, and/or a power greater than oneself* (NANDA-I, 2012, p. 412)

Risk Factors ("related to")

Loss [of any concept of value to the individual]
Low self-esteem
Natural disasters
Physical illness
Depression; anxiety; stress
Separated from support systems
Life changes

Goals/Objectives

Short-term Goal

Client will identify meaning and purpose in life, moving forward with hope for the future.

Long-term Goal

Client will express achievement of support and personal satisfaction from spiritual practices.

Interventions With *Selected Rationales*

1. Be accepting and nonjudgmental when the client expresses anger and bitterness toward God. Stay with the client. *The nurse's presence and nonjudgmental attitude increase the client's feelings of self-worth and promote trust in the relationship.*
2. Encourage the client to ventilate feelings related to meaning of own existence in the face of current loss. *Client may believe he or she cannot go on living without the lost entity. Catharsis can provide relief and put life back into realistic perspective.*
3. Encourage the client as part of grief work to reach out to previously used religious practices for support. Encourage the client to discuss these practices and how they provided support in the past. *Client may find comfort in religious rituals with which he or she is familiar.*
4. Ensure the client that he or she is not alone when feeling inadequate in the search for life's answers. *Validation of client's feelings and assurance that they are shared by others offer encouragement and an affirmation of acceptability.*
5. Contact spiritual leader of client's choice, if he or she requests. *These individuals serve to provide relief from spiritual distress and often can do so when other support persons cannot.*

Outcome Criteria

1. Client verbalizes increased sense of self-concept and hope for the future.
2. Client verbalizes meaning and purpose in life that reinforces hope, peace, and contentment.
3. Client expresses personal satisfaction and support from spiritual practices.

@ INTERNET REFERENCES

- Additional references related to bereavement may be located at the following Web sites:
  a. www.journeyofhearts.org
  b. www.nhpco.org
  c. www.hospicefoundation.org
  d. www.livingwithloss.com
  e. www.caringinfo.org
  f. www.aahpm.org
  g. www.hpna.org

CHAPTER 22

Military Families

■ BACKGROUND ASSESSMENT DATA

There are currently about 1.5 million individuals serving in the U. S. Armed Forces in more than 150 countries around the world (USA.gov, 2013). Because of U.S. involvement in conflicts around the world, perhaps at no time in modern history has so much attention been given to what individuals and families experience as a result of their lives in the military. There is an ongoing effort by organizations that provide services for active duty military personnel and veterans of military combat to keep up with the growing demand, and resources for these services will be required for many years to come. The need for mental health-care practitioners will rise as the increasing number of veterans and their family members struggle to cope with their combat-related experiences.

The Military Family

The military lifestyle offers both positive and negative aspects to those who choose this way of life. Hall (2011) summarizes a number of pros and cons about what has come to be known as The Warrior Society. Some advantages include the following:

- Early retirement compared to civilian counterparts
- The security of a vast system to meet family needs
- Job security with a guaranteed paycheck
- Health-care benefits
- Opportunities to see areas of the world
- Educational opportunities

Some disadvantages include the following:

- Frequent separations and reunions
- Regular household relocations
- Living life under the maxim of "the mission must always come first"
- A pattern of rigidity, regimentation, and conformity in family life
- Feelings of detachment from nonmilitary community
- The social effects of "rank"
- The lack of control over pay, promotion, and other benefits

Mary Wertsch (1996), who conducted a vast amount of research on the culture of the military family, stated, "The great paradox of the military is that its members, the self-appointed frontline guardians of our cherished American democratic values, do not live in democracy themselves" (p. 15). The military is maintained by a rigid authoritarian structure, and these characteristics often extend into the structure of the home.

Isolation and alienation are common facets of military life. To compensate for the extreme mobility, the focus of this lifestyle turns inward to the military world, rather than outward to the local community. Children of military families almost always report that no matter what school they attend, they feel "different" from the other students (Wertsch, 1996). These descriptions apply principally to "career" military families. There is another type of military family that has become a familiar part of the American culture in recent years. The military campaigns of Operation Enduring Freedom (OEF) and Operation Iraqi Freedom (OIF) together make up the longest sustained U.S. military operation since the Vietnam War, and they are the first extended conflicts to depend on an all-volunteer military (Institute of Medicine [IOM], 2012). There has been heavy dependence on the National Guard and Reserves, and an escalation in the pace, duration, and number of deployments and redeployments experienced by these individuals. Many had joined the National Guard or Reserves as a second job for financial reasons or for the educational opportunities available to them. Little thought had been given to the possibility of actually fighting in a war.

Military Spouses and Children

A military spouse inherently knows and lives with the concept of "mission first." Devries and colleagues (2012) state, "While the military works hard to value the family lives of service members and their welfare, the nature of the job is that the mission trumps all other concerns" (p. 11). However, times have changed from the days when life in the military was viewed as a two-person career, in which a woman was expected to "create the right family setting so that her husband's work reflected his life at home, by staying positive, being interested in his duty, and being flexible and adaptable" (Hall, 2012, p. 148). Many of today's military spouses have their own careers or are pursuing higher levels of education. They do not view the military as a joint career with their service member spouse.

The lives of military spouses and children are clearly affected when the active duty assignments of the service member require frequent family moves. Wakefield (2007) has stated, "The many short-term relationships, complications of spousal employment, university transfer issues, escalated misbehavior of the children, day-care arrangements, spousal loneliness, and increased financial obligations are just some of the issues military personnel face that can lead to frustration." In most instances, when the service member receives orders for a new geographical assignment, the spouse's education, career, or both is put on hold, and the entire family is relocated. Other occasions may arise when the family is unable to immediately follow the service member to the new location. In certain instances, such as when a student may be about to complete a semester or is about to graduate, the service member may proceed to the new assignment without the family. This is difficult for the military spouse who is left alone to care for the children, as well as to deal with all aspects of the move.

Military children face unique challenges. They primarily attend civilian public schools in which they form a unique subculture among staff and peers who often do not understand their life experiences. Children who grow up in a career military family learn to adapt to changing situations very quickly and to hide a certain level of fear associated with the nomadic lifestyle.

The Impact of Deployment

Not since the Vietnam War have so many U.S. military families been affected by deployment-related family separation, combat injury, and death. Many service members have been deployed multiple times. Those who are deployed most frequently describe their greatest fear as that of having to leave their spouse and children. Lengthy separations pose many challenges to all members of the family. Spouses undertake all the challenges of managing the household, in addition to assuming the role of the singular parent. The pressure and stress are intense as the spouse attempts to maintain an atmosphere of strength for the children, while experiencing the fears and anxiety associated with the life-threatening conditions facing his or her service member partner.

More than 2 million children have experienced the deployment of a parent to Iraq or Afghanistan, and thousands have either lost a parent or have a parent who was wounded in these conflicts. Children often have difficulty understanding and accepting the changes in appearance, personality, or behavior of a parent upon their return from the combat experience. The following behaviors have been reported in children in response to the deployment of a parent (American Academy of Child & Adolescent Psychiatry, 2013):

- Infants (birth to 12 months): May respond to disruptions in their schedule with decreased appetite, weight loss, irritability, and/or apathy.
- Toddlers (1 to 3 years): May become sullen, tearful, throw temper tantrums, or develop sleep problems.
- Preschoolers (3 to 6 years): May regress in areas such as toilet training, sleep, separation fears, physical complaints, or thumb sucking. May assume blame for parent's departure.
- School-age children (6 to 12 years): Are more aware of potential dangers to parent. May exhibit irritable behavior, aggression, or whininess. May become more regressed and fearful about parent's safety.

- Adolescents (13 to 18 years): May be rebellious, irritable, or more challenging of authority. Parents need to be alert to high-risk behaviors, such as problems with the law, sexual acting out, and drug or alcohol abuse.

Women in the Military

Women make up approximately 15% of the U.S. military and 17% of National Guard and Reserve members (Mathewson, 2011). Women have been serving in the military since the time of the Civil War, mostly in the roles of nurses, spies, and support persons. In recent years, the Pentagon relaxed its ban on women serving in combat roles, and "women began to fly combat aircraft, staff missile placements, drive convoys in the desert, and participate in other roles that involved potential combat exposure" (Mathewson, 2011, p. 217). Early in 2013, the Secretary of Defense lifted the ban on combat jobs to women, gradually opening direct combat units to female troops. At the present time, certain specialty positions continue to remain off-limits, although the plan is to integrate women into these positions. Flexibility in the new law exists for exemptions to occur if further assessment reveals that some jobs are inappropriate for women.

Special Concerns of Women in the Military

- **Sexual Harassment.** Wolfe and associates (1998), in a study of women on active duty during the Persian Gulf War, found that both physical and sexual harassment were higher than those typically found in peacetime military samples. Reports by military therapists convey that these women who were sexually harassed when in the military suffer high rates of a range of problems following discharge, including poor self-image, relationship problems, drug use, depression, and posttraumatic stress disorder (PTSD).
- **Sexual Assault.** Sexual assault is defined as "attempted or completed sexual attack through threat or use of physical force that took place on or off duty during the course of military service" (Mathewson, 2011, p. 221). It is estimated that only about 13% of sexual assaults in the military are reported. Reasons for not reporting include being afraid of causing trouble in their unit, fear that their commanders and fellow soldiers would turn against them, that they would be passed over for well-deserved promotions, or be transferred and removed from duty altogether (Vlahos, 2012).
- **Differential Treatment and Conditions.** Although their numbers have increased, women still constitute a minority in the military. Because of the small number of women in any given unit, officers and enlisted personnel are often housed together. Officers report missing being with other officers to discuss work and to be able to spend time with

their peers, and enlisted women often report feeling uncomfortable with an officer in their presence.

Women's military careers are often limited by their exclusions from occupational specialties. These sanctions often preclude female officers and enlisted personnel from the most prestigious units and occupations in the military, their participation in which is essential to ascending in the ranks should they choose to make the military a career. However, as stated previously, some changes are currently proposed that, when implemented, will decrease occupational discrimination against women in the military.

- **Parenting Issues.** Women's feelings associated with leaving their children often differ from those of men. Women seem to struggle more with guilt feelings for "abandoning" their children, whereas men have stronger emotions tied to a sense of doing their duty. Although men also experience regret at leaving their children, they often rely on the assurance that the children have their mothers to care for them.

Veterans

Most veterans returning from a combat zone undergo a period of adjustment. Although the majority of them do not develop a behavioral health condition, most will experience feelings and reactions that may contribute to difficulties with their reintegration into civilian life. Many veterans suffer from migraine headaches and experience cognitive difficulties, such as memory loss. Hypervigilance, insomnia, and jitteriness are common. The Substance Abuse and Mental Health Services Administration (SAMHSA, 2012) states, "Veterans may struggle to concentrate; engage in aggressive behavior, such as aggressive driving; and use alcohol, tobacco, and drugs excessively. However, the intensity and duration of these and other worrisome behaviors can indicate a more serious problem and the need for professional treatment" (p. 1).

Traumatic Brain Injury

The Departments of Veterans Affairs and Defense (DVA/DoD, 2009) offer the following definition of traumatic brain injury (TBI):

> A traumatically induced structural injury and/or physiological disruption of brain function as a result of an external force that is indicated by new onset or worsening of symptoms such as loss or alteration in consciousness, loss of memory, neurological deficits, or intracranial lesion (p. 16).

Symptoms may be classified as mild, moderate, or severe, according to severity of symptoms. Blasts from explosive devices are the leading cause of TBI for active-duty military personnel in combat. TBI also results from penetrating wounds, severe blows to the head with shrapnel or debris, and falls or bodily collisions with objects following a blast.

Posttraumatic Stress Disorder

Posttraumatic stress disorder (PTSD) is the most common mental disorder among veterans returning from military combat. The disorder can occur when an individual is exposed to an accident or violence in which there is actual or threatened death or serious injury to the self or others. Symptoms of PTSD include the following:

- Re-experiencing the trauma through flashbacks, nightmares, and intrusive thoughts
- Intensive efforts to avoid activities, people, places, situations, or objects that arouse recollections of the trauma
- Chronic negative emotional state and diminished interest or participation in significant activities
- Aggressive, reckless, or self-destructive behavior
- Hypervigilance and exaggerated startle response
- Angry outbursts, problems with concentration, and sleep disturbances

Symptoms of PTSD may be delayed, in some instances for years. When emotions regarding the trauma are constricted, they may suddenly appear at some time in the future following a major life event, stressor, or an accumulation of stressors with time that challenge the person's defenses. Symptoms also may be masked by other physical or mental health problems that the veteran may be experiencing. In some instances, the symptoms do not appear to be problematic until the individual begins a readjustment to routine occupational or social functioning.

Co-occurring disorders are common in individuals with PTSD, including major depressive disorder, substance use disorders, and anxiety disorders. Individuals with TBI also may develop PTSD, depending on the degree of amnesia experienced immediately following the cerebral trauma.

Depression and Suicide

Reports by the DoD and VA indicate that the number of suicides among veterans and active duty military has risen dramatically since 2001, the year that detailed record-keeping began. Suicide among military personnel is closely associated with the diagnoses of substance use disorder, major depressive disorder, PTSD, and TBI. A common theme among investigations of suicide attempts and completed suicides by military service members is marital/relationship distress. A study by Jakupcak and associates (2010) concluded that veterans who are unmarried or those who report lower satisfaction with their social support networks are at increased risk for suicide.

Substance Use Disorder

Substance use disorder is a common co-occurring condition with PTSD. One study reports that almost 22% of veterans with PTSD also receive a diagnosis of substance use disorder (Brancu,

Straits-Troster, & Kudler, 2011). SAMHSA (2012) states that alcohol misuse and abuse, hazardous drinking, and binge drinking are common among OEF and OIF veterans, who often report drinking to numb the agonizing feelings and erase the painful memories related to their combat experiences. One research study of OIF veterans indicated that individuals who were exposed to extreme violence and human trauma were more likely to engage in frequent and heavy drinking than their counterparts who had less exposure to such combat experiences (Killgore et al, 2008).

Substance abuse continues to be a major concern for the military. Although there have been reductions over time in tobacco use and illicit drug use, increases in other areas, such as prescription drug abuse and heavy alcohol use, are an ongoing problem. Alcohol abuse is the most prevalent problem, and referrals for treatment are inadequate (National Institute on Drug Abuse [NIDA], 2011). NIDA (2011) reports, "Research findings highlight the need to improve screening and access to care for alcohol-related problems among service members returning from combat deployments" (p. 1).

■ SYMPTOMATOLOGY (SUBJECTIVE AND OBJECTIVE DATA)

Posttraumatic Stress Disorder

1. Rage reactions
2. Aggression; irritability
3. Substance abuse
4. Flashbacks; nightmares; startle reaction
5. Depression; anxiety; suicidal ideation
6. Feelings of hopelessness
7. Guilt
8. Emotional numbness
9. Panic attacks
10. Confusion, fear, and anxiety among family members

Traumatic Brain Injury

1. Impaired mobility; limited range of motion
2. Decreased muscle strength
3. Perceptual or cognitive impairment
4. Seizures
5. Memory deficits
6. Distractibility; altered attention span or concentration
7. Impaired ability to make decisions, solve problems, reason, or conceptualize
8. Personality changes
9. Inability to perform activities of daily living
10. Confusion, fear, and anxiety among family members

Family Members' Issues

1. Children
   a. Regressive behaviors
   b. Loss of appetite
   c. Temper tantrums
   d. Clinging behaviors
   e. Guilt and self-blame
   f. Sleep problems
   g. Irritability
   h. Aggression
2. Adolescents
   a. Rebelliousness
   b. Irritability
   c. Acting-out behaviors
   d. Promiscuity
   e. Substance abuse
3. Spouse/Partner
   a. Depression
   b. Anxiety
   c. Loneliness
   d. Fear
   e. Feeling overwhelmed and powerless
   f. Anger
4. Spouse/Partner Caregiver
   a. Anger
   b. Anxiety; frustration
   c. Ineffective coping
   d. Sleep deprivation
   e. Somatic symptoms
   f. Fatigue

Common Nursing Diagnoses and Interventions for Military Service Members, Veterans, and Their Families

■ POST-TRAUMA SYNDROME

Definition: *Sustained maladaptive response to a traumatic, overwhelming event* (NANDA International [NANDA-I], 2012, p. 335)

Possible Etiologies ("related to")

War
Witnessing violent death
Witnessing mutilation
Serious threat or injury to self [or others]
Events outside the range of usual human experience

Defining Characteristics ("evidenced by")

Anger; aggression
Depression
Difficulty concentrating
Flashbacks; nightmares; intrusive dreams
Exaggerated startle response
Panic attacks
Hypervigilance
Substance abuse

Goals/Objectives

Short-term Goals

1. Client will begin a healthy grief resolution, initiating the process of psychological healing (within time frame specific to individual).
2. Client will demonstrate ability to deal with emotional reactions in an individually appropriate manner.

Long-term Goal

The client will integrate the traumatic experience into his or her persona, renew significant relationships, and establish meaningful goals for the future.

Interventions With *Selected Rationales*

1. Stay with the client during periods of flashbacks and nightmares. Offer reassurance of safety and security and that these symptoms are not uncommon following a trauma of the magnitude he or she has experienced. *The presence of a trusted individual may help to calm fears for personal safety and reassure the anxious client that he or she is not "going crazy."*
2. Encourage the client to talk about the trauma at his or her own pace. Provide a nonthreatening, private environment, and include a significant other if the client wishes. Acknowledge and validate the client's feelings as they are expressed. *This debriefing process is the first step in the progression toward resolution.*
3. Discuss coping strategies used in response to the trauma. Determine those that have been most helpful, including available support systems and religious and cultural influences. Identify maladaptive coping strategies being used, such as substance abuse or psychosomatic responses, and discuss more adaptive coping strategies. *Resolution of the posttrauma response is largely dependent on the effectiveness of the coping strategies employed.*
4. Help the client understand that *use of substances merely numbs feelings and delays healing.* Refer for treatment of substance use disorder if need is determined.
5. Discuss the use of stress-management techniques, such as deep breathing, meditation, relaxation techniques, and physical exercise.

These interventions help to maintain anxiety at a manageable level and prevent escalation to panic.

6. Administer medications as prescribed, and provide medication education. *A number of medications have been used for clients with PTSD. Some of these include the selective serotonin reuptake inhibitors (SSRIs), trazodone, amitriptyline, imipramine, and phenelzine. Benzodiazepines are sometimes prescribed for their antipanic effects, although their addictive properties make them less desirable. Propranolol and clonidine have been successful in alleviating symptoms such as nightmares, intrusive recollections, hypervigilance, insomnia, startle responses, and angry outbursts.*

Outcome Criteria

1. Client is able to discuss the traumatic experience with trusted nurse/therapist.
2. Client recognizes own position in grief process and demonstrates the initiation of psychological healing.
3. Client has established meaningful, realistic goals and expresses hope for a positive future.

■ RISK FOR SUICIDE

Definition: *At risk for self-inflicted, life-threatening injury* (NANDA International [NANDA-I], 2012, p. 452)

Risk Factors ("related to")

[Depression]
[Perception of lack of social support]
[Physical disabilities from combat injuries]
[Feelings of hopelessness]
Substance abuse
Poor support systems
States desire to die

Goals/Objectives

Short-term Goals

1. Client will seek out staff member when suicidal feelings occur.
2. Client will verbalize adaptive coping strategies for use when suicidal feelings occur.

Long-term Goals

1. Client will demonstrate adaptive coping strategies for use when suicidal feelings occur.
2. Client will not harm self.

Interventions With *Selected Rationales*

1. Assess degree of risk according to seriousness of threat, existence of a plan, and availability and lethality of the means. Ask directly if the person is thinking of acting on thoughts or feelings. *The risk of suicide is greatly increased if the client has developed a plan and particularly if means exist for the client to execute the plan. It is important to get the subject out in the open. This places some of the responsibility for his or her safety with the client.*

2. Ascertain presence of significant others for support. *The presence of a strong support system decreases the risk of suicide.*

3. Determine whether substance abuse is a factor. *The abuse of substances increases the risk of suicide.*

4. Encourage expression of feelings, including appropriate expression of anger. *It is vital that the client express angry feelings, because suicide and other self-destructive behaviors are often viewed as the result of anger turned inward on the self.*

5. Ensure that the environment is safe. Remove all dangerous objects from the client's environment (e.g., sharp items, belts, ties, straps, breakable items, smoking materials). *Client safety is a nursing priority.*

6. Help the client identify more appropriate solutions and offer hope for the future. *In the client's current state of mind, he or she may not be able to see any hope for positive life change. Discussion with a trusted individual may help the client identify options that provide encouragement and hope for improvement.*

7. Negotiate a short-term, no-suicide contract. (Some clinicians question the effectiveness of this intervention; however, it has proved successful with some individuals.)

8. Involve family/significant others in the planning. *This problem affects all members of the family. Outcomes are more successful when all persons involved are allowed input into the plan for intervention.*

Outcome Criteria

1. Client is able to discuss feelings about current situation with nurse or therapist.

2. Client expresses optimism and hope for the future.

3. Client has not harmed self.

■ DISTURBED THOUGHT PROCESSES

Definition: *Disruption in cognitive operations and activities* (Note: This diagnosis has been retired by NANDA-I, but is retained in this text because of its appropriateness in describing these specific behaviors.)

Possible Etiologies ("related to")

[Response to having experienced a trauma outside the range of usual human experience]
[Physical trauma to the brain]

Defining Characteristics ("evidenced by")

[Memory deficits]
[Distractibility]
[Altered attention span or concentration]
[Impaired ability to make decisions, solve problems, reason or conceptualize]
[Personality changes]

Goals/Objectives

Short-term Goal

Client will perform self-care activities with assistance as required.

Long-term Goal

Client will regain cognitive ability to execute mental functions realistic with the extent of the condition or injury.

Interventions With *Selected Rationales*

1. Evaluate mental status. *An accurate assessment of client's strengths and limitations is essential to providing appropriate care and fulfilling client's needs. Consideration should be given to the following issues and concerns:*
   • Extent of impairment in thinking ability
   • Remote and recent memory
   • Orientation to person, place, time, and situation
   • Insight and judgment
   • Changes in personality
   • Attention span, distractibility, and ability to make decisions or solve problems
   • Ability to communicate appropriately
   • Anxiety level
   • Evidence of psychotic behavior
2. Report to the physician any cognitive changes that become obvious. *This is important to ensure that any reversible condition is addressed and that client safety is assured.*
3. Note behavior indicative of potential for violence and take appropriate action *to prevent harm to client and others.*
4. Provide safety measures as required. Institute seizure precautions if indicated. Assist with limited mobility issues. Monitor medication regimen. *Client safety is a nursing priority.*
5. Refer to appropriate rehabilitation providers. *Individuals with traumatic brain injury will require assistance from*

multidisciplinary providers in an effort to achieve his or her highest level of self-care ability.

Outcome Criteria

1. Client is able to assist with aspects of self-care.
2. Client has not experienced injury as a result of cognitive limitations.
3. Client participates in decision-making situations that relate to life situations.

■ INTERRUPTED FAMILY PROCESSES

Definition: *Change in family relationships and/or functioning* (NANDA-I, 2012, p. 311)

Possible Etiologies ("related to")

Situational transition or crisis precipitated by:
[Family member returns from combat with PTSD]
[Family member returns from combat with TBI]

Defining Characteristics ("evidenced by")

[Confusion, fear, and anxiety among family members]
[Inability to adapt to changes associated with veteran member's condition/injury]
[Difficulty accepting/receiving help]
[Inability to express or to accept each other's feelings]

Goals/Objectives

Short-term Goal

Family members will accept assistance from multidisciplinary services in an effort to restore adaptive family functioning.

Long-term Goal

Family will verbalize understanding of trauma-related illness, demonstrate ability to maintain anxiety at a manageable level, and make appropriate decisions to stabilize family functioning.

Interventions With *Selected Rationales*

1. Encourage continuous, open dialogue between family members. *This promotes understanding and assists family members to maintain clear communication and resolve problems effectively.*
2. Assist the family to identify and use previously successful coping strategies. *Most people have developed effective coping skills that when identified can be useful in current situation.*

3. Encourage family participation in multidisciplinary team conference or group therapy. *Participation in family and group therapy for an extended period increases likelihood of success as interactional issues (e.g., marital conflict, scapegoating) can be addressed and dealt with.*

4. Involve family in social support and community activities of their interest and choice. *Involvement with others can help family members to experience new ways of interacting and gain insight into their behavior, providing opportunity for change.*

5. Assist the family to identify situations that may lead to fear or anxiety. Encourage the use of stress-management techniques. *A high level of anxiety and stress interferes with the ability to cope and solve problems effectively.*

6. Make necessary referrals (e.g., Parent Effectiveness, specific disease or disability support groups, self-help groups, clergy, psychological counseling, or family therapy). *Multidisciplinary specialties may be required to effect positive change and enhance conflict resolution. If substance abuse is a problem, all family members should be encouraged to seek support and assistance in dealing with the situation to promote a healthy outcome.*

7. Involve the family in mutual setting of goals to plan for the future. *When all members of the family are involved, commitment to goals and continuation of the plan are more likely to be maintained.*

8. Identify community agencies from which family may seek assistance (e.g., Meals on Wheels, visiting nurse, trauma support group, American Cancer Society, Veterans Administration). *These agencies may provide both immediate and long-term support to individual members and to the family as a group.*

Outcome Criteria

1. Family members verbalize understanding of illness/trauma, treatment regimen, and prognosis.
2. Family members demonstrate ability to express feelings openly and communicate with each other in an appropriate and healthy manner.
3. Family members seek out and accept assistance from community agencies.

■ RISK FOR COMPLICATED GRIEVING

Definition: *At risk for a disorder that occurs after the death of a significant other [or any loss or perceived loss of significance to the individual], in which the experience of distress accompanying bereavement fails to follow normative expectations and manifests in functional impairment* (NANDA-I, 2012, p. 367)

Risk Factors ("related to")

[Military deployment of the individual's spouse/partner, resulting in:
  Depression
  Anxiety
  Loneliness
  Fear
  Feeling overwhelmed
  Powerlessness
  Anger]

Goals/Objectives

Short-term Goal

Client will acknowledge feelings of anger and powerlessness associated with spouse/partner's extended absence.

Long-term Goal

Client will work through stages of grief, achieve a healthy acceptance, and express a sense of control over the present situation and future outcome.

Interventions With *Selected Rationales*

1. Help family members to realize that all of the feelings they are having are a normal part of the grieving process. Validate their feelings of anger, loneliness, fear, powerlessness, dysphoria, and distress at separation from their loved one. *Understanding of the grief process will help prevent feelings of guilt generated by these responses. Individuals need adequate time to accommodate to the loss and all its ramifications.*

2. Help the parent to understand that children's and adolescents' problematic behaviors are symptoms of grieving and that they should not be deemed unacceptable and result in punishment, but rather be recognized as having their basis in grief. *Children and adolescents exhibit grief differently than adults, and they must be allowed to grieve in their own way. Caring support and assistance is required when the behaviors become problematic or maladaptive.*

3. Children should be allowed an appropriate amount of time to grieve. *Some experts believe children need at least 4 weeks to adjust to a parent's deployment (Gabany & Shellenbarger, 2010).* Refer for professional help if improvement is not observed in a reasonable period of time.

4. Assess if maladaptive coping strategies, such as substance abuse, are being used. Assist the client to understand why these are not healthy defenses. *Behaviors that mask the pain of loss delay the process of adaptation.*

5. Suggest caution against spending too much time alone. Encourage resuming involvement in usual activities, and employ previously used successful coping strategies. *Most people have developed effective coping skills that can be useful in the current situation. Keeping busy and receiving support from others eases the burden of loneliness.*

6. Suggest keeping a journal of experiences and feelings. *Journaling can be therapeutic because it helps to get in touch with emotions that are sometimes difficult to express verbally. Writing down thoughts and feelings helps to sort through problems and come to a deeper understanding of oneself or the issues in one's life.*

7. Refer to other resources as needed, such as psychotherapy, family counseling, religious references or pastor, or grief support group. *The individual may require ongoing support to work through the feelings of loss associated with long-term separation issues.*

Outcome Criteria

1. Client recognizes and verbalizes own position in grief process.
2. Client keeps a journal of feelings and emotions.
3. Grieving behaviors of children and adolescents are recognized and accepted. Caring assistance is provided.
4. Family demonstrates ability to adapt to the life change associated with the absence of the service member and to accept assistance and support from others.

■ CAREGIVER ROLE STRAIN

Definition: *Difficulty in performing family/significant other caregiver role* (NANDA-I, 2012, pp. 298–300)

Possible Etiologies ("related to")

24-hour care responsibilities
Severity, chronicity, and unpredictability of illness/[injury] course
Increasing care needs [of care receiver]
Cognitive or psychological problems [of care receiver]

Defining Characteristics ("evidenced by")

Anger
Stress; anxiety
Frustration
Ineffective coping
Sleep deprivation
Somatization

Goals/Objectives

Short-term Goal

Client will identify resources within self and from others to assist with and manage caregiving responsibilities.

Long-term Goal

Caregiver will demonstrate effective problem-solving skills and develop adaptive coping mechanisms to regain equilibrium.

Interventions With *Selected Rationales*

1. Assess the spouse/caregiver's ability to anticipate and fulfill the injured service member's unmet needs. Note caregiver's physical and emotional health, developmental level and abilities, and additional responsibilities of caregiver (e.g., job, raising family). *It is important to ensure that caregiver has realistic self-expectations. Failure in the caregiver role is likely to occur in a situation in which the caregiver is over-burdened and under-supported.*

2. Ensure that the caregiver encourages the injured service member to be as independent as possible. *Not only does this relieve the caregiver of some of the responsibilities, it provides the care receiver with increased feelings of capability, personal control, and self-esteem.*

3. Encourage the caregiver to express feelings and to participate in a support group. *Having others with which to share concerns and fears is therapeutic. Support group members provide ideas for different ways to manage problems, helping caregivers deal more effectively with the situation.*

4. Provide information or demonstrate techniques for dealing with acting out, violent, or disoriented behavior by the injured service member. *The presence of cognitive impairment necessitates learning these techniques or skills to enhance safety of the caregiver and receiver.*

5. Encourage attention to own needs (e.g., eating and sleeping regularly, setting realistic goals, talking with trusted friend, periodic respite from caregiving), accepting own feelings, acknowledging frustrations and limitations, and being realistic about loved one's condition. *This supports and enhances the caregiver's general well-being and coping ability.*

6. Discuss and demonstrate stress management techniques and importance of self-nurturing (e.g., pursuing self-development interests, hobbies, social activities, spiritual enrichment). *Being involved in activities such as these can prevent caregiver burnout.*

Outcome Criteria

1. Caregiver is able to solve problems effectively regarding care of their loved one.
2. Caregiver demonstrates adaptive coping strategies for dealing with stress of the caregiver role.
3. Caregiver openly expresses feelings.
4. Caregiver expresses desire to join a support group of other caregivers.

@ INTERNET REFERENCES

- The following Web sites provide information for and about military service members, their families, and veterans:
  a. www.va.gov
  b. www.bpwfoundation.org/index.php/issues/women_veterans
  c. www.dvnf.org
  d. www.nvf.org
  e. www.ptsd.va.gov
  f. www.ncbi.nlm.nih.gov/pubmedhealth/PMH0001923
  g. www.mayoclinic.com/health/post-traumatic-stress-disorder/DS00246
  h. www.cdc.gov/traumaticbraininjury
  i. www.publichealth.va.gov/vethealthinitiative/traumatic_brain_injury.asp
  j. www.ptsd.va.gov/professional/pages/traumatic-brain-injury-ptsd.asp
  k. www.ninds.nih.gov/disorders/tbi/tbi.htm
  l. www.militaryfamily.org/feature-articles/helping-military-families-is.html
  m. www.woundedwarriorproject.org

Movie Connections

The Best Years of Our Lives (1946) • *The Deer Hunter* (1978) • *Jarhead* (2005) • *In the Valley of Elah* (2007) • *The Lucky Ones* (2008) • *A Walk in My Shoes* (2010)

PSYCHOTROPIC MEDICATIONS

CHAPTER 23

Antianxiety Agents

■ CHEMICAL CLASS: ANTIHISTAMINES
Examples

Generic Name	Trade Name	Half-life	Pregnancy Category	Available Forms (mg)
Hydroxyzine	Vistaril	3 hr	C	CAPS: 25, 50, 100 ORAL SUSP: 25/5 mL SYRUP: 10/5 mL INJ: 25/mL, 50/mL

Indications
- Anxiety disorders
- Temporary relief of anxiety symptoms
- Allergic reactions producing pruritic conditions
- Antiemetic
- Reduction of narcotic requirement, alleviation of anxiety, and control of emesis in preoperative/postoperative clients (parenteral only)

Action
- Exerts central nervous system (CNS) depressant activity at the subcortical level of the CNS
- Has anticholinergic, antihistaminic, and antiemetic properties
- Blocks histamine 1 receptors

Contraindications and Precautions

Contraindicated in: • Hypersensitivity • Pregnancy and lactation

Use Cautiously in: • Elderly or debilitated patients (dosage reduction recommended) • Hepatic or renal dysfunction • Concomitant use of other CNS depressants

Adverse Reactions and Side Effects

- Dry Mouth
- Drowsiness
- Pain at intramuscular site

Interactions

- Additive CNS depression with other **CNS depressants** (e.g., **alcohol, other anxiolytics, opioid analgesics**, and **sedative/hypnotics**) and with **herbal depressants** (e.g., **kava, valerian**).
- Additive anticholinergic effects with other **drugs possessing anticholinergic properties** (e.g., **antihistamines, antidepressants, atropine, haloperidol, phenothiazines**) and **herbal products** such as **angel's trumpet, jimson weed,** and **scopolia.**
- Can antagonize the vasopressor effects of **epinephrine.**

Route and Dosage

INTRAMUSCULAR

- **Anxiety**
  Adults: 50 to 100 mg 4 times/day
- **Pruritus**
  Adults: 25 mg 3 or 4 times/day
- **Pre- and post-operative sedative**
  Adults: 50 to 100 mg
  Children: 0.6 mg/kg
- **Antiemetic/adjunctive therapy to analgesia**
  Adults: 25 to 100 mg q 4 to 6 hr as needed
  Children: 0.5 to 1 mg/kg q 4 to 6 hr as needed

ORAL

- **Anxiety**
  Adults: 50 to 100 mg 4 times/day
  Children (≥6 yr): 50 to 100 mg/day in divided doses
  Children (< 6 yr): 50 mg/day in divided doses
- **Pruritus**
  Adults: 25 mg 3 or 4 times/day
  Children (≥6 yr): 50 to 100 mg/day in divided doses
  Children (< 6 yr): 50 mg/day in divided doses

- **Pre- and post-operative sedative**
  Adults: 50 to 100 mg
  Children: 0.6 mg/kg

■ CHEMICAL CLASS: BENZODIAZEPINES
Examples

Generic (Trade) Name	Controlled/ Pregnancy Categories	Half-life (hr)	Indications	Available Forms (mg)
Alprazolam (Xanax)	C-IV/D	6.3–26.9	• Anxiety disorders • Anxiety symptoms • Anxiety associated with depression • Panic disorder **UNLABELED USES:** • Premenstrual dysphoric disorder • Irritable bowel syndrome and other somatic symptoms associated with anxiety	**TABS:** 0.25, 0.5, 1.0, 2.0 **TABS ER:** 0.5, 1.0, 2.0, 3.0 **TABS (ORALLY DISINTEGRATING):** 0.25, 0.5, 1.0, 2.0 **ORAL SOLU:** 1/mL
Chlordiazepoxide (Librium)	C-IV/D	5–30	• Anxiety disorders • Anxiety symptoms • Acute alcohol withdrawal • Preoperative sedation	**CAPS:** 5, 10, 25
Clonazepam (Klonopin)	C-IV/D	18–50	• Petit mal, akinetic, and myoclonic seizures • Panic disorder **UNLABELED USES:** • Acute manic episodes • Neuralgias • Restless leg syndrome • Adjunct therapy in schizophrenia • Tic disorders	**TABS:** 0.5, 1.0, 2.0 **TABS (ORALLY DISINTEGRATING):** 0.125, 0.25, 0.5, 1.0, 2.0
Clorazepate (Tranxene)	C-IV/D	40–50	• Anxiety disorders • Anxiety symptoms • Acute alcohol withdrawal • Partial seizures	**TABS:** 3.75, 7.5, 15

Generic (Trade) Name	Controlled/ Pregnancy Categories	Half-life (hr)	Indications	Available Forms (mg)
Diazepam (Valium)	C-IV/D	20–80	• Anxiety disorders • Anxiety symptoms • Skeletal muscle relaxant • Acute alcohol withdrawal • Adjunct therapy in convulsive disorders • Status epilepticus • Preoperative sedation	**TABS:** 2, 5, 10 **ORAL SOLU:** 5/5 mL, 5/mL **INJ:** 5/mL **RECTAL GEL:** 2.5, 10, 20
Lorazepam (Ativan)	C-IV/D	10–20	• Anxiety disorders • Anxiety symptoms • Status epilepticus • Preoperative sedation **UNLABELED USES:** • Acute alcohol withdrawal • Insomnia • Chemotherapy-induced nausea and vomiting	**TABS:** 0.5, 1.0, 2.0 **ORAL SOLU:** 2/mL **INJ:** 2/mL, 4/mL
Oxazepam	C-IV/D	5–20	• Anxiety disorders • Anxiety symptoms • Acute alcohol withdrawal	**CAPS:** 10, 15, 30

Action

• Benzodiazepines are thought to potentiate the effects of gamma-aminobutyric acid (GABA), a powerful inhibitory neurotransmitter, thereby producing a calmative effect. The activity may involve the spinal cord, brain stem, cerebellum, limbic system, and cortical areas.

Contraindications and Precautions

Contraindicated in: • Hypersensitivity • Psychoses • Acute narrow-angle glaucoma • Pre-existing CNS depression • Pregnancy and lactation • Shock • Coma

Use Cautiously in: • Elderly or debilitated patients (reduced dosage recommended) • Hepatic/renal/pulmonary impairment • History of drug abuse/dependence • Depressed/suicidal patients • Children

Adverse Reactions and Side Effects

- Drowsiness; dizziness, lethargy
- Nausea and vomiting
- Ataxia
- Dry mouth
- Blurred vision
- Rash
- Hypotension
- Tolerance
- Physical and psychological addiction
- Paradoxical excitation

Interactions

- Additive CNS depression with other **CNS depressants** (e.g., **alcohol, other anxiolytics, opioid analgesics,** and **sedative/ hypnotics**) and with **herbal depressants** (e.g., **kava, valerian**).
- **Cimetidine, oral contraceptives, disulfiram, fluoxetine, iso- niazid, ketoconazole, metoprolol, propoxyphene, propra- nolol,** or **valproic acid** may enhance effects of benzodiazepines.
- Benzodiazepines may decrease the efficacy of **levodopa.**
- Sedative effects of benzodiazepines may be decreased by **theophylline.**
- **Rifampin** and **St. John's Wort** may decrease the efficacy of benzodiazepines.
- Serum concentration of **digoxin** may be increased (and sub- sequent toxicity can occur) with concurrent benzodiazepine therapy.

Route and Dosage

ALPRAZOLAM (XANAX)

Anxiety disorders and anxiety symptoms: **PO** *(Adults)*: 0.25 to 0.5 mg 3 times/day. Maximum daily dose 4 mg in divided doses.

In elderly or debilitated patients: **PO:** 0.25 mg 2 or 3 times/day. Gradually increase if needed and tolerated. Total daily dosages of greater than 2 mg should not be used.

Panic disorder: **PO** *(Adults)*: Initial dose: 0.5 mg 3 times/day. In- crease dose at intervals of 3 to 4 days in increments of no more than 1 mg/day.

Extended-release tablets: **PO** *(Adults)***:** 0.5 to 1 mg once daily. May increase the dose at intervals of 3 to 4 days in increments of no more than 1 mg/day until desired effect has been achieved. Total daily dose range: 3 to 6 mg.

CHLORDIAZEPOXIDE (LIBRIUM)

Mild to Moderate Anxiety: **PO** *(Adults)*: 5 or 10 mg 3 or 4 times/day.

Children (≥6 years): 5 mg 2 to 4 times/day. May be increased to 10 mg 2 or 3 times/day if needed.

Severe Anxiety: **PO** *(Adults)*: 20 or 25 mg 3 or 4 times/day.

Elderly or debilitated patients: **PO**: 5 mg 2 times/day. Increase gradually as needed and tolerated.

Preoperative sedation: **PO** *(Adults)*: 5 to 10 mg 3 or 4 times/day.

Acute alcohol withdrawal: **PO** *(Adults)*: 50 to 100 mg; repeat as needed up to 300 mg/day.

CLONAZEPAM (KLONOPIN)

Seizures: Adults: **PO**: 0.5 mg 3 times/day. May increase by 0.5 to 1 mg every 3 days. Total daily maintenance dose not to exceed 20 mg.

Children **(<10 yr or 30 kg): PO**: Initial daily dose 0.01 to 0.03 mg/kg/day (not to exceed 0.05 mg/kg/day) given in 2 to 3 equally divided doses; increase by not more than 0.25 to 0.5 mg every 3rd day until a daily maintenance dose of 0.1 to 0.2 mg/kg has been reached.

Therapeutic serum concentrations of clonazepam are 20 to 80 mg/ml.

Panic disorder: **PO** *(Adults)*: Initial dose: 0.25 mg 2 times/day. Increase after 3 days toward target dose of 1 mg/day. Some patients may require up to 4 mg/day, in which case the dose may be increased in increments of 0.125 to 0.25 mg twice daily every 3 days until symptoms are controlled.

Acute manic episode: **PO** *(Adults)*: 2 to 16 mg/day.

Tic Disorders: **PO** *(Adults and Children)*: 0.5 to 12 mg/day.

Restless leg syndrome: **PO** *(Adults)*: 0.5 to 2 mg 30 minutes before bedtime.

CLORAZEPATE (TRANXENE)

Anxiety disorders/anxiety symptoms: **PO** *(Adults)*: 7.5 to 15 mg 2 to 4 times/day. Adjust gradually to dose within range of 15 to 60 mg/day. May also be given in a single daily dose at bedtime. The recommended initial dose is 15 mg. Adjust subsequent dosages according to patient response.

Geriatric or debilitated patients: **PO**: 7.5 to 15 mg/day.

Acute alcohol withdrawal: **PO** *(Adults)*: Day 1: 30 mg initially, followed by 15 mg 2 to 4 times/day.

Day 2: 45 to 90 mg in divided doses.

Day 3: 22.5 to 45 mg in divided doses.

Day 4: 15 to 30 mg in divided doses.

Thereafter, gradually reduce the daily dose to 7.5 to 15 mg. Discontinue drug as soon as patient's condition is stable.

Partial seizures: Adults and Children >12 years: **PO**: 7.5 mg 3 times/day. Can increase by no more than 7.5 mg/day at weekly intervals (daily dose not to exceed 90 mg).

Children (9 to 12 yr): **PO**: 7.5 mg 2 times/day initially; may increase by 7.5 mg/week (not to exceed 60 mg/day).

DIAZEPAM (VALIUM)

Antianxiety/adjunct anticonvulsant: **PO** (*Adults*): 2 to 10 mg 2 to 4 times/day.

Antianxiety: **PO** (*Children ≥6 mo*): 1 to 2.5 mg 3 to 4 times/day.

Moderate to severe anxiety: **IM** or **IV** (*Adults*): 2 to 10 mg. Repeat in 3 to 4 hours if necessary.

Skeletal muscle relaxant: **PO** (*Adults*): 2 to 10 mg 3 or 4 times/day.

Children (≥6 mo): **PO**: 0.12 to 0.8 mg/kg/day divided into 3 to 4 equal doses.

Geriatric or debilitated patients: **PO**: 2 to 2.5 mg 1 to 2 times daily initially. Increase gradually as needed and tolerated.

Acute alcohol withdrawal: **PO** (*Adults*): 10 mg 3 to 4 times/day in first 24 hr; decrease to 5 mg 3 or 4 times/day as needed. **IM** or **IV** (*Adults*): 10 mg initially, then 5 to 10 mg in 3 to 4 hours, if necessary.

Status epilepticus/Acute seizure activity: **IV** (*Adults*) (IM route may be used if IV route is unavailable): 5 to 10 mg; may repeat every 10 to 15 minutes to a total of 30 mg; may repeat regimen again in 2 to 4 hours.

Children (≥5 yr): **IM** or **IV**: 0.05 to 0.3 mg/kg/dose given over 3 to 5 minutes every 15 to 30 minutes to a total dose of 10 mg; repeat every 2 to 4 hours.

Children (1 mo to 5 yr): **IM** or **IV**: 0.05 to 0.3 mg/kg/dose given over 3 to 5 minutes every 15 to 30 minutes to a maximum dose of 5 mg; repeat in 2 to 4 hours if needed.

Preoperative sedation: **IM** (*Adults*): 10 mg.

LORAZEPAM (ATIVAN)

Anxiety disorders/anxiety symptoms: **PO** (*Adults*): 2 to 6 mg/day (varies from 1 to10 mg/day) given in divided doses; take the largest dose before bedtime.

Geriatric or debilitated patient: **PO**: 0.5 to 2 mg/day in divided doses; adjust as needed and tolerated.

Children: **PO**: 0.05 mg/kg/dose every 4 to 8 hours. Maximum dose: 2 mg/dose.

Insomnia: **PO** (*Adults*)**:** 2 to 4 mg at bedtime.

Geriatric or debilitated patient: **PO**: 0.25 to 1 mg at bedtime.

Preoperative sedation: **IM** (*Adults*): 0.05 mg/kg (maximum 4 mg) 2 hours before surgery; **IV** (*Adults*): Initial dose is 2 mg or

0.044 mg/kg, whichever is smaller, given 15 to 20 minutes before the procedure.

Status epilepticus: **IV** *(Adults):* 4 mg given slowly (2 mg/min). May be repeated after 10 to 15 minutes if seizures continue or recur.

Neonates and children <18 years: **IV:** 0.05 to 0.1 mg/kg given over 2 to 5 minutes. If needed, a dosage of 0.05 mg/kg may be repeated in 10 to 15 minutes. Maximum dose: 4 mg.

Antiemetic: **IV** *(Adults):* 2 mg 30 minutes prior to chemotherapy; may be repeated every 4 hours as needed

OXAZEPAM

Mild to moderate anxiety: **PO** *(Adults and Children >12 years):* 10 to 15 mg 3 or 4 times/day.

Severe anxiety states: **PO** *(Adults and Children >12 years):* 15 to 30 mg 3 or 4 times/day.

Geriatric patients: **PO:** Initial dosage: 10 mg 3 times/day. If necessary, increase cautiously to 15 mg 3 or 4 times/day.

Acute alcohol withdrawal: **PO** *(Adults):* 15 to 30 mg 3 or 4 times/day.

■ CHEMICAL CLASS: CARBAMATE DRIVATIVE
Examples

Generic Name	Controlled/ Pregnancy Categories	Half-life (hr)	Available Forms (mg)
Meprobamate	C-IV/D	6–17	**TABS:** 200, 400

Indications
• Anxiety disorders
• Temporary relief of anxiety symptoms

Action
• Depresses multiple sites in the CNS, including the thalamus and limbic system.
• May act by blocking the reuptake of adenosine.

Contraindications and Precautions

Contraindicated in: • Hypersensitivity to the drug • Combination with other CNS depressants • Children under age 6 • Pregnancy and lactation • Acute intermittent porphyria

Use Cautiously in: • Elderly or debilitated clients • Hepatic or renal dysfunction • Individuals with a history of drug abuse/addiction

• Clients with a history of seizure disorders • Depressed/suicidal clients

Adverse Reactions and Side Effects

- Palpitations, tachycardia
- Drowsiness, dizziness, ataxia
- Nausea, vomiting, diarrhea
- Tolerance
- Physical and psychological addiction

Interactions

- Additive CNS depression with other **CNS depressants** (e.g., **alcohol, other anxiolytics, opioid analgesics,** and **sedative-hypnotics**) and with **herbal depressants** (e.g., **kava, valerian**).

Route and Dosage

Anxiety disorders/anxiety symptoms: **PO** *(Adults and children >12 yr):* 1200 to 1600 mg/day in 3 or 4 divided doses.
Children (6 to 12 yr): **PO**: 100 to 200 mg 2 or 3 times/day.

■ CHEMICAL CLASS: AZASPIRODECANEDIONES
Examples

Generic Name	Pregnancy Category	Half-life (hr)	Available Forms (mg)
Buspirone HCl	B	2–3	**TABS:** 5, 7.5, 10, 15, 30

Indications

- Anxiety disorders
- Anxiety symptoms

Unlabeled uses:
- Symptomatic management of premenstrual syndrome

Actions

- Unknown
- May produce desired effects through interactions with serotonin, dopamine, and other neurotransmitter receptors
- Delayed onset (a lag time of 7 to 10 days between onset of therapy and subsiding of anxiety symptoms)
- Cannot be used on a prn basis

Contraindications and Precautions

Contraindicated in: • Hypersensitivity to the drug • Severe hepatic or renal impairment • Concurrent use with MAO Inhibitors

Use Cautiously in: • Elderly or debilitated clients • Pregnancy and lactation • Children • Buspirone will not block the withdrawal syndrome in clients with a history of chronic benzodiazepine or other sedative/hypnotic use. Clients should be withdrawn gradually from these medications before beginning therapy with buspirone.

Adverse Reactions and Side Effects

- Drowsiness, dizziness
- Excitement, nervousness
- Fatigue, headache
- Nausea, dry mouth
- Incoordination, numbness
- Palpitations, tachycardia

Interactions

- Increased effects of buspirone with **cimetidine, erythromycin, itraconazole, nefazodone, ketoconazole, clarithromycin, diltiazem, verapamil, fluvoxamine,** and **ritonavir.**
- Decreased effects of buspirone with **rifampin, rifabutin, phenytoin, phenobarbital, carbamazepine, fluoxetine,** and **dexamethasone.**
- Increased serum concentrations of **haloperidol** when used concomitantly with buspirone.
- Use of buspirone with an **MAO inhibitor** may result in elevated blood pressure.
- Increased risk of hepatic effects when used concomitantly with **nefazodone.**
- Additive effects when used with certain **herbal products** (e.g., **kava, valerian**).

Route and Dosage

Anxiety: **PO:** *(Adults):* Initial dosage 7.5 mg 2 times/day. Increase by 5 mg/day every 2 to 3 days as needed. Maximum daily dosage: 60 mg.

■ NURSING DIAGNOSES RELATED TO ALL ANTIANXIETY AGENTS

1. Risk for injury related to seizures, panic anxiety, acute agitation from alcohol withdrawal (indications); abrupt withdrawal from the medication after long-term use; effects of medication intoxication or overdose.
2. Anxiety (specify) related to threat to physical integrity or self-concept.
3. Risk for activity intolerance related to medication side effects of sedation, confusion, and lethargy.

4. Disturbed sleep pattern related to situational crises, physical condition, severe level of anxiety.
5. Deficient knowledge related to medication regimen.
6. Risk for acute confusion related to action of the medication on the CNS.

■ NURSING IMPLICATIONS FOR ANTIANXIETY AGENTS

1. Instruct client not to drive or operate dangerous machinery when taking the medication.
2. Advise client receiving long-term therapy not to quit taking the drug abruptly. Abrupt withdrawal can be life-threatening (with the exception of buspirone). Symptoms include depression, insomnia, increased anxiety, abdominal and muscle cramps, tremors, vomiting, sweating, convulsions, and delirium.
3. Instruct client not to drink alcohol or take other medications that depress the CNS while taking this medication.
4. Assess mood daily. *May aggravate symptoms in depressed persons.* Take necessary precautions for potential suicide.
5. Monitor lying and standing blood pressure and pulse every shift. Instruct client to arise slowly from a lying or sitting position.
6. Withhold drug and notify the physician should paradoxical excitement occur.
7. Have client take frequent sips of water, ice chips, suck on hard candy, or chew sugarless gum to relieve dry mouth.
8. Have client take drug with food or milk to prevent nausea and vomiting.
9. Symptoms of sore throat, fever, malaise, easy bruising, or unusual bleeding should be reported to the physician immediately. They may be indications of blood dyscrasias.
10. Ensure that client taking buspirone understands there is a lag time of 7 to 10 days between onset of therapy and subsiding of anxiety symptoms. Client should continue to take the medication during this time. (Note: This medication is not recommended for PRN administration because of this delayed therapeutic onset. There is no evidence that buspirone creates tolerance or physical dependence as do the CNS depressant anxiolytics.)

■ CLIENT/FAMILY EDUCATION RELATED TO ALL ANTIANXIETY AGENTS

- Do not drive or operate dangerous machinery. Drowsiness and dizziness can occur.
- Do not stop taking the drug abruptly. Can produce serious withdrawal symptoms, such as depression, insomnia, anxiety,

abdominal and muscle cramps, tremors, vomiting, sweating, convulsions, and delirium.

- *(With buspirone only):* Be aware of lag time between start of therapy and subsiding of symptoms. Relief is usually evident within 7 to 10 days. Take the medication regularly, as ordered, so that it has sufficient time to take effect.
- Do not consume other CNS depressants (including alcohol).
- Do not take nonprescription medication without approval from physician.
- Rise slowly from the sitting or lying position to prevent a sudden drop in blood pressure.
- Report to physician immediately symptoms of sore throat, fever, malaise, easy bruising, unusual bleeding, or motor restlessness.
- Be aware of risks of taking these drugs during pregnancy. (Congenital malformations have been associated with use during the first trimester). If pregnancy is suspected or planned, the client should notify the physician of the desirability to discontinue the drug.
- Be aware of possible side effects. Refer to written materials furnished by health-care providers regarding the correct method of self-administration.
- Carry card or piece of paper at all times stating names of medications being taken.

@ INTERNET REFERENCES

   a. http://www.mentalhealth.com/
   b. http://www.nimh.nih.gov/index.shtml
   c. http://www.nimh.nih.gov/health/publications/mental-health-medications/index.shtml
   d. http://www.nlm.nih.gov/medlineplus/druginformation.html

CHAPTER **24**

Antidepressants

■ CHEMICAL CLASS: TRICYCLICS AND RELATED (NONSELECTIVE REUPTAKE INHIBITORS)

Examples

Generic (Trade) Name	Pregnancy Categories/ Half-life (hr)	Indications	Therapeutic Plasma Level Range (mcg/ml)	Available Forms (mg)
TRICYCLICS				
Amitriptyline	C/31–46	• Depression **Unlabeled uses:** • Migraine prevention • Chronic headache prevention • Fibromyalgia • Postherpetic neuralgia	110–250 (including metabolite)	**TABS:** 10, 25, 50, 75, 100, 150
Clomipramine (Anafranil)	C/19–37	• Obsessive-compulsive disorder (OCD) **Unlabeled uses:** • Premenstrual symptoms • Panic disorder	80–100	**CAPS:** 25, 50, 75
Desipramine (Norpramin)	C/12–24	• Depression **Unlabeled uses:** • Alcoholism • Attention-deficit/ hyperactivity disorder (ADHD) • Bulimia nervosa • Diabetic neuropathy • Postherpetic neuralgia • Irritable bowel syndrome	125–300	**TABS:** 10, 25, 50, 75, 100, 150

Generic (Trade) Name	Pregnancy Categories/ Half-life (hr)	Indications	Therapeutic Plasma Level Range (mcg/ml)	Available Forms (mg)
Doxepin (Sinequan)	C/ 8–24	• Depression or anxiety • Depression or anxiety associated with alcoholism • Depression or anxiety associated with organic disease • Psychotic depressive disorders with anxiety **Unlabeled uses:** • Migraine prevention	100–200 (including metabolite)	**CAPS:** 10, 25, 50, 75, 100, 150
Imipramine (Tofranil)	D/11–25	• Depression • Nocturnal enuresis **Unlabeled uses:** • Alcoholism • ADHD • Bulimia nervosa • Migraine prevention • Urinary incontinence	200–350 (including metabolite)	**HCL TABS:** 10, 25, 50 **PAMOATE CAPS:** 75, 100, 125, 150
Nortriptyline (Aventyl; Pamelor)	D/18–44	• Depression **Unlabeled uses:** • ADHD • Postherpetic neuralgia • Irritable bowel syndrome	50–150	**CAPS:** 10, 25, 50, 75 **ORAL SOLUTION:** 10/5 mL
Protriptyline (Vivactil)	C/67–89	• Depression **Unlabeled uses:** • Migraine prevention	100–200	**TABS:** 5, 10
Trimipramine (Surmontil)	C/7–30	• Depression	180 (includes active metabolite)	**CAPS:** 25, 50, 100
DIBENZOXAZEPINE Amoxapine	C/ 8	• Depression • Depression with anxiety	200–500	**TABS:** 25, 50, 100, 150

Continued

Generic (Trade) Name	Pregnancy Categories/ Half-life (hr)	Indications	Therapeutic Plasma Level Range (mcg/ml)	Available Forms (mg)
TETRACYCLICS Maprotiline	B/21–25	• Depression • Depression with anxiety **Unlabeled uses:** • Postherpetic neuralgia	200–300 (including metabolite)	**TABS:** 25, 50, 75
Mirtazapine (Remeron)	C/20–40	• Depression **Unlabeled uses:** • Chronic urticaria • Insomnia associated with depression	Not well established	**TABS:** 7.5, 15, 30, 45 **TABS (ORALLY DISINTEGRATING):** 15, 30, 45

Action
• Inhibit reuptake of norepinephrine or serotonin at the presynaptic neuron

Contraindications and Precautions

Contraindicated in: • Hypersensitivity to any tricyclic or related drug • Concomitant use with monoamine oxidase inhibitors (MAOIs) • Acute recovery period following myocardial infarction • Narrow angle glaucoma • Pregnancy and lactation (safety not established) • Known or suspected seizure disorder (maprotiline)

Use Cautiously in: • Patients with history of seizures (maprotiline contraindicated) • Patients with tendency to have urinary retention • Benign prostatic hypertrophy • Cardiovascular disorders • Hepatic or renal insufficiency • Psychotic patients • Elderly or debilitated patients

Adverse Reactions and Side Effects
• Drowsiness; fatigue
• Dry mouth
• Blurred vision
• Orthostatic hypotension
• Tachycardia; arrhythmias
• Constipation
• Urinary retention
• Blood dyscrasias
• Nausea and vomiting
• Photosensitivity
• Possible QT prolongation (maprotiline)
• Increased risk of suicidality in children and adolescents (black box warning)

Interactions

- Increased effects of tricyclic antidepressants with **bupropion, cimetidine, haloperidol, selective serotonin reuptake inhibitors (SSRIs), and valproic acid**.
- Decreased effects of tricyclic antidepressants with **carbamazepine, barbiturates,** and **rifamycins.**
- Hyperpyretic crisis, convulsions, and death can occur with **MAOIs.**
- Co-administration with **clonidine** may produce hypertensive crisis.
- Decreased effects of **levodopa** and **guanethidine** with tricyclic antidepressants.
- Potentiation of pressor response with direct-acting **sympathomimetics.**
- Increased anti-coagulation effects may occur with **dicumarol.**
- Increased serum levels of **carbamazepine** occur with concomitant use of tricyclics.
- Increased risk of seizures with concomitant use of maprotiline and **phenothiazines.**
- Potential for cardiovascular toxicity of maprotiline when given concomitantly with **thyroid hormones** (e.g., **levothyroxine**).
- Impairment of motor skills is increased with concomitant use of mirtazapine and **CNS depressants** (e.g., **benzodiazepines**).
- Concomitant use of maprotiline and **other drugs that prolong QT interval** may result in life-threatening cardiac arrhythmia because of possible additive effects.
- Increased effects of mirtazapine with concomitant use of **SSRIs.**

Route and Dosage

AMITRIPTYLINE

Depression: **PO** *(Adults)*: 75 mg/day in divided doses. May gradually increase to 150 mg/day. Alternative dosing: May initiate at 50 to 100 mg at bedtime; increase by 25 to 50 mg as necessary, to a total of 150 mg/day.

Hospitalized patients: May require up to 300 mg/day.

Adolescent and elderly patients: 10 mg 3 times/day and 20 mg at bedtime.

Migraine prevention: **PO** *(Adults)*: Common dosage: 50 to 100 mg/day in divided doses. Range: 10 to 300 mg/day.

Prevention of chronic headache: **PO** *(Adults)*: 20 to 100 mg/day.

Fibromyalgia: **PO** *(Adults)*: 10 to 50 mg at bedtime.

Postherpetic neuralgia: **PO** *(Adults)*: 65 to 100 mg/day for at least 3 weeks.

CLOMIPRAMINE (ANAFRANIL)

***Obsessive-compulsive disorder:* PO** (*Adults*): 25 mg/day. Gradually increase to 100 mg/day during first 2 weeks, given in divided doses. May increase gradually over several weeks to maximum of 250 mg/day.

Children and adolescents: 25 mg/day. Gradually increase during first 2 weeks to daily dose of 3 mg/kg or 100 mg, whichever is smaller. Maximum daily dose: 3 mg/kg or 200 mg, whichever is smaller.

***Premenstrual symptoms:* PO** (*Adults*): 25 to 75 mg/day for irritability and dysphoria.

***Panic disorder:* PO** (*Adults*): Initial dosage: 10 mg. Increase to a maximum dose of 150 mg given as multiple daily doses.

DESIPRAMINE (NORPRAMIN)

***Depression:* PO** (*Adults*): 100 to 200 mg/day in divided doses or as a single daily dose. May increase to maximum dose of 300 mg/day.

Elderly and adolescents: 25 to 100 mg/day in divided doses or as a single daily dose. Maximum dose: 150 mg/day.

***Alcoholism:* PO** (*Adults*): 200 to 275 mg/day.

***Attention-deficit/hyperactivity disorder (ADHD):* PO** (*Adults*): 100 to 200 mg/day.

Children and adolescents: Has been studied at dosages of 75 mg/day and 4.6 mg/kg/day. Should be initiated at the lowest dose and then increased according to tolerability and clinical response.

***Bulimia nervosa:* PO** (*Adults*): Initial dose: 25 mg 3 times a day. Titrate dosage up to 200 to 300 mg/day, depending on response and adverse effects.

***Diabetic neuropathy:* PO** (*Adults*): 50 to 250 mg/day.

***Postherpetic neuralgia:* PO** (*Adults*): 94 to 167 mg/day for at least 6 weeks.

***Irritable bowel syndrome:* PO** (*Adults*): 10 to 50 mg/day. May titrate dosage based on response to therapy up to 100 to 200 mg/day.

DOXEPIN (SINEQUAN)

***Depression and/or anxiety:* PO** (*Adults and Children ≥ 12 years*): (Mild to moderate illness) 75 mg/day. May increase to maximum dose of 150 mg/day.

(Mild symptoms associated with organic illness): 25 to 50 mg/day.

(Severe symptoms): 50 mg 3 times/day; may gradually increase to 300 mg/day.

Migraine prevention: **PO** (*Adults*): 75 to 150 mg/day. Occasionally dosages up to 300 mg/day may be required.

IMIPRAMINE (TOFRANIL)

Depression: **PO** (*Adults*): 75 mg/day. May increase to maximum of 200 mg/day. Hospitalized patients may require up to 300 mg/day.

Adolescent and geriatric patients: 30 to 40 mg/day. May increase to maximum of 100 mg/day.

Nocturnal enuresis: **PO** (*Children ≥ 6 years of age*): 25 mg/day 1 hour before bedtime. May increase after 1 week to 50 mg/night if <12 years of age; up to 75 mg/night if >12 years of age. Maximum dose: 2.5 mg/kg/day.

Alcoholism: **PO** (*Adults*): 50 mg/day titrated by 50 mg every 3 to 5 days to a maximum daily dose of 300 mg.

ADHD: **PO** (*Children and adolescents*): 1 mg/kg/day titrated to a maximum dose of 4 mg/kg/day or 200 mg/day, whichever is smaller.

Bulimia nervosa: **PO** (*Adults*): 50 mg/day titrated to 100 mg 2 times a day.

Migraine prevention: **PO** (*Adults*): 10 to 25 mg 3 times a day.

Urinary incontinence: **PO** (*Adults*): 25 mg 2 to 3 times a day.

NORTRIPTYLINE (AVENTYL; PAMELOR)

Depression: **PO** (*Adults*): 25 mg 3 or 4 times a day. The total daily dose may be given at bedtime.

Elderly and adolescent patients: 30 to 50 mg daily in divided doses or total daily dose may be given once/day.

ADHD: **PO** (*Adults*): 25 mg 3 to 4 times/day.

Children and adolescents: 0.5 mg/kg/day, titrated to a maximum dose of 2 mg/kg/day or 100 mg, whichever is less.

Postherpetic neuralgia: **PO** (*Adults*): Dosage range: 58 to 89 mg/day for at least 5 weeks.

Irritable bowel syndrome: **PO** (*Adults*): 10 to 50 mg/day. May titrate dosage based on response to therapy up to 100 to 200 mg/day.

PROTRIPTYLINE (VIVACTIL)

Depression: **PO** (*Adults*): 15 to 40 mg/day divided into 3 or 4 doses. Maximum daily dose: 60 mg.

Adolescent and elderly patients: 5 mg 3 times/day.

TRIMIPRAMINE (SURMONTIL)

Depression: **PO** (*Adults*): 75 mg/day. Increase gradually to 150 to 200 mg/day. Hospitalized patients may require up to 300 mg/day.

Adolescent and elderly patients: Initially, 50 mg/day, with gradual increments up to 100 mg/day.

AMOXAPINE

***Depression and depression with anxiety:* PO** *(Adults)*: 50 mg 2 or 3 times daily. May increase to 100 mg 2 or 3 times daily by end of first week. Maintenance dosage is the lowest dose that will maintain remission.

Elderly patients: 25 mg 2 or 3 times a day. May increase by end of first week to 50 mg 2 or 3 times a day.

MAPROTILINE

***Depression/Depression with anxiety:* PO** *(Adults):* Initial dosage: 75 mg/day. After 2 weeks, may increase gradually in 25 mg increments. Maximum daily dose: 150 mg. *Hospitalized patients with severe depression:* **PO** *(Adults):* Initial dosage: 100 to 150 mg/day. May increase gradually and as tolerated to a maximum dosage of 225 mg/day.

***Elderly patients:* PO:** Initiate dosage at 25 mg/day. 50 to 75 mg/day may be sufficient for maintenance therapy in elderly patients.

***Postherpetic neuralgia:* PO** *(Adults)*: 100 mg/day for 5 weeks.

MIRTAZAPINE (REMERON)

***Depression:* PO** *(Adults)*: Initial dosage: 15 mg/day as a single dose, preferably in the evening before bedtime. The effective dose range is generally 15 to 45 mg/day.

***Chronic urticaria:* PO** *(Adults):* 15 to 30 mg/day.

***Insomnia associated with depression:* PO** *(Adults):* 15 to 45 mg orally once daily before bedtime.

■ CHEMICAL CLASS: SELECTIVE SEROTONIN REUPTAKE INHIBITORS (SSRIs)

Examples

Generic (Trade) Name	Pregnancy Categories/ Half-life	Indications	Available Forms (mg)
Citalopram (Celexa)	C/~ 35 hr	• Treatment of depression **Unlabeled uses:** • Alcoholism • Binge-eating disorder • Generalized anxiety disorder • OCD • Premenstrual Dysphoric Disorder (PMDD)	**TABS:** 10, 20, 40 **ORAL SOLUTION:** 10/5mL
Escitalopram (Lexapro)	C/27–32 hr	• Major Depressive Disorder • Generalized anxiety disorder **Unlabeled uses:** • Posttraumatic stress disorder (PTSD)	**TABS:** 5, 10, 20 **ORAL SOLUTION:** 1/mL

Generic (Trade) Name	Pregnancy Categories/ Half-life	Indications	Available Forms (mg)
Fluoxetine (Prozac; Sarafem; Selfemra)	C/1 to 16 days (including metabolite)	• Depression • Depressive episodes associated with bipolar I disorder and treatment-resistant depression (in combination with olanzapine) • OCD • Bulimia nervosa • Panic disorder • PMDD (Sarafem; Selfemra only) **Unlabeled uses:** • Alcoholism • Borderline Personality Disorder • Fibromyalgia • Hot flashes • PTSD • Migraine prevention • Raynaud phenomenon • Irritable bowel syndrome	**TABS:** 10, 15, 20, 60 **CAPS:** 10, 20, 40 **CAPS, DELAYED-RELEASE:** 90 **ORAL SOLUTION:** 20/5 mL
Fluvoxamine (Luvox)	C/13.6–15.6 hr	• OCD • Social anxiety disorder **Unlabeled uses:** • Panic disorder • PTSD • Bulimia nervosa • Depression and anxiety in children and adolescents	**TABS:** 25, 50, 100 **CAPS (ER):** 100, 150
Paroxetine (Paxil)	C/21 hr (CR: 15–20 hr)	• Major depressive disorder • Panic disorder • OCD • Social anxiety disorder • Generalized anxiety disorder • PTSD • PMDD **Unlabeled uses:** • Hot flashes • Diabetic neuropathy • Irritable bowel syndrome	**TABS:** 10, 20, 30, 40 **ORAL SUSPENSION:** 10/5 mL **TABS (CR):** 12.5, 25, 37.5
Sertraline (Zoloft)	C/26–104 hr (including metabolite)	• Major depressive disorder • OCD • Panic disorder • PTSD • PMDD • Social anxiety disorder	**TABS:** 25, 50, 100 **ORAL CONCENTRATE:** 20/mL
Vilazodone (Viibryd)	C/ 25 hr	• Major depressive disorder	**TABS:** 10, 20, 40
Vortioxetine (Brintellix)	C/ 66 hr	• Major depressive disorder	**TABS:** 5, 10, 15, 20

Action

- Selectively inhibit the central nervous system neuronal uptake of serotonin (5-HT). Vilzodone (Viibryd) is also a partial agonist at serotonergic 5-HT1A receptors. Vortioxetine (Brintellix) also exhibits agonist activity for 5-HT1A receptors, as well as antagonism for 5-HT3 receptors

Contraindications and Precautions

Contraindicated in: • Hypersensitivity to SSRIs • Concomitant use of SSRIs with, or within 14 days' use of, MAO inhibitors • Concomitant use of SSRIs with pimozide • *Fluoxetine:* concomitant use with thioridazine • *Fluvoxamine:* concomitant use with alosetron, astemizole, cisapride, terfenadine, thioridazine, or tizanidine • *Paroxetine:* concomitant use with thioridazine • *Sertraline:* coadministration of oral solution with disulfiram because of alcohol content • *Citalopram:* in clients with congenital long QT syndrome

Use Cautiously in: • Patients with history of seizures • Underweight or anorexic patients • Hepatic or renal insufficiency • Elderly or debilitated patients • Suicidal patients • Clients taking anticoagulants • Pregnancy and lactation

Adverse Reactions and Side Effects

- Headache
- Insomnia
- Nausea
- Anorexia
- Diarrhea
- Constipation
- Sexual dysfunction
- Somnolence
- Dry mouth
- Increased risk of suicidality in children and adolescents (black box warning)
- Serotonin Syndrome. Can occur if taken concurrently with other medications that increase levels of serotonin (e.g., MAOIs, tryptophan, amphetamines, other antidepressants, buspirone, lithium, dopamine agonists, or serotonin 5-HT1 receptor agonists [agents for migraine]). Symptoms of serotonin syndrome include diarrhea, cramping, tachycardia, labile blood pressure, diaphoresis, fever, tremor, shivering, restlessness, confusion, disorientation, mania, myoclonus, hyperreflexia, ataxia, seizures, cardiovascular shock, and death.

Interactions

- Toxic, sometimes fatal, reactions have occurred with concomitant use of **MAOIs.**

- Increased effects of SSRIs with **cimetidine, L-tryptophan, lithium, linezolid**, and **St. John's wort.**
- Serotonin syndrome may occur with concomitant use of SSRIs and **metoclopramide, sibutramine, tramadol, serotonin 5-HT1 receptor agonists** (agents for migraine), or any drug that increases levels of serotonin.
- Concomitant use of SSRIs may increase effects of **hydantoins, tricyclic antidepressants, cyclosporine, benzodiazepines, beta blockers, methadone, carbamazepine, clozapine, olanzapine, pimozide, haloperidol, mexiletine, phenothiazines, St. John's Wort, sumatriptan, trazodone, sympathomimetics, theophylline, procyclidine, propafenone, risperidone, ropivacaine, warfarin,** and **zolpidem.**
- Concomitant use of SSRIs may decrease effects of **buspirone** and **digoxin.**
- **Lithium** levels may be increased or decreased by concomitant use of SSRIs.
- Decreased effects of SSRIs with concomitant use of **carbamazepine** and **cyproheptadine.**
- Increased effects of vortioxetine with concomitant use of **bupropion, fluoxetine, paroxetine,** or **quinidine.**
- Decreased effects of vortioxetine with concomitant use of **CYP inducers** (e.g., **rifampicin, carbamazepine, phenytoin**).

Route and Dosage

CITALOPRAM (CELEXA)

Depression: **PO** *(Adults)*: Initial dosage: 20 mg/day as a single daily dose. May increase in increments of 20 mg at intervals of no less than 1 week. Maximum dose: 40 mg/day.

Elderly clients: 20 mg/day.

Alcoholism: **PO** *(Adults)*: 20 to 40 mg/day.

Binge-eating disorder: **PO** *(Adults)*: 20 to 60 mg/day.

Generalized anxiety disorder: **PO** *(Adults)*: 10 mg/day, titrated up to 40 mg/day.

OCD: **PO** *(Adults)*: Initial dosage: 20 mg/day. Titrate to a target dosage of 40 to 60 mg/day. Maximum dosage: 80 mg/day.

PMDD: **PO** *(Adults)*: 5 mg initiated on estimated day of ovulation. Increase on subsequent days by 5 mg/day to the maximum dose of 30 mg. On the first day of menses, decrease dose to 20 mg and then to 10 mg on second day of menses. Discontinue medication on day 3 of menses. Repeat medication regimen beginning on following initial day of ovulation.

ESCITALOPRAM (LEXAPRO)

Depression: **PO** *(Adults)*: Initial dosage: 10 mg/day as a single daily dose. May increase to 20 mg/day after 1 week.

Elderly clients: **PO:** 10 mg/day.

Children 12 to 17 years: **PO:** Initial dosage: 10 mg/day as a single daily dose. May increase gradually to 20 mg after a minimum of 3 weeks.

Generalized anxiety disorder: **PO** *(Adults):* Initial dosage: 10 mg/day as a single daily dose. May increase to 20 mg/day after 1 week.

PTSD: **PO** *(Adults)*: Initial dose: 10 mg/day as a single daily dose. Increase to 20 mg once daily after 4 weeks.

FLUOXETINE (PROZAC; SARAFEM; SELFEMRA)

Depression: **PO:** *Adults:* Initial dosage: 20 mg/day in the morning. May increase dosage after several weeks if sufficient clinical improvement is not observed. Maximum dose: 80 mg/day.

Children ≥8 years: PO: Initial dosage: 10 mg/day. May increase after 1 week to 20 mg/day.

OCD: **PO:** *Adults:* Initial dosage: 20 mg/day in the morning. May increase dosage after several weeks if sufficient clinical improvement is not observed. Maximum dose: 80 mg/day.

Children 7 to 17 years: **PO** *Adolescents and higher-weight children:* 10 mg/day. May be increased after 2 weeks to 20 mg/day; additional increases may be made after several more weeks (range 20 to 60 mg/day). **PO** *Lower-weight children:* 10 mg/day initially. Dosage may be increased after several more weeks (range 20 to 30 mg/day).

Depressive episodes associated with bipolar I disorder and treatment-resistant depression (in combination with olanzapine): **PO:** *(Adults):* fluoxetine 20 mg and olanzapine 5 mg are administered once daily in the evening without regard to meals. Dosage adjustments, if indicated, should be made with the individual components according to efficacy and tolerability (dosage range fluoxetine 20 to 50 mg and oral olanzapine 5 to 20 mg).

Bulimia nervosa: **PO** *(Adults)*: 60 mg/day administered in the morning. May need to titrate up to this target dose in some clients.

Panic disorder: **PO** *(Adults)*: Initial dose: 10 mg/day. After 1 week, increase dose to 20 mg/day. If no improvement is seen after several weeks, may consider dose increases up to 60 mg/day.

PMDD (Sarafem and Selfemra only): **PO** *(Adults)*: Initial dose: 20 mg/day. Maximum: 80 mg/day. May be given continuously throughout the cycle or intermittently (only during the 14 days prior to anticipated onset of menses).

Alcoholism: **PO** *(Adults)*: Initial dosage: 20 mg/day. Titrate to 40 mg/day after 2 weeks, if needed.

Borderline personality disorder: **PO** *(Adults)*: 20 to 80 mg/day.

Fibromyalgia: **PO** *(Adults):* 20 mg/day (in the morning) for up to 6 weeks.

Hot flashes: **PO** *(Adults):* 20 mg/day for 4 weeks.

PTSD: **PO** *(Adults):* Initial dosage 10 to 20 mg/day. Average target dose: 20 to 50 mg/day in adults and 20 mg in older adults. Highest target dosage: 80 mg/day. Duration of therapy is 6 to 12 months for acute PTSD and 12 to 24 months for chronic PTSD. Dose tapering over 2 to 4 weeks is recommended to avoid withdrawal symptoms.

Children and adolescents: Average target dose: 10 to 20 mg/day. Duration and tapering of therapy is the same as for adults.

Migraine prevention: **PO** *(Adults):* 10 to 40 mg/day.

Raynaud phenomenon: **PO** *(Adults):* 20 to 60 mg/day.

Irritable bowel syndrome: **PO** *(Adults):* 10 to 20 mg/day.

FLUVOXAMINE (LUVOX)

OCD: **PO** *(Adults):* Initial dose: 50 mg (immediate release tabs) or 100 mg (extended-release caps) at bedtime. May increase dose in 50 mg increments every week until therapeutic benefit is achieved. Maximum dose: 300 mg. Administer daily doses of immediate release tabs >100 mg in 2 divided doses. If unequal, give larger dose at bedtime.

Children 8 to 17 years: Initial dose: 25 mg single dose at bedtime. May increase the dose in 25 mg increments every 4 to 7 days to a maximum dose of 200 mg/day. Some adolescents may require up to a maximum dose of 300 mg/day to achieve a therapeutic benefit. Divide daily doses >50 mg into 2 doses. If unequal, give larger dose at bedtime.

Social anxiety disorder: **PO** *(Adults)* (extended release capsules): Initial dose: 100 mg/day as a single daily dose at bedtime. Increase in 50 mg increments every week, as tolerated, until maximum therapeutic benefit is achieved. Maximum dose: 300 mg/day.

Panic disorder: **PO** *(Adults):* Initial dosage: 50 mg/day. Gradually increase after several days to 150 mg/day. For clients who fail to respond after several weeks of treatment, further increases up to 300 mg/day may be considered.

Bulimia nervosa: **PO** *(Adults):* 50 mg/day, titrated up based on therapeutic response to 200 mg/day for up to 12 weeks.

PTSD: **PO** *(Adults):* Initial dosage: 50 mg/day. Increase gradually to target dose of 100 to 250 mg/day in adults, and 100 mg/day in older adults. Maximum recommended dosage: 300 mg/day. Duration of therapy is 6 to 12 months for acute PTSD and 12 to 24 months for chronic PTSD. Dose tapering over 2 to 4 weeks is recommended to avoid withdrawal symptoms.

Children and adolescents: Target dose: 50 mg/day. Duration and tapering of therapy is the same as for adults.

***Depression or anxiety disorder in children and adolescents:* PO** *(≥12 years):* Initial dosage: 25 to 50 mg at bedtime. Maintenance dosage: 150 to 300 mg/day. **PO** *(<12 years):* Initial dosage: 25 mg at bedtime. Maintenance dosage: 100 to 200 mg/day.

PAROXETINE (PAXIL)

***Depression:* PO** *(Adults):* 20 mg/day in the morning. May increase dose in 10 mg increments at intervals of at least 1 week to a maximum of 50 mg/day.

Controlled release: Initial dose: 25 mg/day in the morning. May increase dose in 12.5 mg increments at intervals of at least 1 week to a maximum of 62.5 mg/day.

***Panic disorder:* PO** *(Adults):* 10 mg/day in the morning. May increase dose in 10 mg/day increments at intervals of at least 1 week to a target dose of 40 mg/day. Maximum dose: 60 mg/day. *Controlled release*: Initial dose: 12.5 mg/day. May increase dose in 12.5 mg/day increments at intervals of at least 1 week to a maximum dose of 75 mg/day.

***OCD:* PO** *(Adults):* 20 mg/day. May increase dose in 10 mg/day increments at intervals of at least 1week. Recommended dose: 40 mg/day. Maximum dose: 60 mg/day.

Children and adolescents (7 to 17 years): **PO:** Initial dosage: 10 mg/day. If needed, may increase dosage by 10 mg/day no more frequently than every 7 days, to a maximum dosage of 50 mg/day.

***Social anxiety disorder:* PO** *(Adults):* 20 mg/day. Usual range is 20 to 60 mg/day. *Controlled release:* 12.5 mg/day. May increase dosage at intervals of at least 1 week, in increments of 12.5 mg/day to a maximum of 37.5 mg/day.

Children and adolescents (8 to 17 years): **PO:** Initial dosage: 10 mg/day. If needed, may increase dose by 10 mg/day no more frequently than every 7 days, to a maximum dosage of 50 mg/day.

***GAD and PTSD:* PO** *(Adults)*: Initial dose: 20 mg/day. Usual range is 20 to 50 mg/day. Doses may be increased in increments of 10 mg/day at intervals of at least 1 week.

***PMDD:* PO** *(Adults): Controlled release:* Initial dose: 12.5 mg/day. Usual range: 12.5 to 25 mg/day. Dosage increases may be made at intervals of at least 1 week. May be administered daily throughout the menstrual cycle or limited to luteal phase of menstrual cycle.

***Hot flashes:* PO** *(Adults):* 10 to 20 mg/day. *Controlled release:* 12.5 to 25 mg/day.

Diabetic neuropathy: **PO** *(Adults):* Initial dose: 10 mg/day. Titrate to 20 to 60 mg/day.

Irritable bowel syndrome: **PO** *(Adults):* 20 to 40 mg/day. *Controlled release:* 12.5 to 50 mg/day.

Elderly or debilitated patients: **PO:** Initial dose 10 mg/day. Maximum dose: 40 mg/day. *Controlled release:* Initial dose: 12.5 mg/day. Maximum dose: 50 mg/day.

SERTRALINE (ZOLOFT)

Depression and OCD: **PO** *(Adults):* 50 mg/day (either morning or evening). May increase dosage at 1 week intervals to a maximum of 200 mg/day.

Children and adolescents: **PO** *(≥13 years):* 50 mg/day. May increase by 50 mg at weekly intervals to maximum dosage of 200 mg/day. **PO** *(6 to 12 years):* 25 mg/day. May increase by 25 mg at weekly intervals to maximum dosage of 200 mg/day.

Panic disorder and PTSD: **PO** *(Adults):* Initial dose: 25 mg/day. After 1 week, increase dose to 50 mg/day. If needed, may increase dosage at 1 week intervals to a maximum of 200 mg/day.

PMDD: **PO** *(Adults):* 50 mg/day given on each day of the menstrual cycle or only during each day of the luteal phase of the menstrual cycle. For patients not responding, may increase dosage in 50 mg increments per menstrual cycle up to 150 mg/day when dosing throughout the cycle, or 100 mg/day when dosing only during the luteal phase. If 100 mg/day has been established with luteal phase dosing, titrate at 50 mg/day for first 3 days of each luteal phase dosing period.

Social anxiety disorder: **PO** *(Adults):* Initial dose: 25 mg/day. After 1 week, increase dose to 50 mg/day. May be increased at weekly intervals up to 200 mg/day.

VILAZODONE (VIIBRYD)

Major depressive disorder: **PO** *(Adults):* Initial dosage: 10 mg once daily. After 1 week, increase dosage to 20 mg once daily. After the 2nd week, increase the dosage to 40 mg once daily. Should be taken with food.

VORTIOXETINE (BRINTELLIX)

Major depressive disorder: **PO** *(Adults):* Initial dosage: 10 mg once daily. Dosage may be titrated to 20 mg/day, and may be administered without regard to meals.

■ CHEMICAL CLASS: NOREPINEPHRINE-DOPAMINE REUPTAKE INHIBITORS (NDRIs)

Examples

Generic (Trade) Name	Pregnancy Categories/ Half-life (hr)	Indications	Available Forms (mg)
Bupropion (Wellbutrin; Wellbutrin SR; Wellbutrin XL; Budeprion SR; Budeprion XL; Aplenzin; Zyban)	C/8–24	• Depression (All except Zyban) • Seasonal affective disorder (Wellbutrin XL; Aplenzin) • Smoking cessation (Zyban) **Unlabeled uses:** • ADHD (Wellbutrin; Wellbutrin SR; Wellbutrin XL)	TABS: 75, 100 TABS (SR): 100, 150, 200 TABS (XL): 150, 300 TABS (ER) (APLENZIN): 174, 348, 522

SR=12-hour tablets; XL and ER =24-hour tablets

Action

• Action is unclear. Thought to inhibit the reuptake of norepinephrine and dopamine into presynaptic neurons.

Contraindications and Precautions

Contraindicated in: • Hypersensitivity to the drug • Concomitant use with, or within two weeks use of, MAO inhibitors • Known or suspected seizure disorder • Alcohol or benzodiazepine (or other sedatives) withdrawal • Current or prior diagnosis of bulimia or anorexia nervosa • Concomitant use with more than one bupropion product • Lactation

Use Cautiously in: • Patients with urinary retention • Patients with hepatic or renal function impairment • Patients with suicidal ideation • Patients with recent history of MI or unstable heart disease • Pregnancy (safety not established) • Elderly and debilitated patients

Adverse Reactions and Side Effects

• Dry mouth
• Blurred vision
• Agitation; aggression
• Insomnia
• Tremor
• Sedation; dizziness
• Tachycardia
• Excessive sweating
• Headache
• Nausea/vomiting
• Anorexia; weight loss
• Seizures

- Constipation
- Neuropsychiatric symptoms (e.g., delusions, hallucinations, suicidal ideation)
- Increased risk of suicidality in children and adolescents (black box warning)

Interactions

- Increased effects of bupropion with **amantadine, levodopa, clopidogrel, CYP2B6 inhibitors** (e.g., **cimetidine, ticlopidine, clopidogrel**), **guanfacine,** and **linezolid.**
- Increased risk of acute toxicity with **MAOIs.** Coadministration is contraindicated.
- Coadministration with a **nicotine replacement agent** may cause hypertension.
- Concomitant use with **alcohol** may produce adverse neuropsychiatric events (alcohol tolerance is reduced).
- Decreased effects of bupropion with **carbamazepine, ritonavir,** and **CYP2B6 inducers (e.g., efavirenz, phenobarbital, phenytoin, rifampin).**
- Increased anticoagulant effect of **warfarin** with bupropion.
- Increased effects of drugs metabolized by CYP2D6 isoenzyme (e.g., **nortriptyline, imipramine, desipramine, paroxetine, fluoxetine, sertraline, haloperidol, risperidone, thioridazine, metoprolol, propafenone,** and **flecainide**).
- Increased risk of seizures when bupropion is coadministered with drugs that lower the seizure threshold (e.g., **antidepressants, antipsychotics, systemic steroids, theophylline, tramadol**).

Route and Dosage

Bupropion (Wellbutrin; Budeprion; Aplenzin; Zyban)

Depression (Wellbutrin; Budeprion): **PO** *(Adults) (immediate release tabs):* 100 mg 2 times/day. May increase after 3 days to 100 mg given 3 times/day. For patients who do not show improvement after several weeks of dosing at 300 mg/day, an increase in dosage up to 450 mg/day may be considered. No single dose of bupropion should exceed 150 mg. To prevent the risk of seizures, administer with 4 to 6 hours between doses.

Sustained release tabs (Wellbutrin SR; Budeprion SR): Give as a single 150 mg dose in the morning. May increase to twice a day (total 300 mg), with at least 8 hours between doses. Maximum dose: 400 mg, administered as 200 mg twice a day, with at least 8 hours between doses.

Extended release tabs (Wellbutrin XL; Budeprion XL): Begin dosing at 150 mg/day, given as a single daily dose in the morning. May increase after 3 days to 300 mg/day, given as a single daily dose in the morning. Maximum dose: 450 mg administered as a single daily dose in the morning.

Aplenzin: Initial dose: 174 mg once daily. After 4 days, may increase the dose to 348 mg once daily.

Seasonal affective disorder (Wellbutrin XL): PO *(Adults)*: 150 mg administered each morning beginning in the autumn prior to the onset of depressive symptoms. Dose may be uptitrated to the target dose of 300 mg/day after 1 week. Therapy should continue through the winter season before being tapered to 150 mg/day for 2 weeks prior to discontinuation in early spring.

Aplenzin: **PO** *(Adults):* 174 mg once daily beginning in the autumn prior to the onset of seasonal depressive symptoms. After 1 week, may increase the dose to 348 mg once daily. Continue treatment through the winter season.

Smoking cessation (Zyban): PO *(Adults)*: Begin dosing at 150 mg given once a day in the morning for 3 days. If tolerated well, increase to target dose of 300 mg/day given in doses of 150 mg twice daily with an interval of 8 hours between doses. Continue treatment for 7 to 12 weeks. Some patients may need treatment for as long as 6 months.

ADHD (Wellbutrin; Wellbutrin SR; Wellbutrin XL): PO *(Adults):* 150 to 450 mg/day. Initiate therapy with 150 mg/day and titrate based on tolerability and efficacy. Doses can be given as divided doses or in SR or XL formulations.

Children and adolescents (Wellbutrin; Wellbutrin SR; Wellbutrin XL): Up to 3 mg/kg/day or 150 mg/day initially, titrated to a maximum dosage of up to 6 mg/kg/day or 300 mg/day. Single dose should not exceed 150 mg. Usually given in divided doses for safety and effectiveness: twice daily for children and 3 times daily for adolescents.

■ CHEMICAL CLASS: SEROTONIN-NOREPINEPHRINE REUPTAKE INHIBITORS (SNRIs)

Examples

Generic (Trade) Name	Pregnancy Categories/ Half-life (hr)	Indications	Available Forms (mg)
Desvenlafaxine (Pristiq)	C/ 11–14	• Depression	**TABS ER:** 50, 100
Duloxetine (Cymbalta)	C/ 8–17	• Depression • Chronic musculoskeletal pain • Diabetic peripheral neuropathic pain • Fibromyalgia • Generalized anxiety disorder	**CAPS:** 20, 30, 60

Generic (Trade) Name	Pregnancy Categories/ Half-life (hr)	Indications	Available Forms (mg)
		Unlabeled uses: • Stress urinary incontinence	
Venlafaxine (Effexor)	C/ 5–11 (incl. metabolite)	• Depression • Generalized anxiety disorder (extended release [ER only]) • Social anxiety disorder (ER) • Panic disorder (ER) **Unlabeled uses:** • Hot flashes • PMDD • Diabetic neuropathy • Anxiety and depression in children and adolescents	**TABS:** 25, 37.5, 50, 75, 100 **CAPS XR:** 37.5, 75, 150 **TABS XR:** 37.5, 75, 150, 225
Levomilnacipran (Fetzima)	C/ 12	• Major depressive disorder	**CAPS:** 20, 40, 80, 120

Action

• SNRIs are potent inhibitors of neuronal serotonin and norepinephrine reuptake; weak inhibitors of dopamine reuptake.

Contraindications and Precautions

Contraindicated in: • Hypersensitivity to the drug • Children (safety not established) • Concomitant (or within 14 days) use with MAO inhibitors • Severe renal or hepatic impairment • Pregnancy and lactation (safety not established) • Uncontrolled narrow-angle glaucoma

Use Cautiously in: • Hepatic and renal insufficiency • Elderly and debilitated patients • Patients with history of drug abuse • Patients with suicidal ideation • Patients with history of or existing cardiovascular disease • Patients with history of mania • Patients with history of seizures • Children (Venlafaxine has been used off label with children and adolescents.)

Adverse Reactions and Side Effects

• Headache
• Dry mouth
• Nausea
• Somnolence
• Dizziness
• Insomnia
• Asthenia

- Constipation
- Diarrhea
- Tachycardia; palpitations
- Activation of mania/hypomania
- Abnormal bleeding
- Hypertension
- Mydriasis (venlafaxine)
- Increased risk of suicidality in children and adolescents (black box warning)
- Discontinuation syndrome. Abrupt withdrawal may result in symptoms such as nausea, vomiting, nervousness, dizziness, headache, insomnia, nightmares, paresthesias, agitation, irritability, sensory disturbances, and tinnitus. A gradual reduction in dosage is recommended.

Interactions

- Concomitant use of SNRIs with **MAOIs** results in serious, sometimes fatal, effects resembling neuroleptic malignant syndrome. Coadministration is contraindicated.
- Serotonin syndrome may occur when SNRIs are used concomitantly with **St. John's wort, 5-HT1 receptor agonists (triptans), sibutramine, trazodone,** or other drugs that increase levels of serotonin.
- Increased effects of **haloperidol, clozapine,** and **tricyclic antidepressants** when used concomitantly with venlafaxine.
- Increased effects of venlafaxine with **cimetidine, terbinafine, and azole antifungals.**
- Decreased effects of venlafaxine with **cyproheptadine.**
- Decreased effects of **indinavir** and **metoprolol** with venlafaxine.
- Increased effects of **warfarin and other drugs with anticoagulant effects** with all SNRIs.
- Increased effects of duloxetine with **CYP1A2 inhibitors** (e.g., cimetidine, fluvoxamine, quinolone antibiotics) and **CYP2D6 inhibitors** (e.g., fluoxetine, quinidine, paroxetine).
- Increased risk of liver injury with concomitant use of **alcohol** and duloxetine.
- Increased risk of toxicity or adverse effects from drugs extensively metabolized by CYP2D6 (e.g., **flecainide, phenothiazines, propafenone, tricyclic antidepressants, thioridazine**) when used concomitantly with duloxetine.
- Increased effects of **tricyclic antidepressants** with desvenlafaxine.
- Decreased effects of **midazolam** with desvenlafaxine.
- Increased effects of desvenlafaxine and levomilnacipran with concomitant use of potent **CYP3A4 inhibitors** (e.g., ketoconazole).

Route and Dosage

DESVENLAFAXINE (PRISTIQ)

Depression: **PO** *(Adults):* 50 mg once daily, with or without food.

DULOXETINE (CYMBALTA)

Depression: **PO** *(Adults):* 40 mg/day (given as 20 mg twice a day) to 60 mg/day (given either once a day or as 30 mg twice daily) without regard to meals.

Diabetic peripheral neuropathic pain: **PO** *(Adults):* 60 mg/day given once daily without regard to meals.

Fibromyalgia: **PO** *(Adults):* 30 mg once daily for 1 week and then increase to 60 mg once daily, if needed.

Generalized anxiety disorder: **PO** *(Adults):* 60 mg once daily. For some patients, it may be desirable to start at 30 mg once daily for 1 week to allow the patient to adjust to the medication before increasing to 60 mg once daily. If desired results are not achieved on 60 mg/day, may increase in daily increments of 30 mg to a maximum dosage of 120 mg/day.

Chronic musculoskeletal pain: **PO** *(Adults):* Initial dosage: 30 mg/day for 1 week, then increase to 60 mg/day.

Stress urinary incontinence: **PO** *(Adults):* 80 mg/day in a single dose or two divided doses (range 20 to 120 mg) for 12 weeks.

VENLAFAXINE (EFFEXOR)

Depression: **PO** *(Adults): Immediate-release tabs:* Initial dosage: 75 mg/day in 2 or 3 divided doses, taken with food. May increase in increments up to 75 mg/day at intervals of at least 4 days up to 225 mg/day (not to exceed 375 mg/day in 3 divided doses).

Depression and generalized anxiety disorder: **PO** *(Adults): Extended-release caps:* Initial dosage: 75 mg/day, administered in a single dose. May increase dose in increments of up to 75 mg/day at intervals of at least 4 days to a maximum of 225 mg/day.

Social anxiety disorder: **PO** *(Adults): Extended-release caps:* 75 mg/day as a single dose.

Panic disorder: **PO** *(Adults): Extended-release caps:* Initial dosage: 37.5 mg/day for 7 days. After 7 days, increase dosage to 75 mg/day. May increase dose in increments of up to 75 mg/day at intervals of at least 7 days to a maximum of 225 mg/day.

Hot flashes: **PO** *(Adults): Immediate-release forms:* 12.5 mg 2 times a day for 4 weeks.

Extended-release forms: 37.5 to 150 mg once a day for up to 3 months. Titrate doses.

Premenstrual dysphoric disorder: **PO** *(Adults):* 37.5 to 200 mg/day, starting with either 37.5 mg once daily or 25 mg twice daily during the first menstrual cycle, then decreasing the dose as necessary at the start of subsequent menstrual cycles. Alternatively, intermittent dosing may be used by starting 14 days prior to the start of menses with either 37.5 or 75 mg daily for 2 days, then increasing to either 75 or 112.5 mg daily for 12 days or until the start of menses, followed by 37.5 or 75 mg daily for 2 days.

Diabetic neuropathy: **PO** *(Adults):* Initial dosage: 37.5 mg once or twice daily. May increase by 75 mg each week to a maximum dosage of 225 mg/day.

Anxiety and depression in children and adolescents: **PO** *(Adolescents):* Initial dosage: 37.5 to 75 mg/day. Maintenance dosage: 150 to 300 mg/day. **PO** *(Children):* Initial dosage 37.5 mg/day. Maintenance dosage: 75 to 150 mg/day.

LEVOMILNACIPRAN (FETZIMA)

Major depressive disorder: **PO** *(Adults):* Initial dosage: 20 mg once daily for 2 days, and then increase to 40 mg once daily. May increase dosage in increments of 40 mg at intervals of at least 2 days to the maximum dose of 120 mg once daily.

■ CHEMICAL CLASS: SEROTONIN-2 ANTAGONISTS/REUPTAKE INHIBITORS (SARIs)

Examples

Generic (Trade) Name	Pregnancy Categories/ Half-life	Indications	Therapeutic Plasma Level Ranges	Available Forms (mg)
Nefazodone*	C/ 2–4 hr	• Depression	Not well established	**TABS:** 50, 100, 150, 200, 250
Trazodone (Oleptro [ER])	C/ 4–9 hr	• Depression **Unlabeled uses:** • Aggressive behavior • Insomnia • Migraine prevention • Depression in children and adolescents	800-1600	**TABS:** 50, 100, 150, 300 **TABS (ER):** 150, 300

* Bristol Myers Squibb voluntarily removed their brand of nefazodone (Serzone) from the market in 2004. The generic equivalent is currently available through various other manufacturers.

Action

- Trazodone inhibits neuronal reuptake of serotonin; nefazodone inhibits neuronal reuptake of serotonin and norepinephrine, and acts as antagonist at central 5-HT2 receptors

Contraindications and Precautions

Contraindicated in: • Hypersensitivity • Coadministration with terfenadine, astemizole, cisapride, pimozide, carbamazepine, or triazolam (nefazodone) • Patients with liver disease or baseline increases in serum transaminases (nefazodone) • Concomitant use with, or within 2 weeks of use of, MAO inhibitors • Acute phase of myocardial infarction

Use Cautiously in: • Pregnancy and lactation (safety not established) • Children (safety not established) • Patients with suicidal ideation • Hepatic, renal, or cardiovascular disease • Elderly and debilitated patients

Adverse Reactions and Side Effects

- Drowsiness; dizziness
- Fatigue
- Orthostatic hypotension
- Headache
- Nervousness; insomnia
- Dry mouth
- Nausea
- Somnolence
- Constipation
- Blurred vision
- Priapism (*trazodone*)
- Erectile dysfunction
- Increased risk of suicidality in children and adolescents (black box warning)
- Risk of hepatic failure (*nefazodone*) (black box warning)

Interactions

- Increased effects of **CNS depressants, carbamazepine, digoxin,** and **phenytoin** with trazodone.
- Increased effects of trazodone with **phenothiazines, delavirdine, ginkgo biloba, clarithromycin, azole antifungals,** and **protease inhibitors.**
- Risk of serotonin syndrome with concomitant use of trazodone and **SSRIs** or **SNRIs.**
- Decreased effects of trazodone and nefazodone with **carbamazepine.**
- Increases or decreases in prothrombin time with concurrent use of trazodone and **warfarin.**

- Symptoms of serotonin syndrome and those resembling neuroleptic malignant syndrome may occur with concomitant use of **MAOIs.** Should not be used concurrently or within 2 weeks of use of MAOIs. Nefazodone and trazodone should be discontinued at least 14 days before starting MAOI therapy.
- Risk of serotonin syndrome with concomitant use of trazodone or nefazodone and **sibutramine, triptans, or other drugs that increase serotonin.**
- Increased effects of both drugs with concomitant use of **buspirone** and nefazodone.
- Increased effects of **benzodiazepines, carbamazepine, cisapride, cyclosporine, digoxin,** and **St. John's wort** with nefazodone.
- Risk of rhabdomyolysis with concomitant use of nefazodone and **HMG-CoA reductase inhibitors** (e.g., **simvastatin, atorvastatin, lovastatin**).

Route and Dosage

NEFAZODONE

Depression: **PO** *(Adults):* Initial dosage: 100 mg twice daily. May increase in increments of 100 to 200 mg/day, again on a twice-daily schedule, at intervals of no less than 1 week. Maintenance dosage: 300 to 600 mg/day.

Elderly and debilitated patients: **PO:** 50 mg twice daily.

TRAZODONE

Depression: **PO:** *Adults: Immediate-release tablets:* Initial dosage: 150 mg/day in divided doses. May increase gradually by 50 mg/day every 3 to 4 days. Maximum dose: *Inpatients:* 600 mg/day in divided doses. *Outpatients:* 400 mg/day in divided doses.

Extended-release tablets: Initial dosage: 150 mg once daily. May increase by 75 mg/day every 3 days to maximum dose of 375 mg/day.

Children and adolescents (≥6 years): 1.5 to 2 mg/kg/day in 2 or 3 divided doses. Gradually increase every 3 to 4 days to maximum dose of 6 mg/kg/day in 3 divided doses.

Aggressive behavior: **PO** *(Adults):* 50 mg twice daily. Titrate dose over 1 to 6 weeks based on response and tolerability. Maintenance dosage: 75 to 400 mg/day in 2 to 4 divided dosages.

Children: **PO:** 50 mg once daily at bedtime, titrated up as tolerated and based on response over approximately 1 week. Maintenance dosage: 150 to 200 mg/day in 3 divided doses.

Insomnia: **PO** *(Adults):* 50 to 100 mg at bedtime.

Migraine prevention: **PO** *(Adults):* 100 mg/day.

■ CHEMICAL CLASS: MONOAMINE OXIDASE INHIBITORS (MAOIs)

Examples

Generic (Trade) Name	Pregnancy Categories/ Half-life	Indications	Available Forms (mg)
Isocarboxazid (Marplan)	C/Not Established	• Depression	**TABS:** 10
Phenelzine (Nardil)	C/11.6	• Depression	**TABS:** 15
Tranylcypromine (Parnate)	C/2.4–2.8 hr	• Depression	**TABS:** 10
Selegiline Transdermal System (Emsam)	C/18–25 hr (including metabolites)	• Depression	**TRANSDERMAL PATCHES:** 6, 9, 12

Action

- Inhibition of the enzyme monoamine oxidase, which is responsible for the decomposition of the biogenic amines, epinephrine, norepinephrine, dopamine, and serotonin. This action results in an increase in the concentration of these endogenous amines.

Contraindications and Precautions

Contraindicated in: • Hypersensitivity • Pheochromocytoma • Hepatic or renal insufficiency • History of or existing cardiovascular disease • Hypertension • History of severe or frequent headaches • Concomitant use with other MAOIs, tricyclic antidepressants, carbamazepine, cyclobenzaprine, bupropion, SSRIs, SARIs, buspirone, sympathomimetics, meperidine, dextromethorphan, anesthetic agents, CNS depressants, antihypertensives, caffeine, and food with high tyramine content • Children younger than 16 years of age • Pregnancy and lactation (safety not established)

Use Cautiously in: • Patients with a history of seizures • Diabetes mellitus • Patients with suicidal ideation • Agitated or hypomanic patients • History of angina pectoris or hyperthyroidism

Adverse Reactions and Side Effects

- Dizziness
- Headache
- Orthostatic hypotension
- Constipation or diarrhea
- Nausea
- Disturbances in cardiac rate and rhythm

- Blurred vision
- Dry mouth
- Weight gain
- Hypomania
- Site reactions (itching, irritation) (with selegiline transdermal system)
- Increased risk of suicidality in children and adolescents (black box warning)

Interactions

- Serious, potentially fatal adverse reactions may occur with concurrent use of other **antidepressants, carbamazepine, cyclobenzaprine, bupropion, SSRIs, SARIs, buspirone, sympathomimetics, L-tryptophan, dextromethorphan, anesthetic agents, CNS depressants,** and **amphetamines.** Avoid using within 2 weeks of each other (5 weeks after therapy with **fluoxetine**). (See contraindications.)
- Hypertensive crisis may occur with **amphetamines, methyldopa, levodopa, dopamine, epinephrine, norepinephrine, guanethidine, methylphenidate, guanadrel, reserpine,** or **vasoconstrictors.**
- Hypertension or hypotension, coma, convulsions, and death may occur with **opioids** (avoid use of **meperidine** within 14 to 21 days of MAO inhibitor therapy).
- Additive hypotension may occur with **antihypertensives, thiazide diuretics,** or **spinal anesthesia.**
- MAOIs may inhibit the hypotensive effects of **guanethidine.**
- Additive hypoglycemia may occur with **insulins** or **oral hypoglycemic agents.**
- **Doxapram** may increase pressor response.
- Serotonin syndrome may occur with concomitant use of **St. John's wort.**
- Hypertensive crisis may occur with ingestion of foods or other products containing high concentrations of **tyramine** (see Nursing Implications).
- Consumption of foods or beverages with high **caffeine** content increases the risk of hypertension and arrhythmias.
- Bradycardia may occur with concurrent use of MAOIs and **beta blockers.**
- There is a risk of toxicity from the **5-hydroxytryptamine (5-HT1) receptor agonists** (e.g., **triptans**) with concurrent use of MAOIs.

Route and Dosage

ISOCARBOXAZID (MARPLAN)

Depression: **PO** *(Adults)*: Initial dose: 10 mg twice daily. May increase dosage by 10 mg every 2 to 4 days to 40 mg by end of first week. If needed, may continue to increase dosage by increments of up to 20 mg/week. Maximum dosage: 60 mg/day divided into 2 to 4 doses. Gradually reduce to smallest effective dose.

PHENELZINE (NARDIL)

Depression: **PO** *(Adults)*: Initial dose: 15 mg 3 times/day. Increase to 60 to 90 mg/day in divided doses until therapeutic response is achieved. Then gradually reduce to smallest effective dose (15 mg/day or every other day).

TRANYLCYPROMINE (PARNATE)

Depression: **PO** *(Adults)*: 30 mg/day in divided doses. After 2 weeks, may increase by 10 mg/day, at 1 to 3 week intervals, up to a maximum dose of 60 mg/day.

SELEGILINE TRANSDERMAL SYSTEM (EMSAM)

Depression: **Transdermal patch** *(Adults)*: Initial dose: 6 mg/24 hr. If necessary, dosage may be increased in increments of 3 mg/24 hr at intervals of no less than 2 weeks up to a maximum dose of 12 mg/24 hr.

Elderly clients: The daily recommended dosage is 6 mg/24 hr.

■ PSYCHOTHERAPEUTIC COMBINATIONS*
Examples

Generic (Trade) Name	Indications	Available Forms (mg)
Olanzapine/Fluoxetine (Symbyax)	• For the acute treatment of depressive episodes associated with bipolar I disorder in adults • Treatment-resistant depression	**CAPS:** olanzapine 3/fluoxetine 25; olanzapine 6/fluoxetine 25; olanzapine 6/fluoxetine 50; olanzapine 12/fluoxetine 25; olanzapine 12/fluoxetine 50
Chlordiazepoxide/ Amitriptyline (Limbitrol)	• For the treatment of moderate to severe depression associated with moderate to severe anxiety.	**TABS:** chlordiazepoxide 5/amitriptyline 12.5; chlordiazepoxide 10/amitriptyline 25
Perphenazine/Amitriptyline HCl	• For the treatment of moderate to severe anxiety or agitation and depressed mood • For the treatment of patients with schizophrenia who have associated symptoms of depression	**TABS:** perphenazine 2/amitriptyline 10; perphenazine 2/amitriptyline 25; perphenazine 4/amitriptyline 10; perphenazine 4/amitriptyline 25; perphenazine 4/amitriptyline 50

* These medications are presented for general information only. For detailed information, the reader is directed to the chapters that deal with each of the specific drugs that make up these combinations.

Route and Dosage

OLANZAPINE/FLUOXETINE (SYMBYAX)

Depression associated with Bipolar I disorder and treatment-resistant depression: **PO** *(Adults)*: Initial dosage: olanzapine 6 mg/fluoxetine 25 mg once daily in the evening. Dosage adjustments, if indicated, can be made according to efficacy and tolerability.

Elderly: **PO:** Initial dosage: olanzapine 3 to 6 mg/fluoxetine 25 mg once daily in the evening. Dosage adjustments should be made with caution.

CHLORDIAZEPOXIDE/AMITRIPTYLINE (LIMBITROL)

Moderate to severe depression associated with moderate to severe anxiety: **PO** *(Adults)*: Initial dose: chlordiazepoxide 10 mg/amitriptyline 25 mg given 3 or 4 times a day in divided doses. May increase to 6 times a day, as required. Some patients respond to smaller doses and can be maintained on 2 tablets daily.

PERPHENAZINE/AMITRIPTYLINE HCL (ETRAFON)

Anxiety/Agitation/Depression: **PO** *(Adults)*: Initial dose: perphenazine 2 to 4 mg/amitriptyline 10 to 25 mg administered 3 or 4 times a day, or perphenazine 4 mg/amitriptyline 50 mg administered 2 times a day. Once a satisfactory response is achieved, reduce to smallest amount necessary to obtain relief.

■ NURSING DIAGNOSES RELATED TO ALL ANTIDEPRESSANTS

1. Risk for suicide related to depressed mood.
2. Risk for injury related to possible side effects of sedation, lowered seizure threshold, orthostatic hypotension, priapism, photosensitivity, arrhythmias, hypertensive crisis, or serotonin syndrome.
3. Social isolation related to depressed mood.
4. Risk for constipation related to possible side effects of the medication.
5. Insomnia related to depressed mood and elevated level of anxiety.

■ NURSING IMPLICATIONS FOR ANTIDEPRESSANTS

The plan of care should include monitoring for the following side effects from antidepressant medications. Nursing implications are designated by an asterisk (*).

1. **May occur with all chemical classes:**
   a. **Dry mouth**
      * Offer the client sugarless candy, ice, frequent sips of water.
      * Strict oral hygiene is very important.

b. **Sedation**
   * Request an order from the physician for the drug to be given at bedtime.
   * Request that the physician decrease the dosage or perhaps order a less sedating drug.
   * Instruct the client not to drive or use dangerous equipment when experiencing sedation.
c. **Nausea**
   * Medication may be taken with food to minimize GI distress.
d. **Discontinuation syndrome**
   * All classes of antidepressants have varying potentials to cause discontinuation syndromes. Abrupt withdrawal following long-term therapy with SSRIs and SNRIs may result in dizziness, lethargy, headache, and nausea. Fluoxetine is less likely to result in withdrawal symptoms because of its long half-life. Abrupt withdrawal from tricyclics may produce hypomania, akathisia, cardiac arrhythmias, gastrointestinal upset, and panic attacks. The discontinuation syndrome associated with MAOIs includes flulike symptoms, confusion, hypomania, and worsening of depressive symptoms. All antidepressant medication should be tapered gradually to prevent withdrawal symptoms.
2. **Most commonly occur with tricyclics and related medications and others, such as the SARIs and bupropion:**
   a. **Blurred vision**
      * Offer reassurance that this symptom should subside after a few weeks.
      * Instruct the client not to drive until vision is clear.
      * Clear small items from routine pathway to prevent falls.
   b. **Constipation**
      * Order foods high in fiber; increase fluid intake if not contraindicated; and encourage the client to increase physical exercise, if possible.
   c. **Urinary retention**
      * Instruct the client to report hesitancy or inability to urinate.
      * Monitor intake and output.
      * Try various methods to stimulate urination, such as running water in the bathroom or pouring water over the perineal area.
   d. **Orthostatic hypotension**
      * Instruct the client to rise slowly from a lying or sitting position.
      * Monitor blood pressure (lying and standing) frequently, and document and report significant changes.
      * Avoid long hot showers or tub baths.

e. **Reduction of seizure threshold**
  * Observe clients with history of seizures closely.
  * Institute seizure precautions as specified in hospital procedure manual.
  * Bupropion (Wellbutrin) should be administered in doses of no more than 150 mg and should be given at least 4 hours apart. Bupropion has been associated with a relatively high incidence of seizure activity in anorexic and cachectic clients.

f. **Tachycardia; arrhythmias**
  * Carefully monitor blood pressure and pulse rate and rhythm, and report any significant change to the physician.

g. **Photosensitivity**
  * Ensure that client wears sunblock lotion, protective clothing, and sunglasses when outdoors.

h. **Weight gain**
  * Provide instructions for reduced-calorie diet.
  * Encourage increased level of activity, if appropriate.

3. **Most commonly occur with SSRIs and SNRIs:**
  a. **Insomnia; agitation**
    * Administer or instruct client to take dose early in the day.
    * Instruct client to avoid caffeinated food and drinks.
    * Teach relaxation techniques to use before bedtime.

  b. **Headache**
    * Administer analgesics, as prescribed.
    * If relief is not achieved, physician may order another antidepressant.

  c. **Weight Loss** (may occur early in therapy)
    * Ensure that client is provided with caloric intake sufficient to maintain desired weight.
    * Caution should be taken in prescribing these drugs for anorectic clients.
    * Weigh client daily or every other day, at the same time and on the same scale if possible.
    * After prolonged use, some clients may gain weight on these drugs.

  d. **Sexual dysfunction**
    * Men may report abnormal ejaculation or impotence.
    * Women may experience delay or loss of orgasm.
    * If side effect becomes intolerable, a switch to another antidepressant may be necessary.

  e. **Serotonin Syndrome** (may occur when two drugs that potentiate serotonergic neurotransmission are used concurrently [see "Interactions"]).
    * Most frequent symptoms include changes in mental status, restlessness, myoclonus, hyperreflexia, tachycardia, labile blood pressure, diaphoresis, shivering, and tremors.

* Discontinue offending agent immediately.
* The physician may prescribe medications to block serotonin receptors, relieve hyperthermia and muscle rigidity, and prevent seizures. In severe cases, artificial ventilation may be required. The histamine-1 receptor antagonist, cyproheptadine, is commonly used to treat the symptoms of serotonin syndrome.
* Supportive nursing measures include monitoring vital signs, providing safety measures to prevent injury when muscle rigidity and changes in mental status are resent, cooling blankets and tepid baths to assist with temperature regulation, and monitoring intake and output (Cooper & Sejnowski, 2013).
* The condition will usually resolve on its own once the offending medication has been discontinued. However, if left untreated, the condition may progress to life-threatening complications such as seizures, coma, hypotension, ventricular arrhythmias, disseminated intravascular coagulation, rhabdomyolysis, metabolic acidosis, and renal failure (Cooper & Sejnowski, 2013).

4. **Most commonly occur with MAOIs:**
   a. **Hypertensive crisis**
      * Hypertensive crisis occurs if the individual consumes foods or other substances containing tyramine when receiving MAOI therapy. Foods that should be avoided include aged cheeses, raisins, fava beans, red wines, smoked and processed meats, caviar, pickled herring, soy sauce, monosodium glutamate (MSG), beer, chocolate, yogurt, and bananas. Drugs that should be avoided include other antidepressants, sympathomimetics (including over-the-counter cough and cold preparations), stimulants (including over-the-counter diet drugs), antihypertensives, meperidine and other opioid narcotics, and antiparkinsonian agents, such as levodopa.
      * Symptoms of hypertensive crisis include severe occipital headache, palpitations, nausea and vomiting, nuchal rigidity, fever, sweating, marked increase in blood pressure, chest pain, and coma.
      * Treatment of hypertensive crisis: Discontinue drug immediately; monitor vital signs; administer short-acting antihypertensive medication, as ordered by physician; use external cooling measures to control hyperpyrexia.
      * *Note:* Hypertensive crisis has not shown to be a problem with selegiline transdermal system at the 6 mg/24 hr dosage, and dietary restrictions at this dose are not recommended. Dietary modifications are recommended, however, at the 9 mg/24 hr and 12 mg/24 hr dosages.

　　b. **Application site reactions** (with selegiline transdermal system [Emsam])
　　　* The most common reactions include rash, itching, erythema, redness, irritation, swelling, or urticarial lesions. Most reactions resolve spontaneously, requiring no treatment. However, if reaction becomes problematic, it should be reported to the physician. Topical corticosteroids have been used in treatment.

5. **Miscellaneous side effects:**
　　a. **Priapism (with trazodone)**
　　　* Priapism is a rare side effect, but it has occurred in some men taking trazodone.
　　　* If prolonged or inappropriate penile erection occurs, the medication should be withheld and the physician notified immediately.
　　　* Priapism can become very problematic, requiring surgical intervention, and, if not treated successfully, can result in impotence.
　　b. **Hepatic failure (with nefazodone)**
　　　* Cases of life-threatening hepatic failure have been reported in clients treated with nefazodone.
　　　* Advise clients to be alert for signs or symptoms suggestive of liver dysfunction (e.g., jaundice, anorexia, GI complaints, or malaise) and to report them to the physician immediately.

■ CLIENT/FAMILY EDUCATION RELATED TO ALL ANTIDEPRESSANTS

* Continue to take the medication even though the symptoms have not subsided. The therapeutic effect may not be seen for as long as 4 weeks. If after this length of time no improvement is noted, the physician may prescribe a different medication.
* Use caution when driving or operating dangerous machinery. Drowsiness and dizziness can occur. If these side effects become persistent or interfere with activities of daily living, the client should report them to the physician. Dosage adjustment may be necessary.
* Do not stop taking the drug abruptly. To do so might produce withdrawal symptoms, such as nausea, vertigo, insomnia, headache, malaise, nightmares, and return of symptoms for which the medication was prescribed.
* Use sunblock lotion and wear protective clothing when spending time outdoors. The skin may be sensitive to sunburn.
* Report occurrence of any of the following symptoms to the physician immediately: sore throat, fever, malaise, yellowish skin, unusual bleeding, easy bruising, persistent nausea and

vomiting, severe headache, rapid heart rate, difficulty urinating, anorexia or weight loss, seizure activity, stiff or sore neck, and chest pain.

- Rise slowly from a sitting or lying position to prevent a sudden drop in blood pressure.
- Take frequent sips of water, chew sugarless gum, or suck on hard candy if dry mouth is a problem. Good oral care (frequent brushing, flossing) is very important.
- Do not consume the following foods or medications when taking MAOIs: aged cheese, wine (especially Chianti), beer, chocolate, colas, coffee, tea, sour cream, smoked and processed meats, chicken or beef liver, soy sauce, pickled herring, yogurt, raisins, caviar, broad beans, cold remedies, diet pills. To do so could cause a life-threatening hypertensive crisis.
- Follow the correct procedure for applying the selegiline transdermal patch:
  - Apply to dry, intact skin on upper torso, upper thigh, or outer surface of upper arm.
  - Apply approximately same time each day to new spot on skin, after removing and discarding old patch.
  - Wash hands thoroughly after applying the patch.
  - Avoid exposing application site to direct heat (e.g., heating pads, electric blankets, heat lamps, hot tub, or prolonged direct sunlight).
  - If patch falls off, apply new patch to a new site and resume previous schedule.
- Avoid smoking when receiving tricyclic therapy. Smoking increases the metabolism of tricyclics, requiring an adjustment in dosage to achieve the therapeutic effect.
- Do not drink alcohol when taking antidepressant therapy. These drugs potentiate the effects of each other.
- Avoid the use of other medications (including over-the-counter medications) without the physician's approval when receiving antidepressant therapy. Many medications contain substances that, in combination with antidepressant medication, could precipitate a life-threatening hypertensive crisis.
- Notify the physician immediately if inappropriate or prolonged penile erections occur when taking trazodone. If the erection persists longer than 4 hours, seek emergency department treatment. This condition is rare, but has occurred in some men who have taken trazodone. If measures are not instituted immediately, impotence can result.
- Do not "double up" on medication if a dose of bupropion (Wellbutrin) is missed, unless advised to do so by the physician. Taking bupropion in divided doses will decrease the risk of seizures and other adverse effects.
- Be aware of possible risks of taking antidepressants during pregnancy. Safe use during pregnancy and lactation has not been

fully established. These drugs are believed to readily cross the placental barrier; if so, the fetus could experience adverse effects of the drug. Inform the physician immediately if pregnancy occurs, is suspected, or is planned.

- Be aware of the side effects of antidepressants. Refer to written materials furnished by health care providers for safe self-administration.
- Carry a card or other identification at all times describing the medications being taken.

INTERNET REFERENCES

a. http://www.mentalhealth.com/
b. http://www.nimh.nih.gov/index.shtml
c. http://www.nimh.nih.gov/health/publications/mental-health-medications/index.shtml
d. http://www.nlm.nih.gov/medlineplus/druginformation.html
e. http://www.ndmda.org

CHAPTER 25

Mood-Stabilizing Agents

■ CHEMICAL CLASS: ANTIMANIC

Examples

Generic (Trade) Name	Pregnancy Category/ Half-life	Indications	Therapeutic Plasma Level Range	Available Forms (mg)
Lithium Carbonate (Lithobid) Lithium Citrate	D/20–27 hr	• Manic episodes associated with bipolar disorder • Maintenance therapy to prevent or diminish intensity of subsequent manic episodes **Unlabeled uses:** • Borderline personality disorder • Neutropenia • Cluster headaches (prophylaxis) • Alcohol dependence • Bulimia • Postpartum affective psychosis • Corticosteroid-induced psychosis	Acute mania: 1.0–1.5 mEq/L Mainte- nance: 0.6–1.2 mEq/L	CAPS: 150, 300, 600 TABS: 300 TABS (ER): 300, 450 SYRUP: 8 mEq lithium (as citrate equivalent to 300 mg lithium carbonate)/ 5 mL

Action

• Not fully understood, but lithium may have an influence on the reuptake of norepinephrine and serotonin. Effects on other neurotransmitters have also been noted. Lithium also alters sodium transport in nerve and muscle cells. The subsiding of manic symptoms with lithium may take 1 to 3 weeks.

Contraindications and Precautions

Contraindicated in: • Hypersensitivity • Severe cardiovascular or renal disease • Dehydrated or debilitated patients • Sodium depletion • Pregnancy and lactation

Use Cautiously in: • Elderly patients • Any degree of cardiac, renal, or thyroid disease • Diabetes mellitus • Urinary retention • Children under the age of 12 years (safety not established)

Adverse Reactions and Side Effects

- Drowsiness, dizziness, headache
- Seizures
- Dry mouth, thirst
- Indigestion, nausea, anorexia
- Fine hand tremors
- Hypotension, arrhythmias, ECG changes
- Polyuria, glycosuria
- Weight gain
- Hypothyroidism
- Dehydration
- Leukocytosis

Interactions

- The effects of lithium (and potential for toxicity) are increased with concurrent use of **carbamazepine, fluoxetine, haloperidol, loop diuretics, methyldopa, NSAIDSs,** and **thiazide diuretics.**
- The effects of lithium are decreased with concurrent use of **acetazolamide, osmotic diuretics, theophylline,** and **urinary alkalinizers.**
- Increased effects of **neuromuscular blocking agents** and **tricyclic antidepressants** with concurrent use of lithium.
- Decreased pressor sensitivity of **sympathomimetics** with lithium.
- Neurotoxicity may occur with concurrent use of lithium and **phenothiazines** or **calcium channel blockers.**

Route and Dosage

Acute mania: **PO** *(Adults and children ≥12 years)*: *Immediate release tabs and caps:* Initial dosage: 300 to 600 mg three times/day. Usual maintenance dose is 300 mg 3 to 4 times a day. *Extended release tabs:* 450 to 900 mg twice daily or 300 to 600 mg 3 times daily. Usual maintenance dose is 450 mg twice daily or 300 mg 3 times daily.

Children <12 years: **PO:** Initial dosage: 15 to 20 mg/kg/day in 2 to 3 divided doses. Dosage may be adjusted weekly until therapeutic level has been achieved.

Serum lithium levels should be taken twice weekly at the initiation of therapy and until therapeutic level has been achieved.

Borderline personality disorder: **PO** *(Adults)*: 900 to 2400 mg/day in 3 to 4 divided doses (or 900 to 1800 mg/day [ER tabs] in

2 divided doses). Titrate dosage to maintain serum levels of
0.8 to 1 mEq/L.

■ CHEMICAL CLASS: ANTICONVULSANTS
Examples

Generic (Trade) Name	Pregnancy Categories/ Half-life	Indications	Therapeutic Piasma Level Range	Available Forms (mg)
Carb amazepine* (Tegretol, Epitol, Carbatrol, Equetro, Teril, Tegretol-XR)	D/25–65 hr (initial) 12–17 hr (repeated doses)	• Epilepsy (except *Equetro*) • Trigeminal neuralgia (except *Equetro*) • Bipolar disorder (FDA approved: *Equetro* only) **Unlabeled uses:** • Borderline personality disorder • Management of alcohol withdrawal • Restless legs syndrome • Postherpetic neuralgia	4–12 mcg/mL	**TABS:** 100, 200 **TABS XR:** 100, 200, 400 **CAPS XR:** 100, 200, 300 **ORAL SUSPENSION:** 100/5 mL
Clonazepam (C-IV) (Klonopin)	D/18–60 hr	• Petit mal, akinetic, and myoclonic seizures • Panic disorder **Unlabeled uses:** • Acute manic episodes • Restless leg syndrome • Tic disorders	20–80 ng/mL	**TABS:** 0.5, 1, 2 **TABS (DISIN- TEGRATING ORAL):** 0.125, 0.25, 0.5, 1, 2
Valproic acid* (Depakene; Depakote; Stavzor; Depacon)	D/5–20 hr	• Epilepsy • Manic episodes (FDA approved: *Stavzor* only) • Migraine prophylaxis (FDA approved: *Stavzor* only) **Unlabeled uses:** • Borderline personality disorder	50–150 mcg/mL	**CAPS:** 250 **CAPS (DR):** 125, 250, 500 **SYRUP:** 250/5 mL **TABS (DR):** 125, 250, 500 **TABS (ER):** 250, 500 **CAPS (SPRIN- KLE):** 125 **INJECTION:** 100/mL in 5 mL vial
Lamotrigine* (Lamictal)	C/~ 33 hr	• Epilepsy • Bipolar disorder	Not established	**TABS:** 25, 50, 100, 150, 200, 250 **TABS (CHEW- ABLE, DIS- PERSIBLE):** 2, 5, 25 **TABS (DISIN- TEGRATING ORAL):** 25, *(Continued)*

Generic (Trade) Name	Pregnancy Categories/ Half-life	Indications	Therapeutic Plasma Level Range	Available Forms (mg)
				50, 100, 200 **TABS (ER):** 25, 50, 100, 200, 250, 300
Topiramate* (Topamax)	C/21 hr	• Epilepsy • Migraine prophylaxis **Unlabeled uses:** • Bipolar disorder • Bulimia nervosa	Not established	**TABS:** 25, 50, 100, 200 **CAPS (SPRINKLE):** 15, 25
Oxcarbazepine* (Trileptal)	C/2 hr (metabo- lite 9 hr)	• Epilepsy **Unlabeled uses:** • Alcohol withdrawal • Bipolar disorder • Diabetic neuropathy	Not established	**TABS:** 150, 300, 600 **ORAL SUSP:** 60/mL

*The FDA has issued a warning indicating reports of suicidal behavior or ideation associated with the use of these drugs (and other antiepileptic medications). The FDA now requires that all manufacturers of drugs in this class include a warning in their labeling to this effect. Results of a study published in the December 2009 issue of *Archives of General Psychiatry* indicate that antiepileptic medications "do not increase risk of suicide attempts in patients with bipolar disorder" (Gibbons et al, 2009).

Action
• Action in the treatment of bipolar disorder is unclear.

Contraindications and Precautions

Carbamazepine

Contraindicated in: hypersensitivity, with MAOIs, lactation, history of previous bone marrow depression

Use Cautiously in: elderly, liver/renal/cardiac disease, pregnancy

Clonazepam

Contraindicated in: hypersensitivity to clonazepam or other benzodiazepines, acute narrow-angle glaucoma, liver disease, pregnancy and lactation

Use Cautiously in: elderly, liver/renal disease

Valproic acid

Contraindicated in: hypersensitivity, liver disease

Use Cautiously in: elderly, renal/cardiac diseases, pregnancy and lactation, patients with bleeding disorders or bone marrow depression

Lamotrigine

> **Contraindicated in:** hypersensitivity, lactation
> **Use Cautiously in:** renal/hepatic/cardiac insufficiency, pregnancy

Topiramate

> **Contraindicated in:** hypersensitivity, lactation
> **Use Cautiously in:** renal and hepatic impairment, pregnancy, children, and the elderly

Oxcarbazepine

> **Contraindicated in:** hypersensitivity (cross sensitivity with carbamazepine may occur); lactation
> **Use Cautiously in:** renal impairment, pregnancy, children under the age of 4 years

Adverse Reactions and Side Effects

Carbamazepine

- Drowsiness, ataxia
- Nausea, vomiting
- Blood dyscrasias

Clonazepam

- Drowsiness, ataxia
- Dependence, tolerance
- Blood dyscrasias

Valproic acid

- Drowsiness, dizziness
- Nausea, vomiting
- Prolonged bleeding time
- Tremor

Lamotrigine

- Ataxia, dizziness, headache
- Nausea, vomiting
- Risk of severe rash
- Photosensitivity

Topiramate

- Drowsiness, dizziness, fatigue, ataxia
- Impaired concentration, nervousness
- Vision changes
- Nausea, weight loss
- Decreased efficacy with oral contraceptives

Oxcarbazepine

- Dizziness, drowsiness
- Headache
- Nausea and vomiting

- Abnormal vision, diplopia, nystagmus
- Ataxia
- Tremor

Interactions

The effects of:	Are increased by:	Are decreased by:	Concurrent use may result in:
Carbamazepine	Verapamil, diltiazem, erythromycin, clarithromycin, SSRIs, tricyclic antidepressants, cimetidine, isoniazid, danazol, lamotrigine, niacin, acetazolamide, dalfopristin, valproate, nefazodone	Cisplatin, doxorubicin, felbamate, rifampin, barbiturates, hydantoins, primidone, theophylline	Decreased levels of corticosteroids, doxycycline, felbamate, quinidine, warfarin, estrogen-containing contraceptives, cyclosporine, benzodiazepines, theophylline, lamotrigine, valproic acid, bupropion, haloperidol, olanzapine, tiagabine, topiramate, voriconazole, ziprasidone, felbamate, levothyroxine, antidepressants. Increased levels of lithium; life-threatening hypertensive reaction with MAOIs.
Clonazepam	CNS depressants, cimetidine, hormonal contraceptives, disulfiram, fluoxetine, isoniazid, ketoconazole, metoprolol, propranolol, valproic acid, or probenecid	Rifampin, theophylline (↓sedative effects), phenytoin	Increased phenytoin levels. Decreased efficacy of levodopa.
Valproic Acid	Chlorpromazine, cimetidine, erythromycin, felbamate, salicylates	Rifampin, carbamazepine, cholestyramine, lamotrigine, phenobarbital, ethosuximide, hydantoins	Increased effects of tricyclic antidepressants, carbamazepine, CNS depressants, ethosuximide, lamotrigine, phenobarbital, warfarin, zidovudine, hydantoins.
Lamotrigine	Valproic acid	Primidone, phenobarbital, phenytoin, rifamycin, succinimides, oral contraceptives, oxcarbazepine, carbamazepine, acetaminophen	Decreased levels of valproic acid Increased levels of carbamazepine and topiramate.
Topiramate	Metformin; hydrochlorothiazide	Phenytoin, carbamazepine, valproic acid, lamotrigine	Increased risk of CNS depression with alcohol or other CNS depressants.

The effects of:	Are increased by:	Are decreased by:	Concurrent use may result in:
			Increased risk of kidney stones with carbonic anhydrase inhibitors. Increased effects of phenytoin, metformin, amitriptyline; decreased effects of oral contraceptives, digoxin, lithium, risperidone, and valproic acid.
Oxcarbazepine	Carbamazepine, phenobarbital, phenytoin, valproic acid, verapamil		Increased concentrations of phenobarbital and phenytoin. Decreased effects of oral contraceptives, felodipine, and lamotrigine.

Route and Dosage

CARBAMAZEPINE (TEGRETOL)

Seizure disorders: **PO** *(Adults and children >12 years):* 200 mg 2 times a day (tablets) or 100 mg 4 times a day (suspension). Increase by 200 mg/day every 7 days until therapeutic levels are achieved (range is 600 to 1200 mg/day in divided doses every 6 to 8 hours). Extended-release products are given twice daily. Maximum dose: 1000 mg/day in children 12 to 15 yr; 1200 mg/day in patients >15 yr.

Children 6 to 12 yr: **PO**: 100 mg 2 times a day (tablets) or 50 mg 4 times/day (suspension). Increase by 100 mg weekly until therapeutic levels are obtained. (Usual range: 400 to 800 mg/day). Maximum daily dose: 1000 mg. Extended-release products are given twice daily.

Children <6 yr: **PO**: 10 to 20 mg/kg/day in 2 to 3 divided doses. May increase weekly until optimal response and therapeutic levels are achieved. Usual maintenance dose is 250 to 350 mg/day. Maximum daily dose: 35 mg/kg/day.

Trigeminal neuralgia: **PO** *(Adults):* Initial dose 100 mg 2 times a day (tablets) or 50 mg 4 times a day (suspension). May increase by up to 200 mg/day until pain is relieved, then maintenance dose of 200 to 1200 mg/day in divided doses (usual range, 400 to 800 mg/day).

Bipolar disorder, mania: (Equetro only) **PO** *(Adults):* Initial dose: 200 mg 2 times a day. Dosage may be adjusted in 200 mg daily increments to achieve optimal clinical response. Doses higher than 1600 mg/day have not been studied.

Borderline personality disorder: **PO** *(Adults):* 400 mg/day in 2 divided doses. May increase dose in increments of 200 mg/day depending on response, tolerability, and plasma concentrations. Maximum dosage: 1600 mg/day.

Management of alcohol withdrawal: **PO** *(Adults):* Dosage on day 1: 600 to 1200 mg. Dosage is then tapered over 5 to 10 days to 0 mg.

Restless leg syndrome: **PO** *(Adults):* 100 to 600 mg daily for up to 5 weeks.

Postherpetic neuralgia: **PO** *(Adults):* 100 to 200 mg/day, slowly increased to a maximum of 1200 mg/day.

CLONAZEPAM (KLONOPIN)

Seizures: **PO** *(Adults and children >10 years or more than 30 kg):* 0.5 mg 3 times a day; may increase by 0.5 to 1 mg every 3 days until seizures are adequately controlled. Maximum daily dose: 20 mg.

Children ≤10 years or 30 kg: **PO**: Initial daily dose 0.01 to 0.03 mg/kg/day (not to exceed 0.05 mg/kg/day) given in 2 or 3 divided doses; increase by no more than 0.25 to 0.5 mg every third day until a daily maintenance dose of 0.1 to 0.2 mg/kg (in 3 divided doses) has been reached, unless seizures are controlled or side effects preclude further increase.

Panic disorder: **PO** *(Adults):* Initial dose: 0.25 mg 2 times a day. May increase in increments of 0.125 to 0.25 mg twice daily every 3 days until symptoms are controlled or until side effects preclude further increase. Usual dose: 1 mg/day. Maximum dose: 4 mg/day.

Bipolar disorder, mania: **PO** *(Adults):* 2 to 16 mg/day.

Restless leg syndrome: **PO** *(Adults):* 0.5 to 2 mg administered 30 minutes before bedtime.

Tic disorders: **PO** *(Adults and children):* 0.5 to 12 mg (after dose titration).

VALPROIC ACID (DEPAKENE; DEPAKOTE)

Epilepsy: **PO**: *(Adults and children ≥10 years):* Initial dose: 5 to 15 mg/kg/day. Increase by 5 to 10 mg/kg/week until therapeutic levels are reached. Maximum recommended dosage: 60 mg/kg/day. When daily dosage exceeds 250 mg, give in 2 divided doses.

Manic episodes: **PO** *(Adults):* Initial dose: 750 mg in divided doses. Titrate rapidly to achieve the lowest therapeutic dose that produces the desired response or trough plasma levels of 50 to 125 mcg/mL. Maximum recommended dose: 60/mg/kg/day.

Migraine prophylaxis: **PO** *(Adults and children ≥16 years):* 250 mg twice daily. Some patients may require up to 1000 mg/day.

Borderline personality disorder: **PO** *(Adults):* 750 mg/day in divided doses. Titrate to maintain a therapeutic plasma level of 50 to 100 mcg/mL.

LAMOTRIGINE (LAMICTAL)

Epilepsy: PO (*Adults and children >12 years*):

For patients not taking carbamazepine, valproate, phenobarbital, phenytoin, or primidone: Weeks 1 and 2: 25 mg/day; weeks 3 and 4: 50 mg/day; week 5 onward to maintenance: Increase by 50 mg/day every 1 to 2 weeks; usual maintenance dosage: 225 to 375 mg/day in 2 divided doses.

For patients taking valproate: Weeks 1 and 2: 25 mg every other day; weeks 3 and 4: 25 mg/day; week 5 onward to maintenance: increase by 25 to 50 mg/day every 1 to 2 weeks; usual maintenance dosage: 100 to 400 mg/day in 1 or 2 divided doses (maintenance dose of 100 to 200 mg/day if receiving valproate alone).

For patients taking carbamazepine, phenobarbital, phenytoin, or primidone, but not valproate: Weeks 1 and 2: 50 mg/day; weeks 3 and 4: 100 mg/day in 2 divided doses; week 5 onward to maintenance: increase by 100 mg/day every 1 to 2 weeks; usual maintenance dosage: 300 to 500 mg/day in 2 divided doses.

Children 2 to 12 years: Refer to manufacturer's dosing recommendations.

Bipolar Disorder: Escalation regimen:

For patients not taking carbamazepine, valproate, phenobarbital, phenytoin, or primidone: **PO** (*Adults*): Weeks 1 and 2: 25 mg/day; weeks 3 and 4: 50 mg/day; week 5: 100 mg/day; then 200 mg/day.

For patients taking valproate: **PO** (*Adults*): Weeks 1 and 2: 25 mg every other day; weeks 3 and 4: 25 mg/day; week 5: 50 mg/day; then 100 mg/day.

For patients taking carbamazepine, phenobarbital, phenytoin, or primidone, but not valproate: **PO** (*Adults*): Weeks 1 and 2: 50 mg/day; weeks 3 and 4: 100 mg/day in divided doses; week 5: 200 mg/day in divided doses; week 6: 300 mg/day in divided doses; then up to 400 mg/day in divided doses.

TOPIRAMATE (TOPAMAX)

Epilepsy (monotherapy): *Adults and children ≥10 years):* **PO:** 25 mg twice daily initially, gradually increasing at weekly intervals to 200 mg twice daily over a 6-week period.

Children 2 to <10 years and ≤11 kg: **PO:** 25 mg daily in the evening initially, gradually increasing at weekly intervals to 75 mg twice daily over a 5 to 7 week period; if needed, may continue to titrate dose on a weekly basis up to 150 mg twice daily.

Children 2 to <10 years and 12 to 22 kg: **PO:** 25 mg daily in the evening initially, gradually increasing at weekly intervals to 100 mg twice daily over a 5 to 7 week period; if needed may continue to titrate dose on a weekly basis up to 150 mg twice daily.

Children 2 to <10 years and 23 to 31 kg: **PO:** 25 mg daily in the evening initially, gradually increasing at weekly intervals to 100 mg twice daily over a 5 to 7 week period; if needed may continue to titrate dose on a weekly basis up to 175 mg twice daily.

Children 2 to <10 years and 32 to 38 kg: **PO:** 25 mg daily in the evening initially, gradually increasing at weekly intervals to 125 mg twice daily over a 5 to 7 week period; if needed may continue to titrate dose on a weekly basis up to 175 mg twice daily.

Children 2 to <10 and >38 kg: **PO:** 25 mg daily in the evening initially, gradually increasing at weekly intervals to 125 mg twice daily over a 5 to 7 week period; if needed may continue to titrate dose on a weekly basis up to 200 mg twice daily.

Epilepsy (adjunctive therapy): **PO** *(Adults and children ≥17 years):* 25 to 50 mg/day increasing by 25 to 50 mg/day at weekly intervals up to 200 to 400 mg/day in 2 divided doses (200 to 400 mg day in 2 divided doses for partial seizures and 400 mg/day in 2 divided doses for primary generalized tonic-clonic seizures). Maximum dose: 1600 mg/day.

Bipolar disorder: **PO** *(Adults):* Initial dose: 25 to 50 mg/day. Increase to target range of 100 to 200 mg/day in divided doses. Maximum dosage: 400 mg/day.

Bulimia nervosa: **PO:** *(Adults):* 25 mg/day for the first week, then titrated by 25 to 50 mg/week to the minimal effective dosage or a maximum dosage of 400 mg/day.

OXCARBAZEPINE (TRILEPTAL)

Epilepsy: **PO** *(Adults): Adjunctive therapy:* 300 mg twice daily, may be increased by up to 600 mg/day at weekly intervals up to 1200 mg/day (up to 2400 mg/day may be needed).

Conversion to monotherapy: 300 mg twice daily; may be increased by 600 mg/day at weekly intervals, whereas other antiepileptic drugs are tapered over 3 to 6 weeks; dose of oxcarbazepine should be increased up to 2400 mg/day over a period of 2 to 4 weeks.

Initiation of monotherapy: 300 mg twice daily, increase by 300 mg/day every third day, up to 1200 mg/day. Maximum maintenance dose should be achieved over 2 to 4 weeks.

Children 2 to 16 years: **PO** *Adjunctive therapy:* 4 to 5 mg/kg twice daily (up to 600 mg/day), increased over 2 weeks to achieve 900 mg/day in patients 20 to 29 kg, 1200 mg/day in patients 29.1 to 39 kg, and 1800 mg/day in patients >39 kg (range 6 to 51 mg/kg/day). In patients <20 kg, initial dose of 16 to 20 mg/kg/day may be used, not to exceed 60 mg/kg/day.

Conversion to monotherapy: 8 to 10 mg/kg/day given twice daily; may be increased by 10 mg/kg/day at weekly intervals, whereas other antiepileptic drugs are tapered over 3 to 6 weeks; dose of oxcarbazepine should be increased up to 600 to 900 mg/day in patients ≤ 20 kg, 900 to 1200 mg/day in patients 25 to 30 kg, 900 to 1500 mg/day in patients 35 to 40 kg, 1200 to 1500 mg/day in patients 45 kg, 1200 to 1800 mg/day in patients 50 to 55 kg, 1200 to 2100 mg/day in patients 60 to 65 kg, and 1500 to 2100 mg/day in patients 70 kg. Maximum maintenance dose should be achieved over 2 to 4 weeks.

Alcohol withdrawal: **PO** *(Adults):* 600 to 1800 mg in divided doses for 6 weeks to 6 months.

Bipolar disorder: **PO** *(Adults):* Initial dose: 300 mg/day. Titrate to a maximum dose of 900 to 2400 mg/day.

Diabetic neuropathy: **PO** *(Adults):* Initial dose: 150 to 300 mg/day. Titrate to recommended dose of 900 to 1200 mg/day. Maximum dose: 1800 mg/day.

■ CHEMICAL CLASS: CALCIUM CHANNEL BLOCKERS

Examples

Generic (Trade) Name	Pregnancy Categories/ Half-life	Indications	Therapeutic Plasma Level Range	Available Forms (mg)
Verapamil (Calan; Isoptin; Verelan)	C/3–7 hr (initially) 4.5-12 hr (repeated dosing) ~12 hr (SR) 2–5 hr (IV)	• Angina • Arrhythmias • Hypertension **Unlabeled uses:** • Bipolar mania • Migraine headache prophylaxis	80–300 ng/ml	**TABS:** 40, 80, 120 **TABS (XR):** 120, 180, 240 **CAPS XR:** 100, 120, 180, 200, 240, 300, 360 **INJECTION:** 2.5/mL

Action
• Action in the treatment of bipolar disorder is unclear.

Contraindications and Precautions

Contraindicated in: • Hypersensitivity • Severe left ventricular dysfunction • Heart block • Hypotension • Cardiogenic shock • Congestive heart failure • Patients with atrial flutter or atrial fibrillation and an accessory bypass tract

Use Cautiously in: • Liver or renal disease • Cardiomyopathy • Intracranial pressure • Elderly patients • Pregnancy and lactation (safety not established)

Adverse Reactions and Side Effects
• Drowsiness
• Dizziness
• Headache
• Hypotension
• Bradycardia
• Nausea
• Constipation

Interactions

- Effects of verapamil are increased with concomitant use of **amiodarone, beta blockers, cimetidine, ranitidine,** and **grapefruit juice.**
- Effects of verapamil are decreased with concomitant use of **barbiturates, calcium salts, hydantoins, rifampin** and **antineoplastics.**
- Effects of the following drugs are increased with concomitant use of verapamil: **beta blockers, disopyramide, flecainide, doxorubicin, benzodiazepines, buspirone, carbamazepine, digoxin, dofetilide, ethanol, imipramine, nondepolarizing muscle relaxants, prazosin, quinidine, sirolimus, tacrolimus,** and **theophylline.**
- Serum **lithium** levels may be altered when administered concurrently with verapamil.

Route and Dosage

Angina: **PO** *(Adults):* 80 to 120 mg 3 times/day.

Arrhythmias: **PO** *(Adults):* 240 to 320 mg/day in 3 or 4 divided doses.

Hypertension: **PO** *(Adults):* 40 to 80 mg 3 times/day. Maximum recommended daily dose: 480 mg.

Bipolar mania: **PO** *(Adults):* 80 to 320 mg/day in divided doses.

Migraine prophylaxis: **PO** *(Adults):* 160 to 320 mg/day in 3 to 4 divided doses.

■ CHEMICAL CLASS: ANTIPSYCHOTICS

Examples

Generic (Trade) Name	Pregnancy Categories/ Half-life (hr)	Indications	Available Forms (mg)
Olanzapine (Zyprexa)	C/21–54	• Schizophrenia • Bipolar disorder • Agitation associated with schizophrenia and mania (IM)	**TABS:** 2.5, 5, 7.5, 10, 15, 20 **TABS (ORALLY DISINTE- GRATING):** 5, 10, 15, 20 **POWDER FOR INJECTION (IM):** 10 mg/vial **POWDER FOR SUSPENSION, ER (PER VIAL):** 210, 300, 405
Olanzapine and fluoxetine (Symbyax)*		Symbyax: • For the treatment of depressive episodes associated with bipolar disorder • Treatment-resistant depression	Symbyax: **CAPS:** 3 olanzapine/25 fluoxetine, 6 olanzapine/25 fluoxetine 6 olanzapine/50 fluoxetine, 12 olanzapine/25 fluoxetine, 12 olanzapine/ 50 fluoxetine
Aripiprazole (Abilify)	C/75–94 (including metabolite)	• Bipolar mania • Schizophrenia • Irritability associated with autistic disorder	**TABS:** 2, 5, 10, 15, 20, 30 **TABS (ORALLY DISINTE- GRATING):** 10, 15

Generic (Trade) Name	Pregnancy Categories/ Half-life (hr)	Indications	Available Forms (mg)
		• Major depressive disorder (adjunctive treatment)	ORAL SOLUTION: 1/mL INJECTION: 7.5/mL
Chlorpromazine	C/24	• Bipolar mania • Schizophrenia • Emesis/hiccoughs • Acute intermittent porphyria • Hyperexcitable, combative behavior in children • Preoperative apprehension	TABS: 10, 25, 50, 100, 200 INJECTION: 25/mL
Quetiapine (Seroquel)	C/6	• Schizophrenia • Acute manic episodes • Major depression (adjunctive therapy) • Obsessive-compulsive disorder	TABS: 25, 50, 100, 200, 300, 400 TABS (XR): 50, 150, 200, 300, 400
Risperidone (Risperdal)	C/3–20 (including metabolite)	• Bipolar mania • Schizophrenia • Irritability associated with autistic disorder **Unlabeled uses:** • Obsessive-compulsive disorder	TABS: 0.25, 0.5, 1, 2, 3, 4 TABS (ORALLY DISINTEGRATING): 0.5, 1, 2, 3, 4 ORAL SOLUTION: 1/mL POWDER FOR INJECTION: 12.5/vial, 25/vial, 37.5/vial, 50/vial
Ziprasidone (Geodon)	C/7 (oral); 2–5 (IM)	• Bipolar mania • Schizophrenia • Acute agitation in schizophrenia (IM)	CAPS: 20, 40, 60, 80 POWDER FOR INJECTION: 20/vial
Asenapine (Saphris)	C/24	• Schizophrenia • Bipolar disorder	TABS (SUBLINGUAL): 5, 10

'For information related to action, contraindications/precautions, adverse reactions and side effects, and interactions, refer to the monographs for olanzapine (Chapters 25 and 26) and fluoxetine (Chapter 24).

Action
- Efficacy in schizophrenia is achieved through a combination of dopamine and serotonin type 2 (5HT2) antagonism.
- Mechanism of action in the treatment of acute manic episodes is unknown.

Contraindications and Precautions

Olanzapine:

Contraindicated in: hypersensitivity; lactation. *Orally disintegrating tablets only:* Phenylketonuria (orally disintegrating tablets contain aspartame).

Use Cautiously in: hepatic insufficiency, elderly clients (reduce dosage), pregnancy and children (safety not established), cardiovascular or cerebrovascular disease, history of glaucoma, history of seizures, history of attempted suicide, prostatic hypertrophy, diabetes or risk factors for diabetes, narrow angle glaucoma, history of paralytic ileus; patients with pre-existing low white blood cell count and/or history of drug-induced leukopenia/neutropenia; elderly patients with psychosis related to neurocognitive disorder (NCD) (black box warning).

Aripiprazole:

Contraindicated in: hypersensitivity; lactation

Use Cautiously in: cardiovascular or cerebrovascular disease; conditions that cause hypotension (dehydration, treatment with antihypertensives or diuretics); elderly patients; pregnancy, children, and adolescents (safety not established); patients with diabetes or seizure disorders; elderly patients with NCD-related psychosis (black box warning)

Chlorpromazine:

Contraindicated in: hypersensitivity (cross-sensitivity with other phenothiazines may occur); narrow-angle glaucoma; bone marrow depression; severe liver or cardiovascular disease; concurrent pimozide use

Use Cautiously in: elderly and debilitated patients; children with acute illnesses, infections, gastroenteritis, or dehydration (increased risk of extrapyramidal reactions); diabetes; respiratory disease; prostatic hypertrophy; CNS tumors, epilepsy; intestinal obstruction; pregnancy or lactation (safety not established); elderly patients with NCD-related psychosis (black box warning)

Quetiapine:

Contraindicated in: hypersensitivity; lactation; concurrent use with drugs that prolong the QT interval; patients with history of arrhythmias, including bradycardia

Use Cautiously in: cardiovascular or cerebrovascular disease; dehydration or hypovolemia (increased risk of hypotension); elderly patients; hepatic impairment; hypothyroidism; history of suicide attempt; patients with diabetes or a history of seizures; pregnancy or children (safety not established); elderly patients with NCD-related psychosis (black box warning)

Risperidone:

Contraindicated in: hypersensitivity; lactation

Use Cautiously in: elderly or debilitated patients; renal or hepatic impairment; cardiovascular disease; history of seizures; history of suicide attempt or drug abuse; diabetes or risk factors for diabetes; pregnancy or children (safety not established); elderly patients with NCD-related psychosis (black box warning)

Ziprasidone:

Contraindicated in: hypersensitivity; history of QT prolongation, arrhythmias, recent MI, or uncompensated heart failure; concurrent use of other drugs known to prolong QT interval; hypokalemia or hypomagnesemia; lactation

Use Cautiously in: concurrent diuretic therapy or diarrhea (may increase the risk of hypotension, hypokalemia, or hypomagnesemia); hepatic impairment; cardiovascular or cerebrovascular disease; hypotension, concurrent antihypertensive therapy, dehydration, or hypovolemia (may increase risk of orthostatic hypotension); elderly patients; patients at risk for aspiration pneumonia; history of suicide attempt; pregnancy and children (safety not established); patients with pre-existing low white blood cell count and/or history of drug-induced leukopenia/neutropenia; elderly patients with NCD-related psychosis (black box warning)

Asenapine:

Contraindicated in: hypersensitivity; lactation; history of QT prolongation or arrhythmias; concurrent use of other drugs known to prolong QT interval

Use Cautiously in: patients with hepatic, renal, or cardiovascular insufficiency; diabetes or risk factors for diabetes; history of seizures; history of suicide attempt; patients at risk for aspiration pneumonia; elderly patients; pregnancy and children (safety not established); elderly patients with NCD-related psychosis (black box warning)

Adverse Reactions and Side Effects

Olanzapine

- Drowsiness, dizziness, weakness
- Dry mouth, constipation, increased appetite
- Nausea
- Weight gain or loss
- Orthostatic hypotension, tachycardia
- Restlessness
- Rhinitis
- Tremor
- Headache

Aripiprazole

- Drowsiness, light-headedness
- Headache
- Insomnia, restlessness

- Constipation
- Nausea
- Weight loss

Chlorpromazine

- Sedation
- Blurred vision
- Hypotension
- Constipation
- Dry mouth
- Photosensitivity
- Extrapyramidal symptoms
- Weight gain
- Urinary retention

Quetiapine

- Drowsiness, dizziness
- Hypotension, tachycardia
- Headache
- Constipation
- Dry mouth
- Nausea
- Weight gain

Risperidone

- Agitation, anxiety
- Drowsiness, dizziness
- Extrapyramidal symptoms
- Headache
- Insomnia
- Constipation
- Nausea/vomiting
- Weight gain
- Rhinitis
- Sexual dysfunction
- Diarrhea
- Dry mouth

Ziprasidone

- Drowsiness, dizziness
- Restlessness
- Headache
- Constipation
- Diarrhea
- Dry mouth
- Nausea
- Weight gain
- Prolonged QT interval
- Sexual dysfunction

Asenapine

- Constipation
- Dry mouth
- Nausea and vomiting
- Weight gain
- Restlessness
- QTc interval prolongation
- Tachycardia
- Extrapyramidal symptoms
- Drowsiness, dizziness
- Insomnia
- Headache

Interactions

The effects of	Are increased by:	Are decreased by:	Concurrent use may result in:
Olanzapine	Fluvoxamine and other CYP1A2 inhibitors, fluoxetine	Carbamazepine and other CYP1A2 inducers, omeprazole, rifampin	Decreased effects of levodopa and dopamine agonists. Increased hypotension with antihypertensives. Increased CNS depression with alcohol or other CNS depressants.
Aripiprazole	Ketoconazole and other CYP3A4 inhibitors; quinidine, fluoxetine, paroxetine, or other potential CYP2D6 inhibitors	Carbamazepine, famotidine, valproate	Increased CNS depression with alcohol or other CNS depressants. Increased hypotension with antihypertensives.
Chlorpromazine	Beta blockers; paroxetine	Centrally acting anticholinergics	Increased effects of beta blockers; excessive sedation and hypotension with meperidine; decreased hypotensive effect of guanethidine; decreased effect of oral anticoagulants; decreased or increased phenytoin levels; increased orthostatic hypotension with thiazide diuretics. Increased CNS depression with alcohol or other CNS depressants. Increased hypotension with antihypertensives. Increased anticholinergic effects with anticholinergic agents.

(Continued)

The effects of	Are increased by:	Are decreased by:	Concurrent use may result in:
Quetiapine	Cimetidine; ketoconazole, itraconazole, fluconazole, erythromycin, or other CYP3A4 inhibitors	Phenytoin; thioridazine	Decreased effects of levodopa and dopamine agonists. Increased CNS depression with alcohol or other CNS depressants. Increased hypotension with antihypertensives.
Risperidone	Clozapine, fluoxetine, paroxetine, or ritonavir	Carbamazepine	Decreased effects of levodopa and dopamine agonists. Increased effects of clozapine and valproate. Increased CNS depression with alcohol or other CNS depressants. Increased hypotension with antihypertensives.
Ziprasidone	Ketoconazole and other CYP3A4 inhibitors.	Carbamazepine	Life-threatening prolongation of QT interval with quinidine, dofetilide, other class Ia and III antiarrhythmics, pimozide, sotalol, thioridazine, chlorpromazine, pentamidine, arsenic trioxide, mefloquine, dolasetron, tacrolimus, droperidol, gatifloxacin, or moxifloxacin. Decreased effects of levodopa and dopamine agonists. Increased CNS depression with alcohol or other CNS depressants. Increased hypotension with antihypertensives.
Asenapine	Fluvoxamine; imipramine; valproate	Carbamazepine; cimetidine; paroxetine	Increased effects of paroxetine and dextromethorphan. Increased CNS depression with alcohol or other CNS depressants. Increased hypotension with antihypertensives; additive effect of QT interval prolongation with quinidine, dofetilide, other class Ia and III antiarrhythmics, pimozide, sotalol, thioridazine, chlorpromazine, pentamidine, arsenic trioxide, mefloquine, dolasetron, tacrolimus, droperidol, gatifloxacin, or moxifloxacin.

Route and Dosage

OLANZAPINE (ZYPREXA)

Bipolar disorder: **PO** *(Adults):* 10 to 15 mg once daily initially; may increase every 24 hours by 5 mg/day (not to exceed 20 mg/day).

Children *≥13 years:* **PO:** Initial dosage: 2.5 or 5 mg once daily. May increase in increments of 2.5 or 5 mg. Recommended maintenance dosage: 10 mg/day.

Schizophrenia: **PO** *(Adults):* 5 to 10 mg/day initially; may increase at weekly intervals by 5 mg/day (not to exceed 20 mg/day).

Children *≥13 years:* **PO:** Initial dosage: 2.5 or 5 mg once daily. May increase in increments of 2.5 or 5 mg. Recommended maintenance dosage 10 mg/day.

Agitation associated with schizophrenia or mania: **IM** *(Adults):* 10 mg, administered slowly, deep into muscle mass. May repeat in 2 to 4 hours, as needed. Maximum dose: 30 mg/day IM. (Dosage for elderly or debilitated patients: 2.5 to 5 mg.)

OLANZAPINE AND FLUOXETINE (SYMBYAX)

Depressive episodes associated with bipolar disorder: **PO** *(Adults):* Initial dosage: 6/25 given once daily in the evening. Adjust dosage according to efficacy and tolerability to within a range of 6 to 12 olanzapine/25 to 50 fluoxetine.

ARIPIPRAZOLE (ABILIFY)

Bipolar mania: **PO** *(Adults):* Usual starting dose: 15 mg once daily as monotherapy, or 10 to 15 mg as adjunctive therapy with lithium or valproate given once daily. Dosage may be increased to 30 mg/day based on clinical response. The safety of dosages higher than 30 mg have not been evaluated.

Children 10 to 17 years: **PO:** Initial dosage: 2 mg/day. Titrate to 5 mg/day after 2 days and to the target dosage of 10 mg/day after 2 additional days. Subsequent dosage increases should be administered in 5 mg/day increments. Usual dosage: 10 mg/day as monotherapy, or as adjunctive therapy with lithium or valproate.

Major depressive disorder (adjunctive treatment): **PO** *(Adults):* Initial dosage: 2 to 5 mg/day for patients already taking another antidepressant. May increase dosage by up to 5 mg/day at intervals of at least a week. Maintenance dosage range: 2 to 15 mg/day.

Schizophrenia: **PO** *(Adults):* Initial dosage: 10 or 15 mg/day as a single dose. Doses up to 30 mg have been used. Dosage increases should not be made before 2 weeks, the time required to achieve steady state.

Children 13 to 17 years: **PO:** Initial dosage: 2 mg/day. Titrate to 5 mg after 2 days and to the target dose of 10 mg after 2 additional days. Subsequent dose increases should be administered in 5 mg increments. Maintenance dosage: 10 to 30 mg/day.

Irritability associated with autistic disorder: **PO** *(Children 6 to 17 years):* Initial dosage: 2 mg/day. The dosage should be increased to 5 mg/day, with subsequent increases to 10 or 15 mg/day if needed. Dosage adjustments of up to 5 mg/day should occur gradually, at intervals of no less than 1 week. Usual dosage: 5 to 15 mg/day.

CHLORPROMAZINE

Psychotic disorders: **PO** *(Adults and children ≥12 years):* 10 to 25 mg 2 to 4 times/day. May increase by 20 to 50 mg every 3 to 4 days until effective dose is reached, usually 200 to 400 mg/day (up to 1000 mg/day). **IM** *(Adults and children ≥12 years):* Initial dose: 25 to 50 mg. May give additional 25 to 50 mg in 1 hr. Increase gradually over several days (up to 400 mg every 3 to 12 hr in severe cases—maximum of 1000 mg/day).

Pediatric behavioral disorders: **PO** *(Children 6 months to 12 years):* 0.55 mg/kg every 4 to 6 hr as needed. **IM** *(Outpatients):* 0.55 mg/kg every 6 to 8 hr, as needed. *(Hospitalized patients):* Start with low dosage and increase gradually. In severe behavior disorders, 50 to 100 mg/day, or in older children, 200 mg/day or more may be necessary. Maximum dosage: 40 mg/day in children 6 mo to 4 yr (or weighing 22.7 kg) or 75 mg/day in children 5 to 12 yr (or weighing 22.7 to 45.5 kg).

Nausea and vomiting: **PO** *(Adults and children ≥12 years):* 10 to 25 mg every 4 to 6 hr. **IM** *(Adults and children ≥12 years):* 25 mg initially, may repeat 25 to 50 mg every 3 to 4 hours, as needed, until vomiting stops.

Children >6 mo: **PO:** 0.55 mg/kg every 4 to 6 hr. **IM** 0.55 mg/kg every 6 to 8 hours, not to exceed 40 mg/day in children up to 5 years (or weighing 22.7 kg) or 75 mg/day in children 5 to 12 years (or weighing 22.7 to 45.5 kg).

Intractable hiccoughs: **PO** *(Adults and children ≥12 years):* 25 to 50 mg 3 or 4 times daily. If symptoms persist for 2 to 3 days, give 25 to 50 mg **IM**.

Preoperative sedation: **PO** *(Adults and children ≥12 years):* 25 to 50 mg 2 to 3 hours before surgery; or **IM**: 12.5 to 25 mg 1 to 2 hr before surgery.

Children >6 mo: **PO:** 0.55 mg/kg 2 to 3 hours before surgery, or **IM:** 0.5 mg/kg 1 to 2 hr before surgery.

Acute intermittent porphyria: **PO** *(Adults):* 25 to 50 mg 3 or 4 times/day, or **IM** *(Adults):* 25 mg 3 or 4 times/day until patient can take **PO**.

QUETIAPINE (SEROQUEL)

Schizophrenia: **PO** *(Adults):* *Immediate-release:* 25 mg twice daily initially, increased by 25 to 50 mg 2 to 3 times daily over 3 days, up to 300 to 400 mg/day in 2 to 3 divided doses by the 4th day (not to exceed 800 mg/day). *Extended-release:* 300 mg once daily. Increase by 300 mg/day (not to exceed 800 mg/day).

Children 13 to 17 years: **PO:** *Immediate-release:* 25 mg twice daily on Day 1; increase to 50 mg twice daily on Day 2; then increase to 100 mg twice daily on Day 3; then increase to 150 mg twice daily on Day 4; then increase to 200 mg twice daily on Day 5. May then increase by no more than 100 mg/day (not to exceed 800 mg/day).

Bipolar mania: **PO** *(Adults):* *Immediate-release:* 50 mg twice daily on Day 1; then increase to 100 mg twice daily on Day 2; then increase to 150 mg twice daily on Day 3; then increase to 200 mg twice daily on Day 4. May then increase by no more than 200 mg/day up to 400 mg twice daily on Day 6, if needed. *Extended-release:* 300 mg once daily on Day 1; then 600 mg once daily on Day 2; then 400 to 800 mg once daily starting on Day 3.

Children 10 to 17 years: **PO:** *Immediate release:* 25 mg twice daily on Day 1; then increase to 50 mg twice daily on Day 2; then increase to 100 mg twice daily on Day 3; then increase to 150 mg twice daily on Day 4; then increase to 200 mg twice daily on Day 5. May then increase by no more than 100 mg/day (not to exceed 600 mg/day).

Major depression (adjunctive therapy): **PO** *(Adults):* *Extended-release:* Initial dosage: 50 mg once daily in the evening. On Day 3, the dose may be increased to 150 mg once daily in the evening. Usual dosage: 150 to 300 mg/day.

Obsessive-compulsive disorder: **PO** *(Adults):* Initial dosage: 50 mg/day and increased based on therapeutic effect and tolerance. Dosage range: 25 to 400 mg/day.

RISPERIDONE (RISPERDAL)

Bipolar mania: **PO** *(Adults):* 2 to 3 mg/day as a single daily dose; dose may be increased at 24-hour intervals by 1 mg (range 1 to 6 mg/day). **IM** *(Adults):* 25 mg every 2 weeks; some patients may require larger dose of 37.5 or 50 mg every 2 weeks.

Children 10 to 17 years: **PO:** Initial dosage: 0.5 mg once daily in either morning or evening. May be increased at intervals of at least 24 hours in increments of 0.5 or 1 mg/day, to a recommended dosage of 2.5 mg/day.

Schizophrenia: **PO** *(Adults):* Initial dosage: 2 mg/day administered as a single dose or in two divided doses. May increase dose at 24-hour intervals in increments of 1 to 2 mg/day to a recommended dose of 4 to 8 mg/day. **IM** *(Adults):* 25 mg every 2 weeks; some patients may require larger dose of 37.5 or 50 mg every 2 weeks.

Adolescents (13 to 17 years): **PO:** Initial dosage: 0.5 mg once daily, increased by 0.5 to 1.0 mg no more frequently than every 24 hours to 3 mg daily. May administer half the daily dose twice daily if drowsiness persists.

Irritability associated with autistic disorder: **PO** *(Children and adolescents 5 to 16 years weighing <20 kg):* 0.25 mg/day initially. After at least 4 days of therapy, may increase to 0.5 mg/day. Dose increases in increments of 0.25 mg/day may be considered at 2 week or longer intervals. May be given as a single dose or in divided doses.

Children and adolescents 5 to 16 years weighing ≥20 kg: **PO:** 0.5 mg/day initially. After at least 4 days of therapy, may increase to 1.0 mg/day. Dose increases in increments of 0.5 mg/day may be considered at 2 week or longer intervals. May be given as a single dose or in divided doses.

Obsessive-compulsive disorder: **PO** *(Adults):* Initial dosage: 0.5 or 1 mg/day. May be increased by 0.5 or 1 mg weekly based on therapeutic effect and tolerance. Dosage range: 0.5 to 4 mg/day.

ZIPRASIDONE (GEODON)

Bipolar mania: **PO** *(Adults):* Initial dosage: 40 mg twice daily. Increase dose to 60 or 80 mg twice/day on the 2nd day of treatment. Adjust dose on the basis of toleration and efficacy within the range of 40 to 80 mg twice/day.

Schizophrenia: **PO** *(Adults):* Initial dose: 20 mg twice daily. Dose increments may be made at 2-day intervals up to 80 mg twice daily.

Acute agitation in schizophrenia: **IM** *(Adults):* 10 to 20 mg as needed up to 40 mg/day. May be given as 10 mg every 2 hours or 20 mg every 4 hours. Maximum dosage: 40 mg/day.

ASENAPINE (SAPHRIS)

Schizophrenia: **PO** *(Adults):* Usual dosage: 5 mg twice daily. May increase up to 10 mg twice daily after 1 week based on tolerability.

Bipolar disorder: **PO** *(Adults):* Usual dose: 10 mg twice daily. Decrease to 5 mg twice daily if there are adverse effects or based on individual tolerability. *As adjunctive therapy with lithium or valproate:* Initial dosage: 5 mg twice daily. Increase to 10 mg twice daily depending on the clinical response and tolerability.

■ NURSING DIAGNOSES RELATED TO ALL MOOD-STABILIZING AGENTS

1. Risk for injury related to manic hyperactivity.
2. Risk for self-directed or other-directed violence related to unresolved anger turned inward on the self or outward on the environment.
3. Risk for injury related to lithium toxicity.
4. Risk for injury related to adverse effects of mood stabilizing drugs.
5. Risk for activity intolerance related to side effects of drowsiness and dizziness.

■ NURSING IMPLICATIONS FOR MOOD-STABILIZING AGENTS

The plan of care should include monitoring for the following side effects from mood-stabilizing drugs. Nursing implications are designated by an asterisk (*).

1. **May occur with lithium:**
   a. **Drowsiness, dizziness, headache**
      * Ensure that client does not participate in activities that require alertness or operate dangerous machinery.
   b. **Dry mouth; thirst**
      * Provide sugarless candy, ice, frequent sips of water. Ensure that strict oral hygiene is maintained.
   c. **GI upset; nausea/vomiting**
      * Administer medications with meals to minimize GI upset.
   d. **Fine hand tremors**
      * Report to physician, who may decrease dosage. Some physicians prescribe a small dose of beta-blocker propranolol to counteract this effect.
   e. **Hypotension; arrhythmias; pulse irregularities**
      * Monitor vital signs two or three times a day. Physician may decrease dose of medication.
   f. **Polyuria; dehydration**
      * May subside after initial week or two. Monitor daily intake and output and weight. Monitor skin turgor daily.
   g. **Weight gain**
      * Provide instructions for reduced calorie diet. Emphasize importance of maintaining adequate intake of sodium.
2. **May occur with anticonvulsants:**
   a. **Nausea/vomiting**
      * May give with food or milk to minimize GI upset.
   b. **Drowsiness; dizziness**
      * Ensure that client does not operate dangerous machinery or participate in activities that require alertness.
   c. **Blood dyscrasias**
      * Ensure that client understands the importance of regular blood tests while receiving anticonvulsant therapy.
   d. **Prolonged bleeding time (with valproic acid)**
      * Ensure that platelet counts and bleeding time are determined before initiation of therapy with valproic acid. Monitor for spontaneous bleeding or bruising.
   e. **Risk of severe rash (with lamotrigine)**
      * Ensure that client is informed that he or she must report evidence of skin rash to physician immediately.
   f. **Decreased efficacy of oral contraceptives (with topiramate)**
      * Ensure that client is aware of decreased efficacy of oral contraceptives with concomitant use.

g. **Risk of suicide with all antiepileptic drugs** (warning by FDA, December 2008)
  * Monitor for worsening of depression, suicidal thoughts or behavior, or any unusual changes in mood or behavior.

3. **May occur with calcium channel blocker:**

  a. **Drowsiness; dizziness**
    * Ensure that client does not operate dangerous machinery or participate in activities that require alertness.

  b. **Hypotension; bradycardia**
    * Take vital signs just before initiation of therapy and before daily administration of the medication. Physician will provide acceptable parameters for administration. Report marked changes immediately.

  c. **Nausea**
    * May give with food to minimize GI upset.

  d. **Constipation**
    * Encourage increased fluid (if not contraindicated) and fiber in the diet.

4. **May occur with antipsychotics:**

  a. **Drowsiness; dizziness**
    * Ensure that client does not operate dangerous machinery or participate in activities that require alertness.

  b. **Dry mouth; constipation**
    * Provide sugarless candy or gum, ice, and frequent sips of water. Provide foods high in fiber; encourage physical activity and fluid if not contraindicated.

  c. **Increased appetite; weight gain**
    * Provide calorie-controlled diet; provide opportunity for physical exercise; provide diet and exercise instruction.

  d. **ECG changes**
    * Monitor vital signs. Observe for symptoms of dizziness, palpitations, syncope, or weakness.

  e. **Extrapyramidal symptoms**
    * Monitor for symptoms. Administer prn medication at first sign.

  f. **Hyperglycemia and diabetes**
    * Monitor blood glucose regularly. Observe for the appearance of symptoms of polydipsia, polyuria, polyphagia, and weakness at any time during therapy.

■ CLIENT/FAMILY EDUCATION RELATED TO MOOD-STABILIZING AGENTS

* Do not drive or operate dangerous machinery. Drowsiness or dizziness can occur.
* Do not stop taking the drug abruptly. Can produce serious withdrawal symptoms. The physician will administer orders for tapering the drug when therapy is to be discontinued.

Report the following symptoms to the physician immediately:
- *Client taking anticonvulsant:* unusual bleeding, spontaneous bruising, sore throat, fever, malaise, skin rash, dark urine, and yellow skin or eyes.
- *Client taking calcium channel blocker:* irregular heartbeat, shortness of breath, swelling of the hands and feet, pronounced dizziness, chest pain, profound mood swings, severe and persistent headache.
- *Client taking lithium:* ataxia, blurred vision, severe diarrhea, persistent nausea and vomiting, tinnitus, excessive urine output, increasing tremors, or mental confusion.
- *Client taking antipsychotic:* sore throat, fever, malaise, unusual bleeding, easy bruising, persistent nausea and vomiting, severe headache, rapid heart rate, difficulty urinating, muscle twitching, tremors, darkly colored urine, excessive urination, excessive thirst, excessive hunger, weakness, pale stools, yellow skin or eyes, muscular incoordination, or skin rash.

- For the client on lithium: ensure that the diet contains adequate sodium. Drink 6-8 glasses of water each day. Avoid drinks that contain caffeine (that have a diuretic effect). Have serum lithium level checked every 1 to 2 months, or as advised by physician.
- For the client on asenapine: Place the tablet *under* the tongue and allow to dissolve completely. Do not chew or swallow tablet. Do not eat or drink for 10 minutes.
- Avoid consuming alcoholic beverages and nonprescription medications without approval from physician.
- Carry card at all times identifying the name of medications being taken.

@ INTERNET REFERENCES

a. http://www.mentalhealth.com/
b. http://www.nimh.nih.gov/index.shtml
c. http://www.nimh.nih.gov/health/publications/mental-health-medications/index.shtml
d. http://www.nlm.nih.gov/medlineplus/druginformation.html
e. http://www.ndmda.org

CHAPTER 26

Antipsychotic Agents

■ CHEMICAL CLASS: PHENOTHIAZINES
Examples

Generic (Trade) Name	Pregnancy Categories/ Half-life	Indications	Available Forms (mg)
Chlorpromazine	C/24 hr	• Bipolar mania • Schizophrenia • Emesis/hiccoughs • Acute intermittent porphyria • Hyperexcitable, combative behavior in children • Preoperative apprehension	**TABS:** 10, 25, 50, 100, 200 **INJ:** 25/mL
Fluphenazine	C/HCl: 18 hr Decanoate: 6.8–9.6 days	• Psychotic disorders	**TABS:** 1, 2.5, 5, 10 **ELIXIR:** 0.5/ mL **CONC:** 5/mL **INJ:** 2.5/mL **INJ (DECANOATE):** 25/mL
Perphenazine	C/9–12 hr	• Schizophrenia • Nausea and vomiting	**TABS:** 2, 4, 8, 16
Prochlorperazine	C/3–5 hr (oral) 6.9 hr (IV)	• Schizophrenia • Nonpsychotic anxiety • Nausea and vomiting	**TABS:** 5, 10 **SUPP:** 25 **INJ:** 5/mL
Thioridazine	C/24 hr	• Management of schizophrenia in patients who do not have an acceptable response to other antipsychotic therapy	**TABS:** 10, 25, 50, 100,
Trifluoperazine	C/18 hr	• Schizophrenia • Nonpsychotic anxiety	**TABS:** 1, 2, 5, 10

Action

- These drugs are thought to work by blocking postsynaptic dopamine receptors in the basal ganglia, hypothalamus, limbic system, brainstem, and medulla.
- They also demonstrate varying affinity for cholinergic, alpha$_1$-adrenergic, and histaminic receptors.
- Antipsychotic effects may also be related to inhibition of dopamine-mediated transmission of neural impulses at the synapses.

Contraindications and Precautions

Contraindicated in: • Hypersensitivity (cross-sensitivity may exist among phenothiazines) • In comatose or severely CNS-depressed clients • Poorly-controlled seizure disorders • Clients with blood dyscrasias • Narrow angle glaucoma • Clients with liver, renal, or cardiac insufficiency • Bone marrow depression • Concurrent pimozide use • Coadministration with other drugs that prolong QT interval, or in patients with long QT syndrome or history of cardiac arrhythmias

Use Cautiously in: • Elderly and debilitated patients • Children with acute illnesses, infections, gastroenteritis, or dehydration (increased risk of extrapyramidal reactions) • Diabetes • Respiratory disease • Prostatic hypertrophy • CNS tumors • Epilepsy • Intestinal obstruction • Pregnancy or lactation (safety not established) • Elderly patients with psychosis related to neurocognitive disorder (NCD) (black-box warning)

Adverse Reactions and Side Effects

- Dry mouth
- Blurred vision
- Constipation
- Urinary retention
- Nausea
- Skin rash
- Sedation
- Orthostatic hypotension
- Photosensitivity
- Decreased libido
- Amenorrhea
- Retrograde ejaculation
- Gynecomastia
- Weight gain
- Reduction of seizure threshold
- Agranulocytosis
- Extrapyramidal symptoms
- Tardive dyskinesia
- Neuroleptic malignant syndrome
- Prolongation of QT interval (**thioridazine**)

Interactions

- Coadministration of phenothiazines and **beta-blockers** may increase effects from either or both drugs.
- Increased effects of phenothiazines with **paroxetine.**
- Concurrent administration with **meperidine** may produce excessive sedation and hypotension.
- Therapeutic effects of phenothiazines may be decreased by **centrally-acting anticholinergics.** Anticholinergic effects are increased.
- Concurrent use may result in decreased hypotensive effect of **guanethidine.**
- Phenothiazines may reduce effectiveness of **oral anticoagulants.**
- Concurrent use with phenothiazines may increase or decrease **phenytoin** levels.
- Increased orthostatic hypotension with **thiazide diuretics.**
- Increased CNS depression with **alcohol** or other **CNS depressants.**
- Increased hypotension with **antihypertensives.**
- Concurrent use with **epinephrine** or **dopamine** may result in severe hypotension.

Route and Dosage

CHLORPROMAZINE

Psychotic disorders: **PO** (*Adults and children ≥12 years*): 10 to 25 mg 2 to 4 times/day. May increase by 20 to 50 mg every 3 to 4 days until effective dose is reached, usually 200 to 400 mg/day (up to 1000 mg/day). **IM** *Adults and children ≥12 years:* Initial dose: 25 to 50 mg. May give additional 25 to 50 mg in 1 hr. Increase gradually over several days (up to 400 mg every 3 to 12 hr in severe cases—maximum of 1000 mg/day).

Pediatric behavioral disorders: **PO** (*Children 6 months to 12 years*): 0.55 mg/kg every 4 to 6 hr as needed. **IM** (*Outpatients*): 0.55 mg/kg every 6 to 8 hr, as needed. (*Hospitalized patients*): Start with low dosage and increase gradually. In severe behavior disorders, 50 to 100 mg/day, or in older children, 200 mg/day or more may be necessary. Maximum dosage: 40 mg/day in children 6 mo to 4 yr (or weighing 22.7 kg) or 75 mg/day in children 5 to 12 yr (or weighing 22.7 to 45.5 kg).

Nausea and vomiting: **PO** (*Adults and children ≥12 years*): 10 to 25 mg every 4 to 6 hr. **IM** (*Adults and children ≥12 years*): 25 mg initially, may repeat 25 to 50 mg every 3 to 4 hours, as needed, until vomiting stops.

Children >6 mo: **PO**: 0.55 mg/kg every 4 to 6 hr. **IM** 0.55 mg/kg every 6 to 8 hours, not to exceed 40 mg/day in children up to 5 years (or weighing 22.7 kg) or 75 mg/day in children 5 to 12 years (or weighing 22.7 to 45.5 kg).

Intractable hiccoughs: **PO** *(Adults and children ≥12 years):* 25 to 50 mg 3 or 4 times daily. If symptoms persist for 2 to 3 days, give 25 to 50 mg **IM**.

Preoperative sedation: **PO** *(Adults and children ≥12 years):* 25 to 50 mg 2 to 3 hours before surgery, or **IM**: 12.5 to 25 mg 1 to 2 hr before surgery.

Children >6 mo: **PO**: 0.55 mg/kg 2 to 3 hours before surgery, or **IM**: 0.5 mg/kg 1 to 2 hr before surgery.

Acute intermittent Porphyria: **PO** *(Adults):* 25 to 50 mg 3 or 4 times/day, or **IM** *(Adults):* 25 mg 3 or 4 times/day until patient can take **PO**.

FLUPHENAZINE

Psychotic disorders: **PO** *(Adults):* Initial dose: 2.5 to 10 mg/day in divided doses every 6 to 8 hours. Maintenance dose: 1 to 5 mg/day. **IM** *(Adults):* Initial dose: 1.25 mg. Usual dosage range: 2.5 to 10 mg/day in divided doses at 6 to 8 hour intervals.

Elderly or debilitated patients: **PO**: 1 to 2.5 mg/day initially. Adjust dosage according to response.

Decanoate formulation: **IM, SC** *(Adults):* Initial dose: 12.5 to 25 mg. May be repeated every 3 to 4 weeks. Dosage may be slowly increased in 12.5 mg increments as needed (not to exceed 100 mg/dose).

PERPHENAZINE

Schizophrenia: **PO** *(Adults and children ≥12 years): Outpatients*: 4 to 8 mg 3 times/day initially. Reduce as soon as possible to minimum effective dose. *Hospitalized patients:* 8 to 16 mg 2 to 4 times a day, not to exceed 64 mg/day.

Nausea and vomiting: **PO** *(Adults):* 8 to 16 mg daily in divided doses, up to 24 mg, if necessary.

PROCHLORPERAZINE

Schizophrenia: **PO** *(Adults) Mild conditions:* 5 or 10 mg 3 or 4 times a day. *Moderate conditions:* 10 mg 3 or 4 times/day. Gradually increase dosage by small increments over 2 or 3 days to 50 to 75 mg/day. *Severe conditions:* 100 to 150 mg/day. **IM** *(Adults):* 10 to 20 mg every 2 to 4 hours for up to 4 doses, then 10 to 20 mg every 4 to 6 hours, if needed. When control is achieved, switch to oral dosage.

Children ≥12 years: **PO**: 5 to 10 mg 3 to 4 times/day.

Children 2 to 12 years: **PO**: 2.5 mg 2 to 3 times/day. Maximum dose: 20 mg/day.

Nonpsychotic anxiety: **PO** *(Adults):* 5 mg 3 to 4 times/day, not to exceed 20 mg/day or longer than 12 weeks.

Nausea and vomiting: **PO** *(Adults):* 5 to 10 mg 3 or 4 times a day. **Rectal** *(Adults):* 25 mg twice daily. **IM**: 5 to 10 mg. May repeat every 3 or 4 hours, not to exceed 40 mg/day.

Children 9.1 to 13.2 kg: **PO:** 2.5 mg 1 or 2 times a day, not to exceed 7.5 mg/day.

Children 13.6 to 17.7 kg: **PO:** 2.5 mg 2 or 3 times a day, not to exceed 10 mg/day.

Children 18.2 to 38.6 kg: **PO:** 2.5 mg 3 times a day or 5 mg twice daily, not to exceed 15 mg/day.

Children 2 years and older and at least 9.1 kg: **IM:** 0.132 mg/kg. Usually only 1 dose is required.

THIORIDAZINE

Schizophrenia (intractable to other antipsychotics): **PO** *(Adults):* Initial dose: 50 to 100 mg 3 times a day. May increase gradually to maximum dosage of 800 mg/day. Once effective response has been achieved, may reduce gradually to determine the minimum maintenance dose. Usual daily dosage range: 200 to 800 mg, divided into 2 to 4 doses.

Children: **PO:** Initial dose: 0.5 mg/kg/day given in divided doses. Increase gradually until therapeutic effect has been achieved or maximum dose of 3 mg/kg/day has been reached.

TRIFLUOPERAZINE

Schizophrenia: **PO** *(Adults and children ≥12 years):* 2 to 5 mg twice daily. Usual optimum dosage range: 15 to 20 mg/day, although a few may require 40 mg/day or more.

Children 6 to 12 years: **PO:** Initial dose: 1 mg once or twice daily. May increase dose gradually to a maximum of 15 mg/day.

Nonpsychotic anxiety: **PO** *(Adults):* 1 or 2 mg twice daily. Do not administer more than 6 mg/day or for longer than 12 weeks.

■ CHEMICAL CLASS: THIOXANTHENES

Examples

Generic (Trade) Name	Pregnancy Categories/ Half-life (hr)	Indications	Available Forms (mg)
Thiothixene (Navane)	C/34	• Schizophrenia	CAPS: 1, 2, 5, 10

Action

- Blocks postsynaptic dopamine receptors in the basal ganglia, hypothalamus, limbic system, brainstem, and medulla
- Demonstrates varying affinity for cholinergic, alpha$_1$-adrenergic, and histaminic receptors

Contraindications and Precautions

Contraindicated in: • Hypersensitivity • Comatose or severely CNS-depressed patients • Bone marrow depression or blood dyscrasias • Parkinson's disease • Severe hypotension or hypertension • Circulatory collapse • Children under age 12 • Pregnancy and lactation (safety not established)

Use Cautiously in: • Patients with history of seizures • Respiratory, renal, hepatic, thyroid, or cardiovascular disorders • Elderly or debilitated patients • Patients exposed to extreme environmental heat • Patients taking atropine or atropine-like drugs • Elderly patients with NCD-related psychosis (black-box warning)

Adverse Reactions and Side Effects

• Refer to this section under Phenothiazines.

Interactions

• Additive CNS depression with **alcohol** and other **CNS depressants.**
• Additive anticholinergic effects with other drugs that have anticholinergic properties.
• Possible additive hypotension with **antihypertensive agents.**
• Concurrent use with **epinephrine** or **dopamine** may result in severe hypotension.

ROUTE AND DOSAGE

Schizophrenia: **PO:** *(Adults and children ≥12 years): Mild conditions:* Initial dosage: 2 mg 3 times/day. May increase to 15 mg/day. *Severe conditions:* Initial dosage: 5 mg twice daily. Optimal dose is 20 to 30 mg/day. If needed, may increase gradually, not to exceed 60 mg/day.

■ CHEMICAL CLASS: PHENYLBUTYLPIPERADINES

Examples

Generic (Trade) Name	Pregnancy Categories/ Half-life	Indications	Available Forms (mg)
Haloperidol (Haldol)	C/~18 hr (oral); ~3 wk (IM decanoate)	• Psychotic disorders • Tourette's disorder • Pediatric behavior problems and hyperactivity	**TABS:** 0.5, 1, 2, 5, 10, 20 **CONC:** 2/mL **INJ (LACTATE):** 5/mL **INJ (DECANOATE):** 50/mL; 100/mL
Pimozide (Orap)	C/~ 55 hr	• Tourette's disorder	**TABS:** 1, 2

Action

• Blocks postsynaptic dopamine receptors in the hypothalamus, limbic system, and reticular formation

- Demonstrates varying affinity for cholinergic, alpha$_1$-adrenergic, and histaminic receptors

Contraindications and Precautions

Contraindicated in: • Hypersensitivity to the drug • Coadministration with other drugs that prolong the QT interval • Coadministration with drugs that inhibit CYP3A enzymes (**pimozide**) • Treatment of tics other than those associated with Tourette's disorder (**pimozide**) • Coadministration with other drugs that may cause tics (e.g., pemoline, methylphenidate, amphetamines) until it has been determined whether the tics are caused by the medications or Tourette's disorder (**pimozide**) • Parkinson disease (**haloperidol**) • In comatose or severely CNS-depressed clients • Clients with blood dyscrasias or bone marrow depression • Narrow-angle glaucoma • Clients with liver, renal, or cardiac insufficiency • Pregnancy and lactation (safety not established)

Use Cautiously in: • Elderly and debilitated clients • Diabetic clients • Depressed clients • Clients with history of seizures • Clients with respiratory insufficiency • Prostatic hypertrophy • Children • Elderly patients with NCD-related psychosis (black-box warning)

Adverse Reactions and Side Effects

- Dry mouth
- Blurred vision
- Constipation
- Urinary retention
- Nausea
- Skin rash
- Sedation
- Orthostatic hypotension
- Photosensitivity
- Decreased libido
- Amenorrhea
- Retrograde ejaculation
- Gynecomastia
- Weight gain
- Reduction of seizure threshold
- Agranulocytosis
- Extrapyramidal symptoms
- Tardive dyskinesia
- Neuroleptic malignant syndrome
- Prolongation of QT interval

Interactions

- Decreased serum concentrations of haloperidol, worsening schizophrenic symptoms, and tardive dyskinesia with concomitant use of **anticholinergic agents.**

- Increased plasma concentrations when administered with drugs that inhibit CYP3A enzymes (**azole antifungal agents; macrolide antibiotics**) and CYP1A2 enzymes (**fluoxetine; fluvoxamine**).
- Decreased therapeutic effects of haloperidol with **carbamazepine**; increased effects of **carbamazepine.**
- Additive hypotension with **antihypertensives.**
- Additive CNS depression with **alcohol** or other **CNS depressants.**
- Coadministration of haloperidol and **lithium** may result in alterations in consciousness, encephalopathy, extrapyramidal effects, fever, leukocytosis, and increased serum enzymes.
- Decreased therapeutic effects of haloperidol with **rifamycins.**
- Concurrent use with **epinephrine** or **dopamine** may result in severe hypotension.
- Additive effects with other drugs that prolong QT interval (e.g., **phenothiazines**, **tricyclic antidepressants**, **antiarrhythmic agents**).

Route and Dosage

Haloperidol (Haldol)

Psychotic disorders: **PO** *(Adults and children ≥12 years): Moderate symptoms or geriatric or debilitated patients:* 0.5 to 2 mg 2 or 3 times a day. *Severe symptoms or chronic or resistant patients:* 3 to 5 mg 2 or 3 times a day. Some patients may require dosages up to 100 mg/day.

Children (3 to 12 years; weight range 15 to 40 kg): Initial dose: 0.5 mg/day. May increase in 0.5 mg increments at 5- to 7-day intervals up to 0.15 mg/kg/day or until therapeutic effect is obtained. Administer in 2 or 3 divided doses.

Control of acutely agitated schizophrenic patient: **IM (lactate)** *(Adults):* 2 to 5 mg. May be repeated every 1 to 8 hours, not to exceed 100 mg/day.

Chronic psychosis requiring prolonged antipsychotic therapy: **IM (decanoate)** *(Adults):* 10 to 15 times the previous daily oral dose, not to exceed 100 mg initially. Repeat every 4 weeks, or adjust interval to patient response. For maintenance, titrate dosage upward or downward based on therapeutic response.

Tourette's disorder: **PO** *(Adults and children ≥12 years):* Initial dosage: 0.5 to 2 mg given 2 or 3 times/day.

Children (3 to 12 years; 15 to 40 kg): **PO:** 0.25 to 0.5 mg/day given in 2 to 3 divided doses; may increase by 0.25 to 0.5 mg every 5 to 7 days; maximum dose: 0.15 mg/kg/day.

Behavioral disorders/Hyperactivity: **PO:** *(Children 3 to 12 years; 15 to 40 kg):* 0.25 to 0.5 mg/day given in 2 to 3 divided doses;

may increase by 0.25 to 0.5 mg every 5 to 7 days; maximum dose: 0.15 mg/kg/day.

PIMOZIDE (ORAP)

Tourette's disorder: **PO** *(Adults): Initial dose:* 1 to 2 mg/day in divided doses. Thereafter, increase dose every other day. *Maintenance dose:* Less than 0.2 mg/kg/day or 10 mg/day, whichever is less. Doses greater than 0.2 mg/kg/day or 10 mg/day are not recommended.

Children (12 years and older): **PO:** Initial dose: 0.05 mg/kg, preferably taken once at bedtime. The dose may be increased every third day to a maximum of 0.2 mg/kg, not to exceed 10 mg/day.

■ CHEMICAL CLASS: DIBENZEPINE DERIVATIVES

Examples

Generic (Trade) Name	Pregnancy Categories/ Half-life	Indications	Available Forms (mg)
Asenapine (Saphris)	C/24 hr	• Schizophrenia • Bipolar disorder	**TABS (SUBLINGUAL):** 5, 10
Clozapine (Clozaril)	B/ 8 hr (single dose); 12 hr (at steady state)	• Treatment resistant schizophrenia • Recurrent suicidal behavior	**TABS:** 12.5, 25, 50, 100, 200 **TABS (ORALLY DISINTE-GRATING):** 12.5, 25, 100, 150, 200
Loxapine (Loxitane)	C/8 hr	• Schizophrenia	**CAPS:** 5, 10, 25, 50
Olanzapine (Zyprexa)	C/21–54 hr	• Schizophrenia • Bipolar disorder • Acute agitation associated with schizophrenia and mania (IM)	**TABS:** 2.5, 5, 7.5, 10, 15, 20 **TABS (ORALLY DISINTE-GRATING):** 5, 10, 15, 20 **POWDER FOR INJECTION (IM):** 10/vial **POWDER FOR SUSPEN-SION, ER (PER VIAL):** 210, 300, 405
Quetiapine (Seroquel)	C/6 hr	• Schizophrenia • Acute manic episodes • Major depression (adjunctive therapy) • Obsessive-compulsive disorder	**TABS:** 25, 50, 100, 200, 300, 400 **TABS (XR):** 50, 150, 200, 300, 400

Action

Asenapine

• Efficacy in schizophrenia is achieved through a combination of dopamine and serotonin type 2 (5HT2) antagonism.

- Mechanism of action in the treatment of acute manic episodes is unknown.

Clozapine

- Exerts an antagonistic effect on dopamine receptors, with a particularly high affinity for the D4 receptor.
- It appears to be more active at limbic than at striatal dopamine receptors.
- Also acts as an antagonist at adrenergic, cholinergic, histaminergic, and serotonergic receptors.

Loxapine

- Mechanism of action has not been fully established.
- Exerts strong antagonistic effects on dopamine D2, histamine H1, alpha-adrenergic, and muscarinic M1 receptors.

Olanzapine

- Efficacy in schizophrenia is mediated through a combination of dopamine and 5HT2 antagonism.
- Also shows antagonism for muscarinic, histaminic, and adrenergic receptors.
- The mechanism of action of olanzapine in the treatment of bipolar mania is unknown.

Quetiapine

- Antipsychotic activity is thought to be mediated through a combination of dopamine and serotonin receptor antagonism. Other effects may be due to antagonism of histamine H1 receptors and alpha-adrenergic receptors.

Contraindications and Precautions

Asenapine

Contraindicated in: hypersensitivity; lactation; history of QT prolongation or arrhythmias; concurrent use of other drugs known to prolong QT interval

Use Cautiously in: patients with hepatic, renal, or cardiovascular insufficiency; diabetes or risk factors for diabetes; history of seizures; history of suicide attempt; patients at risk for aspiration pneumonia; elderly patients; pregnancy and children (safety not established); elderly patients with NCD-related psychosis (black box warning)

Clozapine

Contraindicated in: hypersensitivity; myeloproliferative disorders; history of clozapine-induced agranulocytosis or severe granulocytopenia; concomitant use with other drugs that have the potential to suppress bone marrow function; severe CNS depression or comatose states; uncontrolled epilepsy; lactation; children (safety not established)

Use Cautiously in: patients with hepatic, renal, respiratory, or cardiac insufficiency; patients with QT syndrome or risk factors for QT interval prolongation or ventricular arrhythmias; diabetes mellitus or risk factors for diabetes; prostatic enlargement; narrow angle glaucoma; pregnancy; elderly patients with NCD-related psychosis (black box warning)

Loxapine

Contraindicated in: hypersensitivity; comatose or severe drug-induced depressed states; clients with blood dyscrasias; hepatic, renal, or cardiac insufficiency; severe hypotension or hypertension; children, pregnancy, and lactation (safety not established)

Use Cautiously in: patients with epilepsy or history of seizures; glaucoma; urinary retention; respiratory insufficiency; prostatic hypertrophy; elderly patients with NCD-related psychosis (black box warning)

Olanzapine

Contraindicated in: hypersensitivity; lactation. *Orally disintegrating tablets only:* Phenylketonuria (orally disintegrating tablets contain aspartame).

Use Cautiously in: hepatic insufficiency, elderly clients (reduce dosage), pregnancy and children (safety not established), cardiovascular or cerebrovascular disease, history of glaucoma, history of seizures, history of attempted suicide, prostatic hypertrophy, diabetes or risk factors for diabetes, narrow angle glaucoma, history of paralytic ileus; patients with pre-existing low white blood cell count and/or history of drug-induced leukopenia/neutropenia; elderly patients with NCD-related psychosis (black box warning)

Quetiapine

Contraindicated in: hypersensitivity; lactation; concurrent use with drugs that prolong the QT interval; patients with history of arrhythmias, including bradycardia

Use Cautiously in: cardiovascular or cerebrovascular disease; dehydration or hypovolemia (increased risk of hypotension); hepatic impairment; hypothyroidism; history of suicide attempt; pregnancy or children (safety not established); patients with diabetes or risk factors for diabetes; history of seizures; elderly patients with NCD-related psychosis (black box warning)

Adverse Reactions and Side Effects

Aripiprazole

- Drowsiness, light-headedness
- Headache

- Insomnia, restlessness
- Constipation
- Nausea
- Weight loss

Clozapine

- Drowsiness, dizziness, sedation
- Nausea and vomiting
- Dry mouth; blurred vision
- Agranulocytosis
- Seizures (appear to be dose-related)
- Salivation
- Myocarditis; cardiomyopathy
- Tachycardia
- Constipation
- Fever
- Weight gain
- Orthostatic hypotension
- Neuroleptic malignant syndrome
- Hyperglycemia

Loxapine

- Drowsiness, dizziness
- Anticholinergic effects (dry mouth, blurred vision, urinary retention, constipation, paralytic ileus)
- Nausea and vomiting
- Extrapyramidal symptoms
- Seizures
- Hypotension; hypertension; tachycardia
- Blood dyscrasias
- Neuroleptic malignant syndrome

Olanzapine

- Drowsiness, dizziness, weakness
- Dry mouth, constipation, increased appetite
- Nausea; weight gain
- Orthostatic hypotension, tachycardia
- Restlessness; insomnia
- Rhinitis
- Tremor
- Headache
- Hyperglycemia

Quetiapine

- Drowsiness, dizziness
- Hypotension, tachycardia
- Headache
- Nausea, dry mouth, constipation
- Weight gain
- Hyperglycemia

Interactions

The effects of:	Are increased by:	Are decreased by:	Concurrent use may result in:
Asenapine	Fluvoxamine; imipramine; valproate	Carbamazepine; cimetidine; paroxetine	Increased effects of paroxetine and dextromethorphan; Increased CNS depression with alcohol or other CNS depressants. Increased hypotension with antihypertensives; Additive effects on QT interval prolongation with quinidine, dofetilide, other class Ia and III antiarrhythmics, pimozide, sotalol, thioridazine, chlorpromazine, pentamidine, arsenic trioxide, mefloquine, dolasetron, tacrolimus, droperidol, gatifloxacin, or moxifloxacin.
Clozapine	Caffeine, citalopram, cimetidine, fluoxetine, fluvoxamine, sertraline, CYP3A4 inhibiting drugs (e.g., ketoconazole), risperidone, ritonavir	CYP1A2 inducers (e.g., carbamazepine, omeprazole, rifampin), phenobarbital, phenytoin, nicotine	Additive CNS depression with alcohol or other CNS depressants. Increased hypotension with antihypertensive agents. Additive anticholinergic effects with anticholinergic agents. Concomitant use with benzodiazepines may result in respiratory depression, stupor, hypotension, and/or respiratory or cardiac arrest. Increased effects of risperidone with chronic coadministration
Loxapine			Additive CNS depression with alcohol or other CNS depressants. Increased hypotension with antihypertensive agents. Additive anticholinergic effects with anticholinergic agents. Concomitant use with lorazepam (and possibly other benzodiazepines) may result in respiratory depression, stupor, hypotension, and/or respiratory or cardiac arrest.
Olanzapine	Fluvoxamine and other CYP1A2 inhibitors, fluoxetine	Carbamazepine and other CYP1A2 inducers, omeprazole, rifampin	Decreased effects of levodopa and dopamine agonists. Increased hypotension with antihypertensives. Increased CNS depression with alcohol or other CNS depressants. Increased anticholinergic effects with anticholinergic agents.

The effects of:	Are increased by:	Are decreased by:	Concurrent use may result in:
Quetiapine	Cimetidine; keto-conazole, itraconazole, fluconazole, erythromycin, or other CYP3A4 inhibitors	Phenytoin, thioridazine	Decreased effects of levodopa and dopamine agonists. Increased CNS depression with alcohol or other CNS depressants. Increased hypertension with antihypertensives. Additive anticholinergic effects with anticholinergic agents.

Route and Dosage

ASENAPINE (SAPHRIS)

Schizophrenia: Adults: **PO:** Usual starting and target dose: 5 mg twice daily. The safety of doses above 10 mg twice daily has not been evaluated in clinical trials.

Bipolar disorder: Adults: **PO:** Recommended initial dose: 10 mg twice daily. The dose can be decreased to 5 mg twice daily if there are adverse effects. The safety of doses above 10 mg twice daily has not been evaluated in clinical trials.

CLOZAPINE (CLOZARIL)

Schizophrenia and recurrent suicidal behavior: **PO** *(Adults):* Initial dose: 12.5 mg once or twice daily. May increase dosage by 25 to 50 mg/day over a period of 2 weeks to a target dose of 300 to 450 mg/day. If required, make additional increases in increments of 100 mg not more than once or twice weekly to a maximum dosage of 900 mg/day. Titrate dosage slowly to observe for possible seizures and agranulocytosis. Dosage should be maintained at the lowest level effective for controlling symptoms.

NOTE: A baseline white blood cell (WBC) count and absolute neutrophil count (ANC) must be taken before initiation of treatment with clozapine and weekly for the first 6 months of treatment. Because of the risk of agranulocytosis, clozapine is available only in a 1-week supply through the Clozaril Patient Management System, which combines WBC testing, patient monitoring, and controlled distribution through participating pharmacies. If the counts remain within the acceptable levels (i.e., WBC at least 3500/mm³ and the ANC at least 2000/mm³) during the 6-month period, blood counts may be monitored biweekly, and a 2-week supply of medication may then be dispensed. If for a 6-month period the counts remain within the acceptable level for the biweekly period, counts may then be monitored every 4 weeks thereafter. When the medication is discontinued, weekly WBC counts are continued for an additional 4 weeks.

LOXAPINE (LOXITANE)

Schizophrenia: **PO** *(Adults):* Initial dosage: 10 mg twice daily, although some severely disturbed patients may require up to 50 mg/day. Increase dosage fairly rapidly over the first 7 to 10 days until symptoms are controlled. The usual therapeutic and maintenance dosage range is 60 to 100 mg/day. Doses higher than 250 mg/day are not recommended. Dosage should be maintained at the lowest level effective for controlling symptoms.

OLANZAPINE (ZYPREXA)

Bipolar disorder: **PO** *(Adults):* 10 to 15 mg once daily initially; may increase every 24 hours by 5 mg/day (not to exceed 20 mg/day).

Children ≥13 years: **PO:** Initial dosage: 2.5 or 5 mg once daily. May increase in increments of 2.5 or 5 mg. Recommended maintenance dosage: 10 mg/day.

Schizophrenia: **PO** *(Adults):* 5 to 10 mg/day initially; may increase at weekly intervals by 5 mg/day (not to exceed 20 mg/day).

Children ≥13 years: **PO:** Initial dosage: 2.5 or 5 mg once daily. May increase in increments of 2.5 or 5 mg. Recommended maintenance dosage 10 mg/day.

Agitation associated with schizophrenia or mania: **IM** *(Adults):* 10 mg, administered slowly, deep into muscle mass. May repeat in 2 to 4 hours, as needed. Maximum dose: 30 mg/day IM. (Dosage for elderly or debilitated patients: 2.5 to 5 mg.).

QUETIAPINE (SEROQUEL)

Schizophrenia: **PO** *(Adults): Immediate-release:* 25 mg twice daily initially, increased by 25 to 50 mg 2 to 3 times daily over 3 days, up to 300 to 400 mg/day in 2 to 3 divided doses by the 4th day (not to exceed 800 mg/day). *Extended-release:* 300 mg once daily. Increase by 300 mg/day (not to exceed 800 mg/day).

Children 13 to 17 years: **PO:** *Immediate-release:* 25 mg twice daily on Day 1; increase to 50 mg twice daily on Day 2; then increase to 100 mg twice daily on Day 3; then increase to 150 mg twice daily on Day 4; then increase to 200 mg twice daily on Day 5. May then increase by no more than 100 mg/day (not to exceed 800 mg/day).

Acute manic episodes: **PO** *(Adults): Immediate-release:* 50 mg twice daily on Day 1; then increase to 100 mg twice daily on Day 2; then increase to 150 mg twice daily on Day 3; then increase to 200 mg twice daily on Day 4. May then increase by no more than 200 mg/day up to 400 mg twice daily on Day 6, if needed.

Extended-release: 300 mg once daily on Day 1; then 600 mg once daily on Day 2; then 400 to 800 mg once daily starting on Day 3.
Children 10 to 17 years: **PO:** *Immediate release:* 25 mg twice daily on Day 1; then increase to 50 mg twice daily on Day 2; then increase to 100 mg twice daily on Day 3; then increase to 150 mg twice daily on Day 4; then increase to 200 mg twice daily on Day 5. May then increase by no more than 100 mg/day (not to exceed 600 mg/day).

Major depression (adjunctive therapy): **PO** *(Adults):* *Extended-release:* Initial dosage: 50 mg once daily in the evening. On Day 3, the dose may be increased to 150 mg once daily in the evening. Usual dosage: 150 to 300 mg/day.

Obsessive-compulsive disorder: **PO** *(Adults):* Initial dosage: 50 mg/day and increased based on therapeutic effect and tolerance. Dosage range: 25 to 400 mg/day.

■ CHEMICAL CLASS: BENZISOXAZOLE DERIVATIVES
Example

Generic (Trade) Name	Pregnancy Categories/ Half-life	Indications	Available Forms (mg)
Risperidone (Risperdal)	C/3–20 hr (including metabolite)	• Bipolar mania • Schizophrenia • Irritability associated with autistic disorder **Unlabeled uses:** • Obsessive-compulsive disorder	**TABS:** 0.25, 0.5, 1, 2, 3, 4 **TABS (ORALLY DISINTE-GRATING):** 0.5, 1, 2, 3, 4 **ORAL SOLUTION:** 1/mL **POWDER FOR INJECTION:** 12.5/vial, 25/vial, 37.5/vial, 50/vial
Paliperidone (Invega)	C/23 hr (oral) 25–49 days (IM)	• Schizophrenia • Schizoaffective disorder	**TABS (ER):** 1.5, 3, 6, 9 **INJ (ER):** 39/0.25 mL; 78/0.5 mL; 117/ 0.75 mL; 156/mL; 234/1.5 mL
Iloperidone (Fanapt)	C/18–33 hr	• Schizophrenia	**TABS:** 1, 2, 4, 6, 8, 10, 12
Ziprasidone (Geodon)	C/7 hr (oral) 2–5 hr (IM)	• Schizophrenia • Bipolar mania • Acute agitation in schizophrenia (IM)	**CAPS:** 20, 40, 60, 80 **POWDER FOR INJECTION:** 20/vial

Action
• Exerts antagonistic effects on dopamine, serotonin, alpha adrenergic, and histaminergic receptors

Contraindications and Precautions

Contraindicated in: • Known hypersensitivity • Comatose or severely depressed patients • Bradycardia, recent MI, or uncompensated heart failure • Lactation • Patients with history of QT prolongation or cardiac arrhythmias • Concurrent use with drugs know to cause QT prolongation

Use Cautiously in: • Clients with hepatic or renal impairment • Clients with history of seizures • Clients with diabetes or risk factors for diabetes • Clients exposed to temperature extremes • Elderly or debilitated clients • Clients with history of suicide attempt • Pregnancy and children (safety not established) • Elderly patients with NCD-related psychosis (black-box warning) • Conditions that increase risk of hypotension (e.g., dehydration [including from diuretic therapy or diarrhea], hypovolemia, concurrent antihypertensive therapy)

Adverse Reactions and Side Effects

- Anxiety
- Agitation
- Dry mouth
- Weight gain
- Orthostatic hypotension
- Insomnia
- Sedation
- Extrapyramidal symptoms
- Dizziness
- Headache
- Constipation
- Diarrhea
- Nausea
- Rhinitis
- Rash
- Tachycardia
- Hyperglycemia
- Prolonged QT interval

Interactions

- Increased effects of risperidone with **clozapine** or **ritonavir.**
- Increased effects of iloperidone, paliperidone, and risperidone with concomitant use of **CYP2D6 inhibitors** (e.g., **fluoxetine, paroxetine).**
- Decreased effects of **levodopa** and **other dopamine agonists** with risperidone, paliperidone, and ziprasidone.
- Decreased effectiveness of risperidone, paliperidone, and ziprasidone with **carbamazepine.**
- Additive CNS depression with **CNS depressants,** such as **alcohol, antihistamines, sedative/hypnotics,** or **opioid analgesics.**

- Increased effects of **clozapine** and **valproate** with risperidone.
- Additive hypotension with **antihypertensive agents.**
- Additive orthostatic hypotension with coadministration of other drugs that result in this adverse reaction.
- Additive anticholinergic effects with **anticholinergic agents.**
- Serious life-threatening arrhythmias with drugs known to prolong QT interval (e.g., **antiarrhythmics** [such as, **quinidine, procainamide, amiodarone, sotalol**], **chlorpromazine, thioridazine, gatifloxacin, moxifloxacin, pentamidine, levomethadyl**).
- Increased risk of life-threatening arrhythmias with concurrent use of paliperidone and **chloroquine.**
- Increased effects of iloperidone and ziprasidone with concomitant use of **CYP3A4 inhibitors (e.g., ketoconazole).**
- Increased risk of seizures with coadministration of ziprasidone and **tramadol.**

Route and Dosage

RISPERIDONE (RISPERDAL)

Bipolar mania: **PO** *(Adults):* 2 to 3 mg/day as a single daily dose; dose may be increased at 24-hour intervals by 1 mg (range 1 to 6 mg/day). **IM** *(Adults):* 25 mg every 2 weeks; some patients may require larger dose of 37.5 or 50 mg every 2 weeks.

Children 10 to 17 years: **PO:** Initial dosage: 0.5 mg once daily in either morning or evening. May be increased at intervals of at least 24 hours in increments of 0.5 or 1 mg/day, to a recommended dosage of 2.5 mg/day.

Schizophrenia: **PO** *(Adults):* Initial dosage: 2 mg/day administered as a single dose or in two divided doses. May increase dose at 24-hour intervals in increments of 1 to 2 mg/day to a recommended dose of 4 to 8 mg/day. **IM** *(Adults):* 25 mg every 2 weeks; some patients may require larger dose of 37.5 or 50 mg every 2 weeks.

Adolescents (13 to 17 years): **PO:** Initial dosage: 0.5 mg once daily, increased by 0.5 to 1.0 mg no more frequently than every 24 hours to 3 mg daily. May administer half the daily dose twice daily if drowsiness persists.

Irritability associated with autistic disorder: **PO** *(Children and adolescents 5 to 16 years weighing <20 kg):* 0.25 mg/day initially. After at least 4 days of therapy, may increase to 0.5 mg/day. Dose increases in increments of 0.25 mg/day may be considered at 2 week or longer intervals. May be given as a single dose or in divided doses.

Children and adolescents 5 to 16 years weighing ≥20 kg: **PO:** 0.5 mg/day initially. After at least 4 days of therapy, may increase to 1.0 mg/day. Dose increases in increments of 0.5 mg/day may be considered at 2 week or longer intervals. May be given as a single dose or in divided doses.

Obsessive-compulsive disorder: **PO** *(Adults):* Initial dosage: 0.5 or 1 mg/day. May be increased by 0.5 or 1 mg weekly based on therapeutic effect and tolerance. Dosage range: 0.5 to 4 mg/day.

PALIPERIDONE (INVEGA)

Schizophrenia and schizoaffective disorder: **PO** *(Adults):* 6 mg as a single daily dose. For some patients, a lower dosage of 3 mg/day may be sufficient. After clinical assessment, dose increases may be made at intervals of more than 5 days. When dose increases are indicated, small increments of 3 mg/day are recommended. Maximum recommended dose: 12 mg/day.

ILOPERIDONE (FANAPT)

Schizophrenia: **PO** *(Adults):* Initiate treatment with 1 mg twice daily on the first day, then 2 mg twice daily the second day, then increase by 2 mg/day every day until a target dose of 12 to 24 mg/day given in two divided doses is reached.

ZIPRASIDONE (GEODON)

Bipolar mania: **PO** *(Adults):* Initial dosage: 40 mg twice daily. Increase dose to 60 or 80 mg twice/day on the 2nd day of treatment. Adjust dose on the basis of toleration and efficacy within the range of 40 to 80 mg twice/day.

Schizophrenia: **PO** *(Adults):* Initial dose: 20 mg twice daily. Dose increments may be made at 2-day intervals up to 80 mg twice daily.

Acute agitation in schizophrenia: **IM** *(Adults):* 10 to 20 mg as needed up to 40 mg/day. May be given as 10 mg every 2 hours or 20 mg every 4 hours. Maximum dosage: 40 mg/day.

■ CHEMICAL CLASS: QUINOLINONES

Example

Generic (Trade) Name	Pregnancy Categories/ Half-life (hr)	Indications	Available Forms (mg)
Aripiprazole (Abilify)	C/75 (aripiprazole); 94 (metabolite)	• Bipolar mania • Schizophrenia • Irritability associated with autistic disorder • Major depressive disorder (adjunctive treatment)	**TABS:** 2, 5, 10, 15, 20, 30 **TABS (ORALLY DISINTEGRATING):** 10, 15 **ORAL SOLUTION:** 1/mL **INJ:** 7.5/mL

Action

- The efficacy of aripiprazole is thought to occur through a combination of partial agonist activity at D2 and 5-HT1A receptors and antagonist activity at 5-HT2A receptors.
- Also exhibits antagonist activity at adrenergic α_1 receptors.

Contraindications and Precautions

Contraindicated in: • Hypersensitivity • Lactation

Use Cautiously in: • History of seizures • Hepatic or renal impairment • Known cardiovascular or cerebrovascular disease • Conditions that cause hypotension (dehydration, hypovolemia, treatment with antihypertensive medication) • Conditions that increase the core body temperature (excessive exercise, exposure to extreme heat, dehydration) • Patients with diabetes or risk factors for diabetes • Pregnancy (weigh benefits of the drug to potential risk to fetus) • Children and adolescents (safety and effectiveness not established) • Elderly patients with NCD-related psychosis (black-box warning)

Adverse Reactions and Side Effects

- Headache
- Nausea and vomiting
- Constipation
- Anxiety, restlessness
- Insomnia
- Light-headedness
- Drowsiness, sedation, somnolence
- Weight gain
- Blurred vision
- Increased salivation
- Extrapyramidal Symptoms
- Hyperglycemia
- Disruption in the body's ability to reduce core body temperature

Interactions

- Decreased plasma levels of aripiprazole with **carbamazepine** and other **CYP3A4 inducers.**
- Increased plasma levels and potential for aripiprazole toxicity with **CYP2D6 inhibitors,** such as **quinidine, fluoxetine,** and **paroxetine.**
- Decreased metabolism and increased effects of aripiprazole with **ketoconazole** or **other CYP3A4 inhibitors.**
- Additive hypotensive effects with **antihypertensive drugs.**
- Additive CNS effects with **alcohol** and other **CNS depressants.**

Route and Dosage

Aripiprazole (Abilify)

Bipolar mania: **PO** *(Adults):* Usual starting dose: 15 mg once daily as monotherapy, or 10 to 15 mg as adjunctive therapy with lithium or valproate given once daily. Dosage may be increased to 30 mg/day based on clinical response. The safety of dosages higher than 30 mg have not been evaluated.

Children 10 to 17 years: **PO:** Initial dosage: 2 mg/day. Titrate to 5 mg/day after 2 days and to the target dosage of 10 mg/day after 2 additional days. Subsequent dosage increases should be administered in 5 mg/day increments. Usual dosage: 10 mg/day as monotherapy, or as adjunctive therapy with lithium or valproate.

Major depressive disorder (adjunctive treatment): **PO** *(Adults):* Initial dosage: 2 to 5 mg/day for patients already taking another antidepressant. May increase dosage by up to 5 mg/day at intervals of at least a week. Maintenance dosage range: 2 to 15 mg/day.

Schizophrenia: **PO** *(Adults):* Initial dosage: 10 or 15 mg/day as a single dose. Doses up to 30 mg have been used. Dosage increases should not be made before 2 weeks, the time required to achieve steady state.

Children 13 to 17 years: **PO:** Initial dosage: 2 mg/day. Titrate to 5 mg after 2 days and to the target dose of 10 mg after 2 additional days. Subsequent dose increases should be administered in 5 mg increments. Maintenance dosage: 10 to 30 mg/day.

Irritability associated with autistic disorder: **PO** *(Children 6 to 17 years):* Initial dosage: 2 mg/day. The dosage should be increased to 5 mg/day, with subsequent increases to 10 or 15 mg/day if needed. Dosage adjustments of up to 5 mg/day should occur gradually, at intervals of no less than 1 week. Usual dosage: 5 to 15 mg/day.

■ CHEMICAL CLASS: BENZISOTHIAZOLINONE DERIVATIVE

Example

Generic (Trade) Name	Pregnancy Categories/ Half-life (hr)	Indications	Available Forms (mg)
Lurasidone (Latuda)	B/18	• Schizophrenia • Depressive episodes associated with Bipolar I Disorder	**TABS:** 20, 40, 60, 80, 120

Action

• The efficacy of lurasidone in schizophrenia is thought to be mediated through a combination of central dopamine Type 2 (D2) and serotonin Type 2 (5-HT2A) receptor antagonism.

Contraindications and Precautions

Contraindicated in: • Hypersensitivity • Children (safety not established)

Use Cautiously in: • Renal or hepatic impairment • History of suicide • Diabetes mellitus • Overheating/dehydration • History of leukopenia or previous drug-induced leukopenia • Elderly or debilitated patients • Pregnancy • Elderly patients with NCD-related psychosis (black-box warning)

Adverse Reactions and Side Effects

• Akathisia
• Drowsiness
• Parkinsonism
• Agitation
• Dizziness
• Nausea
• Neuroleptic malignant syndrome
• Seizures
• Agranulocytosis

Interactions

• Decreased effects of lurasidone with **CYP3A4 inducers** (e.g., **carbamazepine, dexamethasone, phenobarbital, phenytoin, rifampin**).
• Increased effects of lurasidone with **CYP3A4 inhibitors** (e.g., **ketoconazole**).
• Increased effects of **digoxin** and **midazolam** with concomitant use of lurasidone.
• Coadministration of lurasidone and **lithium** may result in alterations in consciousness, encephalopathy, extrapyramidal effects, fever, leukocytosis, and increased serum enzymes.
• Increased sedation may occur with other **CNS depressants**, including **alcohol, sedative/hypnotics, opioids,** some **antidepressants,** and **antihistamines.**

Route and Dosage

LURASIDONE (LATUDA)

***Schizophrenia:* PO** *(Adults):* Initial dosage: 40 mg once daily. Usual dosage range: 40 to 80 mg/day. Maximum dose: 160 mg/day.

***Depressive episodes associated with Bipolar I Disorder:* PO** *(Adults):* Initial dosage: 20 mg once daily as monotherapy or as adjunctive therapy with lithium or valproate. Usual dosage range: 20 to 120 mg/day. Maximum dose: 120 mg/day.

NOTE: _Lurasidone (Latuda) should be taken with food (at least 350 calories)._ Administration with food substantially increases the absorption of this medication.

■ NURSING DIAGNOSES RELATED TO ALL ANTIPSYCHOTIC AGENTS

1. Risk for other-directed violence related to panic anxiety and mistrust of others.
2. Risk for injury related to medication side effects of sedation, photosensitivity, reduction of seizure threshold, agranulocytosis, extrapyramidal symptoms, tardive dyskinesia, neuroleptic malignant syndrome, and/or QT prolongation.
3. Risk for activity intolerance related to medication side effects of sedation, blurred vision, and/or weakness.
4. Noncompliance with medication regimen related to suspiciousness and mistrust of others.

■ NURSING IMPLICATIONS FOR ANTIPSYCHOTIC AGENTS

The plan of care should include monitoring for the following side effects from antipsychotic medications. Nursing implications related to each side effect are designated by an asterisk (*). A profile of side effects comparing various antipsychotic medications is presented in Table 26-1.

1. Anticholinergic Effects (see Table 26-1 for differences between typical and atypical antipsychotics)
   a. Dry Mouth
      * Provide the client with sugarless candy or gum, ice, and frequent sips of water.
      * Ensure that client practices strict oral hygiene.
   b. Blurred Vision
      * Explain that this symptom will most likely subside after a few weeks.
      * Advise client not to drive a car until vision clears.
      * Clear small items from pathway to prevent falls.
   c. Constipation
      * Order foods high in fiber; encourage increase in physical activity and fluid intake if not contraindicated.
   d. Urinary Retention
      * Instruct client to report any difficulty urinating; monitor intake and output.
2. Nausea; Gastrointestinal (GI) Upset (may occur with all classifications)
      * Tablets or capsules may be administered with food to minimize GI upset.

TABLE 26-1 Comparison of Side Effects Among Antipsychotic Agents

Class	Generic (Trade) Name	EPS†	Sedation	Anti-cholinergic	Orthostatic Hypotension	Weight Gain
Typical Antipsychotic Agents	Chlorpromazine	3	4	3	4	*
	Fluphenazine	5	2	2	2	
	Haloperidol (Haldol)	5	2	2	2	*
	Loxapine	3	2	2	2	*
	Perphenazine	4	2	2	2	*
	Pimozide (Orap)	4	2	3	2	*
	Prochlorperazine	3	2	2	2	*
	Thioridazine	2	4	4	4	*
	Thiothixene (Navane)	4	2	2	2	*
	Trifluoperazine	4	2	2	2	*
Atypical Antipsychotic Agents	Aripiprazole (Abilify)	1	2	1	3	2
	Asenapine (Saphris)	1	3	1	3	2
	Clozapine (Clozaril)	1	5	5	4	5
	Iloperidone (Fanapt)	1	2	1	3	3
	Lurasidone (Latuda)	1	3	1	3	3
	Olanzapine (Zyprexa)	1	3	2	2	5
	Paliperidone (Invega)	1	2	1	3	5
	Quetiapine (Seroquel)	1	2	2	3	4
	Risperidone (Risperdal)	1	2	1	3	4
	Ziprasidone (Geodon)	1	3	1	2	2

Key: 1=Very low; 2=Low; 3=Moderate; 4=High; 5=Very high

†EPS=Extrapyramidal Symptoms

*Weight gain occurs, but incidence is unknown

Source: Adapted from Black and Andreasen (2011); *Drug Facts and Comparisons* (2014); and Schatzberg, Cole, and DeBattista (2010).

* Concentrates may be diluted and administered with fruit juice or other liquid; they should be mixed immediately before administration.

3. Skin Rash (may occur with all classifications)
   * Report appearance of any rash on skin to physician.
   * Avoid spilling any of the liquid concentrate on skin; contact dermatitis can occur.

4. Sedation (see Table 26-1 for differences between typical and atypical antipsychotics)
   * Discuss with physician possibility of administering drug at bedtime.
   * Discuss with physician possible decrease in dosage or order for less sedating drug.
   * Instruct client not to drive or operate dangerous equipment when experiencing sedation.

5. Orthostatic Hypotension (see Table 26-1 for differences between typical and atypical antipsychotics)
   * Instruct client to rise slowly from a lying or sitting position.
   * Monitor blood pressure (lying and standing) each shift; document and report significant changes.

6. Photosensitivity (may occur with all classifications)
   * Ensure that client wears protective sunblock lotion, clothing, and sunglasses when spending time outdoors.

7. Hormonal Effects (may occur with all classifications, but more common with typical antipsychotics)
   a. Decreased libido, retrograde ejaculation, gynecomastia (men)
      * Provide explanation of the effects and reassurance of reversibility. If necessary, discuss with physician possibility of ordering alternate medication.
   b. Amenorrhea (women)
      * Offer reassurance of reversibility; instruct client to continue use of contraception, because amenorrhea does not indicate cessation of ovulation.
   c. Weight Gain (may occur with all classifications; has been problematic with the atypical antipsychotics)
      * Weigh client every other day; order calorie-controlled diet; provide opportunity for physical exercise; provide diet and exercise instruction.

8. ECG Changes. ECG changes, including prolongation of the QT interval, are possible with most of the antipsychotics. This is particularly true with ziprasidone, thioridazine, pimozide, haloperidol, paliperidone, iloperidone, asenapine, and clozapine. Caution is advised in prescribing this medication to individuals with history of arrhythmias. Conditions that produce hypokalemia and/or hypomagnesemia, such as diuretic therapy or diarrhea, should be taken into consideration when prescribing. Routine ECG should be taken before initiation of therapy and periodically during

therapy. Clozapine has also been associated with other cardiac events, such as ischemic changes, arrhythmias, congestive heart failure, myocarditis, and cardiomyopathy.

* Monitor vital signs every shift.
* Observe for symptoms of dizziness, palpitations, syncope, weakness, dyspnea, and peripheral edema.

9. Reduction of seizure threshold (more common with the typical than the atypical antipsychotics, with the exception of clozapine)

* Closely observe clients with history of seizures.
* **NOTE:** This is particularly important with clients taking clozapine (Clozaril), with which seizures have been frequently associated. Dose appears to be an important predictor, with a greater likelihood of seizures occurring at higher doses. Extreme caution is advised in prescribing clozapine for clients with history of seizures.

10. Agranulocytosis (more common with the typical than the atypical antipsychotics, with the exception of clozapine)

* Agranulocytosis usually occurs within the first 3 months of treatment. Observe for symptoms of sore throat, fever, malaise. A complete blood count should be monitored if these symptoms appear.
* **EXCEPTION:** There is a significant risk of agranulocytosis with clozapine (Clozaril). Agranulocytosis is a potentially fatal blood disorder in which the client's white blood cell (WBC) count can drop to extremely low levels. A baseline WBC count and absolute neutrophil count (ANC) must be taken before initiation of treatment with clozapine and weekly for the first 6 months of treatment. Only a 1-week's supply of medication is dispensed at a time. If the counts remain within the acceptable levels (i.e., WBC at least $3,500/mm^3$ and the ANC at least $2,000/mm^3$) during the 6-month period, blood counts may be monitored biweekly, and a 2-week supply of medication may then be dispensed. If for a 6-month period the counts remain within the acceptable level for the biweekly period, counts may then be monitored every 4 weeks thereafter. When the medication is discontinued, weekly WBC counts are continued for an additional 4 weeks.

11. Hypersalivation (most common with clozapine)

* A significant number of clients receiving clozapine (Clozaril) therapy experience extreme salivation. Offer support to the client because this may be an embarrassing situation. It may even be a safety issue (e.g., risk of aspiration), if the problem is very severe. Management has included the use of sugar-free gum to increase the swallowing rate, as well as the prescription of medications

such as an anticholinergic (e.g., scopolamine patch) or alpha$_2$-adrenoceptor agonist (e.g., clonidine).

12. Extrapyramidal symptoms (EPS) (see Table 26-1 for differences between typical and atypical antipsychotics)
    * Observe for symptoms and report; administer antiparkinsonian drugs, as ordered (see Chapter 27)
    a. Pseudoparkinsonism (tremor, shuffling gait, drooling, rigidity)
       * Symptoms may appear 1 to 5 days following initiation of antipsychotic medication; occurs most often in women, the elderly, and dehydrated clients.
    b. Akinesia (muscular weakness)
       * Same as pseudoparkinsonism.
    c. Akathisia (continuous restlessness and fidgeting)
       * This occurs most frequently in women; symptoms may occur 50 to 60 days following initiation of therapy.
    d. Dystonia (involuntary muscular movements [spasms] of face, arms, legs, and neck)
       * This occurs most often in men and in people younger than 25 years of age.
    e. Oculogyric crisis (uncontrolled rolling back of the eyes)
       * This may appear as part of the syndrome described as dystonia. It may be mistaken for seizure activity. Dystonia and oculogyric crisis should be treated as an emergency situation. The physician should be contacted, and intravenous benztropine mesylate (Cogentin) is commonly administered. Stay with the client and offer reassurance and support during this frightening time.

13. Tardive dyskinesia (bizarre facial and tongue movements, stiff neck, and difficulty swallowing) (may occur with all classifications, but more common with typical antipsychotics)
    * All clients receiving long-term (months or years) antipsychotic therapy are at risk.
    * The symptoms are potentially irreversible.
    * The drug should be withdrawn at first sign, which is usually vermiform movements of the tongue; prompt action may prevent irreversibility.
    * The Abnormal Involuntary Movement Scale (AIMS) is a rating scale that was developed in the 1970s by the National Institute of Mental Health to measure involuntary movements associated with tardive dyskinesia. The AIMS aids in early detection of movement disorders and provides a means for ongoing surveillance. The AIMS assessment tool, examination procedure, and interpretation of scoring are presented in Appendix P.

14. Neuroleptic Malignant Syndrome (NMS) (more common with the typical than the atypical antipsychotics)
    * This is a relatively rare, but potentially fatal, complication of treatment with antipsychotic drugs. Routine assessments

should include temperature and observation for parkinsonian symptoms.

* Onset can occur within hours or even years after drug initiation, and progression is rapid over the following 24 to 72 hours.
* Symptoms include severe parkinsonian muscle rigidity, very high fever, tachycardia, tachypnea, fluctuations in blood pressure, diaphoresis, and rapid deterioration of mental status to stupor and coma.
* Discontinue neuroleptic medication immediately.
* Monitor vital signs, degree of muscle rigidity, intake and output, level of consciousness.
* The physician may order bromocriptine (Parlodel) or dantrolene (Dantrium) to counteract the effects of NMS.

15. Hyperglycemia and diabetes (more common with atypical antipsychotics). Studies have suggested an increased risk of treatment-emergent hyperglycemia-related adverse events in clients using atypical antipsychotics (e.g., risperidone, clozapine, olanzapine, quetiapine, ziprasidone, paliperidone, iloperidone, asenapine, lurasidone, and aripiprazole). The U.S. Food and Drug Administration (FDA) recommends that clients with diabetes starting on atypical antipsychotic drugs be monitored regularly for worsening of glucose control. Clients with risk factors for diabetes should undergo fasting blood glucose testing at the beginning of treatment and periodically thereafter. All clients taking these medications should be monitored for symptoms of hyperglycemia (polydipsia, polyuria, polyphagia, and weakness). If these symptoms appear during treatment, the client should undergo fasting blood glucose testing.

16. Increased risk of mortality in elderly patients with psychosis related to neurocognitive disorder (NCD). Studies have indicated that elderly patients with NCD-related psychosis who are treated with antipsychotic drugs are at increased risk of death, compared with placebo. Causes of death are most commonly related to infections or cardiovascular problems. All antipsychotic drugs now carry black-box warnings to this effect. They are not approved for treatment of elderly patients with NCD-related psychosis.

■ CLIENT/FAMILY EDUCATION RELATED TO ALL ANTIPSYCHOTICS

* Use caution when driving or operating dangerous machinery. Drowsiness and dizziness can occur.
* Do not stop taking the drug abruptly after long-term use. To do so might produce withdrawal symptoms, such as nausea, vomiting, dizziness, gastritis, headache, tachycardia, insomnia, and tremulousness.

- Use sunblock lotion and wear protective clothing when spending time outdoors. Skin is more susceptible to sunburn, which can occur in as little as 30 minutes.
- Report weekly (if receiving clozapine therapy) to have blood levels drawn and to obtain a weekly supply of the drug.
- Report occurrence of any of the following symptoms to the physician immediately: sore throat, fever, malaise, unusual bleeding, easy bruising, persistent nausea and vomiting, severe headache, rapid heart rate, fainting, difficulty urinating, muscle twitching, tremors, darkly colored urine, excessive urination, excessive thirst, excessive hunger, weakness, pale stools, yellow skin or eyes, muscular incoordination, or skin rash.
- Rise slowly from a sitting or lying position to prevent a sudden drop in blood pressure.
- Take frequent sips of water, chew sugarless gum, or suck on hard candy, if experiencing a problem with dry mouth. Good oral care (frequent brushing, flossing) is very important.
- Consult the physician regarding smoking when taking this medication. Smoking increases the metabolism of some antipsychotics, possibly requiring adjustment in dosage to achieve therapeutic effect.
- Dress warmly in cold weather and avoid extended exposure to very high or low temperatures. Body temperature is harder to maintain with this medication. Avoid drinking alcohol when on antipsychotic therapy. These drugs potentiate each other's effects.
- Do not consume other medications (including over-the-counter products) without physician's approval. Many medications contain substances that interact with antipsychotics in a way that may be harmful.
- Be aware of possible risks of taking antipsychotic medication during pregnancy. Safe use during pregnancy and lactation has not been established. Antipsychotics are thought to readily cross the placental barrier; if so, a fetus could experience adverse effects of the drug. Inform the physician immediately if pregnancy occurs, is suspected, or is planned.
- Be aware of side effects of antipsychotic drugs. Refer to written materials furnished by health-care providers for safe self-administration.
- Continue to take medication, even if feeling well and as though it is not needed. Symptoms may return if medication is discontinued.
- Carry card or other identification at all times describing medications being taken.

INTERNET REFERENCES

a. http://www.mentalhealth.com/
b. http://www.nimh.nih.gov/index.shtml
c. http://www.nimh.nih.gov/health/publications/mental-health-medications/index.shtml
d. http://www.nlm.nih.gov/medlineplus/druginformation.html
e. http://www.schizophrenia.com

CHAPTER **27**

Antiparkinsonian Agents*

■ CHEMICAL CLASS: ANTICHOLINERGICS
Examples

Generic (Trade) Name	Pregnancy Categories/ Half-life (hr)	Indications	Available Forms (mg)
Benztropine (Cogentin)	C/Unknown	• Parkinsonism • Drug-induced extrapyramidal symptoms	**TABS:** 0.5, 1, 2 **INJ:** 1/mL
Biperiden (Akineton)	C/18.4– 24.3	• Parkinsonism • Drug-induced extrapyramidal symptoms	**TABS:** 2
Trihexyphenidyl	C/5.6–10.2	• Parkinsonism • Drug-induced extrapyramidal symptoms	**TABS:** 2, 5 **ELIXIR:** 2/5 mL
Diphenhydramine (Benadryl)	B/4–15	• Parkinsonism • Drug-induced extrapyramidal symptoms • Motion sickness • Allergy reactions • Insomnia • Cough suppressant	**TABS & CAPS:** 25, 50 **TABS, CHEWABLE:** 12.5 **STRIPS (ORALLY DISINTEGRATING):** 12.5, 25 **ELIXIR/SYRUP/ORAL SOLU:** 12.5/5 mL **ORAL SUSPENSION:** 25/5 mL **INJ:** 50/mL

Action
• Blocks acetylcholine receptors to diminish excess cholinergic effects. May also inhibit the reuptake and storage of dopamine

---

*This chapter includes only those antiparkinsonian agents indicated for treatment of antipsychotic-induced extrapyramidal symptoms or neuroleptic malignant syndrome (bromocriptine).

at central dopamine receptors, thereby prolonging the action of dopamine.

- Diphenhydramine also blocks histamine release by competing with histamine for H1 receptor sites. Decreased allergic response and somnolence are affected by diminished histamine activity.

Contraindications and Precautions

Contraindicated in: • Hypersensitivity • Angle-closure glaucoma • Pyloric or duodenal obstruction • Peptic ulcers • Prostatic hypertrophy • Bladder neck obstructions • Megaesophagus • Megacolon • Myasthenia gravis • Lactation • Children (*except* diphenhydramine)

Use Cautiously in: • Tachycardia • Cardiac arrhythmias • Hypertension • Hypotension • Tendency toward urinary retention • Clients exposed to high environmental temperatures • Pregnancy

Adverse Reactions and Side Effects

- Dry mouth
- Blurred vision
- Constipation
- Paralytic ileus
- Urinary retention
- Tachycardia
- Agitation, nervousness
- Decreased sweating
- Elevated temperature
- Nausea/vomiting
- Sedation
- Dizziness
- Exacerbation of psychoses
- Orthostatic hypotension

Interactions

- *(Diphenhydramine):* Additive sedative effects with **CNS depressants.**
- Increased effects of **beta-blockers** with diphenhydramine.
- Additive anticholinergic effects with other drugs that have anticholinergic properties.
- Anticholinergic drugs counteract the cholinergic effects of **bethanechol.**
- Possible increased **digoxin** levels with anticholinergics.
- Concomitant use of anticholinergics with **haloperidol** may result in worsening of psychotic symptoms, decreased haloperidol serum levels, and development of tardive dyskinesia.

- Possible decreased efficacy of **phenothiazines** and increased incidence of anticholinergic side effects with concomitant use.
- Decreased effects of **levodopa** with concomitant use.

Route and Dosage

BENZTROPINE (COGENTIN)

Parkinsonism: **PO** *(Adults):* 0.5 to 2 mg/day in 1 or 2 divided doses (range 0.5 to 6 mg/day).

Drug-induced extrapyramidal symptoms: **PO, IM, IV** *(Adults):*1 to 4 mg given once or twice daily.

Acute dystonic reactions: **IM, IV** *(Adults):* 1 to 2 mg, then 1 to 2 mg PO twice daily.

BIPERIDEN (AKINETON)

Parkinsonism: **PO** *(Adults):* 2 mg 3 or 4 times/day, not to exceed 16 mg/24 hr.

Drug-induced extrapyramidal symptoms: **PO** *(Adults):* 2 mg 1 to 3 times/day.

TRIHEXYPHENIDYL

Parkinsonism: **PO** *(Adults):* Initial dose: 1 mg the first day; increase by 2 mg increments at 3 to 5 day intervals, up to a daily dose of 6 to 10 mg in 3 divided doses taken at mealtimes.

Drug-induced extrapyramidal symptoms: **PO** *(Adults):* Initial dosage: 1 mg. Repeat dosage every few hours until symptoms are controlled. Maintenance or prophylactic use: 5 to 15 mg/day.

DIPHENHYDRAMINE (BENADRYL)

Parkinsonism and drug-induced extrapyramidal symptoms/Motion sickness/Allergy reactions: **PO:** *(Adults and children ≥12 years):* 25 to 50 mg every 4 to 6 hours. Maximum dosage: 300 mg/day. **IM/IV:** *(Adults):* 10 to 50 mg IV or 100 mg IM. Maximum daily dose: 400 mg.

Children 6 to 12 years: **PO:** 12.5 to 25 mg every 4 to 6 hours, not to exceed 150 mg/day.

Insomnia: **PO:** *(Adults and children ≥12 years):* 50 mg at bedtime.

Cough suppressant: *(Adults and children ≥ 12 years):* **PO Liquid:** 25 to 50 mg every 4 hr, not to exceed 300 mg/day. **PO Syrup:** 25 mg every 4 hours, not to exceed 150 mg/day.

Children 6 to 12 yr: **PO Liquid:** 12.5 to 25 mg every 4 hr, not to exceed 150 mg/day. **PO Syrup:** 12.5 mg every 4 hours, not to exceed 75 mg/day.

Children 2 to 6 yr: **PO Syrup:** 6.25 mg every 4 hr, not to exceed 25 mg/day.

■ CHEMICAL CLASS: DOPAMINERGIC AGONISTS

Examples

Generic (Trade) Name	Pregnancy Categories/ Half-life (hr)	Indications	Available Forms (mg)
Amantadine (Symmetrel)	C/10–25	• Parkinsonism • Drug-induced extrapyramidal symptoms • Prophylaxis and treatment of Influenza A viral infection	**TABS, CAPS:** 100 **SYRUP:** 50/5mL
Bromocriptine (Parlodel)	B/8–20	• Parkinsonism • Hyperprolactinemia • Acromegaly • Neuroleptic malignant syndrome	**TABS:** 2.5 **CAPS:** 5

Action

- Amantadine increases dopamine at the receptor either by releasing intact striatal dopamine stores or by blocking neuronal dopamine reuptake. It also inhibits the replication of influenza A virus isolates from each of the subtypes.
- Bromocriptine increases dopamine by direct stimulation of dopamine receptors.

Contraindications and Precautions

Contraindicated in:

AMANTADINE: • Hypersensitivity to the drug • Pregnancy, lactation, and in children under 1 year (safety not established) • Angle closure glaucoma

BROMOCRIPTINE: • Hypersensitivity to this drug, other ergot alkaloids, or sulfites (contained in some preparations) • Uncontrolled hypertension • Pregnancy, lactation, and children (Has been used in children ages 11 to 16 years in the treatment of prolactin-secreting adenomas.)

Use Cautiously in: • Hepatic or renal impairment • Uncontrolled psychiatric disturbances • History of congestive heart failure, myocardial infarction, or ventricular arrhythmia • Elderly or debilitated clients • Orthostatic hypotension

AMANTADINE: • Clients with a history of seizures • Concurrent use of CNS stimulants

BROMOCRIPTINE: • Clients with history of peptic ulcer or gastrointestinal bleeding

Adverse Reactions and Side Effects

AMANTADINE: • Nausea • Dizziness • Insomnia; somnolence • Depression; anxiety • Hallucinations • Arrhythmia; tachycardia • Dry mouth • Blurred vision

BROMOCRIPTINE: • Nausea and vomiting • Headache; dizziness; drowsiness • Orthostatic hypotension • Confusion • Constipation; diarrhea • Skin mottling • Exacerbation of Raynaud's syndrome • Ataxia

Interactions

The effects of	Are increased by:	Are decreased by:	Concurrent use may result in:
Amantadine	Quinidine, quinine, triamterene, thiazine diuretics, trimethoprim/ sulfamethoxazole, thioridazine		Potentiation of anticholinergic side effects with anticholinergic agents; increased effects of CNS stimulants with concurrent use.
Bromocriptine	Erythromycin, protease inhibitors, isometheptene, phenylpropanolamine (and other sympathomimetics)	Phenothiazines (and other antipsychotics), metoclopramide	Additive vasoconstriction with triptans; increased plasma levels of probenecid, methyldopa, salicylates, and sulfonamides

Route and Dosage

AMANTADINE (SYMMETREL)

Parkinsonism: **PO** *(Adults):* 100 mg 1 to 2 times/day (up to 400 mg/day).

Drug-induced extrapyramidal symptoms: **PO** *(Adults):* 100 mg twice daily (up to 300 mg/day in divided doses).

Influenza A viral infection: **PO:** *(Adults and Children >12 yr):* 200 mg/day as a single dose or 100 mg twice daily.
Children 9 to 12 yr: **PO:** 100 mg twice daily.
Children 1 to 9 yr: **PO:** 4.4 to 8.8 mg/kg/day, not to exceed 150 mg/day.

BROMOCRIPTINE (PARLODEL)

Parkinsonism: **PO** *(Adults):* Initial dose: 1.25 mg twice daily with meals. May increase dosage every 2 to 4 weeks by 2.5 mg/day with meals. Assessments are advised at 2-week intervals to ensure that the lowest dosage producing an optimal therapeutic response is not exceeded.

Hyperprolactinemia: **PO** *(Adults and children ≥16 years):* Initial dose: 1.25 to 2.5 mg/day with meals. May increase by 2.5 mg every 2 to 7 days. Usual therapeutic dosage range: 2.5 to 15 mg/day.

Children 11 to 15 years: **PO:** Initial dosage: 1.25 to 2.5 mg/day. Dosage may be increased as tolerated until a therapeutic response is achieved. Therapeutic dosage range: 2.5 to 10 mg/day.

Acromegaly: **PO** *(Adults):* Initial dosage: 1.25 to 2.5 mg for 3 days (with food) at bedtime. May increase by 1.25 to 2.5 mg/day every 3 to 7 days. Usual therapeutic dosage range: 20 to 30 mg/day. Maximum dosage: 100 mg/day.

Neuroleptic malignant syndrome: **PO** *(Adults):* 5 mg every 4 hours.

■ NURSING DIAGNOSES RELATED TO ANTIPARKINSONIAN AGENTS

1. Risk for injury related to symptoms of Parkinson's disease or drug-induced EPS.
2. Hyperthermia related to anticholinergic effect of decreased sweating.
3. Activity intolerance related to side effects of drowsiness, dizziness, ataxia, weakness, confusion.
4. Deficient knowledge related to medication regimen.

■ NURSING IMPLICATIONS FOR ANTIPARKINSONIAN AGENTS

The plan of care should include monitoring for the following side effects from antiparkinsonian medications. Nursing implications related to each side effect are designated by an asterisk (*).

1. **Anticholinergic Effects.** These side effects are identical to those produced by antipsychotic drugs. Taking both medications compounds these effects. For this reason, the physician may elect to prescribe an antiparkinsonian agent only at the onset of EPS, rather than as routine adjunctive therapy.
   a. **Dry Mouth**
      * Offer sugarless candy or gum, ice, frequent sips of water.
      * Ensure that client practices strict oral hygiene.
   b. **Blurred Vision**
      * Explain that symptom will most likely subside after a few weeks.
      * Offer to assist with tasks requiring visual acuity.
   c. **Constipation**
      * Order foods high in fiber; encourage increase in physical activity and fluid intake, if not contraindicated.
   d. **Paralytic Ileus**
      * A rare, but potentially very serious side effect of anticholinergic drugs. Monitor for abdominal distension, absent bowel sounds, nausea, vomiting, epigastric pain.
      * Report any of these symptoms to physician immediately.
   e. **Urinary Retention**
      * Instruct client to report any difficulty urinating; monitor intake and output.

f. **Tachycardia, Decreased Sweating, Elevated Temperature**
   * Assess vital signs each shift; document and report significant changes to physician.
   * Ensure that client remains in cool environment, because the body is unable to cool itself naturally with this medication.
2. **Nausea, Gastrointestinal (GI) Upset**
   * May administer tablets or capsules with food to minimize GI upset.
3. **Sedation, Drowsiness, Dizziness**
   * Discuss with physician possibility of administering drug at bedtime.
   * Discuss with physician possible decrease in dosage or order for less sedating drug.
   * Instruct client not to drive or use dangerous equipment while experiencing sedation or dizziness.
4. **Exacerbation of Psychoses**
   * Assess for signs of loss of contact with reality.
   * Intervene during a hallucination; talk about real people and real events; reorient client to reality.
   * Stay with client during period of agitation and delirium; remain calm and reassure client of his or her safety.
   * Discuss with physician possible decrease in dosage or change in medication.
5. **Orthostatic Hypotension**
   * Instruct client to rise slowly from a lying or sitting position; monitor blood pressure (lying and standing) each shift; document and report significant changes.

■ **CLIENT/FAMILY EDUCATION RELATED TO ALL ANTIPARKINSONIAN AGENTS**

• Take the medication with food if GI upset occurs.
• Use caution when driving or operating dangerous machinery. Drowsiness and dizziness can occur.
• Do not stop taking the drug abruptly. To do so might produce unpleasant withdrawal symptoms.
• Report occurrence of any of the following symptoms to the physician immediately: pain or tenderness in area in front of ear; extreme dryness of mouth; difficulty urinating; abdominal pain; constipation; fast, pounding heart beat; rash; visual disturbances; mental changes.
• Rise slowly from a sitting or lying position to prevent a sudden drop in blood pressure.
• Stay inside in air-conditioned room when weather is very hot. Perspiration is decreased with antiparkinsonian agents, and the body cannot cool itself as well. There is greater susceptibility to heat stroke. Inform physician if air-conditioned housing is not available.

- Take frequent sips of water, chew sugarless gum, or suck on hard candy if dry mouth is a problem. Good oral care (frequent brushing, flossing) is very important.
- Do not drink alcohol while on antiparkinsonian therapy.
- Do not consume other medications (including over-the-counter products) without physician's approval. Many medications contain substances that interact with antiparkinsonian agents in a way that may be harmful.
- Be aware of possible risks of taking antiparkinsonian agents during pregnancy. Safe use during pregnancy and lactation has not been fully established. It is thought that antiparkinsonian agents readily cross the placental barrier; if so, fetus could experience adverse effects of the drug. Inform physician immediately if pregnancy occurs, is suspected, or is planned.
- Be aware of side effects of antiparkinsonian agents. Refer to written materials furnished by health-care providers for safe self-administration.
- Continue to take medication, even if feeling well and as though it is not needed. Symptoms may return if medication is discontinued.
- Carry card or other identification at all times describing medications being taken.

@ **INTERNET REFERENCES**

    a. http://www.mentalhealth.com/
    b. http://www.nimh.nih.gov/index.shtml
    c. http://www.nimh.nih.gov/health/publications/mental-health-medications/index.shtml
    d. http://www.nlm.nih.gov/medlineplus/druginformation.html

CHAPTER **28**

Sedative-Hypnotics

■ CHEMICAL CLASS: BENZODIAZEPINES
Examples

Generic (Trade) Name	Controlled/ Pregnancy Categories	Half-life (hr)	Indications	Available Forms (mg)
Estazolam	C-IV/X	8–28	Insomnia	**TABS:** 1, 2
Flurazepam	C-IV/ (Contraindicated in pregnancy)	2–3 (active metabolite 47–100)	Insomnia	**CAPS:** 15, 30
Quazepam (Doral)	C-IV/X	39 (active metabolite 73)	Insomnia	**TABS:** 15
Temazepam (Restoril)	C-IV/X	9–15	Insomnia	**CAPS:** 7.5, 15, 22.5, 30
Triazolam (Halcion)	C-IV/X	1.5–5.5	Insomnia	**TABS:** 0.125, 0.25

Action
- Potentiate gamma aminobutyric acid (GABA) neuronal inhibition.
- The sedative effects involve GABA receptors in the limbic, neocortical, and mesencephalic reticular systems.

Contraindications and Precautions

Contraindicated in: • Hypersensitivity to these or other benzodiazepines • Pregnancy and lactation • Respiratory depression and sleep apnea • *(Triazolam):* concurrent use with ketoconazole, itraconazole, or nefazodone, medications that impair the metabolism of triazolam by cytochrome P450 3A (CYP3A) • *(Quazepam):* established or suspected sleep apnea • *(Flurazepam):* Children younger than age 15 • *(Estazolam, quazepam, temazepam, triazolam):* Children younger than age 18

Use Cautiously in: • Elderly and debilitated patients • Hepatic or renal dysfunction • Patients with history of drug abuse and dependence • Depressed or suicidal patients • Patients with compromised respiratory function.

Adverse Reactions and Side Effects

- Drowsiness
- Headache
- Confusion
- Lethargy
- Tolerance
- Physical and psychological dependence
- Potentiates the effects of other CNS depressants
- May aggravate symptoms in depressed persons
- Palpitations; tachycardia; hypotension
- Paradoxical excitement
- Dry mouth
- Nausea and vomiting
- Blood dyscrasias

Interactions

- Additive CNS depression with **alcohol** and other **CNS depressants.**
- Decreased clearance and increased effects of benzodiazepines with **cimetidine, oral contraceptives, disulfiram,** and **isoniazid.**
- Increased effects of benzodiazepines with **azole antifungals** and **nefazodone** (contraindicated with *triazolam*).
- More rapid onset or more prolonged benzodiazepine effect with **probenecid.**
- Increased clearance and decreased half-life of benzodiazepines with **rifampin.**
- Increased benzodiazepine clearance with **cigarette smoking.**
- Decreased pharmacological effects of benzodiazepines with **theophylline, carbamazepine,** and **St. John's Wort.**
- Increased bioavailability of triazolam with **macrolides.**
- Benzodiazepines may increase serum levels of **digoxin** and **phenytoin,** and increase risk of toxicity.
- Potentiation of respiratory depression with **methadone.**

Route and Dosage

ESTAZOLAM
Insomnia: **PO** *(Adults):* 1 to 2 mg at bedtime.
Healthy elderly: **PO:** 1 mg at bedtime. Increase with caution.
Debilitated or small elderly patients: **PO:** 0.5 mg at bedtime.

FLURAZEPAM
Insomnia: **PO** *(Adults):* 15 to 30 mg at bedtime.
Elderly or debilitated: **PO:** 15 mg at bedtime.

QUAZEPAM (DORAL)
Insomnia: **PO** *(Adults):* 7.5 to 15 mg at bedtime.
Elderly or debilitated: **PO:** Initial dose: 7.5 mg at bedtime. If not effective after 1 or 2 nights, may increase to 15 mg.

TEMAZEPAM (RESTORIL)
Insomnia: **PO** *(Adults):* 15 to 30 mg at bedtime; 7.5 mg may be sufficient for some patients.
Elderly or debilitated: **PO:** 7.5 mg at bedtime.

TRIAZOLAM (HALCION)
Insomnia: **PO** *(Adults):* 0.125 to 0.5 mg at bedtime.
Elderly or debilitated: **PO:** 0.125 to 0.25 mg at bedtime.

■ CHEMICAL CLASS: BARBITURATES
Examples

Generic (Trade) Name	Controlled/ Pregnancy Categories	Half-life (hr)	Indications	Available Forms (mg)
Amobarbital	C-II/D	16–40	• Sedation • Insomnia	**INJECTION:** powder, 500/vial
Butabarbital (Butisol)	C-III/D	66–140	• Sedation • Insomnia	**TABS:** 15, 30, 50 **ELIXIR:** 30/5 mL
Pentobarbital (Nembutal)	C-II/D	15–50	• Insomnia • Preanesthetic in pediatric patients • Acute convulsive episodes	**INJ:** 50/mL
Phenobarbital (Solfoton; Luminal)	C-IV/D	53–118	• Sedation • Anticonvulsant	**TABS:** 15, 16, 30, 60, 90, 100 **CAPS:** 16 **ELIXIR:** 15/5 mL; 20/5 mL **INJ (MG/ML):** 30, 60, 65, 130
Secobarbital (Seconal)	C-II/D	15–40	• Preoperative sedation • Insomnia	**CAPS:** 100

Action

• Depress the sensory cortex, decrease motor activity, and alter cerebellar function.
• All levels of CNS depression can occur, from mild sedation to hypnosis to coma to death.
• Can induce anesthesia in sufficiently high therapeutic doses.

Contraindications and Precautions

Contraindicated in: • Hypersensitivity to barbiturates • Severe hepatic, renal, cardiac, or respiratory disease • Individuals with history of drug abuse or dependence • Porphyria • Uncontrolled severe pain • Intra-arterial or subcutaneous administration • Lactation

Use Cautiously in: • Elderly and debilitated patients • Patients with hepatic, renal, cardiac, or respiratory impairment • Depressed or suicidal patients • Pregnancy • Children

Adverse Reactions and Side Effects

- Bradycardia
- Hypotension
- Somnolence
- Agitation
- Confusion
- Nausea, vomiting
- Constipation
- Skin rashes
- Respiratory depression
- Physical and psychological dependence

Interactions

- Additive CNS depression with **alcohol** and other **CNS depressants.**
- Decreased effects of barbiturates with **rifampin.**
- Increased effects of barbiturates with **MAO Inhibitors** or **valproic acid.**
- Decreased effects of the following drugs with concurrent use of barbiturates: **anticoagulants, beta blockers, carbamazepine, clonazepam, oral contraceptives, corticosteroids, digitoxin, doxorubicin, doxycycline, felodipine, fenoprofen, griseofulvin, metronidazole, phenylbutazone, quinidine, theophylline, chloramphenicol,** and **verapamil.**
- Concomitant use with **methoxyflurane** may enhance renal toxicity.

Route and Dosage

AMOBARBITAL
Sedation: **IM** *(Adults):* 30 to 50 mg, 2 or 3 times/day.
Insomnia: **IM** *(Adults):* 65 to 200 mg at bedtime.
NOTE: Do not inject a volume >5 mL IM at any one site regardless of drug concentration. Tissue irritation can occur.

BUTABARBITAL (BUTISOL)
Daytime sedation: **PO** *(Adults):* 15 to 30 mg, 3 or 4 times/day.
Insomnia: **PO** *(Adults):* 50 to 100 mg at bedtime.
Preoperative sedation: **PO** *(Adults):* 50 to 100 mg, 60 to 90 minutes before surgery.
Children: **PO:** 2 to 6 mg/kg; maximum dose: 100 mg.

PENTOBARBITAL (NEMBUTAL)
Insomnia: **IM** *(Adults):* Usual dosage: 150 to 200 mg.
Preanesthetic sedation: **IM:** *(Children):* 2 to 6 mg/kg, not to exceed
  100 mg.
NOTE: Inject deeply into large muscle mass. Do not exceed
  a volume of 5 mL at any one site because of possible tissue
  irritation.

PHENOBARBITAL (LUMINAL; SOLFOTON)
Sedation: **PO, IM** *(Adults):* 30 to 120 mg/day in 2 to 3 divided
  doses not to exceed 400 mg/day.
Children: **PO:** 2 mg/kg 3 times daily.
Preoperative sedation: **IM** *(Adults):* 100 to 200 mg, 60 to 90 min
  before the procedure.
Children: **PO, IM, or IV:** 1 to 3 mg/kg 60 to 90 min before the
  procedure.
Insomnia: **PO, IM, or IV** *(Adults):* 100 to 320 mg at bedtime.

SECOBARBITAL (SECONAL)
Preoperative sedation: **PO** *(Adults):* 200 to 300 mg 1 to 2 hr before
  surgery.
Children: **PO:** 2 to 6 mg/kg, not to exceed 100 mg.
Insomnia: **PO** *(Adults):* 100 mg at bedtime.

■ CHEMICAL CLASS: MISCELLANEOUS (NONBARBITURATE)
Examples

Generic (Trade) Name	Controlled/ Pregnancy Categories	Half-life (hr)	Indications	Available Forms (mg)
Chloral hydrate	C-IV/C	7–10	• Insomnia • Preoperative sedation • Alcohol withdrawal	**CAPS:** 500 **SYRUP:** 250/5 mL; 500/5 mL
Eszopiclone (Lunesta)	C-IV/C	6	• Insomnia	**TABS:** 1, 2, 3
Ramelteon (Rozerem)	Not controlled/C	1–2.6	• Insomnia	**TABS:** 8
Zaleplon (Sonata)	C-IV/C	1	• Insomnia	**CAPS:** 5, 10
Zolpidem (Ambien)	C-IV/C	2–3	• Insomnia	**TABS:** 5, 10 **TABS CR:** 6.25, 12.5 **TABS SUBLINGUAL:** 1.75, 3.5, 5, 10 **SPRAY SOLUTION, LINGUAL:** 5 per actuation

Action

Zolpidem and zaleplon:
- Bind to GABA receptors in the central nervous system. Appear to be selective for the omega1-receptor subtype.

Eszopiclone:
- Action as a hypnotic is unclear, but thought to interact with GABA-receptor complexes near benzodiazepine receptors.

Chloral hydrate:
- Action unknown. Produces a calming effect through depression of the central nervous system.
- Has generally been replaced by safer and more effective agents.

Ramelteon:
- Ramelteon is a melatonin receptor agonist with high affinity for melatonin MT1 and MT2 receptors.

Contraindications and Precautions

Contraindicated in: • Hypersensitivity • In combination with other CNS depressants • Pregnancy and lactation
Zolpidem, zaleplon, eszopiclone, ramelteon: • Children (safety not established)
Chloral hydrate: • Severe hepatic, renal, or cardiac impairment • Esophagitis, gastritis, or peptic ulcer disease
Ramelteon: • Severe hepatic function impairment • Concomitantly with fluvoxamine
Use Cautiously in: • Elderly or debilitated patients • Depressed or suicidal patients • Patients with history of drug abuse or dependence • Patients with hepatic, renal or respiratory dysfunction • Patients susceptible to acute intermittent porphyria (**chloral hydrate**)

Adverse Reactions and Side Effects
- Headache
- Drowsiness
- Dizziness
- Lethargy
- Amnesia
- Nausea
- Dry mouth
- Rash
- Paradoxical excitement
- Physical and/or psychological dependence
- Abnormal thinking and behavioral changes

Chloral hydrate, eszopiclone: • Unpleasant taste

Interactions

The effects of:	Are increased by:	Are decreased by:	Concurrent use may result in:
Chloral Hydrate	**Alcohol** and other **CNS depressants** including **antihistamines, antidepressants, opioids, sedative/hypnotics,** and **antipsychotics**		Increased effects of **oral anticoagulants;** symptoms of sweating, hot flashes, tachycardia, hypertension, weakness, and nausea with **IV furosemide;** decreased effects of **phenytoin**
Eszopiclone	Drugs that inhibit the CYP3A4 enzyme system, including **ketoconazole, itraconazole, clarithromycin, nefazodone, ritonavir** and **nelfinavir**	**Lorazepam**; drugs that induce the CYP3A4 enzyme system, such as **rifampin**; taking eszopiclone with or immediately after a **high-fat or heavy meal**	Additive CNS depression with **alcohol** and other **CNS depressants**, including **antihistamines, antidepressants, opioids, sedative/hypnotics,** and **antipsychotics;** decreased effects of **lorazepam**
Ramelteon	**Alcohol, azole antifungals,** and **fluvoxamine**	**Rifampin**; taking ramelteon with or immediately after a **high fat or heavy meal**	
Zaleplon	**Cimetidine**	Drugs that induce the CYP3A4 enzyme system, including **rifampin, phenytoin, carbamazepine,** and **phenobarbital;** taking zaleplon with or immediately after a **high-fat or heavy meal**	Additive CNS depression with **alcohol** and other **CNS depressants,** including **antihistamines, antidepressants, opioids, sedative/hypnotics,** and **antipsychotics**
Zolpidem	**Ritonavir, SSRIs**	**Flumazenil; rifampin;** Administration with **food**	Risk of life-threatening cardiac arrhythmias with **amiodarone;** additive CNS depression with **alcohol** and other **CNS depressants,** including **antihistamines, antidepressants, opioids, sedative/hypnotics,** and **antipsychotics**

Route and Dosage

CHLORAL HYDRATE

Daytime sedation: **PO** *(Adults):* 250 mg 3 times a day after meals. Maximum daily dose: 2 g.

Children: **PO:** 25 to 50 mg/kg/day given in divided doses every 6 to 8 hours, not to exceed 500 mg per single dose.

Preoperative sedation: **PO** *(Adults):* 500 to 1000 mg 30 minutes before surgery.

Preprocedural sedation: **PO** *(Children):* 50 to 75 mg/kg 30 to 60 minutes before procedure. May repeat the dose in 30 minutes if needed. Single dose should not exceed 1 g total for infants or 2 g total for children.

Insomnia: **PO** *(Adults):* 500 mg to 1 g 15 to 30 minutes before bedtime.

Children: **PO:** 50 mg/kg/day, up to 1 g per single dose. May give in divided doses.

Alcohol withdrawal: **PO** *(Adults):* 500 mg to 1 g repeated at 6-hour intervals if needed. Maximum daily dose: 2 g.

ESZOPICLONE (LUNESTA)

Insomnia: **PO** *(Adults):* 2 mg immediately before bedtime; may be increased to 3 mg if needed (3 mg dose is more effective for sleep maintenance).

Elderly patients: **PO:** 1 mg immediately before bedtime for patients who have difficulty falling asleep; 2 mg immediately before bedtime for patients who have difficulty staying asleep.

RAMELTEON (ROZEREM)

Insomnia: **PO** *(Adults):* 8 mg within 30 minutes of bedtime. It is recommended that ramelteon not be taken with or immediately after a high-fat meal.

ZALEPLON (SONATA)

Insomnia: **PO** *(Adults):* 10 mg (range 5 to 20 mg) at bedtime.

Elderly and debilitated patients: **PO:** 5 mg at bedtime, not to exceed 10 mg.

ZOLPIDEM (AMBIEN)

Insomnia: **PO** *(Adults):* 10 mg at bedtime. *Extended-release tablets:* 12.5 mg at bedtime.

Elderly or debilitated patients and patients with hepatic impairment: **PO:** 5 mg at bedtime. *Extended-release tablets:* 6.25 mg at bedtime.

■ NURSING DIAGNOSES RELATED TO ALL SEDATIVE-HYPNOTICS

1. Risk for injury related to abrupt withdrawal from long-term use or decreased mental alertness caused by residual sedation.
2. Disturbed sleep pattern/insomnia related to situational crises, physical condition, or severe level of anxiety.

3. Risk for activity intolerance related to side effects of lethargy, drowsiness, dizziness.
4. Risk for acute confusion related to action of the medication on the central nervous system.

■ NURSING IMPLICATIONS FOR SEDATIVE-HYPNOTICS

The nursing care plan should include monitoring for the following side effects from sedative-hypnotics. Nursing implications related to each side effect are designated by an asterisk (*):

1. **Drowsiness, dizziness, lethargy (most common side effects)**
   * Instruct client not to drive or operate dangerous machinery while taking the medication.
2. **Tolerance, physical and psychological addiction**
   * Instruct client to take the medication exactly as directed. Do not take more than the amount prescribed because of the habit-forming potential. Recommended for short-term use only. Abrupt withdrawal after long-term use may result in serious, even life-threatening, symptoms. *Exception:* **Ramelteon** is not considered to be a drug of abuse or dependence. It is not classified as a controlled substance. It has, however, been associated with cases of rebound insomnia after abrupt discontinuation following long-term use.
3. **Potentiates the effects of other CNS depressants**
   * Instruct client not to drink alcohol or take other medications that depress the CNS when taking this medication.
4. **May aggravate symptoms in depressed persons**
   * Assess mood daily.
   * Take necessary precautions for potential suicide.
5. **Orthostatic hypotension; palpitations; tachycardia**
   * Monitor lying and standing blood pressure and pulse every shift.
   * Instruct client to arise slowly from a lying or sitting position.
   * Monitor pulse rate and rhythm and report any significant change to the physician.
6. **Paradoxical excitement**
   * Withhold drug and notify the physician.
7. **Dry mouth**
   * Have client take frequent sips of water, ice chips, suck on hard candy, or chew sugarless gum.
8. **Nausea and vomiting**
   * Have client take drug with food or milk (unless it is a drug in which taking with food is not recommended).
9. **Blood dyscrasias**
   * Symptoms of sore throat, fever, malaise, easy bruising, or unusual bleeding should be reported to the physician immediately.

10. **Abnormal thinking and behavioral changes**
    * Unusual changes in behavior, including aggressiveness, hallucinations, and suicidal ideation, have been reported. Certain complex behaviors, such as sleep-driving, preparing and eating food, and making phone calls, with amnesia for the behavior, have occurred. Although a direct correlation to the behavior with use of sedative/hypnotics cannot be made, the emergence of any new behavioral sign or symptom of concern requires careful and immediate evaluation.

■ CLIENT/FAMILY EDUCATION RELATED TO ALL SEDATIVE-HYPNOTICS

- Do not drive or operate dangerous machinery. Drowsiness and dizziness can occur.
- Do not stop taking the drug abruptly after prolonged use. Can produce serious withdrawal symptoms, such as depression, insomnia, anxiety, abdominal and muscle cramps, tremors, vomiting, sweating, convulsions, and delirium.
- Do not consume other CNS depressants (including alcohol).
- Do not take nonprescription medication without approval from physician.
- Rise slowly from the sitting or lying position to prevent a sudden drop in blood pressure.
- Report to physician immediately symptoms of sore throat, fever, malaise, easy bruising, unusual bleeding, motor restlessness, or any thinking or behavior that is outside the usual range of thinking or characterization for the individual taking the medication.
- Be aware of risks of taking these drugs during pregnancy. (Congenital malformations have been associated with use during the first trimester). If pregnancy is suspected or planned, notify the physician of the desirability to discontinue the drug.
- Be aware of possible side effects. Refer to written materials furnished by health-care providers regarding the correct method of self-administration.
- Carry card or piece of paper at all times stating names of medications being taken.

@ INTERNET REFERENCES

   a. http://www.mentalhealth.com/
   b. http://www.nimh.nih.gov/index.shtml
   c. http://www.nimh.nih.gov/health/publications/mental-health-medications/index.shtml
   d. http://www.nlm.nih.gov/medlineplus/druginformation.html

CHAPTER 29

Agents Used to Treat Attention-Deficit/ Hyperactivity Disorder

■ CHEMICAL CLASS: CENTRAL NERVOUS SYSTEM (CNS) STIMULANTS (AMPHETAMINES)

Examples

Generic (Trade) Name	Controlled/ Pregnancy Categories	Half-life (hr)	Indications	Available Forms (mg)
Amphetamine/ dextroamphetamine mixtures (Adderall; Adderall XR)	C-II/C	9–13	• ADHD • Narcolepsy	**TABS:** 5, 7.5, 10, 12.5, 15, 20, 30 **CAPS (XR):** 5, 10, 15, 20, 25, 30
Dextroamphetamine sulfate (Dexedrine; Dextrostat)	C-II/C	~12	• ADHD • Narcolepsy	**TABS:** 5, 10 **CAPS (ER):** 5, 10, 15 **ORAL SOLU:** 5 mg/ 5 mL
Methamphetamine (Desoxyn)	C-II/C	4–5	• ADHD • Exogenous obesity	**TABS:** 5
Lisdexamfetamine (Vyvanse)	C-II/C	<1	• ADHD	**CAPS:** 20, 30, 40 50, 60, 70

Action

- CNS stimulation is mediated by release of norepinephrine from central noradrenergic neurons in cerebral cortex, reticular activating system, and brainstem.
- At higher doses, dopamine may be released in the mesolimbic system.
- Action in the treatment of ADHD is unclear. Recent research indicates that their effectiveness in the treatment of hyperactivity disorders is based on the activation of dopamine D4

receptors in the basal ganglia and thalamus, which depress, rather than enhance, motor activity (Erlij et al, 2012).

Contraindications and Precautions

Contraindicated in: • Advanced arteriosclerosis • Symptomatic cardiovascular disease • Moderate to severe hypertension • Hyperthyroidism • Hypersensitivity or idiosyncrasy to the sympathomimetic amines • Glaucoma • Agitated states • History of drug abuse • During or within 14 days following administration of MAO inhibitors (hypertensive crisis may occur) • Children younger than 3 years (dextroamphetamine; amphetamine; mixtures) • Children younger than 6 years (methamphetamine; lisdexamfetamine) • Pregnancy and lactation

Use Cautiously in: • Patients with mild hypertension • Children with psychoses (may exacerbate symptoms) • Tourette's disorder (may exacerbate tics) • Anorexia • Insomnia • Elderly, debilitated, or asthenic patients • Patients with suicidal or homicidal tendencies

Adverse Reactions and Side Effects

- Overstimulation
- Restlessness
- Dizziness
- Insomnia
- Headache
- Palpitations
- Tachycardia
- Elevation of blood pressure
- Anorexia
- Weight loss
- Dry mouth
- Tolerance
- New or worsened psychiatric symptoms
- Physical and psychological addiction
- Suppression of growth in children (with long-term use)

Interactions

- Increased sensitivity to amphetamines with **furazolidone.**
- Use of amphetamines with **MAO inhibitors** can result in hypertensive crisis.
- Increased effects of amphetamines and risk of serotonin syndrome with **selective serotonin reuptake inhibitors (SSRIs).**
- Prolonged effects of amphetamines with **urinary alkalinizers.**
- Hastened elimination of amphetamines with **urinary acidifiers.**
- Amphetamines may reverse the hypotensive effects of **guanethidine and other antihypertensives.**

- Concomitant use of amphetamines and **tricyclic antidepressants** may increase blood levels of both drugs.
- Patients with diabetes mellitus who take amphetamines may require **insulin** adjustment.
- **Adrenergic blockers** are inhibited by amphetamines.

Route and Dosage

AMPHETAMINE/DEXTROAMPHETAMINE MIXTURES (ADDERALL; ADDERALL XR)

***ADHD:* PO:** *(Adults and children ≥6 years):* Initial dose: 5 mg once or twice daily. May be increased in increments of 5 mg at weekly intervals until optimal response is obtained. Maximum dose: 40 mg/day. *Extended-release caps:* Initial dosage: 10 mg once daily in the morning. May increase in increments of 10 mg at weekly intervals. Maximum dose: 30 mg/day.

Children 3 to 5 years: **PO:** Initial dose: 2.5 mg/day. May increase in increments of 2.5 mg/day at weekly intervals until optimal response is obtained.

***Narcolepsy:* PO:** *(Adults and children ≥12 years):* Initial dose: 10 mg/day; may increase in increments of 10 mg/day at weekly intervals up to a maximum of 60 mg/day.

Children 6 to 12 years of age: **PO:** Narcolepsy is rare in children younger than 12 years. When it does occur, initial dose is 5 mg/day. May increase in increments of 5 mg/day at weekly intervals up to a maximum of 60 mg/day.

DEXTROAMPHETAMINE SULFATE (DEXEDRINE; DEXTROSTAT)

***ADHD:* PO:** *(Adults and children ≥6 years):* Initial dosage: 5 mg once or twice daily. May be increased in increments of 5 mg at weekly intervals. More than 40 mg/day is seldom required. (Sustained-release capsules should not be used as initial therapy.)

Children 3 to 5 years: **PO:** Initial dose: 2.5 mg/day. May increase in increments of 2.5 mg/day at weekly intervals until optimal response is achieved.

***Narcolepsy:* PO** *(Adults):* 5 to 60 mg/day in single or divided doses. Sustained-release capsules should not be used as initial therapy.

Children ≥12 years: **PO:** 10 mg/day. May increase by 10 mg/day at weekly intervals until response is obtained or 60 mg is reached.

Children 6 to 12 years: **PO:** 5 mg/day. May increase by 5 mg/day at weekly intervals until response is obtained or 60 mg is reached.

METHAMPHETAMINE (DESOXYN)

***ADHD:* PO:** *(Adults and children ≥6 years):* 5 mg once or twice daily. May increase in increments of 5 mg at weekly intervals. Usual effective dose is 20 to 25 mg/day in divided doses.

***Exogenous obesity:* PO:** *(Adults and children ≥12 years):* Usual dosage: One 5-mg tablet taken 30 minutes before each meal.

LISDEXAMFETAMINE (VYVANSE)

ADHD: **PO:** *(Adults and children ≥6 years):* Initial dosage: 30 mg once daily in the morning. Dosage may be increased in increments of 10 or 20 mg/day at weekly intervals, up to a maximum of 70 mg/day.

■ CHEMICAL CLASS: CNS STIMULANTS (MISCELLANEOUS AGENTS)

Examples

Generic (Trade) Name	Controlled/ Pregnancy Categories	Half-life	Indications	Available Forms (mg)
Dexmethylphenidate (Focalin; Focalin XR)	C-II/C	2.2 hr	• ADHD	**TABS:** 2.5, 5, 10 **CAPS (ER):** 5, 10, 15, 20, 25, 30, 35, 40
Methylphenidate (Ritalin; Ritalin-SR; Ritalin LA; Methylin; Methylin ER; Metadate ER; Metadate CD; Concerta; Daytrana)	C-II/C	2-4 hr	• ADHD • Narcolepsy (except Concerta, Metadate CD, and Ritalin LA)	**IMMEDIATE RELEASE TABS (METHYLIN, RITALIN):** 5, 10, 20 **CHEWABLE TABS (METHYLIN):** 2.5, 5, 10 **TABS ER (METADATE ER; METHYLIN ER):** 10, 20 **TABS ER (CONCERTA):** 18, 27, 36, 54 **TABS SR (RITALIN-SR):** 20 **CAPS ER (METADATE CD; RITALIN LA):** 10, 20, 30, 40, (50, 60— *METADATE CD ONLY)* **ORAL SOLU (METHYLIN):** 5/5 mL, 10/5 mL **TRANSDERMAL PATCH (DAYTRANA):** 10, 15, 20, 30 (based on 9-hour delivery system)

ER, CD, LA=extended release forms; SR=sustained release

Actions

- Dexmethylphenidate blocks the reuptake of norepinephrine and dopamine into the presynaptic neuron and increases the release of these monoamines into the extraneuronal space.
- Methylphenidate activates the brainstem arousal system and cortex to produce its stimulant effect.
- Recent research indicates that the effectiveness of CNS stimulants in the treatment of hyperactivity disorders is based on the activation of dopamine D4 receptors in the basal ganglia and thalamus, which depress, rather than enhance, motor activity (Erlij et al, 2012).

Contraindications and Precautions

Contraindicated in: • Hypersensitivity • Pregnancy, lactation, and children younger than 6 years (safety has not been established) • Clients with marked anxiety, tension, or agitation • Glaucoma • Hyperthyroidism • Motor tics or family history or diagnosis of Tourette's syndrome • During or within 14 days of treatment with MAO inhibitors (hypertensive crisis can occur) • Clients with structural cardiac abnormalities, cardiomyopathy, arrhythmias, recent MI, or other serious cardiac problems • Clients with pre-existing psychotic disorder

Use Cautiously in: • Patients with history of seizure disorder and/or EEG abnormalities • Hypertension • History of drug or alcohol dependence • Emotionally unstable patients • Renal or hepatic insufficiency • Diabetes mellitus

Adverse Reactions and Side Effects

- Headache
- Nausea
- Rhinitis
- Fever
- Anorexia
- Insomnia
- Tachycardia; palpitations; hypertension
- Nervousness
- Abdominal pain
- Growth suppression in children (with long-term use)
- Skin redness or itching at site of transdermal patch (*Daytrana*)

Interactions

- Decreased effectiveness of **antihypertensive agents.**
- Increased serum levels of anticonvulsants (e.g., **phenobarbital, phenytoin,** and **primidone**), **tricyclic antidepressants, SSRIs, warfarin.**
- Increased effects of **vasopressor agents** with concurrent use.
- Hypertensive crisis may occur with concurrent use (or within 2 weeks use) of **MAO inhibitors.**
- Concurrent use with **clonidine** may result in serious adverse reactions.
- Increased sympathomimetic effects with other **adrenergics,** including **vasoconstrictors** and **decongestants.**

Route and Dosage

DEXMETHYLPHENIDATE (FOCALIN; FOCALIN XR)
ADHD: (Immediate release tabs): **PO** *(Adults and Children ≥6 years): Patients not previously taking methylphenidate:* 2.5 mg 2 times a day. May be increased weekly as needed up to 10 mg 2 times a day.

Patients currently taking methylphenidate: Starting dose is one-half of the methylphenidate dose, up to 10 mg 2 times a day.

(Extended-release capsules): **PO** *(Adults): Patients not previously taking methylphenidate:* 10 mg once daily. May be increased by 10 mg after 1 week to 40 mg/day. *Patients currently taking methylphenidate:* Starting dose is one-half of the methylphenidate dose, up to 40 mg/day given as a single daily dose. *Patients currently taking dexmethylphenidate:* Give same daily dose as a single dose.

PO *(Children ≥6 years): Patients not previously taking methylphenidate:* 5 mg once daily. May be increased by 5 mg weekly up to 30 mg/day. *Patients currently taking methylphenidate:* Starting dose is one-half of the methylphenidate dose, up to 30 mg/day, given as a single daily dose. *Patients currently taking dexmethylphenidate:* Give same daily dose as a single dose.

METHYLPHENIDATE (RITALIN; RITALIN-SR; RITALIN LA; METHYLIN; METHYLIN ER; METADATE ER; METADATE CD; CONCERTA; DAYTRANA)

ADHD: (Immediate release forms): **PO** *(Adults):* 5 to 20 mg 2 or 3 times/day preferably 30 to 45 min before meals. Average dose is 20 to 30 mg/day. To prevent interruption of sleep, take last dose of the day before 6 p.m.

PO *(Children ≥6 years):* Individualize dosage. May start with low dose of 2.5 to 5 mg twice daily before breakfast and lunch. May increase dosage in 5 to 10 mg increments at weekly intervals. Maximum daily dosage: 60 mg.

(Extended-release forms):

Ritalin-SR, Methylin ER, and Metadate ER: **PO** *(Adults and Children ≥6 years):* May be used in place of the immediate release tablets when the 8-hour dosage corresponds to the titrated 8-hour dosage of the immediate release tablets. Must be swallowed whole.

Ritalin LA and Metadate CD: **PO** *(Adults and Children ≥6 years):* Initial dosage: 20 mg once daily in the morning before breakfast. May increase dosage in 10 mg increments at weekly intervals to a maximum of 60 mg taken once daily in the morning. Capsules may be swallowed whole with liquid or opened and contents sprinkled on soft food (e.g., applesauce). Ensure that entire contents of capsule are consumed when taken in this manner. *Note:* Ritalin LA may be used in place of twice daily regimen given once daily at same total dose, or in place of SR product at same dose.

Concerta: Should be taken once daily in the morning. Must be swallowed whole and not chewed, divided, or crushed.

PO *(Adults 18 to 65 years):* Initial dosage: 18 or 36 mg/day for patients who are not currently taking methylphenidate or for patients who are on stimulants other than methylphenidate. May be increased in

18 mg increments at weekly intervals to a maximum dose of 72 mg/day.

PO *(Children 13 to 17 years):* Initial dosage: 18 mg/day for patients who are not currently taking methylphenidate or for patients who are on stimulants other than methylphenidate. May be increased in 18 mg increments at weekly intervals to a maximum dose of 72 mg/day, not to exceed 2 mg/kg/day.

PO *(Children 6 to 12 years):* Initial dosage: 18 mg/day for patients who are not currently taking methylphenidate or for patients who are on stimulants other than methylphenidate. May be increased in 18 mg increments at weekly intervals to a maximum dose of 54 mg/day.

Clients currently using methylphenidate: Should use following conversion table:

Previous methylphenidate dose	Recommended Concerta dose
5 mg 2 or 3 times/day or 20 mg (SR)	18 mg every morning
10 mg 2 or 3 times/day or 40 mg (SR)	36 mg every morning
15 mg 2 or 3 times/day or 60 mg (SR)	54 mg every morning

Daytrana: Transdermal Patch *(Adults and children ≥6 years):* Patch should be applied to hip area 2 hours before an effect is needed and should be removed 9 hours after application. Alternate hips with additional doses. Dosage for patients new to methylphenidate should be titrated to desired effect according to the following recommended schedule:

	Week 1	Week 2	Week 3	Week 4
Nominal Delivered Dose (mg/9 hours)	10 mg	15 mg	20 mg	30 mg
Delivery Rate (based on 9-hr wear period)	(1.1 mg/hr)	(1.6 mg/hr)	(2.2 mg/hr)	(3.3 mg/hr)

Patients converting from another formulation of methylphenidate should follow the above titration schedule due to differences in bioavailability of Daytrana compared to other products.

Narcolepsy: **PO** *(Adults): Ritalin, Methylin, Methylin ER, Ritalin-SR, and Metadate ER* indicated for this use. 10 mg 2 to 3 times a day. Maximum dose 60 mg/day.

■ **CHEMICAL CLASS: ALPHA-ADRENERGIC AGONISTS**

Examples

Generic (Trade) Name	Pregnancy Categories/ Half-life	Indications	Available Forms (mg)
Clonidine (Catapress; Kapvay [ER])	C/12–22	• Hypertension • ADHD in children (ER only) **Unlabeled use:** • ADHD (immediate release) • Tourette's disorder	**TABS:** 0.1, 0.2, 0.3 **TABS (MODIFIED-RELEASE):** 0.1 **TABS (EXTENDED-RELEASE):** 0.1, 0.2 **SUSP (EXTENDED-RELEASE):** 0.09/mL **TRANSDERMAL PATCHES:** 0.1/24 hr, 0.2/24 hr, 0.3/24 hr
Guanfacine (Tenex; Intuniv)	B/16–18	• Hypertension *(Tenex)* • ADHD *(Intuniv)* **Unlabeled use:** • Tourette's disorder	**TABS** *(TENEX)*: 1, 2 **TABS (ER)** *(INTUNIV)*: 1, 2, 3, 4

Action

- Stimulates alpha-adrenergic receptors in the brain, thereby reducing sympathetic outflow from the CNS resulting in decreases in peripheral vascular resistance, heart rate, and blood pressure.
- Mechanism of action in the treatment of ADHD is unknown.

Contraindications and Precautions

Contraindicated in: • Hypersensitivity to the drug or any of its inactive ingredients

Use Cautiously in: • Coronary insufficiency • Recent myocardial infarction • Cerebrovascular disease • History of hypotension, bradycardia, or syncope • Chronic renal or hepatic failure • Elderly • Pregnancy and lactation

Adverse Reactions and Side Effects

- Orthostatic hypotension
- Bradycardia
- Palpitations
- Syncope
- Dry mouth
- Constipation

- Nausea
- Fatigue
- Sedation
- Erectile dysfunction
- Rebound syndrome with abrupt withdrawal

Interactions

- Increased effects of clonidine with **verapamil** and **beta-blockers.**
- Decreased effects of clonidine with **prazosin** and **tricyclic antidepressants.**
- Decreased effects of **levodopa** with clonidine.
- Additive CNS effects with **CNS depressants,** including **alcohol, antihistamines, opioid analgesics,** and **sedative/ hypnotics.**
- Additive hypotensive effects with other **antihypertensives** and **nitrates.**
- Decreased effects of guanfacine with **barbiturates, carbamazepine, rifampin, tricyclic antidepressants,** or **phenytoin.**
- Increased effects of guanfacine with **ketoconazole.**
- Increased effects of **valproic acid** with guanfacine.

Route and Dosage

CLONIDINE (CATAPRES; KAPVAY)

Hypertension: **PO** *(Adults):* Initial dosage: 0.1 mg twice daily (immediate release), 0.1 mg at bedtime (modified release) or 0.17 mg once daily (suspension). May increase dosage in increments of 0.1 mg/day (0.09 mg for suspension) at weekly intervals until desired response is achieved. Maximum dose: 2.4 mg/day (immediate release or 0.52 mg/day (suspension).

Transdermal system: Transdermal system delivering 0.1 mg to 0.3 mg/24 hr applied every 7 days. Initiate with 0.1 mg/24 hr system. Dosage increments may be made every 1 to 2 weeks when system is changed.

ADHD: **PO** *(Children ≥6 years): Extended release:* Initial dose: 0.1 mg at bedtime. May increase in increments of 0.1 mg/day at weekly intervals to maximum dose of 0.4 mg/day.

Immediate release: Initial dose: 0.05 mg at bedtime. May increase dosage over several weeks to 0.15 to 0.3 mg/day in 3 or 4 divided doses.

Tourette's disorder: **PO** *(Children and adolescents):* 0.0025 to 0.015 mg/kg/day for 6 weeks to 3 months.

GUANFACINE (TENEX; INTUNIV)

Hypertension (Immediate release): **PO** *(Adults):* 1 mg daily at bedtime. If satisfactory results are not achieved after 3 to 4 weeks, may increase to 2 mg.

ADHD (Extended release): **PO** *(Children 6 to 17 years):* Initial dosage: 1 mg once daily. May increase dose in increments of 1 mg/day at weekly intervals until desired response is achieved. Maximum dose: 4 mg/day. Tablets should not be chewed, crushed, or broken before swallowing, and should not be administered with high-fat meals.

Tourette's disorder: **PO** *(Children and adolescents):* Initial dosage: 0.5 mg at bedtime. May increase dose by 0.5 mg every 3 to 7 days to maximum dosage of 4 mg/day.

■ CHEMICAL CLASS: MISCELLANEOUS AGENTS FOR ADHD

Examples

Generic (Trade) Name	Pregnancy Categories/ Half-life	Indications	Available Forms (mg)
Atomoxetine (Strattera)	C/5 hr	• ADHD	**CAPS:** 10, 18, 25, 40, 60, 80, 100
Bupropion (Wellbutrin; Wellbutrin SR; Wellbutrin XL; Budeprion SR; Budeprion XL; Aplenzin; Zyban)	B/8–24 hr	• Depression (All except Zyban) • Seasonal affective disorder (Wellbutrin XL; Aplenzin) • Smoking cessation (Zyban) **Unlabeled use:** • ADHD (Wellbutrin; Wellbutrin SR; Wellbutrin XL)	**TABS:** 75, 100 **TABS SR:** 100, 150, 200 **TABS XL:** 150, 300 **TABS (ER) (APLENZIN):** 174, 348, 522

SR=12-hour tablets; XL=24-hour tablets

Action

- Atomoxetine selectively inhibits the reuptake of the neurotransmitter norepinephrine.
- Bupropion is a weak inhibitor of the neuronal uptake of norepinephrine, serotonin, and dopamine.
- Action in the treatment of ADHD is unclear.

Contraindications and Precautions

Contraindicated in: • Hypersensitivity • Coadministration with or within 2 weeks after discontinuing an MAO inhibitor • Lactation

Atomoxetine: • Narrow-angle glaucoma • Current or prior history of pheochromocytoma

Bupropion: • Known or suspected seizure disorder • Acute phase of myocardial infarction • Clients with current or prior diagnosis of bulimia or anorexia nervosa • Clients undergoing abrupt discontinuation of alcohol or sedatives (increased risk of seizures)

Use Cautiously in: • Clients with suicidal ideation • Clients with urinary retention • Hypertension • Hepatic, renal, or cardiovascular insufficiency • Pregnancy (use only if benefits outweigh possible risks to fetus) • Children and adolescents (may increase suicidal risk) • Elderly and debilitated patients

Atomoxetine: • Children younger than 6 years (safety not established)

Adverse Reactions and Side Effects

- Dry mouth
- Anorexia
- Nausea and vomiting
- Constipation
- Urinary retention
- Sexual dysfunction
- Headache
- Dizziness
- Insomnia or sedation
- Palpitations; tachycardia
- Weight loss
- Abdominal pain
- Increased sweating

Atomoxetine:
- Fatigue
- Cough
- New or worsened psychiatric symptoms
- Severe liver damage

Bupropion:
- Weight gain
- Tremor
- Seizures
- Blurred vision

Interactions

The effects of:	Are increased by:	Are decreased by:	Concurrent use may result in:
Atomoxetine	Concomitant use of **CYP2D6 inhibitors** (paroxetine, fluoxetine, quinidine)		Risk of additive hypertensive effects with pressor agents, such as **dobutamine** or **dopamine;** potentially fatal reactions with concurrent use (or use within 2 weeks of discontinuation) of **MAOIs;** increased cardiovascular effects of

The effects of:	Are increased by:	Are decreased by:	Concurrent use may result in:
			albuterol with concurrent use
Bupropion	Amantadine, levodopa, cimetidine, clopidogrel, ticlopidine, guanfacine	Carbamazepine, ritonavir	Increased risk of acute toxicity with **MAOIs**; increased risk of hypertension with **nicotine replacement agent**; adverse neuropsychiatric events with **alcohol** (alcohol tolerance is reduced); increased anticoagulant effect of **warfarin**; increased effects of drugs metabolized by CYP2D6 (e.g., **nortriptyline, imipramine, desipramine, paroxetine, fluoxetine, sertraline, haloperidol, risperidone, thioridazine metoprolol, propafenone,** and **flecainide**); increased risk of seizures with drugs that lower the seizure threshold (antidepressants, antipsychotics, theophylline, corticosteroids, stimulants/anorectics)

Route and Dosage

ATOMOXETINE (STRATTERA)

ADHD: PO *(Adults, adolescents, and children weighing more than 70 kg):* Initial dose: 40 mg/day. Increase after a minimum of 3 days to a target total daily dose of 80 mg, as a single dose in the morning or 2 evenly divided doses in the morning and late afternoon or early evening. After 2 to 4 weeks, total dosage may be increased to a maximum of 100 mg, if needed.

PO *(Children weighing 70 kg or less):* Initial dose: 0.5 mg/kg/day. May be increased every 3 days to a daily target dose of 1.2 mg/kg taken either as a single dose in the morning or 2 evenly divided doses in the morning and late afternoon or early evening. Maximum daily dose: 1.4 mg/kg or 100 mg daily, whichever is less.

Adjusted Dosing: Hepatic impairment: In clients with moderate hepatic impairment, reduce to 50% of usual dose. In clients with severe hepatic impairment, reduce to 25% of usual dose.

Adjusted Dosing: Coadministration with strong CYP2D6 inhibitors (e.g., quinidine, fluoxetine, paroxetine): **PO** *(Adults, adolescents, and children weighing more than 70 kg body weight):* Initiate dosage at 40 mg/day and only increase to the usual target dose of 80 mg/day if symptoms fail to improve after 4 weeks and the initial dose is well tolerated. **PO** *(Children and adolescents up to 70 kg body weight):* Initiate dosage at 0.5 mg/kg/day and only increase to the usual target dose of 1.2 mg/kg/day if symptoms fail to improve after 4 weeks and the initial dose is well tolerated.

BUPROPION (WELLBUTRIN; BUDEPRION; APLENZIN; ZYBAN)

***Depression (Wellbutrin; Budeprion):* PO** *(Adults) (immediate release tabs):* 100 mg 2 times/day. May increase after 3 days to 100 mg given 3 times/day. For patients who do not show improvement after several weeks of dosing at 300 mg/day, an increase in dosage up to 450 mg/day may be considered. No single dose of bupropion should exceed 150 mg. To prevent the risk of seizures, administer with 4 to 6 hours between doses.

Sustained release tabs (Wellbutrin SR; Budeprion SR): Give as a single 150 mg dose in the morning. May increase to twice a day (total 300 mg), with at least 8 hours between doses. Maximum dose: 400 mg, administered as 200 mg twice a day, with at least 8 hours between doses.

Extended release tabs (Wellbutrin XL; Budeprion XL): Begin dosing at 150 mg/day, given as a single daily dose in the morning. May increase after 3 days to 300 mg/day, given as a single daily dose in the morning. Maximum dose: 450 mg administered as a single daily dose in the morning.

Aplenzin: Initial dose: 174 mg once daily. After 4 days, may increase the dose to 348 mg once daily.

***Seasonal affective disorder (Wellbutrin XL):* PO** *(Adults):* 150 mg administered each morning beginning in the autumn prior to the onset of depressive symptoms. Dose may be uptitrated to the target dose of 300 mg/day after 1 week. Therapy should continue through the winter season before being tapered to 150 mg/day for 2 weeks prior to discontinuation in early spring.

Aplenzin: **PO** *(Adults):* 174 mg once daily beginning in the autumn prior to the onset of seasonal depressive symptoms. After 1 week, may increase the dose to 348 mg once daily. Continue treatment through the winter season.

***Smoking cessation (Zyban):* PO** *(Adults):* Begin dosing at 150 mg given once a day in the morning for 3 days. If tolerated well, increase to target dose of 300 mg/day given in doses of 150 mg twice daily with an interval of 8 hours between doses. Continue treatment for 7 to 12 weeks. Some patients may need treatment for as long as 6 months.

***ADHD (Wellbutrin; Wellbutrin SR; Wellbutrin XL):* PO** *(Adults):* 150 to 450 mg/day. Initiate therapy with 150 mg/day and titrate based on tolerability and efficacy. Doses can be given as divided doses or in SR or XL formulations.

Children and adolescents (Wellbutrin; Wellbutrin SR; Wellbutrin XL):
Up to 3 mg/kg/day or 150 mg/day initially, titrated to a maximum dosage of up to 6 mg/kg/day or 300 mg/day. Single dose should not exceed 150 mg. Usually given in divided doses for safety and effectiveness: twice daily for children and 3 times daily for adolescents.

■ NURSING DIAGNOSES RELATED TO AGENTS FOR ADHD

1. Risk for injury related to overstimulation and hyperactivity (CNS stimulants [or seizures] possible side effect of bupropion).
2. Risk for suicide secondary to major depression related to abrupt withdrawal after extended use (CNS stimulants).
3. Risk for suicide (children and adolescents) as a side effect of atomoxetine and bupropion (black-box warning).
4. Imbalanced nutrition, less than body requirements, related to side effects of anorexia and weight loss (CNS stimulants).
5. Disturbed sleep pattern related to side effects of overstimulation or insomnia.
6. Nausea related to side effects of atomoxetine or bupropion.
7. Pain related to side effect of abdominal pain (atomoxetine, bupropion) or headache (all agents).
8. Risk for activity intolerance related to side effects of sedation or dizziness (atomoxetine or bupropion).

■ NURSING IMPLICATIONS FOR ADHD AGENTS

The plan of care should include monitoring for the following side effects from agents for ADHD. Nursing implications related to each side effect are designated by an asterisk (*).

1. **Overstimulation, restlessness, insomnia** (with CNS stimulants)
   * Assess mental status for changes in mood, level of activity, degree of stimulation, and aggressiveness.
   * Ensure that the client is protected from injury.
   * Keep stimuli low and environment as quiet as possible to discourage overstimulation.
   * To prevent insomnia, administer the last dose at least 6 hours before bedtime. Administer sustained release forms in the morning.
2. **Palpitations, tachycardia** (with CNS stimulants; atomoxetine; bupropion; clonidine) or bradycardia (clonidine, guanfacine)
   * Monitor and record vital signs at regular intervals (two or three times a day) throughout therapy. Report significant changes to the physician immediately.

NOTE: The FDA has issued warnings associated with CNS stimulants and atomoxetine of the risk for sudden death in patients who have cardiovascular disease. A careful personal and family history of heart disease, heart defects, or hypertension should be obtained before these medications are prescribed. Careful monitoring of cardiovascular function during administration must be ongoing.

3. **Anorexia, weight loss** (with CNS stimulants, atomoxetine, and bupropion)
   * To reduce anorexia, the medication may be administered immediately after meals. The client should be weighed regularly (at least weekly) when receiving therapy with CNS stimulants, atomoxetine, or bupropion because of the potential for anorexia and weight loss, and temporary interruption of growth and development.

4. **Tolerance, physical and psychological dependence** (with CNS stimulants)
   * Tolerance develops rapidly.
   * In children with ADHD, a drug "holiday" should be attempted periodically under direction of the physician to determine the effectiveness of the medication and the need for continuation.
   * The drug should not be withdrawn abruptly. To do so could initiate the following syndrome of symptoms: nausea, vomiting, abdominal cramping, headache, fatigue, weakness, mental depression, suicidal ideation, increased dreaming, and psychotic behavior.

5. **Nausea and vomiting** (with atomoxetine and bupropion)
   * May be taken with food to minimize GI upset.

6. **Constipation** (with atomoxetine, bupropion, clonidine, and guanfacine)
   * Increase fiber and fluid in diet, if not contraindicated.

7. **Dry Mouth** (with clonidine and guanfacine)
   * Offer the client sugarless candy, ice, frequent sips of water.
   * Strict oral hygiene is very important.

8. **Sedation** (with clonidine and guanfacine)
   * Warn client that this effect is increased by concomitant use of alcohol and other CNS drugs.
   * Warn clients to refrain from driving or performing hazardous tasks until response has been established.

9. **Potential for seizures** (with bupropion)
   * Protect client from injury if seizure should occur. Instruct family and significant others of clients on bupropion therapy how to protect client during a seizure if one should occur. Ensure that doses of the immediate release medication are administered 4 to 6 hours apart, and doses of the sustained release medication at least 8 hours apart.

10. **Severe liver damage** (with atomoxetine)
    * Monitor for the following side effects and report to physician immediately: itching, dark urine, right upper quadrant pain, yellow skin or eyes, sore throat, fever, malaise.

11. **New or worsened psychiatric symptoms** (with CNS stimulants and atomoxetine)
    * Monitor for psychotic symptoms (e.g., hearing voices, paranoid behaviors, delusions.
    * Monitor for manic symptoms, including aggressive and hostile behaviors.
12. **Rebound Syndrome** (with clonidine and guanfacine)
    * Client should be instructed not to discontinue therapy abruptly. To do so may result in symptoms of nervousness, agitation, headache, and tremor, and a rapid rise in blood pressure. Dosage should be tapered gradually under the supervision of the physician.

■ CLIENT/FAMILY EDUCATION RELATED TO AGENTS FOR ADHD

- Use caution in driving or operating dangerous machinery. Drowsiness, dizziness and blurred vision can occur.
- Do not stop taking CNS stimulants abruptly. To do so could produce serious withdrawal symptoms.
- Avoid taking CNS stimulants late in the day to prevent insomnia. Take no later than 6 hours before bedtime.
- Do not take other medications (including over-the-counter drugs) without physician's approval. Many medications contain substances that, in combination with agents for ADHD, can be harmful.
- Diabetic clients should monitor blood sugar two or three times a day or as instructed by the physician. Be aware of need for possible alteration in insulin requirements because of changes in food intake, weight, and activity.
- Avoid consumption of large amounts of caffeinated products (coffee, tea, colas, chocolate), as they may enhance the CNS stimulant effect.
- Notify physician if symptoms of restlessness, insomnia, anorexia, or dry mouth become severe or if rapid, pounding heartbeat becomes evident. Report any of the following side effects to the physician immediately: shortness of breath; chest pain; jaw/left arm pain; fainting; seizures; sudden vision changes; weakness on one side of the body; slurred speech; confusion; itching; dark urine; right upper quadrant pain; yellow skin or eyes; sore throat; fever; malaise; increased hyperactivity; believing things that are not true; or hearing voices.
- Be aware of possible risks of taking agents for ADHD during pregnancy. Safe use during pregnancy and lactation has not been established. Inform the physician immediately if pregnancy is suspected or planned.

- Be aware of potential side effects of agents for ADHD. Refer to written materials furnished by health care providers for safe self-administration.
- Carry a card or other identification at all times describing medications being taken.

@ **INTERNET REFERENCES**

  a. http://www.mentalhealth.com/
  b. http://www.nimh.nih.gov/index.shtml
  c. http://www.nimh.nih.gov/health/publications/mental-health-medications/index.shtml
  d. http://www.nlm.nih.gov/medlineplus/druginformation.html
  e. http://www.chadd.org
  f. http://www.nimh.nih.gov/health/topics/attention-deficit-hyperactivity-disorder-adhd/index.shtml

Comparison of Developmental Theories

Age	Stage	Major Developmental Tasks
Freud's Stages of Psychosexual Development		
Birth–18 months	Oral	Relief from anxiety through oral gratification of needs
18 months–3 years	Anal	Learning independence and control, with focus on the excretory function
3–6 years	Phallic	Identification with parent of same gender; development of sexual identity; focus is on genital organs
6–12 years	Latency	Sexuality is repressed; focus is on relationships with same-gender peers
13–20 years	Genital	Libido is reawakened as genital organs mature; focus is on relationships with members of the opposite gender

Stages Of Development in H. S. Sullivan's Interpersonal Theory

Birth–18 months	Infancy	Relief from anxiety through oral gratification of needs
18 months–6 years	Childhood	Learning to experience a delay in personal gratification without undue anxiety
6–9 years	Juvenile	Learning to form satisfactory peer relationships
9–12 years	Preadolescence	Learning to form satisfactory relationships with persons of the same gender; the initiation of feelings of affection for another person
12–14 years	Early adolescence	Learning to form satisfactory relationships with persons of the opposite gender; developing a sense of identity
14–21 years	Late adolescence	Establishing self-identity; experiencing satisfying relationships; working to develop a lasting, intimate opposite-gender relationship

Stages of Development in Eric Erikson's Psychosocial Theory

Infancy (Birth–18 months)	Trust vs. mistrust	To develop a basic trust in the mothering figure and be able to generalize it to others
Early childhood (18 months–3 years)	Autonomy vs. shame and doubt	To gain some self-control and independence within the environment
Late childhood (3–6 years)	Initiative vs. guilt	To develop a sense of purpose and the ability to initiate and direct own activities
School age (6–12 years)	Industry vs. inferiority	To achieve a sense of self-confidence by learning, competing, performing successfully, and receiving recognition from significant others, peers, and acquaintances
Adolescence (12–20 years)	Identity vs. role confusion	To integrate the tasks mastered in the previous stages into a secure sense of self
Young adulthood (20–30 years)	Intimacy vs. isolation	To form an intense, lasting relationship or a commitment to another person, a cause, an institution, or a creative effort
Adulthood (30–65 years)	Generativity vs. stagnation	To achieve the life goals established for oneself, while also considering the welfare of future generations
Old age (65 years–death)	Ego integrity vs. despair	To review one's life and derive meaning from both positive and negative events, while achieving a positive sense of self-worth

Stages of Development in M. Mahler's Theory of Object Relations

Birth–1 month	I. Normal autism	Fulfillment of basic needs for survival and comfort
1–5 months	II. Symbiosis	Developing awareness of external source of need fulfillment
	III. Separation–Individuation	
5–10 months	A. Differentiation	Commencement of a primary recognition of separateness from the mothering figure
10–16 months	B. Practicing	Increased independence through locomotor functioning; increased sense of separateness of self
16–24 months	C. Rapprochement	Acute awareness of separateness of self; learning to seek "emotional refueling" from mothering figure to maintain feeling of security
24–36 months	D. Consolidation	Sense of separateness established; on the way to object constancy (i.e., able to internalize a sustained image of loved object/person when it is out of sight); resolution of separation anxiety

Piaget's Stages of Cognitive Development

Birth–2 years	Sensorimotor	With increased mobility and awareness, develops a sense of self as separate from the external environment; the concept of object permanence emerges as the ability to form mental images evolves
2–6 years	Preoperational	Learning to express self with language; develops understanding of symbolic gestures; achievement of object permanence
6–12 years	Concrete operations	Learning to apply logic to thinking; development of understanding of reversibility and spatiality; learning to differentiate and classify; increased socialization and application of rules
12–15+ years	Formal operations	Learning to think and reason in abstract terms; making and testing hypotheses; capability of logical thinking and reasoning expand and are refined; cognitive maturity achieved

Kohlberg's Stages of Moral Development

I. Preconventional (common from ages 4–10 years)	1. Punishment and obedience orientation	Behavior is motivated by fear of punishment
	2. Instrumental relativist orientation	Behavior is motivated by egocentrism and concern for self
II. Conventional (common from ages 10–13 years and into adulthood)	3. Interpersonal concordance orientation	Behavior is motivated by the expectations of others; strong desire for approval and acceptance
	4. Law and order orientation	Behavior is motivated by respect for authority
III. Postconventional (can occur from adolescence on)	5. Social contract legalistic orientation	Behavior is motivated by respect for universal laws and moral principles and guided by an internal set of values
	6. Universal ethical principle orientation	Behavior is motivated by internalized principles of honor, justice, and respect for human dignity and guided by the conscience

Stages of Development in H. Peplau's Interpersonal Theory

Infancy	Learning to count on others	Learning to communicate in various ways with the primary caregiver to have comfort needs fulfilled
Toddlerhood	Learning to delay gratification	Learning the satisfaction of pleasing others by delaying self-gratification in small ways
Early childhood	Identifying oneself	Learning appropriate roles and behaviors by acquiring the ability to perceive the expectations of others
Late childhood	Developing skills in participation	Learning the skills of compromise, competition, and cooperation with others; establishing a more realistic view of the world and a feeling of one's place in it.

SOURCE: Adapted from Townsend, M.C. (2015). *Psychiatric/Mental Health Nursing: Concepts of Care in Evidence-Based Practice* (8th ed.) Philadelphia: FA Davis, pp. 28–46.

Ego Defense Mechanisms

Defense Mechanisms	Example	Defense Mechanisms	Example
Compensation: Covering up a real or perceived weakness by emphasizing a trait one considers more desirable	A physically handicapped boy is unable to participate in football, so he compensates by becoming a great scholar.	**Rationalization:** Attempting to make excuses or formulate logical reasons to justify unacceptable feelings or behaviors	John tells the rehab nurse, "I drink because it's the only way I can deal with my bad marriage and my worse job."
Denial: Refusing to acknowledge the existence of a real situation or the feelings associated with it	A woman who drinks alcohol every day and cannot stop fails to acknowledge that she has a problem.	**Reaction Formation:** Preventing unacceptable or undesirable thoughts or behaviors from being expressed by exaggerating opposite thoughts or types of behaviors	Jane hates nursing. She attended nursing school to please her parents. During career day, she speaks to prospective students about the excellence of nursing as a career.
Displacement: The transfer of feelings from one target to another that is	A client is angry at his physician, does not express it, but	**Regression:** Responding to stress by retreating to an earlier level of	When 2-year-old Jay is hospitalized for tonsillitis he will drink only

Continued

Defense Mechanisms	Example	Defense Mechanisms	Example
considered less threatening or that is neutral	becomes verbally abusive with the nurse.	development and the comfort measures associated with that level of functioning	from a bottle, even though his mom states he has been drinking from a cup for 6 months.
Identification: An attempt to increase self-worth by acquiring certain attributes and characteristics of an individual one admires	A teenager who required lengthy rehabilitation after an accident decides to become a physical therapist as a result of his experiences.	**Repression:** Involuntarily blocking unpleasant feelings and experiences from one's awareness	An accident victim can remember nothing about the accident.
Intellectualization: An attempt to avoid expressing actual emotions associated with a stressful situation by using the intellectual processes of logic, reasoning, and analysis	S's husband is being transferred with his job to a city far away from her parents. She hides anxiety by explaining to her parents the advantages associated with the move.	**Sublimation:** Rechanneling of drives or impulses that are personally or socially unacceptable into activities that are constructive	A mother whose son was killed by a drunk driver channels her anger and energy into being the president of the local chapter of Mothers Against Drunk Driving.
Introjection: Integrating the beliefs and values of another individual into one's own ego structure	Children integrate their parents' value system into the process of conscience formation. A child says to friend, "Don't cheat. It's wrong."	**Suppression:** The voluntary blocking of unpleasant feelings and experiences from one's awareness	Scarlett O'Hara says, "I don't want to think about that now. I'll think about that tomorrow."

Defense Mechanisms	Example	Defense Mechanisms	Example
Isolation: Separating a thought or memory from the feeling tone or emotion associated with it	A young woman describes being attacked and raped, without showing any emotion.	**Undoing:** Symbolically negating or canceling out an experience that one finds intolerable	Joe is nervous about his new job and yells at his wife. On his way home he stops and buys her some flowers.
Projection Attributing feelings or impulses unacceptable to one's self to another person	Sue feels a strong sexual attraction to her track coach and tells her friend, "He's coming on to me!"		

SOURCE: Townsend, M.C. (2015). *Psychiatric/Mental Health Nursing: Concepts of Care in Evidence-Based Practice* (8th ed.) Philadelphia: FA Davis, p. 19.

APPENDIX C

Levels of Anxiety

Level	Perceptual Field	Ability to Learn	Physical Characteristics	Emotional/Behavioral Characteristics
Mild	Heightened perception (e.g., noises may seem louder; details within the environment are clearer). Increased awareness. Increased alertness.	Learning is enhanced.	Restlessness Irritability	May remain superficial with others. Rarely experienced as distressful. Motivation is increased.
Moderate	Reduction in perceptual field. Reduced alertness to environmental events (e.g., someone talking may not be heard; part of the room may not be noticed).	Learning still occurs, but not at optimal ability. Decreased attention span. Decreased ability to concentrate.	Increased restlessness. Increased heart and respiration rate. Increased perspiration. Gastric discomfort Increased muscular tension. Increase in speech rate, volume, and pitch.	A feeling of discontent May lead to a degree of impairment in interpersonal relationships as individual begins to focus on self and the need to relieve personal discomfort.
Severe	Greatly diminished. Only extraneous details are perceived, or fixation on a single detail may occur. May not take notice of	Extremely limited attention span. Unable to concentrate or problem-solve. Effective learning cannot occur.	Headaches Dizziness Nausea Trembling Insomnia Palpitations Tachycardia	Feelings of dread, loathing, horror Total focus on self and intense desire to relieve the anxiety.

Continued

Level	Perceptual Field	Ability to Learn	Physical Characteristics	Emotional/Behavioral Characteristics
	an event even when attention is directed by another.		Hyperventilation Urinary frequency Diarrhea	
Panic	Unable to focus on even one detail within the environment. Misperceptions of the environment are common (e.g., a perceived detail may be elaborated and out of proportion).	Learning cannot occur. Unable to concentrate. Unable to comprehend even simple directions.	Dilated pupils Labored breathing Severe trembling Sleeplessness Palpitations Diaphoresis and pallor Muscular incoordination Immobility or purposeless hyperactivity Incoherence or inability to verbalize	Sense of impending doom Terror Bizarre behavior, including shouting, screaming, running about wildly, or clinging to anyone or anything from which a sense of safety and security is derived. Hallucinations; delusions Extreme withdrawal into self

SOURCE: From Townsend, M.C. (2015). *Psychiatric/Mental Health Nursing: Concepts of Care in Evidence-Based Practice* (8th ed.) Philadelphia: FA Davis, pp. 18–19.

Stages of Grief

A Comparison of Models by Elisabeth Kübler-Ross, John Bowlby, George Engel, and William Worden

	Stages/Tasks				Possible Time Dimension	Behaviors
Kübler-Ross	Bowlby	Engel	Worden			
I. Denial	I. Numbness/protest	I. Shock/disbelief	I. Accepting the reality of the loss		Occurs immediately on experiencing the loss. Usually lasts no more than a few weeks.	Individual has difficulty believing that the loss has occurred
II. Anger	II. Disequilibrium	II. Developing awareness			In most cases begins within hours of the loss. Peaks within a few weeks.	Anger is directed toward self or others. Ambivalence and guilt may be felt toward the lost object.
III. Bargaining		III. Restitution				The individual fervently seeks alternatives to improve current situation. Attends to various rituals associated with the culture in which the loss has occurred.
IV. Depression	III. Disorganization and despair	IV. Resolution of the loss	II. Processing the pain of grief		Very individual. Commonly 6 to 12 months. Longer for some.	The actual work of grieving. Preoccupation with the lost entity. Feelings of helplessness and loneliness occur in response to realization of the loss. Feelings associated the loss are confronted.

V. Acceptance		How the environment changes depends on the roles the lost entity played in the life of the bereaved person. Adaptations will have to be made as the changes are presented in daily life. New coping skills will have to be developed.
IV. Reorganization	III. Adjusting to a world without the lost entity	Ongoing
V. Recovery		Resolution is complete. The bereaved person experiences a reinvestment in new relationships and new goals. The lost entity is not purged or replaced, but relocated in the life of the bereaved. At this stage, terminally ill persons express a readiness to die.
	IV. Finding an enduring connection with the lost entity in the midst of embarking on a new life.	

SOURCE: Adapted from Townsend, M.C. (2015), *Psychiatric/Mental Health Nursing: Concepts of Care in Evidence-Based Practice* (8th ed.) Philadelphia: FA Davis.

Relationship Development and Therapeutic Communication

■ PHASES OF A THERAPEUTIC NURSE-CLIENT RELATIONSHIP

Psychiatric nurses use interpersonal relationship development as the primary intervention with clients in various psychiatric and mental health settings. This is congruent with Peplau's (1962) identification of counseling as the major subrole of nursing in psychiatry. If Sullivan's (1953) belief is true—that is, that all emotional problems stem from difficulties with interpersonal relationships—then this role of the nurse in psychiatry becomes especially meaningful and purposeful. It becomes an integral part of the total therapeutic regimen.

The therapeutic interpersonal relationship is the means by which the nursing process is implemented. Through the relationship, problems are identified and resolution is sought. Tasks of the relationship have been categorized into four phases: the pre-interaction phase, the orientation (introductory) phase, the working phase, and the termination phase. Although each phase is presented as specific and distinct from the others, there may be some overlapping of tasks, particularly when the interaction is limited.

The Pre-interaction Phase

The pre-interaction phase involves preparation for the first encounter with the client. Tasks include the following:

1. Obtaining available information about the client from the chart, significant others, or other health team members. From this information, the initial assessment is begun. From this initial information, the nurse may also become aware of personal responses to knowledge about the client.
2. Examining one's feelings, fears, and anxieties about working with a particular client. For example, the nurse may have been

reared in an alcoholic family and have ambivalent feelings about caring for a client who is alcohol dependent. All individuals bring attitudes and feelings from prior experiences to the clinical setting. The nurse needs to be aware of how these preconceptions may affect his or her ability to care for individual clients.

The Orientation (Introductory) Phase

During the orientation phase, the nurse and client become acquainted. Tasks include the following:

1. Creating an environment for the establishment of trust and rapport.
2. Establishing a contract for intervention that details the expectations and responsibilities of both the nurse and client.
3. Gathering assessment information to build a strong client data base.
4. Identifying the client's strengths and limitations.
5. Formulating nursing diagnoses.
6. Setting goals that are mutually agreeable to the nurse and client.
7. Developing a plan of action that is realistic for meeting the established goals.
8. Exploring feelings of both the client and the nurse in terms of the introductory phase. Introductions are often uncomfortable, and the participants may experience some anxiety until a degree of rapport has been established. Interactions may remain on a superficial level until anxiety subsides. Several interactions may be required to fulfill the tasks associated with this phase.

The Working Phase

The therapeutic work of the relationship is accomplished during this phase. Tasks include the following:

1. Maintaining the trust and rapport that was established during the orientation phase.
2. Promoting the client's insight and perception of reality.
3. Problem solving in an effort to bring about change in the client's life.
4. Overcoming resistance behaviors on the part of the client as the level of anxiety rises in response to discussion of painful issues.
5. Continuously evaluating progress toward goal attainment.

The Termination Phase

Termination of the relationship may occur for a variety of reasons: the mutually agreed-upon goals may have been reached, the client may be discharged from the hospital, or in the case of a student nurse, the clinical rotation may come to an end. Termination can be a difficult phase for both the client and nurse. Tasks include the following:

1. Bringing a therapeutic conclusion to the relationship. This occurs when:
   a. Progress has been made toward attainment of mutually set goals.
   b. A plan for continuing care or for assistance during stressful life experiences is mutually established by the nurse and client.
   c. Feelings about termination of the relationship are recognized and explored. Both the nurse and client may experience feelings of sadness and loss. The nurse should share his or her feelings with the client. Through these interactions, the client learns that it is acceptable to undergo these feelings at a time of separation. Through this knowledge, the client experiences growth during the process of termination.

NOTE: When the client feels sadness and loss, behaviors to delay termination may become evident. If the nurse experiences the same feelings, he or she may allow the client's behaviors to delay termination. For therapeutic closure, the nurse must establish the reality of the separation and resist being manipulated into repeated delays by the client.

Therapeutic Communication Techniques

Technique	Explanation/ Rationale	Examples
Using silence	Gives the client the opportunity to collect and organize thoughts, to think through a point, or to consider introducing a topic of greater concern than the one being discussed.	
Accepting	Conveys an attitude of reception and regard.	"Yes, I understand what you said." Eye contact; nodding.
Giving recognition	Acknowledging; indicating awareness; better than complimenting, which reflects the nurse's judgment.	"Hello, Mr. J. I notice that you made a ceramic ash tray in OT." "I see you made your bed."

Therapeutic Communication Techniques—cont'd

Technique	Explanation/ Rationale	Examples
Offering self	Making oneself available on an unconditional basis, increasing client's feelings of self-worth.	"I'll stay with you awhile." "We can eat our lunch together." "I'm interested in you."
Giving broad openings	Allows the client to take the initiative in introducing the topic; emphasizes the importance of the client's role in the interaction.	"What would you like to talk about today?" "Tell me what you are thinking."
Offering general leads	Offers the client encouragement to continue.	"Yes, I see." "Go on." "And after that?"
Placing the event in time or sequence	Clarifies the relationship of events in time so that the nurse and client can view them in perspective.	"What seemed to lead up to...?" "Was this before or after...?" "When did this happen?"
Making observations	Verbalizing what is observed or perceived. This encourages the client to recognize specific behaviors and compare perceptions with the nurse.	"You seem tense." "I notice you are pacing a lot." "You seem uncomfortable when you...."
Encouraging description of perceptions	Asking the client to verbalize what is being perceived; often used with clients experiencing hallucinations.	"Tell me what is happening now." "Are you hearing the voices again?" "What do the voices seem to be saying?"
Encouraging comparison	Asking the client to compare similarities and differences in ideas, experiences, or interpersonal relationships. Helps the client recognize life experiences that tend to recur as well as those aspects of life that are changeable.	"Was this something like...?" "How does this compare with the time when...?" "What was your response the last time this situation occurred?"

Continued

Therapeutic Communication Techniques—cont'd

Technique	Explanation/ Rationale	Examples
Restating	Repeating the main idea of what the client has said. This lets the client know whether an expressed statement has been understood and gives him or her the chance to continue, or to clarify if necessary.	Cl: "I can't study. My mind keeps wandering." Ns: "You have difficulty concentrating." Cl: "I can't take that new job. What if I can't do it?" Ns: "You're afraid you will fail in this new position."
Reflecting	Questions and feelings are referred back to the client so that they may be recognized and accepted, and so that the client may recognize that his or her point of view has value. This is a good technique to use when the client asks the nurse for advice.	Cl: "What do you think I should do about my wife's drinking problem?" Ns: "What do *you* think you should do?" Cl: "My sister won't help a bit toward my mother's care. I have to do it all!" Ns: "You feel angry when she doesn't help."
Focusing	Taking notice of a single idea or even a single word. Works especially well with a client who is moving rapidly from one thought to another. This technique is *not* therapeutic, however, with the client who is very anxious. Focusing should not be pursued until the anxiety level has subsided.	"This point seems worth looking at more closely. Perhaps you and I can discuss it together."

Therapeutic Communication Techniques—cont'd

Technique	Explanation/ Rationale	Examples
Exploring	Delving further into a subject, idea, experience, or relationship. Especially helpful with clients who tend to remain on a superficial level of communication. However, if the client chooses not to disclose further information, the nurse should refrain from pushing or probing in an area that obviously creates discomfort.	"Please explain that situation in more detail." "Tell me more about that particular situation."
Seeking clarification and validation	Striving to explain that which is vague or incomprehensible and searching for mutual understanding; clarifying the meaning of what has been said facilitates and increases understanding for both client and nurse.	"I'm not sure that I understand. Would you please explain?" "Tell me if my understanding agrees with yours." "Do I understand correctly that you said...?"
Presenting reality	When the client has a misperception of the environment, the nurse defines reality or indicates his or her perception of the situation for the client.	"I understand that the voices seem real to you, but I do not hear any voices." "There is no one else in the room but you and me."
Voicing doubt	Expressing uncertainty as to the reality of the client's perceptions. Often used with clients experiencing delusional thinking.	"I understand that you believe that to be true, but I see the situation differently." "I find that hard to believe (or accept)." "That seems rather doubtful to me."

Continued

Therapeutic Communication Techniques—cont'd

Technique	Explanation/ Rationale	Examples
Verbalizing the implied	Putting into words what the client has only implied or said indirectly; can also be used with the client who is mute or is otherwise experiencing impaired verbal communication. This clarifies that which is *implicit* rather than *explicit*.	Cl: "It's a waste of time to be here. I can't talk to you or anyone." Ns: "Are you feeling that no one understands?" Cl: (Mute) Ns: "It must have been very difficult for you when your husband died in the fire."
Attempting to translate words into feelings	When feelings are expressed indirectly, the nurse tries to "desymbolize" what has been said and to find clues to the underlying true feelings.	Cl: "I'm way out in the ocean." Ns: "You must be feeling very lonely now."
Formulating a plan of action	When a client has a plan in mind for dealing with what is considered to be a stressful situation, it may serve to prevent anger or anxiety from escalating to an unmanageable level.	"What could you do to let your anger out harmlessly?" "Next time this comes up, what might you do to handle it more appropriately?"

SOURCE: Adapted from Hays, J.S. & Larson, K.H. (1963). *Interacting with Patients*. New York: Holt, Rinehart, and Winston.

Nontherapeutic Communication Techniques

Technique	Explanation/ Rationale	Examples
Giving reassurance	Indicates to the client that there is no cause for anxiety, thereby devaluing the client's feelings. May discourage the client from further expression of feelings if he or	"I wouldn't worry about that if I were you." "Everything will be all right." **Better to say:** "We will work on that together."

Nontherapeutic Communication Techniques—cont'd

Technique	Explanation/Rationale	Examples
	she believes they will only be downplayed or ridiculed.	
Rejecting	Refusing to consider or showing contempt for the client's ideas or behavior. This may cause the client to discontinue interaction with the nurse for fear of further rejection.	"Let's not discuss...." "I don't want to hear about...." **Better to say:** "Let's look at that a little closer."
Giving approval or disapproval	Sanctioning or denouncing the client's ideas or behavior. Implies that the nurse has the right to pass judgment on whether the client's ideas or behaviors are "good" or "bad," and that the client is expected to please the nurse. The nurse's acceptance of the client is then seen as conditional depending on the client's behavior.	"That's good. I'm glad that you...." "That's bad. I'd rather you wouldn't...." **Better to say:** "Let's talk about how your behavior invoked anger in the other clients at dinner."
Agreeing/disagreeing	Indicating accord with or opposition to the client's ideas or opinions. Implies that the nurse has the right to pass judgment on whether the client's ideas or opinions are "right" or "wrong." Agreement prevents the client from later modifying his or her point	"That's right. I agree." "That's wrong. I disagree." "I don't believe that." **Better to say:** "Let's discuss what you feel is unfair about the new community rules."

Continued

Nontherapeutic Communication Techniques—cont'd

Technique	Explanation/ Rationale	Examples
	of view without admitting error. Disagreement implies inaccuracy, provoking the need for defensiveness on the part of the client.	
Giving advice	Telling the client what to do or how to behave implies that the nurse knows what is best and that the client is incapable of any self-direction. It nurtures the client in the dependent role by discouraging independent thinking.	"I think you should...." "Why don't you...." **Better to say:** "What do you think you should do?" or "What do you think would be best for you?"
Probing	Persistent questioning of the client; pushing for answers to issues the client does not wish to discuss. This causes the client to feel used and valued only for what is shared with the nurse, and places the client on the defensive.	"Tell me how your mother abused you when you were a child." "Tell me how you feel toward your mother now that she is dead." "Now tell me about...." **Better technique:** The nurse should be aware of the client's response and discontinue the interaction at the first sign of discomfort.
Defending	Attempting to protect someone or something from verbal attack. To defend what the client has criticized is to imply that he or she has no right to express ideas, opinions, or feelings. Defending does not change the client's feelings and may cause the client to	"No one here would lie to you." "You have a very capable physician. I'm sure he only has your best interests in mind." **Better to say:** "I will try to answer your questions and clarify some issues regarding your treatment."

Nontherapeutic Communication Techniques—cont'd

Technique	Explanation/ Rationale	Examples
	think the nurse is taking sides against the client.	
Requesting an explanation	Asking the client to provide the reasons for thoughts, feelings, behavior, and events. Asking "why" a client did something or feels a certain way can be very intimidating, and implies that the client must defend his or her behavior or feelings.	"Why do you think that?" "Why do you feel this way?" "Why did you do that?" **Better to say:** "Describe what you were feeling just before that happened."
Indicating the existence of an external source of power	Attributing the source of thoughts, feelings, and behavior to others or to outside influences. This encourages the client to project blame for his or her thoughts or behaviors on others rather than accepting the responsibility personally.	"What makes you say that?" "What made you do that?" "What made you so angry last night?" **Better to say:** "You became angry when your brother insulted your wife."
Belittling feelings expressed	When the nurse misjudges the degree of the client's discomfort, a lack of empathy and understanding may be conveyed. The nurse may tell the client to "perk up" or "snap out of it." This causes the client to feel insignificant or unimportant. When one is experiencing discomfort, it is no relief to hear	Cl: "I have nothing to live for. I wish I were dead." Ns: "Everybody gets down in the dumps at times. I feel that way myself sometimes." **Better to say:** "You must be very upset. Tell me what you are feeling right now."

Continued

Nontherapeutic Communication Techniques—cont'd

Technique	Explanation/ Rationale	Examples
	that others are or have been in similar situations.	
Making stereotyped comments	Clichés and trite expressions are meaningless in a nurse-client relationship. When the nurse makes empty conversation, it encourages a like response from the client.	"I'm fine, and how are you?" "Hang in there. It's for your own good." "Keep your chin up." **Better to say:** "The therapy must be difficult for you at times. How do you feel about your progress at this point?"
Using denial	Denying that a problem exists blocks discussion and avoids helping the client identify and explore areas of difficulty.	Cl: "I'm nothing." Ns: "Of course you're something. Everybody is somebody." **Better to say:** "You're feeling like no one cares about you right now."
Interpreting	With this technique the therapist seeks to make conscious that which is unconscious, to tell the client the meaning of his or her experience.	"What you really mean is...." "Unconsciously you're saying...." **Better technique:** The nurse must leave interpretation of the client's behavior to the psychiatrist. The nurse has not been prepared to perform this technique and, in attempting to do so, may endanger other nursing roles with the client.
Introducing an unrelated topic	Changing the subject causes the nurse to take over the direction of the discussion. This may occur in order to get to something that the nurse wants to discuss with the client or to get away from a topic that he or she would prefer not to discuss.	Cl: "I don't have anything to live for." Ns: "Did you have visitors this weekend?" **Better technique:** The nurse must remain open and free to hear the client, to take in all that is being conveyed, both verbally and nonverbally.

SOURCE: Adapted from Hays, J.S. & Larson, K.H. (1963). *Interacting with Patients*. New York: Holt, Rinehart, and Winston.

Psychosocial Therapies

■ GROUP THERAPY

Group therapy is a type of psychosocial therapy with a number of clients at one time. The group is founded in a specific theoretical framework, with the goal being to encourage improvement in interpersonal functioning.

Nurses often lead "therapeutic groups," which are based to a lesser degree in theory. The focus of therapeutic groups is more on group relations, interactions among group members, and the consideration of a selected issue.

Types of groups include *task groups*, in which the function is to accomplish a specific outcome or task; *teaching groups*, in which knowledge or information is conveyed to a number of individuals; *supportive-therapeutic* groups, which help prevent future upsets by teaching participants effective ways of dealing with emotional stress arising from situational or developmental crises; and *self-help groups* of individuals with similar problems who meet to help each other with emotional distress associated with those problems.

Yalom (2005) identified 11 curative factors that individuals can achieve through interpersonal interactions within the group. They include the following:

1. The instillation of hope.
2. Universality (individuals come to understand that they are not alone in the problems they experience).
3. The imparting of information.
4. Altruism (mutual sharing and concern for each other).
5. The corrective recapitulation of the primary family group.
6. The development of socializing techniques.
7. Imitative behavior.
8. Interpersonal learning.
9. Group cohesiveness.
10. Catharsis (open expression of feelings).
11. Existential factors (the group is able to help individual members take direction of their own lives and to accept responsibility for the quality of their existence).

■ PSYCHODRAMA

Psychodrama is a specialized type of therapeutic group that employs a dramatic approach in which clients become "actors" in life-situation scenarios.

The group leader is called the *director*, group members are the *audience*, and the *set*, or *stage*, may be specially designed or may just be any room or part of a room selected for this purpose. Actors are members from the audience who agree to take part in the "drama" by role-playing a situation about which they have been informed by the director. Usually the situation is an issue with which one individual client has been struggling. The client plays the role of himself or herself and is called the *protagonist*. In this role, the client is able to express true feelings toward individuals (represented by group members) with whom he or she has unresolved conflicts.

In some instances, the group leader may ask for a client to volunteer to be the protagonist for that session. The client may choose a situation he or she wishes to enact and select the audience members to portray the roles of others in the life situation. The psychodrama setting provides the client with a safer and less threatening atmosphere than the real situation in which to express true feelings. Resolution of interpersonal conflicts is facilitated.

When the drama has been completed, group members from the audience discuss the situation they have observed, offer feedback, express their feelings, and relate their own similar experiences. In this way, all group members benefit from the session, either directly or indirectly.

Nurses often serve as actors, or role players, in psychodrama sessions. Leaders of psychodrama have graduate degrees in psychology, social work, nursing, or medicine with additional training in group therapy and specialty preparation to become a psychodramatist.

■ FAMILY THERAPY

In family therapy, the nurse-therapist works with the family as a group to improve communication and interaction patterns. Areas of assessment include communication, manner of self-concept reinforcement, family members' expectations, handling differences, family interaction patterns, and the "climate" of the family (a blend of feelings and experiences that are the result of sharing and interacting).

The Family as a System

General systems theory is a way of organizing thought according to the holistic perspective. A system is considered greater than the sum of its parts. A family can be viewed as a system composed of various subsystems. The systems approach to family therapy is composed of eight major concepts: (1) differentiation of self; (2) triangles; (3) nuclear family emotional process; (4) family projection process; (5) multigenerational transmission process; (6) sibling position profiles; (7) emotional cutoff; and (8) societal regression. The goal is to increase the level of differentiation of self, while remaining in touch with the family system.

The Structural Model

In this model, the family is viewed as a social system within which the individual lives and to which the individual must adapt. The individual both contributes to and responds to stresses within the family. Major concepts include systems, subsystems, transactional patterns, and boundaries. The goal of therapy is to facilitate change in the family structure. The therapist does this by joining the family, evaluating the family system, and restructuring the family.

The Strategic Model

This model uses the interactional or communications approach. Functional families are open systems in which clear and precise messages, congruent with the situation, are sent and received. Healthy communication patterns promote nurturance and individual self-worth. In dysfunctional families, viewed as partially closed systems, communication is vague, and messages are often inconsistent and incongruent with the situation. Destructive patterns of communication tend to inhibit healthful nurturing and decrease individual feelings of self-worth. Concepts of this model include double-bind communication, pseudomutuality and pseudohostility, marital schism, and marital skew. The goal of therapy is to create change in destructive behavior and communication patterns among family members. This is accomplished by using paradoxical intervention (prescribing the symptom) and reframing (changing the setting or viewpoint in relation to which a situation is experienced and placing it in another more positive frame of reference).

■ MILIEU THERAPY

In psychiatry, milieu therapy, or a therapeutic community, constitutes a manipulation of the environment in an effort to create behavioral changes and to improve the psychological health and functioning of the individual. The goal of therapeutic community is for the client to learn adaptive coping, interaction, and relationship skills that can be generalized to other aspects of his or her life. The community environment itself serves as the primary tool of therapy.

According to Skinner (1979), a therapeutic community is based on seven basic assumptions:

1. The health in each individual is to be realized and encouraged to grow.
2. Every interaction is an opportunity for therapeutic intervention.

3. The client owns his or her own environment.
4. Each client owns his or her behavior.
5. Peer pressure is a useful and a powerful tool.
6. Inappropriate behaviors are dealt with as they occur.
7. Restrictions and punishment are to be avoided.

Since the goals of milieu therapy relate to helping the client learn to generalize that which is learned to other aspects of his or her life, the conditions that promote a therapeutic community in the hospital setting are similar to the types of conditions that exist in real-life situations. They include the following:

1. The fulfillment of basic physiological needs.
2. Physical facilities that are conducive to the achievement of the goals of therapy.
3. The existence of a democratic form of self-government.
4. The assignment of unit responsibilities according to client capabilities.
5. A structured program of social and work-related activities.
6. The inclusion of community and family in the program of therapy in an effort to facilitate discharge from the hospital.

The program of therapy on the milieu unit is conducted by the interdisciplinary treatment (IDT) team. The team includes some, or all, of the following disciplines, and may include others that are not specified here: psychiatrist, clinical psychologist, psychiatric clinical nurse specialist, psychiatric nurse, mental health technician, psychiatric social worker, occupational therapist, recreational therapist, art therapist, music therapist, psychodramatist, dietitian, and chaplain.

Nurses play a crucial role in the management of a therapeutic milieu. They are involved in the assessment, diagnosis, outcome identification, planning, implementation, and evaluation of all treatment programs. They have significant input into the IDT plans that are developed for all clients. They are responsible for ensuring that clients' basic needs are fulfilled, for continual assessment of physical and psychosocial status, for medication administration, for the development of trusting relationships, for setting limits on unacceptable behaviors, for client education, and ultimately, for helping clients, within the limits of their capability, become productive members of society.

Milieu therapy came into its own during the 1960s through early 1980s. During this period, psychiatric inpatient treatment provided sufficient time to implement programs of therapy that were aimed at social rehabilitation. Currently, care in inpatient psychiatric facilities is shorter and more biologically based, limiting clients' benefit from the socialization that occurs in a milieu as treatment program. Although strategies for milieu therapy are still used, they have been modified to conform to the short-term approach to care or to outpatient treatment programs.

■ CRISIS INTERVENTION

A *crisis* is "a sudden event in one's life that disturbs homeostasis, during which usual coping mechanisms cannot resolve the problem" (Lagerquist, 2012). All individuals experience crises at one time or another. This does not necessarily indicate psychopathology.

Crises are precipitated by specific, identifiable events and are determined by an individual's personal perception of the situation. They are acute, not chronic, and generally last no more than 4 to 6 weeks.

Crises occur when an individual is exposed to a stressor and previous problem-solving techniques are ineffective. This causes the level of anxiety to rise. Panic may ensue when new techniques are employed and resolution fails to occur.

Six types of crises have been identified. They include dispositional crises, crises of anticipated life transitions, crises resulting from traumatic stress, maturational or developmental crises, crises reflecting psychopathology, and psychiatric emergencies. The type of crisis determines the method of intervention selected.

Crisis intervention is designed to provide rapid assistance for individuals who have an urgent need. Aguilera (1998) suggests that the "focus is on the supportive, with the restoration of the individual to his precrisis level of functioning or possibly to a higher level of functioning." (p. 24)

Nurses regularly respond to individuals in crisis in all types of settings. Nursing process is the vehicle by which nurses assist individuals in crisis with a short-term, problem-solving approach to change. A four-phase technique is used: assessment/analysis; planning of therapeutic intervention; intervention; and evaluation of crisis resolution and anticipatory planning. Through this structured method of assistance, nurses assist individuals in crisis to develop more adaptive coping strategies for dealing with stressful situations in the future.

■ RELAXATION THERAPY

Stress is a part of our everyday lives. It can be positive or negative, but it cannot be eliminated. Keeping stress at a manageable level is a lifelong process.

Individuals under stress respond with a physiological arousal that can be dangerous over long periods. Indeed, the stress response has been shown to be a major contributor, either directly or indirectly, to coronary heart disease, cancer, lung ailments, accidental injuries, cirrhosis of the liver, and suicide—six of the leading causes of death in the United States.

Relaxation therapy is an effective means of reducing the stress response in some individuals. The degree of anxiety that an individual experiences in response to stress is related to certain predisposing factors, such as characteristics of temperament with which he or she was born, past experiences resulting in learned patterns of responding, and existing conditions, such as health status, coping strategies, and adequate support systems.

Deep relaxation can counteract the physiological and behavioral manifestations of stress. Various methods of relaxation include the following:

Deep-Breathing Exercises: Tension is released when the lungs are allowed to breathe in as much oxygen as possible. Deep-breathing exercises involve inhaling slowly and deeply through the nose, holding the breath for a few seconds, and then exhaling slowly through the mouth, pursing the lips as if trying to whistle.

Progressive Relaxation: This method of deep-muscle relaxation is based on the premise that the body responds to anxiety-provoking thoughts and events with muscle tension. Each muscle group is tensed for 5 to 7 seconds and then relaxed for 20 to 30 seconds, during which time the individual concentrates on the difference in sensations between the two conditions. Soft, slow background music may facilitate relaxation. A modified version of this technique (called passive progressive relaxation) involves relaxation of the muscles by concentrating on the feeling of relaxation within the muscle, rather than the actual tensing and relaxing of the muscle.

Meditation: The goal of meditation is to gain mastery over attention. It brings on a special state of consciousness as attention is concentrated solely on one thought or object. During meditation, as the individual becomes totally preoccupied with the selected focus, the respiration rate, heart rate, and blood pressure decrease. The overall metabolism declines, and the need for oxygen consumption is reduced.

Mental Imagery: Mental imagery uses the imagination in an effort to reduce the body's response to stress. The frame of reference is very personal, based on what each individual considers a relaxing environment. The relaxing scenario is most useful when taped and played back at a time when the individual wishes to achieve relaxation.

Biofeedback: Biofeedback is the use of instrumentation to become aware of processes in the body that usually go unnoticed and to help bring them under voluntary control. Biological conditions, such as muscle tension, skin surface temperature, blood pressure, and heart rate, are monitored by the biofeedback equipment. With special training, the individual learns to use relaxation and voluntary control to modify the biological condition, in turn indicating a modification of the autonomic function it represents. Biofeedback is often used together with other relaxation techniques such as deep breathing, progressive relaxation, and mental imagery.

■ ASSERTIVENESS TRAINING

Assertive behavior helps individuals feel better about themselves by encouraging them to stand up for their own basic human rights. These rights have equal representation for all individuals. But along with rights comes an equal number of responsibilities. Part of being assertive includes living up to these responsibilities.

Assertive behavior increases self-esteem and the ability to develop satisfying interpersonal relationships. This is accomplished through honesty, directness, appropriateness, and respecting one's own rights, as well as the rights of others.

Individuals develop patterns of responding in various ways, such as role modeling, by receiving positive or negative reinforcement, or by conscious choice. These patterns can take the form of nonassertiveness, assertiveness, aggressiveness, or passive-aggressiveness.

Nonassertive individuals seek to please others at the expense of denying their own basic human rights. *Assertive* individuals stand up for their own rights while protecting the rights of others. Those who respond *aggressively* defend their own rights by violating the basic rights of others. Individuals who respond in a *passive-aggressive* manner defend their own rights by expressing resistance to social and occupational demands.

Some important behavioral considerations of assertive behavior include eye contact, body posture, personal distance, physical contact, gestures, facial expression, voice, fluency, timing, listening, thoughts, and content. Various techniques have been developed to assist individuals in the process of becoming more assertive. Some of these include the following:

1. **Standing up for one's basic human rights.**
   Example: "I have the right to express my opinion."
2. **Assuming responsibility for one's own statements.**
   Example: "I *don't want* to go out with you tonight," instead of "I *can't* go out with you tonight." The latter implies a lack of power or ability.
3. **Responding as a "broken record."** Persistently repeating in a calm voice what is wanted.
   Example:

Telephone salesperson:	"I want to help you save money by changing long-distance services."
Assertive response:	"I don't want to change my long-distance service."
Telephone salesperson:	"I can't believe you don't want to save money!"
Assertive response:	"I don't want to change my long-distance service."

4. **Agreeing assertively.** Assertively accepting negative aspects about oneself. Admitting when an error has been made.
   Example:
   Ms. Jones: "You sure let that meeting get out of hand. What a waste of time."
   Ms. Smith: "Yes, I didn't do a very good job of conducting the meeting today."

5. **Inquiring assertively.** Seeking additional information about critical statements.
   Example:
   Male board member: "You made a real fool of yourself at the board meeting last night."
   Female board member: "Oh, really? Just what about my behavior offended you?"
   Male board member: "You were so damned pushy!"
   Female board member: "Were you offended that I spoke up for my beliefs, or was it because my beliefs are in direct opposition to yours?"

6. **Shifting from content to process.** Changing the focus of the communication from discussing the topic at hand to analyzing what is actually going on in the interaction.
   Example:
   Wife: "Would you please call me if you will be late for dinner?"
   Husband: "Why don't you just get off my back! I always have to account for every minute of my time with you!"
   Wife: "Sounds to me like we need to discuss some other things here. What are you *really* angry about?"

7. **Clouding/fogging.** Concurring with the critic's argument without becoming defensive and without agreeing to change.
   Example:
   Nurse No. 1: "You make so many mistakes. I don't know how you ever got this job!"
   Nurse No. 2: "You're right. I have made some mistakes since I started this job."

8. **Defusing.** Putting off further discussion with an angry individual until he or she is calmer.
   Example: "You are very angry right now. I don't want to discuss this matter with you while you are so upset. I will discuss it with you in my office at 3 o'clock this afternoon."

9. **Delaying assertively.** Putting off further discussion with another individual until one is calmer.
   Example: "That's a very challenging position you have taken, Mr. Brown. I'll need time to give it some thought. I'll call you later this afternoon."

10. **Responding assertively with irony.**
    Example:
    Man: "I bet you're one of them so-called 'women's libbers,' aren't you?"
    Woman: "Yes, thank you for noticing."

11. **Using "I" statements.**
    "I" statements allow an individual to take ownership for his or her feelings rather than saying they are caused by another person. "I" statements are sometimes called "feeling" statements. They express directly what an individual is feeling. "You" statements are accusatory and put the receiver on the defensive. "I" statements have four parts:
    a. How I feel: *these are my feelings and I accept ownership of them.*
    b. When: *describe in a neutral manner the behavior that is the problem.*
    c. Why: *describe what it is about the behavior that is objectionable.*
    d. Suggest change: *offer a preferred alternative to the behavior.*
    Example:
    John has just returned from a hunting trip and walked into the living room in his muddy boots leaving a trail of mud on the carpet. His wife, Mary, may respond as follows:
    With a "you" statement: "You are such a jerk! Can't you see the trail of mud you are leaving on the carpet? I just cleaned this carpet. You make me so angry!"
    With an "I" statement: "I feel so angry when you walk on the carpet in your muddy boots. I just cleaned it, and now I will have to clean it again. I would appreciate it if you would remove your boots on the porch before you come in the house."

    "You" statements are negative and focus on what the person has done wrong. They don't explain what is being requested of the person. "I" statements are more positive. They explain *how* one is feeling, *why* he or she is feeling that way, and *what* the individual wants instead.

■ COGNITIVE THERAPY

Cognitive therapy, developed by Aaron Beck, is commonly used in the treatment of mood disorders. In cognitive therapy, the individual is taught to control thought distortions that are considered to be a factor in the development and maintenance of mood disorders. In the cognitive model, depression is characterized by a triad of negative distortions related to expectations of the environment, self, and future. The environment and activities within it are viewed as unsatisfying, the self is unrealistically devalued, and the future is perceived as hopeless. In the same model, mania is characterized by a positive cognitive triad—the self is seen as highly valued and powerful, experiences within the environment are viewed as overly positive, and the future is seen as one of unlimited opportunity.

The general goals in cognitive therapy are to obtain symptom relief as quickly as possible, to assist the client in identifying dysfunctional patterns of thinking and behaving, and to guide the client to evidence and logic that effectively test the validity of the dysfunctional thinking. Therapy focuses on changing "automatic thoughts" that occur spontaneously and contribute to the distorted affect. Examples of "automatic thoughts" in depression include the following:

1. **Personalizing**: "I'm the only one who failed."
2. **All or nothing**: "I'm a complete failure."
3. **Mind reading**: "He thinks I'm foolish."
4. **Discounting positives**: "The other questions were so easy. Any dummy could have gotten them right."

Examples of "automatic thoughts" in mania include the following:

1. **Personalizing**: "She's this happy only when she's with me."
2. **All or nothing**: "Everything I do is great."
3. **Mind reading**: "She thinks I'm wonderful."
4. **Discounting negatives**: "None of those mistakes are really important."

The client is asked to describe evidence that both supports and disputes the automatic thought. The logic underlying the inferences is then reviewed with the client. Another technique involves evaluating what would most likely happen if the client's automatic thoughts were true. Implications of the consequences are then discussed.

Clients should not become discouraged if one technique seems not to be working. There is no single technique that works with all clients. He or she should be reassured that there are a number of techniques that may be used, and both therapist and client may explore these possibilities. Cognitive therapy has been shown to be an effective treatment for mood disorders, particularly in conjunction with psychopharmacological intervention.

Electroconvulsive Therapy

■ DEFINED

Electroconvulsive therapy (ECT) is a type of somatic treatment in which electric current is applied to the brain through electrodes placed on the temples. The current is sufficient to induce a grand mal seizure, from which the desired therapeutic effect is achieved.

■ INDICATIONS

ECT is primarily used in the treatment of severe depression. It is sometimes administered in conjunction with antidepressant medication, but most physicians prefer to perform this treatment only after an unsuccessful trial of drug therapy.

ECT may also be used as a fast-acting treatment for very hyperactive manic clients in danger of physical exhaustion and for individuals who are extremely suicidal.

ECT was originally attempted in the treatment of schizophrenia but with little success in most instances. There has been evidence, however, of its effectiveness in the treatment of acute schizophrenia, particularly if it is accompanied by catatonic or affective (depression or mania) symptomatology (Black & Andreasen, 2011).

■ CONTRAINDICATIONS

ECT should not be used if there is increased intracranial pressure (from brain tumor, recent cardiovascular accident, or other cerebrovascular lesion). Other conditions, although not considered absolute contraindications, may render clients at high risk for the treatment. They are largely cardiovascular in nature and include myocardial infarction or cerebrovascular accident within the preceding 3 to 6 months, aortic or cerebral aneurysm, severe underlying hypertension, and congestive heart failure.

■ MECHANISM OF ACTION

The exact mechanism of action is unknown. However, it is thought that ECT produces biochemical changes in the brain—an increase in the levels of norepinephrine, serotonin, and dopamine—similar to the effects of antidepressant medications. One recent study

573

revealed that the therapeutic response from ECT may be related to the modulation of white matter microstructure in pathways connecting frontal and limbic areas, which are altered in major depression (Lyden, et al., 2014). The results of studies relating to the mechanism underlying the effectiveness of ECT are still ongoing and continue to be controversial.

■ SIDE EFFECTS AND NURSING IMPLICATIONS
Temporary Memory Loss and Confusion

* These are the most common side effects of ECT. It is important for the nurse to be present when the client awakens in order to alleviate the fears that accompany this loss of memory.
* Provide reassurance that memory loss is only temporary.
* Describe to the client what has occurred.
* Reorient the client to time and place.
* Allow the client to verbalize fears and anxieties related to receiving ECT.
* To minimize confusion, provide a good deal of structure for the client's routine activities.

■ RISKS ASSOCIATED WITH ECT

1. **Mortality**. The mortality rate from ECT is about 2 per 100,000 treatments (Marangell et al., 2003; Sadock & Sadock, 2007). The major cause is cardiovascular complications, such as acute myocardial infarction or cerebrovascular accident.
2. **Brain Damage.** Although the risk of brain damage is an area for continuing study, there is currently no evidence to substantiate that ECT produces any permanent changes in brain structure or functioning (McClintock & Husain, 2011).
3. **Permanent Memory Loss.** Most individuals report no problems with their memory, aside from the time immediately surrounding the ECT treatments. However, some clients have reported retrograde amnesia extending back to months before treatment. In rare instances, more extensive amnesia has occurred, resulting in memory gaps dating back years (Joska & Stein, 2008). They report gaps in recollections of specific personal memories. Black and Andreasen (2011) suggest that all clients receiving ECT should be informed of the possibility for some degree of permanent memory loss.

Although the potential for these effects appears to be minimal, the client must be made aware of the risks involved before consenting to treatment.

■ POTENTIAL NURSING DIAGNOSES ASSOCIATED WITH ECT

1. Risk for injury related to risks associated with ECT.
2. Risk for aspiration related to altered level of consciousness immediately following treatment.

3. Decreased cardiac output related to vagal stimulation occurring during the ECT.
4. Impaired memory/acute confusion related to side effects of ECT.
5. Deficient knowledge related to necessity for and side effects and risks of ECT.
6. Anxiety (moderate to severe) related to impending therapy.
7. Self-care deficit related to incapacitation during postictal stage.
8. Risk for activity intolerance related to post-ECT confusion and memory loss.

■ NURSING INTERVENTIONS FOR CLIENT RECEIVING ECT

1. Ensure that the physician has obtained informed consent and that a signed permission form is on the chart.
2. Ensure that the most recent laboratory reports (complete blood count [CBC], urinalysis) and results of electrocardiogram (ECG) and x-ray examination are available.
3. Client should receive nothing by mouth (NPO) on the morning of the treatment.
4. Prior to the treatment, client should void, dress in night clothes (or other loose clothing), and remove dentures and eyeglasses or contact lenses. Bedrails should be raised.
5. Take baseline vital signs and blood pressure.
6. Administer cholinergic blocking agent (e.g., atropine sulfate, glycopyrrolate) approximately 30 minutes before treatment, as ordered by the physician, to decrease secretions (to prevent aspiration) and increase heart rate (which is suppressed in response to vagal stimulation caused by the ECT).
7. Assist physician and/or anesthesiologist as necessary in the administration of intravenous medications. A short-acting anesthetic, such as methohexital sodium (Brevital sodium), is given along with the muscle relaxant succinylcholine chloride (Anectine).
8. Administer oxygen and provide suctioning as required.
9. After the procedure, take vital signs and blood pressure every 15 minutes for the first hour. Position the client on his or her side to prevent aspiration.
10. Stay with the client until he or she is fully awake, oriented, and able to perform self-care activities without assistance.
11. Describe to the client what has occurred.
12. Allow the client to verbalize fears and anxieties associated with the treatment.
13. Reassure the client that memory loss and confusion are only temporary.
14. Provide the client with a highly structured schedule of routine activities in order to minimize confusion.

APPENDIX **H**

Medication Assessment Tool

Date _____ Client's Name _____ Age _____

Marital Status _____ Children _____

Occupation _____

Presenting Symptoms (subjective & objective) _____

_____

Diagnosis (*DSM-5*) _____

Current Vital Signs: Blood Pressure: Sitting ___/___; Standing ___/___; Pulse _____; Respirations _____

Height _____ Weight _____

CURRENT/PAST USE OF PRESCRIPTION DRUGS (Indicate with "c" or "p" beside name of drug whether current or past use):

Name	Dosage	How Long Used	Why Prescribed	By Whom	Side Effects/Results

CURRENT/PAST USE OF OVER-THE-COUNTER DRUGS (Indicate with "c" or "p" beside name of drug whether current or past use):

Name	Dosage	How Long Used	Why Prescribed	By Whom	Side Effects/Results
___	___	___	___	___	___
___	___	___	___	___	___
___	___	___	___	___	___

CURRENT/PAST USE OF STREET DRUGS, ALCOHOL, NICOTINE, AND/OR CAFFEINE (Indicate with "c" or "p" beside name of drug):

Name	Amount Used	How Often Used	When Last Used	Effects Produced
___	___	___	___	___
___	___	___	___	___
___	___	___	___	___

Any allergies to food or drugs? _____

Any special diet considerations? _____

Do you have (or have you ever had) any of the following? If yes, provide explanation on the back of this sheet.

	Yes	No		Yes	No
1. Difficulty swallowing			13. Blood clots/pain in legs		
2. Delayed wound healing			14. Fainting spells		
3. Constipation problems			15. Swollen ankles/legs/hands		
4. Urination problems			16. Asthma		
5. Recent change in elimination patterns			17. Varicose veins		
6. Weakness or tremors			18. Numbness/tingling (location?)		
7. Seizures			19. Ulcers		
8. Headaches			20. Nausea/vomiting		
9. Dizziness			21. Problems with diarrhea		
10. High blood pressure			22. Shortness of breath		
11. Palpitations			23. Sexual dysfunction		
12. Chest pain			24. Lumps in your breasts		
			25. Blurred or double vision		
			26. Ringing in the ears		
			27. Insomnia		
			28. Skin Rashes		
			29. Diabetes		
			30. Hepatitis (or other liver disease)		
			31. Kidney disease		
			32. Glaucoma		

Are you pregnant or breast feeding? _____ Date of last menses _____ Type of contraception used _____

Describe any restrictions/limitations that might interfere with your use of medication for your current problem. _____

Prescription orders: _____

Patient teaching related to medications prescribed: _____

Lab work or referrals prescribed: _____

Nurse's signature _____

Client's signature _____

Cultural Assessment Tool

Client's name _____ Ethnic origin _____

Address _____ Birthdate _____

Name of significant other _____ Relationship _____

Primary language spoken _____

Second language spoken _____

How does client usually communicate with people who speak a different
language? _____

Is an interpreter required? _____

Available? _____

Highest level of education achieved: _____

Occupation: _____

Presenting problem: _____

_____

Has this problem ever occurred before? _____

If so, in what manner was it handled previously? _____

_____

What is the client's usual manner of coping with stress? _____

_____

Who is (are) the client's main support system(s)? _____

_____

Describe the family living arrangements: _____

_____

Who is the major decision maker in the family? _____

Describe client's/family members' roles within the family. _____

_____

_____

Describe religious beliefs and practices: _____

_____

Are there any religious requirements/restrictions that place limitations on the
client's care? _____

If so, describe: _____

_____

Who in the family takes responsibility for health concerns?

_____

Describe any special health beliefs and practices: _____

_____

_____

From whom does family usually seek medical assistance in time of need?

_____

Describe client's usual emotional/behavioral response to: _____
Anxiety: _____
Anger: _____
Loss/change/failure: _____
Pain: _____
Fear: _____

Describe any topics that are particularly sensitive or that the client is unwilling to discuss (because of cultural taboos): _____

_____

_____

Describe any activities in which the client is unwilling to participate (because of cultural customs or taboos): _____

_____

_____

What are the client's personal feelings regarding touch? _____
What are the client's personal feelings regarding eye contact?

_____

What is the client's personal orientation to time? (past, present, future)

_____

Describe any particular illnesses to which the client may be bioculturally susceptible (e.g., hypertension and sickle cell anemia in African Americans):

_____

_____

Describe any nutritional deficiencies to which the client may be bioculturally susceptible (e.g., lactose intolerance in Native and Asian Americans)

_____

_____

Describe client's favorite foods: _____

_____

Are there any foods the client requests or refuses because of cultural beliefs related to this illness (e.g., "hot" and "cold" foods for Latino Americans and Asian Americans)? If so, please describe: _____

_____

Describe client's perception of the problem and expectations of health care:

_____

_____

DSM-5 Classification*

ICD-9-CM codes are provided, followed by ICD-10-CM codes in parentheses.

■ NEURODEVELOPMENTAL DISORDERS

Intellectual Disabilities

319	(__.__)	Intellectual Disability (Intellectual Developmental Disorder)
		Specify current severity:
317	(70)	Mild
318.0	(71)	Moderate
318.1	(72)	Severe
318.2	(73)	Profound
315.8	(F88)	Global Developmental Delay
319	(F79)	Unspecified Intellectual Disability (Intellectual Developmental Disorder)

Communication Disorders

315.39	(F80.9)	Language Disorder
315.39	(F80.0)	Speech Sound Disorder
315.35	(F80.81)	Childhood-Onset Fluency Disorder (Stuttering)
		Note: Later-onset cases are diagnosed as 307.0 (F98.5) adult-onset fluency disorder.
315.39	(F80.89)	Social (Pragmatic) Communication Disorder
307.9	(F80.9)	Unspecified Communication Disorder

Autism Spectrum Disorder

299.00	(F84.0)	Autism Spectrum Disorder
		Specify if: Associated with a known medical or genetic condition or environmental factor; Associated with another neurodevelopmental, mental, or behavioral disorder
		Specify current severity for Criterion A and Criterion B: Requiring very substantial support, Requiring substantial support, Requiring support

Specify if: With or without accompanying intellectual impairment, With or without accompanying language impairment, With catatonia (use additional code 293.89 [F06.1])

Attention-Deficit/Hyperactivity Disorder

___.__	(___.__)	Attention-Deficit/Hyperactivity Disorder
		Specify whether:
314.01	(F90.2)	Combined presentation
314.00	(F90.0)	Predominantly inattentive presentation
314.01	(F90.1)	Predominantly hyperactive/impulsive presentation
		Specify if: In partial remission
		Specify current severity: Mild, Moderate, Severe
314.01	(F90.8)	Other Specified Attention-Deficit/Hyperactivity Disorder
314.01	(F90.9)	Unspecified Attention-Deficit/Hyperactivity Disorder

Specific Learning Disorder

___.__	(___.__)	Specific Learning Disorder
		Specify if:
315.00	(F81.0)	With impairment in reading (*specify* if with word reading accuracy, reading rate or fluency, reading comprehension)
315.2	(F81.81)	With impairment in written expression (*specify* if with spelling accuracy, grammar and punctuation accuracy, clarity or organization of written expression)
315.1	(F81.2)	With impairment in mathematics (*specify* if with number sense, memorization of arithmetic facts, accurate or fluent calculation, accurate math reasoning)
		Specify current severity: Mild, Moderate, Severe

Motor Disorders

315.4	(F82)	Developmental Coordination Disorder
307.3	(F98.4)	Stereotypic Movement Disorder
		Specify if: With self-injurious behavior, Without self-injurious behavior
		Specify if: Associated with a known medical or genetic condition, neurodevelopmental disorder, or environmental factor
		Specify current severity: Mild, Moderate, Severe

Tic Disorders

307.23	(F95.2)	Tourette's Disorder
307.22	(F95.1)	Persistent (Chronic) Motor or Vocal Tic Disorder
		Specify if: With motor tics only, With vocal tics only

307.21	(F95.0)	Provisional Tic Disorder
307.20	(F95.8)	Other Specified Tic Disorder
307.20	(F95.9)	Unspecified Tic Disorder

Other Neurodevelopmental Disorders

| 315.8 | (F88) | Other Specified Neurodevelopmental Disorder |
| 315.9 | (F89) | Unspecified Neurodevelopmental Disorder |

■ SCHIZOPHRENIA SPECTRUM AND OTHER PSYCHOTIC DISORDERS

The following specifiers apply to Schizophrenia Spectrum and Other Psychotic Disorders where indicated:

[a] *Specify* if: The following course specifiers are only to be used after a 1-year duration of the disorder: First episode, currently in acute episode; First episode, currently in partial remission; First episode, currently in full remission; Multiple episodes, currently in acute episode; Multiple episodes, currently in partial remission; Multiple episodes, currently in full remission; Continuous; Unspecified

[b] *Specify* if: With catatonia (use additional code 293.89 [F06.1])

[c] *Specify* current severity of delusions, hallucinations, disorganized speech, abnormal psychomotor behavior, negative symptoms, impaired cognition, depression, and mania symptoms

301.22	(F21)	Schizotypal (Personality) Disorder
297.1	(F22)	Delusional Disorder[a, c]
		Specify whether: Erotomanic type, Grandiose type, Jealous type, Persecutory type, Somatic type, Mixed type, Unspecified type
		Specify if: With bizarre content
298.8	(F23)	Brief Psychotic Disorder[b, c]
		Specify if: With marked stressor(s), Without marked stressor(s), With postpartum onset
295.40	(F20.81)	Schizophreniform Disorder[b, c]
		Specify if: With good prognostic features, Without good prognostic features
295.90	(F20.9)	Schizophrenia[a, b, c]
__.__	(__.__)	Schizoaffective Disorder[a, b, c]
		Specify whether:
295.70	(F25.0)	Bipolar type
295.70	(F25.1)	Depressive type
__.__	(__.__)	Substance/Medication-Induced Psychotic Disorder[c]
		Note: See the criteria set and corresponding recording procedures for substance- specific codes and ICD-9-CM and ICD-10-CM coding.
		Specify if: With onset during intoxication, With onset during withdrawal

___.___	(___.___)	Psychotic Disorder Due to Another Medical Condition[c]
		Specify whether:
293.81	(F06.2)	With delusions
293.82	(F06.0)	With hallucinations
293.89	(F06.1)	Catatonia Associated With Another Mental Disorder (Catatonia Specifier)
293.89	(F06.1)	Catatonic Disorder Due to Another Medical Condition
293.89	(F06.1)	Unspecified Catatonia
		Note: Code first 781.99 (R29.818) other symptoms involving nervous and musculoskeletal systems.
298.8	(F28)	Other Specified Schizophrenia Spectrum and Other Psychotic Disorder
298.9	(F29)	Unspecified Schizophrenia Spectrum and Other Psychotic Disorder

---

■ BIPOLAR AND RELATED DISORDERS

The following specifiers apply to Bipolar and Related Disorders where indicated:

[a] *Specify*: With anxious distress (*specify* current severity: mild, moderate, moderate-severe, severe); With mixed features; With rapid cycling; With melancholic features; With atypical features; With mood-congruent psychotic features; With mood-incongruent psychotic features; With catatonia (use additional code 293.89 [F06.1]); With peripartum onset; With seasonal pattern

___.___	(___.___)	Bipolar I Disorder[a]
___.___	(___.___)	Current or most recent episode manic
296.41	(F31.11)	Mild
296.42	(F31.12)	Moderate
296.43	(F31.13)	Severe
296.44	(F31.2)	With psychotic features
296.45	(F31.73)	In partial remission
296.46	(F31.74)	In full remission
296.40	(F31.9)	Unspecified
296.40	(F31.0)	Current or most recent episode hypomanic
296.45	(F31.73)	In partial remission
296.46	(F31.74)	In full remission
296.40	(F31.9)	Unspecified
___.___	(___.___)	Current or most recent episode depressed
296.51	(F31.31)	Mild
296.52	(F31.32)	Moderate
296.53	(F31.4)	Severe
296.54	(F31.5)	With psychotic features
296.55	(F31.75)	In partial remission
296.56	(F31.76)	In full remission
296.50	(F31.9)	Unspecified
296.7	(F31.9)	Current or most recent episode unspecified

296.89	(F31.81)	Bipolar II Disorder[a]
		Specify current or most recent episode: Hypomanic, Depressed
		Specify course if full criteria for a mood episode are not currently met: In partial remission, In full remission
		Specify severity if full criteria for a mood episode are not currently met: Mild, Moderate, Severe
301.13	(F34.0)	Cyclothymic Disorder
		Specify if: With anxious distress
___.__	(___.__)	Substance/Medication-Induced Bipolar and Related Disorder
		Note: See the criteria set and corresponding recording procedures for substance-specific codes and ICD-9-CM and ICD-10-CM coding.
		Specify if: With onset during intoxication, With onset during withdrawal
293.83	(___.__)	Bipolar and Related Disorder Due to Another Medical Condition
		Specify if:
	(F06.33)	With manic features
	(F06.33)	With manic- or hypomanic-like episode
	(F06.34)	With mixed features
296.89	(F31.89)	Other Specified Bipolar and Related Disorder
296.80	(F31.9)	Unspecified Bipolar and Related Disorder

■ DEPRESSIVE DISORDERS

The following specifiers apply to Depressive Disorders where indicated:

> [a] *Specify*: With anxious distress (*specify* current severity: mild, moderate, moderate-severe, severe); With mixed features; With melancholic features; With atypical features; With mood-congruent psychotic features; With mood-incongruent psychotic features; With catatonia (use additional code 293.89 [F06.1]); With peripartum onset; With seasonal pattern

296.99	(F34.8)	Disruptive Mood Dysregulation Disorder
___.__	(___.__)	Major Depressive Disorder[a]
___.__	(___.__)	Single episode
296.21	(F32.0)	Mild
296.22	(F32.1)	Moderate
296.23	(F32.2)	Severe
296.24	(F32.3)	With psychotic features
296.25	(F32.4)	In partial remission
296.26	(F32.5)	In full remission
296.20	(F32.9)	Unspecified
___.__	(___.__)	Recurrent episode
296.31	(F33.0)	Mild
296.32	(F33.1)	Moderate

296.33	(F33.2)	Severe
296.34	(F33.3)	With psychotic features
296.35	(F33.41)	In partial remission
296.36	(F33.42)	In full remission
296.30	(F33.9)	Unspecified
300.4	(F34.1)	Persistent Depressive Disorder (Dysthymia)a
		Specify if: In partial remission, In full remission
		Specify if: Early onset, Late onset
		Specify if: With pure dysthymic syndrome; With persistent major depressive episode; With intermittent major depressive episodes, with current episode; With intermittent major depressive episodes, without current episode
		Specify current severity: Mild, Moderate, Severe
625.4	(N94.3)	Premenstrual Dysphoric Disorder
___.___	(___.___)	Substance/Medication-Induced Depressive Disorder
		Note: See the criteria set and corresponding recording procedures for substance-specific codes and ICD-9-CM and ICD-10-CM coding.
		Specify if: With onset during intoxication, With onset during withdrawal
293.83	(___.___)	Depressive Disorder Due to Another Medical Condition
		Specify if:
	(F06.31)	With depressive features
	(F06.32)	With major depressive-like episode
	(F06.34)	With mixed features
311	(F32.8)	Other Specified Depressive Disorder
311	(F32.9)	Unspecified Depressive Disorder

■ ANXIETY DISORDERS

309.21	(F93.0)	Separation Anxiety Disorder
312.23	(F94.0)	Selective Mutism
300.29	(___.___)	Specific Phobia
		Specify if:
	(F40.218)	Animal
	(F40.228)	Natural environment
	(___.___)	Blood-injection injury
	(F40.230)	Fear of blood
	(F40.231)	Fear of injections and transfusions
	(F40.232)	Fear of other medical care
	(F40.233)	Fear of injury
	(F40.248)	Situational
	(F40.298)	Other
300.23	(F40.10)	Social Anxiety Disorder (Social Phobia)
		Specify if: Performance only
300.01	(F41.0)	Panic Disorder
___.___	(___.___)	Panic Attack Specifier

300.22	(F40.00)	Agoraphobia
300.02	(F41.1)	Generalized Anxiety Disorder
__.__	(__.__)	Substance/Medication-Induced Anxiety Disorder
		Note: See the criteria set and corresponding recording procedures for substance-specific codes and ICD-9-CM and ICD-10-CM coding.
		Specify if: With onset during intoxication, With onset during withdrawal, With onset after medication use
293.84	(F06.4)	Anxiety Disorder Due to Another Medical Condition
300.00	(F41.9)	Unspecified Anxiety Disorder

■ OBSESSIVE-COMPULSIVE AND RELATED DISORDERS

The following specifier applies to Obsessive-Compulsive and Related Disorders where indicated:

a *Specify* if: With good or fair insight, With poor insight, With absent insight/delusional beliefs

300.3	(F42)	Obsessive-Compulsive Disorder^a
		Specify if: Tic-related
300.7	(F45.22)	Body Dysmorphic Disorder^a
		Specify if: With muscle dysmorphia
300.3	(F42)	Hoarding Disorder^a
		Specify if: With excessive acquisition
312.39	(F63.3)	Trichotillomania (Hair-Pulling Disorder)
698.4	(L98.1)	Excoriation (Skin-Picking) Disorder
__.__	(__.__)	Substance/Medication-Induced Obsessive-Compulsive and Related Disorder
		Note: See the criteria set and corresponding recording procedures for substance-specific codes and ICD-9-CM and ICD-10-CM coding.
		Specify if: With onset during intoxication, With onset during withdrawal, With onset after medication use
294.8	(F06.8)	Obsessive-Compulsive and Related Disorder Due to Another Medical Condition
		Specify if: With obsessive-compulsive disorder-like symptoms, With appearance preoccupations, With hoarding symptoms, With hair-pulling symptoms, With skin-picking symptoms
300.3	(F42)	Other Specified Obsessive-Compulsive and Related Disorder
300.3	(F42)	Unspecified Obsessive-Compulsive and Related Disorder

■ TRAUMA- AND STRESSOR-RELATED DISORDERS

313.89	(F94.1)	Reactive Attachment Disorder
		Specify if: Persistent
		Specify current severity: Severe
313.89	(F94.2)	Disinhibited Social Engagement Disorder
		Specify if: Persistent
		Specify current severity: Severe
309.81	(F43.10)	Posttraumatic Stress Disorder (includes Post-traumatic Stress Disorder for Children 6 Years and Younger)
		Specify whether: With dissociative symptoms
		Specify if: With delayed expression
308.3	(F43.0)	Acute Stress Disorder
__.__	(__.__)	Adjustment Disorders
		Specify whether:
309.0	(F43.21)	With depressed mood
309.24	(F43.22)	With anxiety
309.28	(F43.23)	With mixed anxiety and depressed mood
309.3	(F43.24)	With disturbance of conduct
309.4	(F43.25)	With mixed disturbance of emotions and conduct
309.9	(F43.20)	Unspecified
309.89	(F43.8)	Other Specified Trauma- and Stressor-Related Disorder
309.9	(F43.9)	Unspecified Trauma- and Stressor-Related Disorder

■ DISSOCIATIVE DISORDERS

300.14	(F44.81)	Dissociative Identity Disorder
300.12	(F44.0)	Dissociative Amnesia
		Specify if:
300.13	(F44.1)	With dissociative fugue
300.6	(F48.1)	Depersonalization/Derealization Disorder
300.15	(F44.89)	Other Specified Dissociative Disorder
300.15	(F44.9)	Unspecified Dissociative Disorder

■ SOMATIC SYMPTOM AND RELATED DISORDERS

300.82	(F45.1)	Somatic Symptom Disorder
		Specify if: With predominant pain
		Specify if: Persistent
		Specify current severity: Mild, Moderate, Severe
300.7	(F45.21)	Illness Anxiety Disorder
		Specify whether: Care seeking type, Care avoidant type
300.11	(__.__)	Conversion Disorder (Functional Neurological Symptom Disorder)
		Specify symptom type:
	(F44.4)	With weakness or paralysis
	(F44.4)	With abnormal movement

	(F44.4)	With swallowing symptoms
	(F44.4)	With speech symptom
	(F44.5)	With attacks or seizures
	(F44.6)	With anesthesia or sensory loss
	(F44.6)	With special sensory symptom
	(F44.7)	With mixed symptoms
		Specify if: Acute episode, Persistent
		Specify if: With psychological stressor (specify stressor), Without psychological stressor
316	(F54)	Psychological Factors Affecting Other Medical Conditions
		Specify current severity: Mild, Moderate, Severe, Extreme
300.19	(F68.10)	Factitious Disorder (includes Factitious Disorder Imposed on Self, Factitious Disorder Imposed on Another)
		Specify Single episode, Recurrent episodes
300.89	(F45.8)	Other Specified Somatic Symptom and Related Disorder
300.82	(F45.9)	Unspecified Somatic Symptom and Related Disorder

■ FEEDING AND EATING DISORDERS

The following specifiers apply to Feeding and Eating Disorders where indicated:

  a *Specify* if: In remission
  b *Specify* if: In partial remission, In full remission
  c *Specify* current severity: Mild, Moderate, Severe, Extreme

307.52	(___.__)	Pica[a]
	(F98.3)	In children
	(F50.8)	In adults
307.53	(F98.21)	Rumination Disorder[a]
307.59	(F50.8)	Avoidant/Restrictive Food Intake Disorder[a]
307.1	(___.__)	Anorexia Nervosa[b, c]
		Specify whether:
	(F50.01)	Restricting type
	(F50.02)	Binge-eating/purging type
307.51	(F50.2)	Bulimia Nervosa[b, c]
307.51	(F50.8)	Binge-Eating Disorder[b, c]
307.59	(F50.8)	Other Specified Feeding or Eating Disorder
307.50	(F50.9)	Unspecified Feeding or Eating Disorder

■ ELIMINATION DISORDERS

307.6	(F98.0)	Enuresis
		Specify whether: Nocturnal only, Diurnal only, Nocturnal and diurnal
307.7	(F98.1)	Encopresis
		Specify whether: With constipation and overflow incontinence, Without constipation and overflow incontinence

__.__	(__.__)	Other Specified Elimination Disorder
788.39	(N39.498)	With urinary symptoms
787.60	(R15.9)	With fecal symptoms
__.__	(__.__)	Unspecified Elimination Disorder
788.30	(R32)	With urinary symptoms
787.60	(R15.9)	With fecal symptoms

■ SLEEP-WAKE DISORDERS

The following specifiers apply to Sleep-Wake Disorders where indicated:

[a] *Specify* if: Episodic, Persistent, Recurrent
[b] *Specify* if: Acute, Subacute, Persistent
[c] *Specify* current severity: Mild, Moderate, Severe

780.52	(G47.00)	Insomnia Disorder[a]
		Specify if: With nonsleep disorder mental co-morbidity, With other medical comorbidity, With other sleep disorder
780.54	(G47.10)	Hypersomnolence Disorder[b, c]
		Specify if: With mental disorder, With medical condition, With another sleep disorder
__.__	(__.__)	Narcolepsy[c]
		Specify whether:
347.00	(G47.419)	Narcolepsy without cataplexy but with hypocretin deficiency
347.01	(G47.411)	Narcolepsy with cataplexy but without hypocretin deficiency
347.00	(G47.419)	Autosomal dominant cerebellar ataxia, deafness, and narcolepsy
347.00	(G47.419)	Autosomal dominant narcolepsy, obesity, and type 2 diabetes
347.10	(G47.429)	Narcolepsy secondary to another medical condition

■ Breathing-Related Sleep Disorders

327.23	(G47.33)	Obstructive Sleep Apnea Hypopnea[c]
__.__	(__.__)	Central Sleep Apnea
		Specify whether:
327.21	(G47.31)	Idiopathic central sleep apnea
786.04	(R06.3)	Cheyne-Stokes breathing
780.57	(G47.37)	Central sleep apnea comorbid with opioid use
		Note: First code opioid use disorder, if present.
		Specify current severity
__.__	(__.__)	Sleep-Related Hypoventilation
		Specify whether:
327.24	(G47.34)	Idiopathic hypoventilation
327.25	(G47.35)	Congenital central alveolar hypoventilation
327.26	(G47.36)	Comorbid sleep-related hypoventilation
		Specify current severity
__.__	(__.__)	Circadian Rhythm Sleep-Wake Disorders[a]
		Specify whether:

307.45	(G47.21)	Delayed sleep phase type
		Specify if: Familial, Overlapping with non-24-hour sleep-wake type
307.45	(G47.22)	Advanced sleep phase type
		Specify if: Familial
307.45	(G47.23)	Irregular sleep-wake type
307.45	(G47.24)	Non-24-hour sleep-wake type
307.45	(G47.26)	Shift work type
307.45	(G47.20)	Unspecified type

■ Parasomnias

__.__	(__.__)	Nonrapid Eye Movement Sleep Arousal Disorders
		Specify whether:
307.46	(F51.3)	Sleepwalking type
		Specify if: With sleep-related eating, With sleep-related sexual behavior (sexsomnia)
307.46	(F51.4)	Sleep terror type
307.47	(F51.5)	Nightmare Disorder[b, c]
		Specify if: During sleep onset
		Specify if: With associated nonsleep disorder, With associated other medical condition, With associated other sleep disorder
327.42	(G47.52)	Rapid Eye Movement Sleep Behavior Disorder
333.94	(G25.81)	Restless Legs Syndrome
__.__	(__.__)	Substance/Medication-Induced Sleep Disorder
		Note: See the criteria set and corresponding recording procedures for substance-specific codes and ICD-9-CM and ICD-10-CM coding.
		Specify whether: Insomnia type, Daytime sleepiness type, Parasomnia type, Mixed type
		Specify if: With onset during intoxication, With onset during discontinuation/withdrawal
780.52	(G47.09)	Other Specified Insomnia Disorder
780.52	(G47.00)	Unspecified Insomnia Disorder
780.54	(G47.19)	Other Specified Hypersomnolence Disorder
780.54	(G47.10)	Unspecified Hypersomnolence Disorder
780.59	(G47.8)	Other Specified Sleep-Wake Disorder
780.59	(G47.9)	Unspecified Sleep-Wake Disorder

■ SEXUAL DYSFUNCTIONS

The following specifiers apply to Sexual Dysfunctions where indicated:

   [a] *Specify* whether: Lifelong, Acquired
   [b] *Specify* whether: Generalized, Situational
   [c] *Specify* current severity: Mild, Moderate, Severe

| 302.74 | (F52.32) | Delayed Ejaculation[a, b, c] |
| 302.72 | (F52.21) | Erectile Disorder[a, b, c] |

302.73	(F52.31)	Female Orgasmic Disorder[a, b, c]
		Specify if: Never experienced an orgasm under any situation
302.72	(F52.22)	Female Sexual Interest/Arousal Disorder[a, b, c]
302.76	(F52.6)	Genito-Pelvic Pain/Penetration Disorder[a, c]
302.71	(F52.0)	Male Hypoactive Sexual Desire Disorder[a, b, c]
302.75	(F52.4)	Premature (Early) Ejaculation[a, b, c]
___.__	(___.__)	Substance/Medication-Induced Sexual Dysfunction[c]
		Note: See the criteria set and corresponding recording procedures for substance-specific codes and ICD-9-CM and ICD-10-CM coding.
		Specify if: With onset during intoxication, With onset during withdrawal, With onset after medication use
302.79	(F52.8)	Other Specified Sexual Dysfunction
302.70	(F52.9)	Unspecified Sexual Dysfunction

■ GENDER DYSPHORIA

___.__	(___.__)	Gender Dysphoria
302.6	(F64.2)	Gender Dysphoria in Children
		Specify if: With a disorder of sex development
302.85	(F64.1)	Gender Dysphoria in Adolescents and Adults
		Specify if: With a disorder of sex development
		Specify if: Posttransition
		Note: Code the disorder of sex development if present, in addition to gender dysphoria.
302.6	(F64.8)	Other Specified Gender Dysphoria
302.6	(F64.9)	Unspecified Gender Dysphoria

■ DISRUPTIVE, IMPULSE-CONTROL, AND CONDUCT DISORDERS

313.81	(F91.3)	Oppositional Defiant Disorder
		Specify current severity: Mild, Moderate, Severe
312.34	(F63.81)	Intermittent Explosive Disorder
___.__	(___.__)	Conduct Disorder
		Specify whether:
312.81	(F91.1)	Childhood-onset type
312.82	(F91.2)	Adolescent-onset type
312.89	(F91.9)	Unspecified onset
		Specify if: With limited prosocial emotions
		Specify current severity: Mild, Moderate, Severe
301.7	(F60.2)	Antisocial Personality Disorder
312.33	(F63.1)	Pyromania
312.32	(F63.2)	Kleptomania
312.89	(F91.8)	Other Specified Disruptive, Impulse-Control, and Conduct Disorder
312.9	(F91.9)	Unspecified Disruptive, Impulse-Control, and Conduct Disorder

■ SUBSTANCE-RELATED AND ADDICTIVE DISORDERS

The following specifiers and note apply to Substance-Related and Addictive Disorders where indicated:

[a] *Specify* if: In early remission, In sustained remission
[b] *Specify* if: In a controlled environment
[c] *Specify* if: With perceptual disturbances
[d] The ICD-10-CM code indicates the comorbid presence of a moderate or severe substance use disorder, which must be present in order to apply the code for substance withdrawal.

Substance-Related Disorders

Alcohol-Related Disorders

___.__	(___.__)	Alcohol Use Disorder[a, b]
		Specify current severity:
305.00	(F10.10)	Mild
303.90	(F10.20)	Moderate
303.90	(F10.20)	Severe
303.00	(___.__)	Alcohol Intoxication
	(F10.129)	With use disorder, mild
	(F10.229)	With use disorder, moderate or severe
	(F10.929)	Without use disorder
291.81	(___.__)	Alcohol Withdrawal[c, d]
	(F10.239)	Without perceptual disturbances
	(F10.232)	With perceptual disturbances
___.__	(___.__)	Other Alcohol-Induced Disorders
291.9	(F10.99)	Unspecified Alcohol-Related Disorder

Caffeine-Related Disorders

305.90	(F15.929)	Caffeine Intoxication
292.0	(F15.93)	Caffeine Withdrawal
___.__	(___.__)	Other Caffeine-Induced Disorders
292.9	(F15.99)	Unspecified Caffeine-Related Disorder

Cannabis-Related Disorders

___.__	(___.__)	Cannabis Use Disorder[a, b]
		Specify current severity
305.20	(F12.10)	Mild
304.30	(F12.20)	Moderate
304.30	(F12.20)	Severe
292.89	(___.__)	Cannabis Intoxication[c]
		Without perceptual disturbances
	(F12.129)	With use disorder, mild
	(F12.229)	With use disorder, moderate or severe
	(F12.929)	Without use disorder
		With perceptual disturbances
	(F12.122)	With use disorder, mild
	(F12.222)	With use disorder, moderate or severe
	(F12.922)	Without use disorder
292.0	(F12.288)	Cannabis Withdrawal[d]

__.__	(__.__)	Other Cannabis-Induced Disorders
292.9	(F12.99)	Unspecified Cannabis-Related Disorder

Hallucinogen-Related Disorders

__.__	(__.__)	Phencyclidine Use Disorder[a, b]
		Specify current severity:
305.90	(F16.10)	Mild
304.60	(F16.20)	Moderate
304.60	(F16.20)	Severe
__.__	(__.__)	Other Hallucinogen Use Disorder[a, b]
		Specify the particular hallucinogen
		Specify current severity:
305.30	(F16.10)	Mild
304.50	(F16.20)	Moderate
304.50	(F16.20)	Severe
292.89	(__.__)	Phencyclidine Intoxication
	(F16.129)	With use disorder, mild
	(F16.229)	With use disorder, moderate or severe
	(F16.929)	Without use disorder
292.89	(__.__)	Other Hallucinogen Intoxication
	(F16.129)	With use disorder, mild
	(F16.229)	With use disorder, moderate or severe
	(F16.929)	Without use disorder
292.89	(F16.983)	Hallucinogen Persisting Perception Disorder
__.__	(__.__)	Other Phencyclidine-Induced Disorders
__.__	(__.__)	Other Hallucinogen-Induced Disorders
292.9	(F16.99)	Unspecified Phencyclidine-Related Disorder
292.9	(F16.99)	Unspecified Hallucinogen-Related Disorder

Inhalant-Related Disorders

__.__	(__.__)	Inhalant Use Disorder[a, b]
		Specify the particular inhalant
		Specify current severity:
305.90	(F18.10)	Mild
304.60	(F18.20)	Moderate
304.60	(F18.20)	Severe
292.89	(__.__)	Inhalant Intoxication
	(F18.129)	With use disorder, mild
	(F18.229)	With use disorder, moderate or severe
	(F18.929)	Without use disorder
__.__	(__.__)	Other Inhalant-Induced Disorders
292.9	(F18.99)	Unspecified Inhalant-Related Disorder

Opioid-Related Disorders

__.__	(__.__)	Opioid Use Disorder[a]
		Specify if: On maintenance therapy, In a controlled environment
		Specify current severity:
305.50	(F11.10)	Mild
304.00	(F11.20)	Moderate
304.00	(F11.20)	Severe

292.89	(___.___)	Opioid Intoxication[c]
		Without perceptual disturbances
	(F11.129)	With use disorder, mild
	(F11.229)	With use disorder, moderate or severe
	(F11.922)	Without use disorder
292.0	(F11.23)	Opioid Withdrawal[d]
___.___	(___.___)	Other Opioid-Induced Disorders
292.9	(F11.99)	Unspecified Opioid-Related Disorder

Sedative-, Hypnotic-, or Anxiolytic-Related Disorders

___.___	(___.___)	Sedative, Hypnotic, or Anxiolytic Use Disorder[a, b]
		Specify current severity:
305.40	(F13.10)	Mild
304.10	(F13.20)	Moderate
304.10	(F13.20)	Severe
292.89	(___.___)	Sedative, Hypnotic, or Anxiolytic Intoxication
	(F13.129)	With use disorder, mild
	(F13.229)	With use disorder, moderate or severe
	(F13.929)	Without use disorder
292.0	(___.___)	Sedative, Hypnotic, or Anxiolytic Withdrawal[c, d]
	(F13.239)	Without perceptual disturbances
	(F13.232)	With perceptual disturbances
___.___	(___.___)	Other Sedative-, Hypnotic-, or Anxiolytic-Induced Disorders
292.9	(F13.99)	Unspecified Sedative-, Hypnotic-, or Anxiolytic-Related Disorder

Stimulant-Related Disorders

___.___	(___.___)	Stimulant Use Disorder[a, b]
		Specify current severity:
___.___	(___.___)	Mild
305.70	(F15.10)	Amphetamine-type substance
305.60	(F14.10)	Cocaine
305.70	(F15.10)	Other or unspecified stimulant
___.___	(___.___)	Moderate
304.40	(F15.20)	Amphetamine-type substance
304.20	(F14.20)	Cocaine
304.40	(F15.20)	Other or unspecified stimulant
___.___	(___.___)	Severe
304.40	(F15.20)	Amphetamine-type substance
304.20	(F14.20)	Cocaine
304.40	(F15.20)	Other or unspecified stimulant
292.89	(___.___)	Stimulant Intoxication[c]
		Specify the specific intoxicant
292.89	(___.___)	Amphetamine or other stimulant, Without perceptual disturbances
	(F15.129)	With use disorder, mild
	(F15.229)	With use disorder, moderate or severe
	(F15.929)	Without use disorder
292.89	(___.___)	Cocaine, Without perceptual disturbances
	(F14.129)	With use disorder, mild

	(F14.229)	With use disorder, moderate or severe
	(F14.929)	Without use disorder
292.89	(___.__)	Amphetamine or other stimulant, With perceptual disturbances
	(F15.122)	With use disorder, mild
	(F15.222)	With use disorder, moderate or severe
	(F15.922)	Without use disorder
292.89	(___.__)	Cocaine, With perceptual disturbances
	(F14.122)	With use disorder, mild
	(F14.222)	With use disorder, moderate or severe
	(F14.922)	Without use disorder
292.0	(___.__)	Stimulant Withdrawal[d]
		Specify the specific substance causing the withdrawal syndrome
	(F15.23)	Amphetamine or other stimulant
	(F14.23)	Cocaine
___.__	(___.__)	Other Stimulant-Induced Disorders
292.9	(___.__)	Unspecified Stimulant-Related Disorder
	(F15.99)	Amphetamine or other stimulant
	(F14.99)	Cocaine

Tobacco-Related Disorders

___.__	(___.__)	Tobacco Use Disorder[a]
		Specify if: On maintenance therapy, In a controlled environment
		Specify current severity:
305.1	(Z72.0)	Mild
305.1	(F17.200)	Moderate
305.1	(F17.200)	Severe
292.0	(F17.203)	Tobacco Withdrawal[d]
___.__	(___.__)	Other Tobacco-Induced Disorders
292.9	(F17.209)	Unspecified Tobacco-Related Disorder

Other (or Unknown) Substance-Related Disorders

___.__	(___.__)	Other (or Unknown) Substance Use Disorder[a, b]
		Specify current severity:
305.90	(F19.10)	Mild
304.90	(F19.20)	Moderate
304.90	(F19.20)	Severe
292.89	(___.__)	Other (or Unknown) Substance Intoxication
	(F19.129)	With use disorder, mild
	(F19.229)	With use disorder, moderate or severe
	(F19.929)	Without use disorder
292.0	(F19.239)	Other (or Unknown) Substance Withdrawal[d]
___.__	(___.__)	Other (or Unknown) Substance-Induced Disorders
292.9	(F19.99)	Unspecified Other (or Unknown) Substance-Related Disorder

■ Nonsubstance-Related Disorders

312.31	(F63.0)	Gambling Disorder[a]
		Specify if: Episodic, Persistent
		Specify current severity: Mild, Moderate, Severe

■ NEUROCOGNITIVE DISORDERS

___.__	(___.__)	Delirium
		[a]Note: See the criteria set and corresponding recording procedures for substance-specific codes and ICD-9-CM and ICD-10-CM coding.
		Specify whether:
___.__	(___.__)	Substance intoxication delirium[a]
___.__	(___.__)	Substance withdrawal delirium[a]
292.81	(___.__)	Medication-induced delirium[a]
293.0	(F05)	Delirium due to another medical condition
293.0	(F05)	Delirium due to multiple etiologies
		Specify if: Acute, Persistent
		Specify if: Hyperactive, Hypoactive, Mixed level of activity
780.09	(R41.0)	Other Specified Delirium
780.09	(R41.0)	Unspecified Delirium

Major and Mild Neurocognitive Disorders

Specify whether due to: Alzheimer's disease, Frontotemporal lobar degeneration, Lewy body disease, Vascular disease, Traumatic brain injury, Substance/medication use, HIV infection, Prion disease, Parkinson's disease, Huntington's disease, Another medical condition, Multiple etiologies, Unspecified

  [a] *Specify* Without behavioral disturbance, With behavioral disturbance. *For possible major neurocognitive disorder and for mild neurocognitive disorder, behavioral disturbance cannot be coded but should still be indicated in writing.*

  [b] *Specify* current severity: Mild, Moderate, Severe. *This specifier applies only to major neurocognitive disorders (including probable and possible).*

NOTE: As indicated for each subtype, an additional medical code is needed for probable major neurocognitive disorder or major neurocognitive disorder. An additional medical code should *not* be used for possible major neurocognitive disorder or mild neurocognitive disorder.

Major or Mild Neurocognitive Disorder Due to Alzheimer's Disease

___.__	(___.__)	Probable Major Neurocognitive Disorder Due to Alzheimer's Disease[b]
		Note: Code first 331.0 (G30.9) Alzheimer's disease.
294.11	(F02.81)	With behavioral disturbance
294.10	(F02.80)	Without behavioral disturbance
331.9	(G31.9)	Possible Major Neurocognitive Disorder Due to Alzheimer's Disease[a, b]
331.83	(G31.84)	Mild Neurocognitive Disorder Due to Alzheimer's Disease[a]

Major or Mild Frontotemporal Neurocognitive Disorder

___.___	(___.___)	Probable Major Neurocognitive Disorder Due to Frontotemporal Lobar Degeneration[b]
		Note: Code first 331.19 (G31.09) frontotemporal disease.
294.11	(F02.81)	With behavioral disturbance
294.10	(F02.80)	Without behavioral disturbance
331.9	(G31.9)	Possible Major Neurocognitive Disorder Due to Frontotemporal Lobar Degeneration[a, b]
331.83	(G31.84)	Mild Neurocognitive Disorder Due to Frontotemporal Lobar Degeneration[a]

Major or Mild Neurocognitive Disorder With Lewy Bodies

___.___	(___.___)	Probable Major Neurocognitive Disorder With Lewy Bodies[b]
		Note: Code first 331.82 (G31.83) Lewy body disease.
294.11	(F02.81)	With behavioral disturbance
294.10	(F02.80)	Without behavioral disturbance
331.9	(G31.9)	Possible Major Neurocognitive Disorder With Lewy Bodies[a, b]
331.83	(G31.84)	Mild Neurocognitive Disorder With Lewy Bodies[a]

Major or Mild Vascular Neurocognitive Disorder

___.___	(___.___)	Probable Major Vascular Neurocognitive Disorder[b]
		Note: No additional medical code for vascular disease.
290.40	(F01.51)	With behavioral disturbance
290.40	(F01.50)	Without behavioral disturbance
331.9	(G31.9)	Possible Major Vascular Neurocognitive Disorder[a, b]
331.83	(G31.84)	Mild Vascular Neurocognitive Disorder[a]

Major or Mild Neurocognitive Disorder Due to Traumatic Brain Injury

___.___	(___.___)	Major Neurocognitive Disorder Due to Traumatic Brain Injury[b]
		Note: For ICD-9-CM, code first 907.0 late effect of intracranial injury without skull fracture. For ICD-10-CM, code first S06.2X9S diffuse traumatic brain injury with loss of consciousness of unspecified duration, sequela
294.11	(F02.81)	With behavioral disturbance
294.10	(F02.80)	Without behavioral disturbance
331.83	(G31.84)	Mild Neurocognitive Disorder Due to Traumatic Brain Injury[a]

*Substance/Medication-Induced Major or Mild
Neurocognitive Disorder[a]*

NOTE: No additional medical code. See the criteria set and corresponding recording procedures for substance-specific codes and ICD-9-CM and ICD-10-CM coding.

Specify if: Persistent

Major or Mild Neurocognitive Disorder Due to HIV Infection

__.__	(__.__)	Major Neurocognitive Disorder Due to HIV Infection[b]
		Note: Code first 042 (B20) HIV infection.
294.11	(F02.81)	With behavioral disturbance
294.10	(F02.80)	Without behavioral disturbance
331.83	(G31.84)	Mild Neurocognitive Disorder Due to HIV Infection[a]

Major or Mild Neurocognitive Disorder Due to Prion Disease

__.__	(__.__)	Major Neurocognitive Disorder Due to Prion Disease[b]
		Note: Code first 046.79 (A81.9) prion disease.
294.11	(F02.81)	With behavioral disturbance
294.10	(F02.80)	Without behavioral disturbance
331.83	(G31.84)	Mild Neurocognitive Disorder Due to Prion Disease[a]

Major or Mild Neurocognitive Disorder Due to Parkinson's Disease

__.__	(__.__)	Major Neurocognitive Disorder Probably Due to Parkinson's Disease[b]
		Note: Code first 332.0 (G20) Parkinson's disease.
294.11	(F02.81)	With behavioral disturbance
294.10	(F02.80)	Without behavioral disturbance
331.9	(G31.9)	Major Neurocognitive Disorder Possibly Due to Parkinson's Disease[a, b]
331.83	(G31.84)	Mild Neurocognitive Disorder Due to Parkinson's Disease[a]

Major or Mild Neurocognitive Disorder Due to Huntington's Disease

__.__	(__.__)	Major Neurocognitive Disorder Due to Huntington's Disease[b]
		Note: Code first 333.4 (G10) Huntington's disease.
294.11	(F02.81)	With behavioral disturbance
294.10	(F02.80)	Without behavioral disturbance
331.83	(G31.84)	Mild Neurocognitive Disorder Due to Huntington's Disease[a]

Major or Mild Neurocognitive Disorder Due to Another Medical Condition

___.___	(___.___)	Major Neurocognitive Disorder Due to Another Medical Condition[b]
		Note: Code first the other medical condition.
294.11	(F02.81)	With behavioral disturbance
294.10	(F02.80)	Without behavioral disturbance
331.83	(G31.84)	Mild Neurocognitive Disorder Due to Another Medical Condition[a]

Major or Mild Neurocognitive Disorder Due to Multiple Etiologies

___.___	(___.___)	Major Neurocognitive Disorder Due to Multiple Etiologies[b]
		Note: Code first all the etiological medical conditions (with the exception of vascular disease).
294.11	(F02.81)	With behavioral disturbance
294.10	(F02.80)	Without behavioral disturbance
331.83	(G31.84)	Mild Neurocognitive Disorder Due to Multiple Etiologies[a]

Unspecified Neurocognitive Disorder

| 799.59 | (R41.9) | Unspecified Neurocognitive Disorder[a] |

■ PERSONALITY DISORDERS
Cluster A Personality Disorders

301.0	(F60.0)	Paranoid Personality Disorder
301.20	(F60.1)	Schizoid Personality Disorder
301.22	(F21)	Schizotypal Personality Disorder

Cluster B Personality Disorders

301.7	(F60.2)	Antisocial Personality Disorder
301.83	(F60.3)	Borderline Personality Disorder
301.50	(F60.4)	Histrionic Personality Disorder
301.81	(F60.81)	Narcissistic Personality Disorder

Cluster C Personality Disorders

301.82	(F60.6)	Avoidant Personality Disorder
301.6	(F60.7)	Dependent Personality Disorder
301.4	(F60.5)	Obsessive-Compulsive Personality Disorder

Other Personality Disorders

| 310.1 | (F07.0) | Personality Change Due to Another Medical Condition |
| | | *Specify* whether: Labile type, Disinhibited type, Aggressive type, Apathetic type, Paranoid |

		type, Other type, Combined type, Unspecified type
301.89	(F60.89)	Other Specified Personality Disorder
301.9	(F60.9)	Unspecified Personality Disorder

■ PARAPHILIC DISORDERS

The following specifier applies to Paraphilic Disorders where indicated:

ᵃ *Specify* if: In a controlled environment, In full remission

302.82	(F65.3)	Voyeuristic Disorderᵃ
302.4	(F65.2)	Exhibitionistic Disorderᵃ
		Specify whether: Sexually aroused by exposing genitals to prepubertal children, Sexually aroused by exposing genitals to physically mature individuals, Sexually aroused by exposing genitals to prepubertal children and to physically mature individuals.
302.89	(F65.81)	Frotteuristic Disorderᵃ
302.83	(F65.51)	Sexual Masochism Disorderᵃ
		Specify if: With asphyxiophilia
302.84	(F65.52)	Sexual Sadism Disorderᵃ
302.2	(F65.4)	Pedophilic Disorder
		Specify whether: Exclusive type, Nonexclusive type
		Specify if: Sexually attracted to males, Sexually attracted to females, Sexually attracted to both
		Specify if: Limited to incest
302.81	(F65.0)	Fetishistic Disorderᵃ
		Specify: Body part(s), Nonliving object(s), Other
302.3	(F65.1)	Transvestic Disorderᵃ
		Specify if: With fetishism, With autogynephilia
302.89	(F65.89)	Other Specified Paraphilic Disorder
302.9	(F65.9)	Unspecified Paraphilic Disorder

■ OTHER MENTAL DISORDERS

294.8	(F06.8)	Other Specified Mental Disorder Due to Another Medical Condition
294.9	(F09)	Unspecified Mental Disorder Due to Another Medical Condition
300.9	(F99)	Other Specified Mental Disorder
300.9	(F99)	Unspecified Mental Disorder

■ MEDICATION-INDUCED MOVEMENT DISORDERS AND OTHER ADVERSE EFFECTS OF MEDICATION

332.1	(G21.11)	Neuroleptic-Induced Parkinsonism
332.1	(G21.19)	Other Medication-Induced Parkinsonism
333.92	(G21.0)	Neuroleptic Malignant Syndrome

333.72	(G24.02)	Medication-Induced Acute Dystonia
333.99	(G25.71)	Medication-Induced Acute Akathisia
333.85	(G24.01)	Tardive Dyskinesia
333.72	(G24.09)	Tardive Dystonia
333.99	(G25.71)	Tardive Akathisia
333.1	(G25.1)	Medication-Induced Postural Tremor
333.99	(G25.79)	Other Medication-Induced Movement Disorder
___.__	(___.__)	Antidepressant Discontinuation Syndrome
995.29	(T43.205A)	Initial encounter
995.29	(T43.205D)	Subsequent encounter
995.29	(T43.205S)	Sequelae
___.__	(___.__)	Other Adverse Effect of Medication
995.20	(T50.905A)	Initial encounter
995.20	(T50.905D)	Subsequent encounter
995.20	(T50.905S)	Sequelae

■ OTHER CONDITIONS THAT MAY BE A FOCUS OF CLINICAL ATTENTION

Relational Problems

Problems Related to Family Upbringing

V61.20	(Z62.820)	Parent-Child Relational Problem
V61.8	(Z62.891)	Sibling Relational Problem
V61.8	(Z62.29)	Upbringing Away From Parents
V61.29	(Z62.898)	Child Affected by Parental Relationship Distress

Other Problems Related to Primary Support Group

V61.10	(Z63.0)	Relationship Distress With Spouse or Intimate Partner
V61.03	(Z63.5)	Disruption of Family by Separation or Divorce
V61.8	(Z63.8)	High Expressed Emotion Level Within Family
V62.82	(Z63.4)	Uncomplicated Bereavement

Abuse and Neglect

Child Maltreatment and Neglect Problems

Child Physical Abuse, Confirmed

| 995.54 | (T74.12XA) | Initial encounter |
| 995.54 | (T74.12XD) | Subsequent encounter |

Child Physical Abuse, Suspected

| 995.54 | (T76.12XA) | Initial encounter |
| 995.54 | (T76.12XD) | Subsequent encounter |

Other Circumstances Related to Child Physical Abuse

| V61.21 | (Z69.010) | Encounter for mental health services for victim of child abuse by parent |
| V61.21 | (Z69.020) | Encounter for mental health services for victim of nonparental child abuse |

V15.41	(Z62.810)	Personal history (past history) of physical abuse in childhood
V61.22	(Z69.011)	Encounter for mental health services for perpetrator of parental child abuse
V62.83	(Z69.021)	Encounter for mental health services for perpetrator of nonparental child abuse

Child Sexual Abuse, Confirmed
| 995.53 | (T74.22XA) | Initial encounter |
| 995.53 | (T74.22XD) | Subsequent encounter |

Child Sexual Abuse, Suspected
| 995.53 | (T76.22XA) | Initial encounter |
| 995.53 | (T76.22XD) | Subsequent encounter |

Other Circumstances Related to Child Sexual Abuse
V61.21	(Z69.010)	Encounter for mental health services for victim of child sexual abuse by parent
V61.21	(Z69.020)	Encounter for mental health services for victim of nonparental child sexual abuse
V15.41	(Z62.810)	Personal history (past history) of sexual abuse in childhood
V61.22	(Z69.011)	Encounter for mental health services for perpetrator of parental child sexual abuse
V62.83	(Z69.021)	Encounter for mental health services for perpetrator of nonparental child sexual abuse

Child Neglect, Confirmed
| 995.52 | (T74.02XA) | Initial encounter |
| 995.52 | (T74.02XD) | Subsequent encounter |

Child Neglect, Suspected
| 995.52 | (T76.02XA) | Initial encounter |
| 995.52 | (T76.02XD) | Subsequent encounter |

Other Circumstances Related to Child Neglect
V61.21	(Z69.010)	Encounter for mental health services for victim of child neglect by parent
V61.21	(Z69.020)	Encounter for mental health services for victim of nonparental child neglect
V15.42	(Z62.812)	Personal history (past history) of neglect in childhood
V61.22	(Z69.011)	Encounter for mental health services for perpetrator of parental child neglect
V62.83	(Z69.021)	Encounter for mental health services for perpetrator of nonparental child neglect

Child Psychological Abuse, Confirmed
| 995.51 | (T74.32XA) | Initial encounter |
| 995.51 | (T74.32XD) | Subsequent encounter |

Child Psychological Abuse, Suspected
| 995.51 | (T76.32XA) | Initial encounter |
| 995.51 | (T76.32XD) | Subsequent encounter |

Other Circumstances Related to Child Psychological Abuse

V61.21	(Z69.010)	Encounter for mental health services for victim of child psychological abuse by parent
V61.21	(Z69.020)	Encounter for mental health services for victim of nonparental child psychological abuse
V15.42	(Z62.811)	Personal history (past history) of psychological abuse in childhood
V61.22	(Z69.011)	Encounter for mental health services for perpetrator of parental child psychological abuse
V62.83	(Z69.021)	Encounter for mental health services for perpetrator of nonparental child psychological abuse

Adult Maltreatment and Neglect Problems

Spouse or Partner Violence, Physical, Confirmed

995.81	(T74.11XA)	Initial encounter
995.81	(T74.11XD)	Subsequent encounter

Spouse or Partner Violence, Physical, Suspected

995.81	(T76.11XA)	Initial encounter
995.81	(T76.11XD)	Subsequent encounter

Other Circumstances Related to Spouse or Partner Violence, Physical

V61.11	(Z69.11)	Encounter for mental health services for victim of spouse or partner violence, physical
V15.41	(Z91.410)	Personal history (past history) of spouse or partner violence, physical
V61.12	(Z69.12)	Encounter for mental health services for perpetrator of spouse or partner violence, physical

Spouse or Partner Violence, Sexual, Confirmed

995.83	(T74.21XA)	Initial encounter
995.83	(T74.21XD)	Subsequent encounter

Spouse or Partner Violence, Sexual, Suspected

995.83	(T76.21XA)	Initial encounter
995.83	(T76.21XD)	Subsequent encounter

Other Circumstances Related to Spouse or Partner Violence, Sexual

V61.11	(Z69.81)	Encounter for mental health services for victim of spouse or partner violence, sexual
V15.41	(Z91.410)	Personal history (past history) of spouse or partner violence, sexual
V61.12	(Z69.12)	Encounter for mental health services for perpetrator of spouse or partner violence, sexual

Spouse or Partner Neglect, Confirmed

995.85	(T74.01XA)	Initial encounter
995.85	(T74.01XD)	Subsequent encounter

Spouse or Partner Neglect, Suspected
995.85	(T76.01XA)	Initial encounter
995.85	(T76.01XD)	Subsequent encounter

Other Circumstances Related to Spouse or Partner Neglect
V61.11	(Z69.11)	Encounter for mental health services for victim of spouse or partner neglect
V15.42	(Z91.412)	Personal history (past history) of spouse or partner neglect
V61.12	(Z69.12)	Encounter for mental health services for perpetrator of spouse or partner neglect

Spouse or Partner Abuse, Psychological, Confirmed
995.82	(T74.31XA)	Initial encounter
995.82	(T74.31XD)	Subsequent encounter

Spouse or Partner Abuse, Psychological, Suspected
995.82	(T76.31XA)	Initial encounter
995.85	(T76.31XD)	Subsequent encounter

Other Circumstances Related to Spouse or Partner Abuse, Psychological
V61.11	(Z69.11)	Encounter for mental health services for victim of spouse or partner psychological abuse
V15.42	(Z91.411)	Personal history (past history) of spouse or partner psychological abuse
V61.12	(Z69.12)	Encounter for mental health services for perpetrator of spouse or partner psychological abuse

Adult Physical Abuse by Nonspouse or Nonpartner, Confirmed
995.81	(T74.11XA)	Initial encounter
995.81	(T74.11XD)	Subsequent encounter

Adult Physical Abuse by Nonspouse or Nonpartner, Suspected
995.81	(T76.11XA)	Initial encounter
995.81	(T76.11XD)	Subsequent encounter

Adult Sexual Abuse by Nonspouse or Nonpartner, Confirmed
995.83	(T74.21XA)	Initial encounter
995.83	(T74.21XD)	Subsequent encounter

Adult Sexual Abuse by Nonspouse or Nonpartner, Suspected
995.83	(T76.21XA)	Initial encounter
995.83	(T76.21XD)	Subsequent encounter

Adult Psychological Abuse by Nonspouse or Nonpartner, Confirmed
995.82	(T74.31XA)	Initial encounter
995.82	(T74.31XD)	Subsequent encounter

Adult Psychological Abuse by Nonspouse or Nonpartner, Suspected
995.82	(T76.31XA)	Initial encounter
995.82	(T76.31XD)	Subsequent encounter

Other Circumstances Related to Adult Abuse by Nonspouse or Nonpartner

| V65.49 | (Z69.81) | Encounter for mental health services for victim of nonspousal adult abuse |
| V62.83 | (Z69.82) | Encounter for mental health services for perpetrator of nonspousal adult abuse |

Educational and Occupational Problems

Educational Problems

| V62.3 | (Z55.9) | Academic or Educational Problem |

Occupational Problems

| V62.21 | (Z56.82) | Problem Related to Current Military Deployment Status |
| V62.29 | (Z56.9) | Other Problem Related to Employment |

Housing and Economic Problems

Housing Problems

V60.0	(Z59.0)	Homelessness
V60.1	(Z59.1)	Inadequate Housing
V60.89	(Z59.2)	Discord With Neighbor, Lodger, or Landlord
V60.6	(Z59.3)	Problem Related to Living in a Residential Institution

Economic Problems

V60.2	(Z59.4)	Lack of Adequate Food or Safe Drinking Water
V60.2	(Z59.5)	Extreme Poverty
V60.2	(Z59.6)	Low Income
V60.2	(Z59.7)	Insufficient Social Insurance or Welfare Support
V60.9	(Z59.9)	Unspecified Housing or Economic Problem

Other Problems Related to the Social Environment

V62.89	(Z60.0)	Phase of Life Problem
V60.3	(Z60.2)	Problem Related to Living Alone
V62.4	(Z60.3)	Acculturation Difficulty
V62.4	(Z60.4)	Social Exclusion or Rejection
V62.4	(Z60.5)	Target of (Perceived) Adverse Discrimination or Persecution
V62.9	(Z60.9)	Unspecified Problem Related to Social Environment

Problems Related to Crime or Interaction With the Legal System

V62.89	(Z65.4)	Victim of Crime
V62.5	(Z65.0)	Conviction in Civil or Criminal Proceedings Without Imprisonment
V62.5	(Z65.1)	Imprisonment or Other Incarceration

| V62.5 | (Z65.2) | Problems Related to Release From Prison |
| V62.5 | (Z65.3) | Problems Related to Other Legal Circumstances |

Other Health Service Encounters for Counseling and Medical Advice

| V65.49 | (Z70.9) | Sex Counseling |
| V65.40 | (Z71.9) | Other Counseling or Consultation |

Problems Related to Other Psychosocial, Personal, and Environmental Circumstances

V62.89	(Z65.8)	Religious or Spiritual Problem
V61.7	(Z64.0)	Problems Related to Unwanted Pregnancy
V61.5	(Z64.1)	Problems Related to Multiparity
V62.89	(Z64.4)	Discord With Social Service Provider, Including Probation Officer, Case Manager, or Social Services Worker
V62.89	(Z65.4)	Victim of Terrorism or Torture
V62.22	(Z65.5)	Exposure to Disaster, War, or Other Hostilities
V62.89	(Z65.8)	Other Problem Related to Psychosocial Circumstances
V62.9	(Z65.9)	Unspecified Problem Related to Unspecified Psychosocial Circumstances

Other Circumstances of Personal History

V15.49	(Z91.49)	Other Personal History of Psychological Trauma
V15.59	(Z91.5)	Personal History of Self-Harm
V62.22	(Z91.82)	Personal History of Military Deployment
V15.89	(Z91.89)	Other Personal Risk Factors
V69.9	(Z72.9)	Problem Related to Lifestyle
V71.01	(Z72.811)	Adult Antisocial Behavior
V71.02	(Z72.810)	Child or Adolescent Antisocial Behavior

Problems Related to Access to Medical and Other Health Care

| V63.9 | (Z75.3) | Unavailability or Inaccessibility of Health Care Facilities |
| V63.8 | (Z75.4) | Unavailability or Inaccessibility of Other Helping Agencies |

Nonadherence to Medical Treatment

V15.81	(Z91.19)	Nonadherence to Medical Treatment
278.00	(E66.9)	Overweight or Obesity
V65.2	(Z76.5)	Malingering
V40.31	(Z91.83)	Wandering Associated With a Mental Disorder
V62.89	(R41.83)	Borderline Intellectual Functioning

*Reprinted with permission from the *Diagnostic and Statistical Manual of Mental Disorders, Fifth Edition*. (2013). American Psychiatric Association.

APPENDIX K

Mental Status Assessment

Gathering the correct information about the client's mental status is essential to the development of an appropriate plan of care. The mental status examination is a description of all the areas of the client's mental functioning. The following are the components that are considered critical in the assessment of a client's mental status. Examples of interview questions and criteria for assessment are included.

◼ IDENTIFYING DATA
1. Name
2. Gender
3. Age
   a. How old are you?
   b. When were you born?
4. Race/culture
   a. What country did you (your ancestors) come from?
5. Occupational/financial status
   a. How do you make your living?
   b. How do you obtain money for your needs?
6. Educational level
   a. What was the highest grade level you completed in school?
7. Significant other
   a. Are you married?
   b. Do you have a significant relationship with another person?
8. Living arrangements
   a. Do you live alone?
   b. With whom do you share your home?
9. Religious preference
   a. Do you have a religious preference?
10. Allergies
    a. Are you allergic to anything?
    b. Foods? Medications?
11. Special diet considerations
    a. Do you have any special diet requirements?
    b. Diabetic? Low sodium?

12. Chief complaint
    a. For what reason did you come for help today?
    b. What seems to be the problem?
13. Medical diagnosis

■ GENERAL DESCRIPTION

Appearance

1. Grooming and dress
    a. Note unusual modes of dress.
    b. Evidence of soiled clothing?
    c. Use of makeup?
    d. Neat; unkempt?
2. Hygiene
    a. Note evidence of body or breath odor.
    b. Condition of skin, fingernails.
3. Posture
    a. Note if standing upright, rigid, slumped over.
4. Height and weight
    a. Perform accurate measurements.
5. Level of eye contact
    a. Intermittent?
    b. Occasional and fleeting?
    c. Sustained and intense?
    d. No eye contact?
6. Hair color and texture
    a. Is hair clean and healthy-looking?
    b. Greasy, matted, tangled?
7. Evidence of scars, tattoos, or other distinguishing skin marks
    a. Note any evidence of swelling or bruises.
    b. Birth marks?
    c. Rashes?
8. Evaluation of client's appearance compared with chronological age.

Motor Activity

1. Tremors
    a. Do hands or legs tremble?
       • Continuously?
       • At specific times?
2. Tics or other stereotypical movements
    a. Any evidence of facial tics?
    b. Jerking or spastic movements?
3. Mannerisms and gestures
    a. Specific facial or body movements during conversation?
    b. Nail biting?
    c. Covering face with hands?
    d. Grimacing?

4. Hyperactivity
   a. Gets up and down out of chair.
   b. Paces.
   c. Unable to sit still.
5. Restlessness or agitation
   a. Lots of fidgeting.
   b. Clenching hands.
6. Aggressiveness
   a. Overtly angry and hostile.
   b. Threatening.
   c. Uses sarcasm.
7. Rigidity
   a. Sits or stands in a rigid position.
   b. Arms and legs appear stiff and unyielding.
8. Gait patterns
   a. Any evidence of limping?
   b. Limitation of range of motion?
   c. Ataxia?
   d. Shuffling?
9. Echopraxia
   a. Evidence of mimicking the actions of others?
10. Psychomotor retardation
    a. Movements are very slow.
    b. Thinking and speech are very slow.
    c. Posture is slumped.
11. Freedom of movement (range of motion)
    a. Note any limitation in ability to move.

Speech Patterns

1. Slowness or rapidity of speech
   a. Note whether speech seems very rapid or slower than normal.
2. Pressure of speech
   a. Note whether speech seems frenzied.
   b. Unable to be interrupted?
3. Intonation
   a. Are words spoken with appropriate emphasis?
   b. Are words spoken in monotone, without emphasis?
4. Volume
   a. Is speech very loud? Soft?
   b. Is speech low-pitched? High-pitched?
5. Stuttering or other speech impairments
   a. Hoarseness?
   b. Slurred speech?
6. Aphasia
   a. Difficulty forming words.
   b. Use of incorrect words.
   c. Difficulty thinking of specific words.
   d. Making up words (neologisms).

General Attitude

1. Cooperative/uncooperative
   a. Answers questions willingly.
   b. Refuses to answer questions.
2. Friendly/hostile/defensive
   a. Is sociable and responsive.
   b. Is sarcastic and irritable.
3. Uninterested/apathetic
   a. Refuses to participate in interview process.
4. Attentive/interested
   a. Actively participates in interview process.
5. Guarded/suspicious
   a. Continuously scans the environment.
   b. Questions motives of interviewer.
   c. Refuses to answer questions.

■ EMOTIONS

Mood

1. Depressed; despairing
   a. An overwhelming feeling of sadness.
   b. Loss of interest in regular activities.
2. Irritable
   a. Easily annoyed and provoked to anger.
3. Anxious
   a. Demonstrates or verbalizes feeling of apprehension.
4. Elated
   a. Expresses feelings of joy and intense pleasure.
   b. Is intensely optimistic.
5. Euphoric
   a. Demonstrates a heightened sense of elation.
   b. Expresses feelings of grandeur ("Everything is wonderful!").
6. Fearful
   a. Demonstrates or verbalizes feeling of apprehension associated with real or perceived danger.
7. Guilty
   a. Expresses a feeling of discomfort associated with real or perceived wrongdoing.
   b. May be associated with feelings of sadness and despair.
8. Labile
   a. Exhibits mood swings that range from euphoria to depression or anxiety.

Affect

1. Congruence with mood
   a. Outward emotional expression is consistent with mood (e.g., if depressed, emotional expression is sadness, eyes downcast, may be crying).

2. Constricted or blunted
   a. Minimal outward emotional expression is observed.
3. Flat
   a. There is an absence of outward emotional expression.
4. Appropriate
   a. The outward emotional expression is what would be expected in a certain situation (e.g., crying upon hearing of a death).
5. Inappropriate
   a. The outward emotional expression is incompatible with the situation (e.g., laughing upon hearing of a death).

■ THOUGHT PROCESSES
Form of Thought

1. Flight of ideas
   a. Verbalizations are continuous and rapid, and flow from one to another.
2. Associative looseness
   a. Verbalizations shift from one unrelated topic to another.
3. Circumstantiality
   a. Verbalizations are lengthy and tedious, and because of numerous details, are delayed reaching the intended point.
4. Tangentiality
   a. Verbalizations that are lengthy and tedious, and never reach an intended point.
5. Neologisms
   a. The individual is making up nonsensical-sounding words, which only have meaning to him or her.
6. Concrete thinking
   a. Thinking is literal; elemental.
   b. Absence of ability to think abstractly.
   c. Unable to translate simple proverbs.
7. Clang associations
   a. Speaking in puns or rhymes; using words that sound alike but have different meanings.
8. Word salad
   a. Using a mixture of words that have no meaning together; sounding incoherent.
9. Perseveration
   a. Persistently repeating the last word of a sentence spoken to the client (e.g., Ns: "George, it's time to go to lunch." George: "lunch, lunch, lunch, lunch").
10. Echolalia
    a. Persistently repeating what another person says.
11. Mutism
    a. Does not speak (either cannot or will not).

12. Poverty of speech
    a. Speaks very little; may respond in monosyllables.
13. Ability to concentrate and disturbance of attention
    a. Does the person hold attention to the topic at hand?
    b. Is the person easily distractible?
    c. Is there selective attention (e.g., blocks out topics that create anxiety)?

Content of Thought

1. Delusions (Does the person have unrealistic ideas or beliefs?)
    a. Persecutory: A belief that someone is out to get him or her is some way (e.g., "The FBI will be here at any time to take me away.").
    b. Grandiose: An idea that he or she is all-powerful or of great importance (e.g., "I am the king...and this is my kingdom! I can do anything!").
    c. Reference: An idea that whatever is happening in the environment is about him or her (e.g., "Just watch the movie on TV tonight. It is about my life.").
    d. Control or influence: A belief that his or her behavior and thoughts are being controlled by external forces (e.g., "I get my orders from Channel 27. I do only what the forces dictate.").
    e. Somatic: A belief that he or she has a dysfunctional body part (e.g., "My heart is at a standstill. It is no longer beating.").
    f. Nihilistic: A belief that he or she, or a part of the body, or even the world does not exist or has been destroyed (e.g., "I am no longer alive.").
2. Suicidal or homicidal ideas
    a. Is the individual expressing ideas of harming self or others?
3. Obsessions
    a. Is the person verbalizing about a persistent thought or feeling that he or she is unable to eliminate from their consciousness?
4. Paranoia/suspiciousness
    a. Continuously scans the environment.
    b. Questions motives of interviewer.
    c. Refuses to answer questions.
5. Magical thinking
    a. Is the person speaking in a way that indicates his or her words or actions have power (e.g., "If you step on a crack, you break your mother's back!")?
6. Religiosity
    a. Is the individual demonstrating obsession with religious ideas and behavior?

7. Phobias
   a. Is there evidence of irrational fears (of a specific object, or a social situation)?
8. Poverty of content
   a. Is little information conveyed by the client because of vagueness or stereotypical statements or clichés?

■ PERCEPTUAL DISTURBANCES

1. Hallucinations. (Is the person experiencing unrealistic sensory perceptions?)
   a. Auditory. (Is the individual hearing voices or other sounds that do not exist?)
   b. Visual. (Is the individual seeing images that do not exist?)
   c. Tactile. (Does the individual feel unrealistic sensations on the skin?)
   d. Olfactory. (Does the individual smell odors that do not exist?)
   e. Gustatory. (Does the individual have a false perception of an unpleasant taste?)
2. Illusions
   a. Does the individual misperceive or misinterpret real stimuli within the environment? (Sees something and thinks it is something else?)
3. Depersonalization (altered perception of the self)
   a. The individual verbalizes feeling "outside the body;" visualizing himself or herself from afar.
4. Derealization (altered perception of the environment)
   a. The individual verbalizes that the environment feels "strange or unreal." A feeling that the surroundings have changed.

■ SENSORIUM AND COGNITIVE ABILITY

1. Level of alertness/consciousness
   a. Is the individual clear-minded and attentive to the environment?
   b. Or is there disturbance in perception and awareness of the surroundings?
2. Orientation. Is the person oriented to the following?
   a. Time.
   b. Place.
   c. Person.
   d. Circumstances.
3. Memory
   a. Recent. (Is the individual able to remember occurrences of the past few days?)
   b. Remote. (Is the individual able to remember occurrences of the distant past?)

   c. Confabulation. (Does the individual fill in memory gaps with experiences that have no basis in fact?)
4. Capacity for abstract thought
   a. Can the individual interpret proverbs correctly?
      • "What does 'no use crying over spilled milk' mean?"

■ IMPULSE CONTROL

1. Ability to control impulses. (Does psychosocial history reveal problems with any of the following?)
   a. Aggression.
   b. Hostility.
   c. Fear.
   d. Guilt.
   e. Affection.
   f. Sexual feelings.

■ JUDGMENT AND INSIGHT

1. Ability to solve problems and make decisions
   a. What are your plans for the future?
   b. What do you plan to do to reach your goals?
2. Knowledge about self
   a. Awareness of limitations.
   b. Awareness of consequences of actions.
   c. Awareness of illness.
      • "Do you think you have a problem?"
      • "Do you think you need treatment?"
3. Adaptive/maladaptive use of coping strategies and ego defense mechanisms (e.g., rationalizing maladaptive behaviors, projection of blame, displacement of anger)

Assigning Nursing Diagnoses to Client Behaviors

Following is a list of client behaviors and the NANDA nursing diagnoses that correspond to the behaviors and that may be used in planning care for the client exhibiting the specific behavioral symptoms.

Behaviors	NANDA Nursing Diagnoses
Aggression; hostility	Risk for injury; Risk for other-directed violence
Anorexia or refusal to eat	Imbalanced nutrition: Less than body requirements
Anxious behavior	Anxiety (Specify level)
Confusion; memory loss	Confusion, acute/chronic; Impaired memory; Disturbed thought processes*
Delusions	Disturbed thought processes*
Denial of problems	Ineffective denial
Depressed mood or anger turned inward	Complicated grieving
Detoxification; withdrawal from substances	Risk for injury
Difficulty accepting new diagnosis or recent change in health status	Risk-prone health behavior
Difficulty making important life decision	Decisional conflict
Difficulty sleeping	Insomnia; Disturbed sleep pattern
Difficulty with interpersonal relationships	Impaired social interaction; ineffective relationship
Disruption in capability to perform usual responsibilities	Ineffective role performance
Dissociative behaviors (depersonalization; derealization)	Disturbed sensory perception (kinesthetic)*
Expresses feelings of disgust about body or body part	Disturbed body image

Behaviors	NANDA Nursing Diagnoses
Expresses anger at God	Spiritual distress
Expresses lack of control over personal situation	Powerlessness
Fails to follow prescribed therapy	Ineffective self-health management; Noncompliance
Flashbacks, nightmares, obsession with traumatic experience	Post-trauma syndrome
Hallucinations	Disturbed sensory perception (auditory; visual)*
Highly critical of self or others	Low self-esteem (chronic; situational)
HIV positive; altered immunity	Ineffective protection
Inability to meet basic needs	Self-care deficit (feeding; bathing; dressing; toileting)
Loose associations or flight of ideas	Impaired verbal communication
Loss of a valued entity, recently experienced	Risk for complicated grieving
Manic hyperactivity	Risk for injury
Manipulative behavior	Ineffective coping
Multiple personalities; gender dysphoria	Disturbed personal identity
Orgasm, problems with; lack of sexual desire; erectile dysfunction	Sexual dysfunction
Overeating, compulsive	Risk for imbalanced nutrition: More than body requirements
Phobias	Fear
Physical symptoms as coping behavior	Ineffective coping
Potential or anticipated loss of significant entity	Grieving
Projection of blame; rationalization of failures; denial of personal responsibility	Defensive coping
Ritualistic behaviors	Anxiety (severe); ineffective coping
Seductive remarks; inappropriate sexual behaviors	Impaired social interaction
Self-inflicted injuries (non-life-threatening)	Self-mutilation; Risk for self-mutilation
Sexual behaviors (difficulty, limitations, or changes in; reported dissatisfaction)	Ineffective sexuality pattern
Stress from caring for chronically ill person	Caregiver role strain
Stress from locating to new environment	Relocation stress syndrome

Behaviors	NANDA Nursing Diagnoses
Substance use as a coping behavior	Ineffective coping
Substance use (denies use is a problem)	Ineffective denial
Suicidal gestures/threats; suicidal ideation	Risk for suicide; Risk for self-directed violence
Suspiciousness	Ineffective coping; Disturbed thought processes[*]
Vomiting, excessive, self-induced	Risk for deficient fluid volume
Withdrawn behavior	Social isolation

[*]These diagnoses have been retired from the NANDA-I list of approved nursing diagnoses.

Brief Mental Status Evaluation

Area of Mental Function Evaluated	Evaluation Activity
Orientation to time	"What year is it? What month is it? What day is it?" (3 points)
Orientation to place	"Where are you now?" (1 point)
Attention and immediate recall	"Repeat these words now: bell, book, & candle." (3 points) "Remember these words and I will ask you to repeat them in a few minutes."
Abstract thinking	"What does this mean: No use crying over spilled milk." (3 points)
Recent memory	"Say the three words I asked you to remember earlier." (3 points)
Naming objects	Point to eyeglasses and ask, "What is this?" Repeat with one other item (e.g., calendar, watch, pencil). (2 points possible)
Ability to follow simple verbal command	"Tear this piece of paper in half and put it in the trash container." (2 points)
Ability to follow simple written command	Write a command on a piece of paper (e.g., TOUCH YOUR NOSE), give the paper to the patient and say, "Do what it says on this paper." (1 point for correct action)
Ability to use language correctly	Ask the patient to write a sentence. (3 points if sentence has a subject, a verb, and has valid meaning)
Ability to concentrate	"Say the months of the year in reverse, starting with December." (1 point each for correct answers from November through August; 4 points possible)

Continued

Area of Mental Function Evaluated	Evaluation Activity
Understanding spatial relationships	Instruct client to draw a clock; put in all the numbers; and set the hands on 3 o'clock. (clock circle = 1 point; numbers in correct sequence = 1 point; numbers placed on clock correctly = 1 point; two hands on the clock = 1 point; hands set at correct time = 1 point. (5 points possible)

Scoring: 21–30 = normal; 11–20 = mild cognitive impairment; 0–10 = severe cognitive impairment (scores are not absolute and must be considered within the comprehensive diagnostic assessment).

Sources: The Merck Manual of Health & Aging (2005); Folstein, Folstein, & McHugh (1975); Kaufman & Zun (1995); Kokman, et al. (1991); and Pfeiffer (1975).

FDA Pregnancy Categories

Category A	Adequate, well-controlled studies in pregnant women have not shown an increased risk of fetal abnormalities.
Category B	Animal studies have revealed no evidence of harm to the fetus; however, there are no adequate and well-controlled studies in pregnant women. **OR** Animal studies have shown an adverse effect, but adequate and well-controlled studies in pregnant women have failed to demonstrate a risk to the fetus.
Category C	Animal studies have shown an adverse effect and there are no adequate and well-controlled studies in pregnant women. **OR** No animal studies have been conducted and there are no adequate and well-controlled studies in pregnant women.
Category D	Studies, adequate well-controlled or observational, in pregnant women have demonstrated a risk to the fetus. However, the benefits of therapy may outweigh the potential risk.
Category X	Studies, adequate well-controlled or observational, in animals or pregnant women have demonstrated positive evidence of fetal abnormalities. The use of the product is contraindicated in women who are or may become pregnant.

SOURCE: Vallerand, A.H., Sanoski, C.A., & Deglin, J.H. (2013). *Davis's Drug Guide for Nurses* (13th ed.). Philadelphia: F.A. Davis. With permission.

APPENDIX O

DEA Controlled Substances Schedules

Classes or schedules are determined by the Drug Enforcement Agency (DEA), an arm of the U.S. Justice Department, and are based on the potential for abuse and dependence liability (physical and psychological) of the medication. Some states may have stricter prescription regulations. Physicians, dentists, podiatrists, and veterinarians may prescribe controlled substances. Nurse practitioners and physician's assistants may prescribe controlled substances with limitations that vary from state to state.

Schedule I (C-I)

Potential for abuse is so high as to be unacceptable. May be used for research with appropriate limitations. Examples are LSD and heroin.

Schedule II (C-II)

High potential for abuse and extreme liability for physical and psychological dependence (amphetamines, opioid analgesics, dronabinol, certain barbiturates). Outpatient prescriptions must be in writing. In emergencies, telephone orders may be acceptable if a written prescription is provided within 72 hours. No refills are allowed.

Schedule III (C-III)

Intermediate potential for abuse (less than C-II) and intermediate liability for physical and psychological dependence (certain non-barbiturate sedatives, certain nonamphetamine CNS stimulants, and certain opioid analgesics). Outpatient prescriptions can be re-filled five times within 6 months from date of issue if authorized by prescriber. Telephone orders are acceptable.

Schedule IV (C-IV)

Less abuse potential than Schedule III with minimal liability for physical or psychological dependence (certain sedative/hypnotics, certain antianxiety agents, some barbiturates, benzodiazepines, chloral hydrate, pentazocine, and propoxyphene). Outpatient prescriptions can be refilled six times within 6 months from date of issue if authorized by prescriber. Telephone orders are acceptable.

Schedule V (C-V)

Minimal abuse potential. Number of outpatient refills determined by prescriber. Some products (cough suppressants with small amounts of codeine, antidiarrheals containing paregoric) may be available without prescription to patients older than 18 years of age.

SOURCE: Vallerand, A.H., Sanoski, C.A., & Deglin, J.H. (2013). *Davis's Drug Guide for Nurses* (13th ed.). Philadelphia: F.A. Davis. With permission.

APPENDIX P

Abnormal Involuntary Movement Scale (AIMS)

Name_____ Rater Name_____
Date_____

Instructions: Complete the examination procedure before making ratings. For movement ratings, circle the highest severity observed. Rate movements that occur upon activation one *less* than those observed spontaneously. Circle movement as well as code number that applies.

   Code: 0 = None
          1 = Minimal, may be normal
          2 = Mild
          3 = Moderate
          4 = Severe

Facial and Oral Movements		
	1. **Muscles of Facial Expression** (e.g., movements of forehead, eyebrows, periorbital area, cheeks, including frowning, blinking, smiling, grimacing)	0 1 2 3 4
	2. **Lips and Perioral Area** (e.g., puckering, pouting, smacking)	0 1 2 3 4
	3. **Jaw** (e.g., biting, clenching, chewing, mouth opening, lateral movement)	0 1 2 3 4
	4. **Tongue** (Rate only increases in movement both in and out of mouth. NOT inability to sustain movement. Darting in and out of mouth.)	0 1 2 3 4

Extremity Movements	5. **Upper (arms, wrists, hands, fingers)** (Include choreic movements [i.e., rapid, objectively purposeless, irregular, spontaneous] and athetoid movements [i.e., slow, irregular, complex serpentine]. *Do not include tremor* [i.e., repetitive, regular, rhythmic].)	0 1 2 3 4
	6. **Lower (legs, knees, ankles, toes)** (e.g., lateral knee movement, foot tapping, heel dropping, foot squirming, inversion and eversion of foot)	0 1 2 3 4
Trunk Movements	7. **Neck, shoulders, hips** (e.g., rocking, twisting, squirming, pelvic gyrations)	0 1 2 3 4
Global Judgments	8. **Severity of abnormal movements overall**	0 1 2 3 4
	9. **Incapacitation due to abnormal movements**	0 1 2 3 4
Dental Status	10. **Patient's awareness of abnormal movements** (Rate only the client's report)	0 No awareness 1 Aware, no distress 2 Aware, mild distress 3 Aware, moderate distress 4 Aware, severe distress
	11. **Current problems with teeth and/or dentures?**	No Yes
	12. **Are dentures usually worn?**	No Yes
	13. **Edentia?**	No Yes
	14. **Do movements disappear in sleep?**	No Yes

Either before or after completing the Examination Procedure, observe the client unobtrusively, at rest (e.g. in waiting room). The chair to be used in this examination should be a hard, firm one without arms.

1. Ask client to remove shoes and socks.
2. Ask client whether there is anything in his/her mouth (i.e., gum, candy, etc.) and if there is, to remove it.

3. Ask client about the current condition of his/her teeth. Ask client if he/she wears dentures. Do teeth or dentures bother client now?

4. Ask client whether he/she notices any movements in mouth, face, hands, or feet. If yes, ask to describe and to what extent they currently bother client or interfere with his/her activities.

5. Have client sit in chair with both hands on knees, legs slightly apart, and feet flat on floor. (Look at entire body for movements while in this position.)

6. Ask client to sit with hands hanging unsupported. If male, between legs, if female and wearing a dress, hanging over knees. (Observe hands and other body areas.)

7. Ask client to open mouth. (Observe tongue at rest within mouth.) Do this twice.

8. Ask client to protrude tongue. (Observe abnormalities of tongue movement.) Do this twice.

9. Ask client to tap thumb with each finger as rapidly as possible for 10 to 15 seconds; separately with right hand, then with left hand. (Observe facial and leg movements.)

10. Flex and extend client's left and right arms (one at a time). (Note any rigidity.)

11. Ask client to stand up. (Observe in profile. Observe all body areas again, hips included.)

12. Ask client to extend both arms outstretched in front with palms down. (Observe trunk, legs, and mouth.)

13. Have client walk a few paces, turn, and walk back to chair. (Observe hands and gait.) Do this twice.

Interpretation of AIMS Score

Add client scores and note areas of difficulty.
Score of:

- 0 to 1 = Low risk
- 2 in only ONE of the areas assessed = borderline/observe closely
- 2 in TWO or more of the areas assessed **or** 3 to 4 in ONLY ONE area = indicative of TD

SOURCE: From U.S. Department of Health and Human Services. Available for use in the public domain.

Hamilton Depression Rating Scale (HDRS)

Instructions: For each item, circle the number to select the one "cue" that best characterizes the patient.

1. **Depressed Mood** (sadness, hopeless, helpless, worthless)
   0 = Absent
   1 = These feeling states indicated only on questioning.
   2 = These feeling states spontaneously reported verbally.
   3 = Communicates feeling states nonverbally; i.e., through facial expression, posture, voice, tendency to weep
   4 = Patient reports virtually only these feeling states in spontaneous verbal and nonverbal communication.

2. **Feelings of Guilt**
   0 = Absent
   1 = Self-reproach; feels he/she has let people down.
   2 = Ideas of guilt or rumination over past errors or sinful deeds
   3 = Present illness is a punishment. Delusions of guilt.
   4 = Hears accusatory or denunciatory voices and/or experiences threatening visual hallucinations.

3. **Suicide**
   0 = Absent
   1 = Feels life is not worth living.
   2 = Wishes he/she were dead or any thoughts of possible death to self.
   3 = Suicidal ideas or gesture.
   4 = Attempts at suicide (any serious attempt rates 4)

4. **Insomnia: Early in the Night**
   0 = No difficulty falling asleep
   1 = Complains of occasional difficulty falling asleep; i.e., more than one-half hour.
   2 = Complains of nightly difficulty falling asleep.

5. **Insomnia: Middle of the Night**
   0 = No difficulty
   1 = Complains of being restless and disturbed during the night.
   2 = Waking during the night— any getting out of bed rates as 2 (except for purposes of voiding)

6. **Insomnia: Early Hours of the Morning**
   0 = No difficulty.
   1 = Waking in early hours of the morning, but goes back to sleep.
   2 = Unable to fall asleep again if he/she gets out of bed.

7. **Work and Activities**
   0 = No difficulty
   1 = Thoughts and feelings of incapacity, fatigue, or weakness related to activities, work, or hobbies.
   2 = Loss of interest in activity, hobbies, or work—either directly reported by patient, or indirectly in listlessness, indecision, and vacillation (feels he/she has to push self to work or activities).
   3 = Decrease in actual time spent in activities or decrease in productivity. Rate 3 if patient

does not spend at least 3 hours a day in activities (job or hobbies), excluding routine chores.

4 = Stopped working because of present illness. Rate 4 if patient engages in no activities except routine chores, or if does not perform routine chores unassisted.

8. **Psychomotor Retardation** (slowness of thought and speech, impaired ability to concentrate, decreased motor activity)

0 = Normal speech and thought.

1 = Slight retardation during the interview.

2 = Obvious retardation during the interview.

3 = Interview difficult.

4 = Complete stupor.

9. **Agitation**

0 = None.

1 = Fidgetiness.

2 = Playing with hands, hair, etc.

3 = Moving about, can't sit still.

4 = Hand wringing, nail biting, hair pulling, biting of lips

10. **Anxiety (Psychic)**

0 = No difficulty.

1 = Subjective tension and irritability.

2 = Worrying about minor matters.

3 = Apprehensive attitude apparent in face or speech.

4 = Fears expressed without questioning.

11. **Anxiety (Somatic):** Physiological concomitants of anxiety (e.g., dry mouth, indigestion, diarrhea, cramps, belching, palpitations, headache, tremor, hyperventilation, sighing, urinary frequency, sweating, flushing)

0 = Absent

1 = Mild

2 = Moderate

3 = Severe

4 = Incapacitating

12. **Somatic Symptoms (Gastrointestinal)**

0 = None

1 = Loss of appetite, but eating without encouragement. Heavy feelings in abdomen.

2 = Difficulty eating without urging from others. Requests or requires medication for constipation or gastrointestinal symptoms.

13. **Somatic Symptoms (General)**

0 = None

1 = Heaviness in limbs, back or head. Backaches, headache, muscle aches. Loss of energy and fatigability.

2 = Any clear-cut symptom rates 2.

14. **Genital Symptoms** (e.g., loss of libido, impaired sexual performance, menstrual disturbances)

0 = Absent

1 = Mild

2 = Severe

15. **Hypochondriasis**

0 = Not present.

1 = Self-absorption (bodily)

2 = Preoccupation with health

3 = Frequent complaints, requests for help, etc.

4 = Hypochondriacal delusions

16. **Loss of Weight (Rate *either* A *or* B)**

A. *According to subjective patient history:*

0 = No weight loss

1 = Probably weight loss associated with present illness

2 = Definite weight loss associated with present illness

B. *According to objective weekly measurements:*

0 = Less than 1 lb. weight loss in week

1 = Greater than 1 lb. weight loss in week

2 = Greater than 2 lb. weight loss in week

17. **Insight**

0 = Acknowledges being depressed and ill.

1 = Acknowledges illness but attributes cause to bad food, climate, overwork, virus, need for rest, etc.

2 = Denies being ill at all

SCORING:

0–6 = No evidence of depressive illness

7–17 = Mild depression

18–24 = Moderate depression

>24 = Severe depression

TOTAL SCORE_____

SOURCE: Hamilton, M. (1960). A rating scale for depression. *Journal of Neurology, Neurosurgery, & Psychiatry, 23,* 56–62. The HDRS is in the public domain.

Hamilton Anxiety Rating Scale (HAM-A)

Below are descriptions of symptoms commonly associated with anxiety. Assign the client the rating between 0 and 4 (for each of the 14 items) that best describes the extent to which he/she has these symptoms.

0 = Not present
1 = Mild
2 = Moderate
3 = Severe
4 = Very severe

Rating

1. **Anxious mood** _____
Worries, anticipation
of the worst, fearful
anticipation, irritability

2. **Tension** _____
Feelings of tension,
fatigability, startle
response, moved
to tears easily,
trembling, feelings
of restlessness,
inability to relax

3. **Fears** _____
Of dark, of strangers,
of being left alone,
of animals, of traffic,
of crowds

4. **Insomnia** _____
Difficulty in falling
asleep, broken sleep,
unsatisfying sleep and
fatigue on waking,
dreams, nightmares,
night terrors

Rating

5. **Intellectual** _____
Difficulty in
concentration, poor
memory

6. **Depressed mood** _____
Loss of interest,
lack of pleasure in
hobbies, depression,
early waking, diurnal
swing

7. **Somatic (muscular)** _____
Pains and aches,
twitching, stiffness,
myoclonic jerks,
grinding of teeth,
unsteady voice,
increased muscular
tone

Rating

Rating

8. **Somatic (sensory)** _____
   Tinnitus, blurred
   vision, hot/cold
   flushes, feelings of
   weakness, tingling
   sensation

9. **Cardiovascular** _____
   symptoms
   Tachycardia, palpi-
   tations, pain in chest,
   throbbing of ves-
   sels, feeling faint

10. **Respiratory** _____
    symptoms
    Pressure or con-
    striction in chest,
    choking feelings,
    sighing, dyspnea

11. **Gastrointestinal** _____
    symptoms
    Difficulty swallow-
    ing, flatulence, ab-
    dominal pain and
    fullness, burning
    sensations, nausea/
    vomiting, borbo-
    rygmi, diarrhea,
    constipation,
    weight loss

12. **Genitourinary** _____
    symptoms
    Urinary frequency,
    urinary urgency,
    amenorrhea,
    menorrhagia, loss
    of libido, premature
    ejaculation,
    impotence

13. **Autonomic** _____
    symptoms
    Dry mouth, flush-
    ing, pallor, tendency
    to sweat, giddiness,
    tension headache,

14. **Behavior at** _____
    interview
    Fidgeting, restless-
    ness or pacing,
    tremor of hands,
    furrowed brow,
    strained face,
    sighing or rapid
    respiration, facial
    pallor, swallowing,
    clearing throat

Client's Total Score _____
SCORING:
   14–17 = Mild Anxiety
   18–24 = Moderate Anxiety
   25–30 = Severe Anxiety

SOURCE: Hamilton, M. (1959). The assessment of anxiety states by rating.
   British Journal of Medical Psychology, 32, 50–55. The HAM-A is in the public
   domain.

NANDA Nursing Diagnoses: Taxonomy II

■ DOMAINS, CLASSES, AND DIAGNOSES

Domain 1: Health Promotion

Class 1: Health Awareness

Deficient diversional activity
Sedentary lifestyle

Class 2: Health Management

Deficient community health
Risk-prone health behavior
Ineffective health maintenance
Readiness for enhanced immunization status
Ineffective protection
Ineffective self-health management
Readiness for enhanced self health management
Ineffective family therapeutic regimen management

Domain 2: Nutrition

Class 1: Ingestion

Insufficient breast milk
Ineffective infant feeding pattern
Imbalanced nutrition: Less than body requirements
Imbalanced nutrition: More than body requirements
Readiness for enhanced nutrition
Risk for imbalanced nutrition: More than body requirements
Impaired swallowing

Class 2: Digestion

Class 3: Absorption

Class 4: Metabolism

Risk for unstable blood glucose level
Neonatal jaundice
Risk for neonatal jaundice
Risk for impaired liver function

Class 5: Hydration

>Risk for electrolyte imbalance
>Readiness for enhanced fluid balance
>Deficient fluid volume
>Risk for deficient fluid volume
>Excess fluid volume
>Risk for imbalanced fluid volume

Domain 3: Elimination and Exchange

Class 1: Urinary Function

>Functional urinary incontinence
>Overflow urinary incontinence
>Reflex urinary incontinence
>Stress urinary incontinence
>Urge urinary incontinence
>Risk for urge urinary incontinence
>Impaired urinary elimination
>Readiness for enhanced urinary elimination
>Urinary retention

Class 2: Gastrointestinal Function

>Constipation
>Perceived constipation
>Risk for constipation
>Diarrhea
>Dysfunctional gastrointestinal motility
>Risk for dysfunctional gastrointestinal motility
>Bowel incontinence

Class 3: Integumentary Function

Class 4: Respiratory Function

>Impaired gas exchange

Domain 4: Activity/Rest

Class 1: Sleep/Rest

>Insomnia
>Sleep deprivation
>Readiness for enhanced sleep
>Disturbed sleep pattern

Class 2: Activity/Exercise

>Risk for disuse syndrome
>Impaired physical mobility
>Impaired bed mobility
>Impaired wheelchair mobility
>Impaired transfer ability
>Impaired walking

Class 3: Energy Balance

Disturbed energy field
Fatigue
Wandering

Class 4: Cardiovascular/Pulmonary Responses

Activity intolerance
Risk for activity intolerance
Ineffective breathing pattern
Decreased cardiac output
Risk for ineffective gastrointestinal perfusion
Risk for ineffective renal perfusion
Impaired spontaneous ventilation
Ineffective peripheral tissue perfusion
Risk for decreased cardiac tissue perfusion
Risk for ineffective cerebral tissue perfusion
Risk for ineffective peripheral tissue perfusion
Dysfunctional ventilatory weaning response

Class 5: Self-Care

Impaired home maintenance
Readiness for enhanced self-care
Bathing self-care deficit
Dressing self-care deficit
Feeding self-care deficit
Toileting self-care deficit
Self-neglect

Domain 5: Perception/Cognition

Class 1: Attention

Unilateral neglect

Class 2: Orientation

Impaired environmental interpretation syndrome

Class 3: Sensation/Perception

Class 4: Cognition

Acute confusion
Chronic confusion
Risk for acute confusion
Ineffective impulse control
Deficient knowledge
Readiness for enhanced knowledge
Impaired memory

Class 5: Communication

Readiness for enhanced communication
Impaired verbal communication

Domain 6: Self-Perception

Class 1: Self-Concept

Hopelessness
Risk for compromised human dignity
Risk for loneliness
Disturbed personal identity
Risk for disturbed personal identity
Readiness for enhanced self-concept

Class 2: Self-Esteem

Chronic low self-esteem
Situational low self-esteem
Risk for chronic low self-esteem
Risk for situational low self-esteem

Class 3: Body Image

Disturbed body image

Domain 7: Role Relationships

Class 1: Caregiving Roles

Ineffective breastfeeding
Interrupted breastfeeding
Readiness for enhanced breastfeeding
Caregiver role strain
Risk for caregiver role strain
Impaired parenting
Risk for impaired parenting
Readiness for enhanced parenting

Class 2: Family Relationships

Risk for impaired attachment
Interrupted family processes
Readiness for enhanced family processes
Dysfunctional family processes

Class 3: Role Performance

Ineffective relationship
Readiness for enhanced relationship
Risk for ineffective relationship
Ineffective role performance
Parental role conflict
Impaired social interaction

Domain 8: Sexuality

Class 1: Sexual Identity

Class 2: Sexual Function

Sexual dysfunction
Ineffective sexuality pattern

Class 3: Reproduction

    Ineffective childbearing process
    Readiness for enhanced childbearing process
    Risk for ineffective childbearing process
    Risk for disturbed maternal/fetal dyad

Domain 9: Coping/Stress Tolerance

Class 1: Post-trauma Responses

    Post-trauma syndrome
    Risk for post-trauma syndrome
    Rape-trauma syndrome
    Relocation stress syndrome
    Risk for relocation stress syndrome

Class 2: Coping Responses

    Ineffective activity planning
    Risk for ineffective activity planning
    Anxiety
    Defensive coping
    Ineffective coping
    Readiness for enhanced coping
    Ineffective community coping
    Readiness for enhanced community coping
    Compromised family coping
    Disabled family coping
    Readiness for enhanced family coping
    Death anxiety
    Ineffective denial
    Adult failure to thrive
    Fear
    Grieving
    Complicated grieving
    Risk for complicated grieving
    Readiness for enhanced power
    Powerlessness
    Risk for powerlessness
    Impaired individual resilience
    Readiness for enhanced resilience
    Risk for compromised resilience
    Chronic sorrow
    Stress overload

Class 3: Neurobehavioral Stress

    Autonomic dysreflexia
    Risk for autonomic dysreflexia
    Disorganized infant behavior
    Risk for disorganized infant behavior

Readiness for enhanced organized infant behavior
Decreased intracranial adaptive capacity

Domain 10: Life Principles

Class 1: Values

Readiness for enhanced hope

Class 2: Beliefs

Readiness for enhanced spiritual wellbeing

Class 3: Value/Belief/Action Congruence

Readiness for enhanced decision making
Decisional conflict
Moral distress
Noncompliance
Impaired religiosity
Readiness for enhanced religiosity
Risk for impaired religiosity
Spiritual distress
Risk for spiritual distress

Domain 11: Safety/Protection

Class 1: Infection

Risk for infection

Class 2: Physical Injury

Ineffective airway clearance
Risk for aspiration
Risk for bleeding
Impaired dentition
Risk for dry eye
Risk for falls
Risk for injury
Impaired oral mucous membrane
Risk for perioperative positioning injury
Risk for peripheral neurovascular dysfunction
Risk for shock
Impaired skin integrity
Risk for impaired skin integrity
Risk for sudden infant death syndrome
Risk for suffocation
Delayed surgical recovery
Risk for thermal injury
Impaired tissue integrity
Risk for trauma
Risk for vascular trauma

Class 3: Violence
    Risk for other-directed violence
    Risk for self-directed violence
    Self-mutilation
    Risk for self-mutilation
    Risk for suicide

Class 4: Environmental Hazards
    Contamination
    Risk for contamination
    Risk for poisoning

Class 5: Defensive Processes
    Risk for adverse reaction to iodinated contrast media
    Latex allergy response
    Risk for latex allergy response
    Risk for allergy response

Class 6: Thermoregulation
    Risk for imbalanced body temperature
    Ineffective thermoregulation
    Hypothermia
    Hyperthermia

Domain 12: Comfort

Class 1: Physical Comfort
    Acute pain
    Chronic pain
    Nausea
    Readiness for enhanced comfort
    Impaired comfort

Class 2: Environmental Comfort
    Readiness for enhanced comfort
    Impaired comfort

Class 3: Social Comfort
    Social isolation
    Impaired comfort
    Readiness for enhanced comfort

Domain 13: Growth/Development

Class 1: Growth
    Risk for disproportionate growth

Class 2: Development
    Delayed growth and development
    Risk for delayed development

SOURCE: *NANDA International.* (2012). *Nursing Diagnoses: Definitions & Classification 2012–2014.* Hoboken, NJ: Wiley-Blackwell. With permission.

Bibliography

Aguilera, D.C. (1998). *Crisis intervention: Theory and methodology* (8th ed.). St. Louis: C.V. Mosby.

American Academy of Child and Adolescent Psychiatry. (2011). *Children of alcoholics*. Retrieved from www.aacap.org/cs/root/facts_for_families/children_of_alcoholics

American Academy of Child and Adolescent Psychiatry. (2013). *Military families resource center*. Retrieved from http://www.aacap.org/AACAP/Families_and_Youth/Resource_Centers/Military_Families_Resource_Center/FAQ.aspx

American Medical Association (AMA). (2010). *Unconventional medical care in the United States*. Policy #H-480-973. Advocacy Resource Center. Chicago, IL: AMA.

American Nurses Association (ANA). (2008). *Home health nursing: Scope and standards of practice*. Silver Spring, MD: ANA.

American Nurses Association (ANA). (2010a). *Nursing's social policy statement: The essence of the profession*. Silver Spring, MD: ANA.

American Nurses Association (2010b). *Scope and standards of practice* (2nd ed.) Silver Spring, MD: ANA.

American Nurses Association (ANA) and International Association of Forensic Nurses (IAFN). (2009). *Forensic nursing: Scope and standards of practice*. Silver Spring, MD: ANA.

American Psychiatric Association. (2013). *Diagnostic and statistical manual of mental disorders* (5th ed.). Washington, DC: American Psychiatric Publishing.

Avants, S.K., Margolin, A., Holford, T.R., & Kosten, T.R. (2000). A randomized controlled trial of auricular acupuncture for cocaine dependence. *Archives of Internal Medicine, 160*(15), 2305–2312.

Bagley, C. & Mallick, K. (2000). Spiraling up and spiraling down: Implications of a long-term study of temperament and conduct disorder for social work with children. *Child & Family Social Work 5*(4), 291–301.

Banks, M.R. & Banks, W.A. (2002). The effects of animal-assisted therapy on loneliness in an elderly population in long-term care facilities. *The Journals of Gerontology Series A: Biological Sciences and Medical Sciences, 57*(7), M428–M432.

Beck, A., Rush, A.J., Shaw, B. F., & Emery, G. (1979). *Cognitive theory of depression*. New York: Guilford Press.

Becker, J.V. & Johnson, B.R. (2008). Gender identity disorders and paraphilias. In R.E. Hales, S.C. Yudofsky, & G.O. Gabbard (Eds.), *The American Psychiatric Publishing textbook of clinical psychiatry* (5th ed.). Washington, DC: American Psychiatric Publishing, pp. 729–754.

Becker, J.V. & Stinson, J.D. (2008). Human sexuality and sexual dysfunctions. In R.E. Hales, S.C. Yudofsky, & G.O. Gabbard (Eds.), *The American Psychiatric Publishing textbook of clinical psychiatry* (5th ed.). Washington, DC: American Psychiatric Publishing, pp. 711–728.

Bellfield, B. & Catalano, J.T. (2012). Developments in current nursing practice. In J.T. Catalano (Ed.), *Nursing now! Today's issues, tomorrow's trends* (6th ed.). Philadelphia: F.A. Davis, pp. 450–466.

Black, D.W. & Andreasen, N.C. (2011). *Introductory textbook of psychiatry* (5th ed.). Washington, DC: American Psychiatric Publishing.

Blumenthal, M. (Ed.). (1998). *The complete German Commission E monographs: Therapeutic guide to herbal medicines.* Austin, TX: American Botanical Garden.

Bourgeois, J.A., Seaman, J.S., & Servis, M.E. (2008). Delirium, dementia, and amnestic and other cognitive disorders. In R.E. Hales, S.C. Yudofsky, & G.O. Gabbard (Eds.), *The American Psychiatric Publishing textbook of psychiatry,* (5th ed.). Washington DC: American Psychiatric Publishing, pp. 303–364.

Bowlby, J. (1961). Processes of mourning. *International Journal of Psycho-analysis, 42,* 317–322.

Brancu, M., Straits-Troster, K., & Kudler, H. (2011). Behavioral health conditions among military personnel and veterans: Prevalence and best practices for treatment. *North Carolina Medical Journal, 72*(1), 54–60.

Breslau, N. (2009, July). The epidemiology of trauma, PTSD, and other posttrauma disorders. *Trauma, Violence, & Abuse, 10*(3), 198–210.

Burgess, A. (2010). *Rape violence.* Gannett Education Course #60025. Retrieved from http://ce.nurse.com/60025/Rape-Violence

Catalano, J.T. (2012). *Nursing now! Today's issues, tomorrow's trends* (6th ed.). Philadelphia: FA Davis.

Centers for Disease Control and Prevention (CDC). (2011, August). Attention deficit hyperactivity disorder among children aged 5–17 in the United States 1998–2009. *NCHS Data Brief, 70.* Hyattsville, MD: National Center for Health Statistics.

Chess, S., Thomas, A., & Birch, H. (1970). The origins of personality. *Scientific American 223,*102.

Child Welfare Information Gateway (CWIG). (2013). *What is child abuse and neglect? Recognizing the signs and symptoms.* Retrieved from www .childwelfare.gov/pubs/factsheets/whatiscan.pdf

Coeytaux, R.R., Kaufman, J.S., Kaptchuk, T.J., Chen, W., Miller, W.M., Callahan, L.F., & Mann, D. (2005). A randomized, controlled trial of acupuncture for chronic daily headache. *Headache, 45*(9), 1113–1123.

College and Association of Registered Nurses of Alberta (CARNA). (2005). *Professional boundaries for registered nurses: Guidelines for the nurse-client relationship.* Edmonton, AB: CARNA.

Constantino, R.E., Crane, P.A., & Young, S.E. (2013). *Forensic nursing: Evidence-based principles and practice.* Philadelphia: F.A. Davis.

Cooper, B.E. & Sejnowski, C.A. (2013). Serotonin syndrome: Recognition and treatment. *AACN Advanced Critical Care, 24*(1), 15–20.

Corr, C.A. & Corr, D.M. (2013). *Death & dying: Life & living* (7th ed.). Belmont, CA: Wadsworth.

Council of Acupuncture and Oriental Medicine Associations (CAOMA). (2013). *Conditions treated by acupuncture and oriental medicine.* Retrieved from http://www.acucouncil.org/conditions_treated.htm

Cummings, J.L. & Mega, M.S. (2003). *Neuropsychiatry and behavioral neuroscience.* New York: Oxford University Press.

Curtis, C.M., Fegley, A.B., & Tuzo, C.N. (2009). *Psychiatric mental health nursing success.* Philadelphia: F.A. Davis.

Davis, C.P. (2012). *Dementia: Treatable causes*. Retrieved from www .emedicinehealth.com/script/main/art.asp?articlekey=59089&pf=3&page3

Delemarre-van de Waal, H.A. & Cohen-Kettenis, P.T. (2006). Clinical management of gender identity disorder in adolescents: A protocol on psychological and pediatric endocrinology aspects. *European Journal of Endocrinology, 155*(1), 131–137.

Department of Veterans Affairs. (2012). How common is PTSD? Retrieved from www.ptsd.va.gov/public/pages/how-common-is-ptsd.asp

Department of Veterans Affairs & Department of Defense (DVA/DoD). (2009). *Clinical practice guideline for management of concussion/mild traumatic brain injury*. Retrieved from http://www.healthquality.va.gov/guidelines/Rehab/mtbi/concussion_mtbi_full_1_0.pdf

Devries, M.R., Hughes, H.K., Watson, H., & Moore, B.A. (2012). Understanding the military culture. In B.A. Moore (Ed.), *Handbook of counseling military couples*. New York: Routledge, pp. 7–18.

Dion, Y., Annable, L., Sandor, P., & Chouinard, G. (2002). Risperidone in the treatment of Tourette syndrome: A double-blind, placebo-controlled trial. *Journal of Clinical Psychopharmacology, 22*(1), 31–39.

Doenges, M.E., Moorhouse, M.F., & Murr, A.C. (2013). *Nurse's pocket guide: Diagnoses, prioritized interventions, and rationales* (13th ed.). Philadelphia: F.A. Davis.

Doenges, M.E., Moorhouse, M.F., & Murr, A.C. (2013). *Nursing diagnosis manual: Planning, individualizing, and documenting client care* (4th ed.). Philadelphia: F.A. Davis.

Dopheide, J.A. & Pliszka, S.R. (2009). Attention deficit/hyperactivity disorder: An Update. *Pharmacotherapy, 29*(6), 656–679.

Dougherty, C.M. (2011). Evidence collection in the emergency department. In V.A. Lynch (Ed.), *Forensic nursing science* (2nd ed.). St. Louis: Mosby, pp. 155–167.

Dreyfus, E.A. (2012). *Sexuality and sex therapy, Part II*. Retrieved from www .selfhelpmagazine.com/node/5025

Drug Facts and Comparisons. (2014). St. Louis, MO: Wolters Kluwer.

Eisendrath, S.J. & Lichtmacher, J.E. (2012). Psychiatric disorders. In S.J. McPhee, M.A. Papadakis, & M.W. Rabow (Eds.), *Current medical diagnosis and treatment 2012*. New York: McGraw-Hill, pp. 1010–1064.

Engel, G. (1964). Grief and grieving. *American Journal of Nursing, 64*, 93.

Epstein, S. (1991). Beliefs and symptoms in maladaptive resolutions of the traumatic neurosis. In D. Ozer, J.M. Healy, Jr., & A.J. Stewart (Eds.), *Perspectives on personality* (Vol. 3). London: Jessica Kingsley.

Erikson, E.H. (1963). *Childhood and Society*. New York: W.W. Norton.

Erlij, D., Acosta-Garcia, J., Rojas-Marquez, M., Gonzalez-Hernandez, B., Escartin-Perez, E., Aceves, J., & Floran, B. (2012). Dopamine D4 receptor stimulation in GABAergic projections of the globus pallidus to the reticular thalamic nucleus and the substantia nigra reticulate of the rat decreases locomotor activity. *Neuropharmacology, 62*(2), 1111–1118.

Ernst, L.S. (2012, October). Animal-assisted therapy: Using animals to promote healing. *Nursing 2012, 42*(10), 54–58.

Fohrman, D.A. & Stein, M.T. (2006). Psychosis: Six steps rule out medical causes in kids. *The Journal of Family Practice Online, 5*(2). Retrieved from http://www.jfponline.com/pages.asp?aid=3887

Foley, D.L., Eaves, L.J., Wormley, B., Silberg, J.L., Maes, H.H., Kuh, J., & Riley, B. (2004). Childhood adversity, monoamine oxidase A genotype, and risk for conduct disorder. *Archives of General Psychiatry*, 61, 738–744.

Folstein, M.F., Folstein, S.E., & McHugh, P.R. (1975). Mini-mental state: A practical method for grading the cognitive state of patients for the clinician. *Journal of Psychiatric Research*, *12*(3), 189–198.

Foroud, T., Gray, J., Ivashina, J., & Conneally, P.M. (1999). Differences in duration of Huntington's disease based on age at onset. *Journal of Neurology, Neurosurgery and Psychiatry*, *66*(1), 52–56.

Freud, S. (1962). The neuro-psychoses of defense. In J. Strachey (Ed.), *Standard edition of the complete psychological works of Sigmund Freud, Vol 3*. London: Hogarth Press (original work published 1894).

Freudenreich, O. (2010). Differential diagnosis of psychotic symptoms: Medical "mimics." *Psychiatric Times*, *27*(12), 52–61.

Friedmann, E. & Thomas, S.A. (1995). Pet ownership, social support, and one-year survival after acute myocardial infarction in the cardiac arrhythmia suppression trial. *American Journal of Cardiology*, *76*(17), 1213.

Gabany, E. & Shellenbarger, T. (2010). Caring for families with deployment stress: How nurses can make a difference in the lives of military families. *American Journal of Nursing*, *110*(11), 36–41.

Gibbons, R.D., Hur, K., Brown, C.H., & Mann, J.J. (2009). Relationship between antiepileptic drugs and suicide attempts in patients with bipolar disorder. *Archives of General Psychiatry*, *66*(12), 1354–1360.

Gibson, B. & Catlin, A.J. (2010). Care of the child with the desire to change gender–Part I. *Pediatric Nursing*, *36*(1), 53–59.

Godenne, G. (2001). The role of pets in nursing homes . . . and psychotherapy. *The Maryland Psychiatrist*, *27*(3), 5–6.

Gordon, M. (1994). *Nursing diagnosis: Process and application* (3rd ed.). St. Louis: Mosby-Year Book.

Gunderson, J.G. (2011). An introduction to borderline personality disorder: Diagnosis, origins, course, and treatment. *National Education Alliance—Borderline Personality Disorder*. Retrieved from www.borderlinepersonalitydisorder.com/understading-bpd/a-bpd-brief/

Haddad, P.M. (2001). Antidepressant discontinuation syndromes: Clinical relevance, prevention, and management. *Drug Safety*, *24*(3), 183–197.

Hall, L.K. (2012). The military lifestyle and the relationship. In B.A. Moore (Ed.), *Handbook of counseling military couples*. New York: Routledge, pp. 137–156.

Halmi, K.A. (2008). Eating disorders: Anorexia nervosa, bulimia nervosa, and obesity. In R.E. Hales, S.C. Yudofsky, & G.O. Gabbard (Eds.), *Textbook of psychiatry* (5th ed.). Washington, DC: American Psychiatric Publishing, pp. 971–997.

Halstead, H. L. (2005). Spirituality in older adults. In M. Stanley, K.A. Blair, & P. G. Beare (Eds.), *Gerontological nursing: A health promotion/protection approach* (3rd ed.). Philadelphia: F. A. Davis, pp. 285–292.

Harvard Medical School. (2001, April). Bipolar disorder—Part I. *The Harvard Mental Health Letter*. Boston, MA: Harvard Medical School Publications Group.

Harvard Medical School. (2005). The homeless mentally ill. *Harvard Mental Health Letter*, *21*(11), 4–7.

Hays, J.S. & Larson, K.H. (1963). *Interacting with patients*. New York: Holt, Rinehart, & Winston.

Hazlett, H.C., Poe, M.D., Gerig, G., Styner, M., Chappell, C., Smith, R.G., Vachet, C., & Piven, J. (2011). Early brain overgrowth in autism associated with an increase in cortical surface area before age 2 years. *Archives of General Psychiatry, 68*(5), 467–476.

Hill, J. (2003). Early identification of individuals at risk for antisocial personality disorder. *British Journal of Psychiatry, 182*(suppl. 44), s11–s14.

Hodgins, D.C., Stea, J.N., & Grant, J.E. (2011). Gambling disorders. *The Lancet, 378*(9806), 1874–1888.

Hollander, E., Berlin, H.A., & Stein, D.J. (2008). Impulse-control disorders not elsewhere classified. In R.E. Hales, S.C. Yudofsky, & G.O. Gabbard (Eds.), *Textbook of psychiatry* (5th ed.). Washington, DC: American Psychiatric Publishing, pp. 777–820.

Holt, G.A. & Kouzi, S. (2002). Herbs through the ages. In M.A. Bright (Ed.), *Holistic health and healing*. Philadelphia: F.A. Davis, 135–160.

Hornor, G. (2005). Domestic violence and children. *Journal of Pediatric Health Care, 19*(4), 206–212.

Institute of Medicine (IOM). (2012). *Returning home from Iraq and Afghanistan: Preliminary assessment of readjustment needs of veterans, service members, and their families*. Washington, DC: The National Academies Press.

Jakupcak, M., Vannoy, S., Imel., Z., Cook, J.W., Fontana, A., Rosenheck, R., & McFall, M. (2010). Does PTSD moderate the relationship between social support and suicide risk in Iraq and Afghanistan war veterans seeking mental health treatment? *Depression and Anxiety, 27*(11), 1001–1005.

James, D.J. & Glaze, L.E. (2006, September). *Mental health problems of prison and jail inmates*. Bureau of Justice Statistics Special Report.

Jaret, P. (2010). *Eating disorders and depression*. Retrieved from www.webmd.com/depression/features/eating-disorders

Jeffreys, J.S. (2010, Winter). Understanding grief in older adults. In *Living With Loss Magazine*. Eckert, CO: Bereavement Publications, Inc., pp. 18–19.

Jensen, J.E. & Miller, B. (2004). *Home health psychiatric care: A guide to understanding home health psychiatric care as covered under Medicare Part A*. Seattle, WA: The Washington Institute for Mental Illness Research & Training.

Jonsson, S.A., Luts, A., Guldberg-Kjaer, N., & Brun, A. (1997). Hippocampal pyramidal cell disarray correlates negatively to cell number: Implications for the pathogenesis of schizophrenia. *European Archives of Psychiatry and Clinical Neuroscience, 247*(3), 120–127.

Joska, J.A. & Stein, D.J. (2008). Mood disorders. In R.E. Hales, S.C. Yudofsky, & G.O. Gabbard (Eds.), *Textbook of psychiatry* (5th ed.). Washington, DC: American Psychiatric Publishing, pp. 457–504.

Kaufman, D.M., & Zun, L. (1995). A quantifiable, brief mental status examination for emergency patients. *Journal of Emergency Medicine, 13*(4), 440–456.

Killgore, W.D., Cotting, D.I., Thomas, J.L., Cox, A.L., McGurk, D., Vo, A.H., Castro, C.A., & Hoge, C.W. (2008). Post-combat invincibility: Violent combat experiences are associated with increased risk-taking propensity following deployment. *Journal of Psychiatric Research, 42*(13), 1112–1121.

King, B.M. (2011). *Human sexuality today* (7th ed.). Upper Saddle River, NJ: Pearson Education.

Knoll, J. (2011). The suicide prevention contract: Contracting for comfort. *Psychiatric Times*. Retrieved from www.psychiatrictimes.com/suicide/suicide-prevention-contract-contracting-comfort

Kokman, E., Smith, G.E., Petersen, R.C., Tangalos, E., & Ivnik, R.C. (1991). The short test of mental status: Correlations with standardized psychometric testing. *Archives of Neurology*, *48*(7), 725–728.

Kübler-Ross, E. (1969). *On death and dying*. New York: Macmillan.

Ladd, G.W. (1999). Peer relationships and social competence during early and middle childhood. *Annual Review of Psychology*, *50*, 333–359.

Lagerquist, S.L. (2012). *Davis's NCLEX-RN Success* (3rd ed.). Philadelphia: F.A. Davis.

Ledray, L. E. (2009). Evidence collection and care of the sexual assault survivor: The SANE-SART response. *Minnesota Center Against Violence and Abuse*. Retrieved from http://www.mincava.umn.edu/documents/commissioned/2forensicevidence/2forensicevidence.html

Leiblum, S.R. (1999). Sexual problems and dysfunction: Epidemiology, classification, and risk factors. *The Journal of Gender-Specific Medicine*, *2*(5), 41–45.

Levenson, J.L. (2009). Medical aspects of catatonia. *Primary Psychiatry*, *16*(3), 23–26.

Levine, G.N., Allen, K., Braun, L.T., Christian, H.E., Friedmann, E., Taubert, K.A., Thomas, S.A., Wells, D.L., & Lange, R.A. (2013). Pet ownership and cardiovascular risk: A scientific statement from the American Heart Association. *Circulation Journal of the American Heart Association*. Published online before print at http://circ.ahajournals.org/content/early/2013/05/09/CIR.0b013e31829201e1.citation

Linnet, K.M., Wisborg, K., Obel, C., Secher, N.J., Thomsen, P.H., Agerbo, E., & Henriksen, T.B. (2005). Smoking during pregnancy and the risk for hyperkinetic disorder in offspring. *Pediatrics*, *116*(2), 462–467.

Lochner, C., duToit, P.L., Zungu-Dirwayi, N., Marais, A., vanKradenburg, J., Curr, B., Seedat, S., Niehaus, D.J.H., & Stein, D.J. (2002). Childhood trauma in obsessive-compulsive disorder, trichotillomania, and controls. *Depression and Anxiety*, *15*(2), 66–68.

Lubit, R.H. (2013). Oppositional defiant disorder. Retrieved from http://emedicine.medscape.com/article/918095-overview

Lubit, R.H. (2013). Borderline personality disorder. *eMedicine Psychiatry*. Retrieved from http://emedicine.medscape.com/article/913575-overview

Lutz, C.A. & Przytulski, K.R. (2011). *Nutrition and diet therapy evidence-based applications* (5th ed.). Philadelphia: F.A. Davis.

Lyden, H., Espinoza, R.T., Pirnia, T., Clark, K., Joshi, S.H., Leaver, A.M., Woods, R.P., & Narr, K.L. (2014). Electroconvulsive therapy mediates neuroplasticity of white matter microstructure in major depression. *Translational Psychiatry 4*, e380; doi: 10.1038/tp.2014.21.

Lynch, V.A. (2011). *Forensic nursing science* (2nd ed.). St. Louis: Mosby.

Lynch, V.A. & Koehler, S.A. (2011). Forensic investigation of death. In V.A. Lynch (Ed.), *Forensic nursing science* (2nd ed.). St. Louis: Mosby, pp. 179–194.

Mack, A.H., Franklin, J.E., & Frances, R.J. (2003). Substance Use Disorders. In R.E. Hales & S.C. Yudofsky (Eds.), *Textbook of clinical psychiatry* (4th ed.). Washington, DC: American Psychiatric Publishing, pp. 309–378.

Mahler, M., Pine, F., & Bergman, A. (1975). *The psychological birth of the human infant*. New York: Basic Books.

Maldonado, J.R. & Spiegel, D. (2008). Dissociative Disorders. In R.E. Hales, S.C. Yudofsky, & G.O. Gabbard (Eds.), *Textbook of psychiatry* (5th ed.). Washington, DC: American Psychiatric Publishing, pp. 665–710.

Marangell, L.B., Silver, J.M., Goff, D.C., & Yudofsky, S.C. (2003). Psychopharmacology and electroconvulsive therapy. In R.E. Hales & S.C. Yudofsky (Eds.), *Textbook of clinical psychiatry* (4th ed.). Washington, DC: American Psychiatric Publishing, pp. 1047–1150.

Mathewson, J. (2011). In support of military women and families. In R.B. Everson & C.R. Figley (Eds.), *Families under fire*. New York: Routledge, pp. 215–235.

McClintock, S.M. & Husain, M.M. (2011). Electroconvulsive therapy does not damage the brain. *Journal of the American Psychiatric Nurses Association, 17*(3), 212–213.

Merck manual of health & aging. (2005). New York: Random House.

Minzenberg, M.J., Yoon, J.H., & Stein, D.J. (2008). Schizophrenia. In R.E. Hales, S.C. Yudofsky, & G.O. Gabbard (Eds.), *Textbook of psychiatry* (5th ed.). Washington, DC: American Psychiatric Publishing, pp. 407–456.

Moreyra, P., Ibanez, A., Saiz-Ruiz, J., Nissenson, K., & Blanco, C. (2000). Review of the phenomenology, etiology, and treatment of pathological gambling. *German Journal of Psychiatry, 3*, 37–52.

Murray, R. B., Zentner, J. P., & Yakimo, R. (2009). *Health promotion strategies through the life span* (8th ed.). Upper Saddle River, NJ: Prentice-Hall.

Nahin, R.L., Barnes, P.M., Stussman, B.J., & Bloom, B. (2009, July 20). Costs of complementary and alternative medicine (CAM) and frequency of visits to CAM practitioners. *National Health Statistics Reports, 18*. Hyattsville, MD: National Center for Health Statistics.

NANDA International (NANDA-I). (2012). *Nursing diagnoses: Definitions and classification, 2012–2014*. Hoboken, NJ: Wiley-Blackwell.

National Center for Complementary and Alternative Medicine (NCCAM). (2008). *The use of complementary and alternative medicine in the United States*. NCCAM Publication No. D424. Bethesda, MD: National Institutes of Health.

National Center for Complementary and Alternative Medicine (NCCAM). (2012a). *Acupuncture: An introduction*. NCCAM Publication No. D404. Bethesda, MD: National Institutes of Health.

National Center for Complementary and Alternative Medicine (NCCAM). (2012b). *Chiropractic: An introduction*. NCCAM Publication No. D403. Bethesda, MD: National Institutes of Health.

National Center for Complementary and Alternative Medicine (NCCAM). (2012c). *What is complementary and alternative medicine?* NCCAM Publication No. D347. Bethesda, MD: National Institutes of Health.

National Coalition for the Homeless (NCH). (2009). *HIV/AIDS and homelessness*. Retrieved from http://www.nationalhomeless.org/

National Coalition for the Homeless (NCH). (2009). *Homeless families with children*. Retrieved from http://www.nationalhomeless.org/

National Coalition for the Homeless (NCH). (2009). *How many people experience homelessness?* Retrieved from http://www.nationalhomeless.org/

National Coalition for the Homeless (NCH). (2009). *Who is homeless?* Retrieved from http://www.nationalhomeless.org/

National Coalition for the Homeless (NCH). (2009). *Why are people homeless?* Retrieved from http://www.nationalhomeless.org/

National Council of State Boards of Nursing (NCSBN). (2013). *Test plan for the National Council Licensure Examination for Registered Nurses.* Retrieved from http://www.ncsbn.org

National Institute of Mental Health (NIMH). (2013). *Mental disorders in America: The numbers count.* Bethesda, MD: National Institutes of Health.

National Institute on Drug Abuse (NIDA). (2011). *Substance abuse among the military, veterans, and their families.* Washington, DC: National Institutes of Health. Retrieved from www.drugabuse.gov/sites/default/files/veterans.pdf

Neddermeyer, D.M. (2006). Holistic health care increasing in popularity worldwide. EzineArticles. Retrieved from http://ezinearticles.com/?Holistic-Health-Care-Increasing-in-Popularity-Worldwide&id=373550

Oldham, J.M., Gabbard, G.O., Goin, M.K., Gunderson, J., Soloff, P., Spiegel, D., Stone, M., & Phillips, K.A. (2006). Practice guideline for the treatment of patients with borderline personality disorder. In *The American Psychiatric Association practice guidelines for the treatment of psychiatric disorders, Compendium 2006.* Washington, DC: American Psychiatric Publishing.

Parcell, S. (2008). Biochemical and nutritional influences on pain. In J.F. Audette & A. Bailey (Eds.), *Integrative pain medicine.* New York: Springer-Verlag, 133–172.

PDR for herbal medicines (4th ed.). (2007). Montvale, NJ: Thomson Healthcare Inc.

Peplau, H.E. (1962). Interpersonal techniques: The crux of psychiatric nursing. *American Journal of Nursing 62*(6), 50–54.

Peplau, H.E. (1991). *Interpersonal relations in nursing.* New York: Springer.

Pfeiffer, E. (1975). A short portable mental status questionnaire for the assessment of organic brain deficit in elderly patients. *Journal of the American Geriatric Society, 23*(10), 433–441.

Phillips, K.A. (2009). *Understanding body dysmorphic disorder.* New York: Oxford University Press.

Phillips, N.A. (2000, July). Female sexual dysfunction: Evaluation and treatment. *American Family Physician, 62*(1), 127–136, 141–142.

Piaget, J. & Inhelder, B. (1969). *The Psychology of the child.* New York: Basic Books.

Pies, R.W. (2013, April 29). Grief and depression: The sages knew the difference. *Psychiatric Times.* Retrieved from www.psychiatrictimes.com/display/article/10168/2140230

Popper, C.W., Gammon, G.D., West, S.A., & Bailey, C.E. (2003). Disorders usually first diagnosed in infancy, childhood, or adolescence. In R.E. Hales & S.C. Yudofsky (Eds.), Textbook of clinical psychiatry (4th ed.). Washington, DC: The American Psychiatric Publishing, pp. 833–974.

Pranthikanti, S. (2007). Ayurvedic treatments. In J.H. Lake & D. Spiegel (Eds.), *Complementary and alternative treatments in mental health care.* Washington, DC: American Psychiatric Publishing, 225–272.

Prator, B.C. (2006). Serotonin syndrome. *Journal of Neuroscience Nursing, 38*(2), 102–105.

Presser, A.M. (2000). *Pharmacist's guide to medicinal herbs.* Petaluma, CA: Smart Publications.

Puri, B.K. & Treasaden, I.H. (2012). *Textbook of psychiatry* (3rd ed.). Philadelphia: Churchill Livingstone Elsevier.

Rabins, P., Bland, W., Bright-Long, L., Cohen, E., Katz, I., Rovner, B., Schneider, L., & Blacker, D. (2006). Practice guideline for the treatment of patients with Alzheimer's disease and other dementias of late life. *American Psychiatric Association practice guidelines for the treatment of psychiatric disorders, Compendium 2006.* Washington, DC: American Psychiatric Association.

Ramsland, K. (2009). *The childhood psychopath: Bad seed or bad parents?* Retrieved from www.trutv.com/library/crime/criminal_mind/psychology/psychopath/2.html

Regard, M., Knoch, D., Gutling, E., & Landis, T. (2003). Brain damage and addictive behavior: A neuropsychological and electroencephalogram investigation with pathologic gamblers. *Cognitive and Behavioral Neurology, 16*(1), 47–53.

Registered Nurses Association of British Columbia (RNABC). (2003). *Nurse-Client relationships.* Vancouver, BC: RNABC.

Research Center for Human-Animal Interaction (ReCHAI). (2008). *Veterans and shelter dogs initiative.* Retrieved from http://vabenefitblog.com/rechai-veterans-and-shelter-dogs-initiative

Rizwan, S., Manning, J.T., & Brabin, B.J. (2007). Maternal smoking during pregnancy and possible effects of in utero testosterone: Evidence from the 2D:4D finger length ratio. *Early Human Development, 83*(2), 87–90.

Sadock, B.J. & Sadock, V.A. (2007). Synopsis of psychiatry: Behavioral sciences/clinical psychiatry (10th ed.). Philadelphia: Lippincott Williams & Wilkins.

Substance Abuse and Mental Health Services Administration (SAMHSA). (2012). Behavioral health issues among Afghanistan and Iraq U.S. war veterans. *SAMHSA In Brief, 7*(1).

Substance Abuse and Mental Health Services Administration (SAMHSA). (2011). *Current statistics on the prevalence and characteristics of people experiencing homelessness in the United States.* Retrieved from http://homeless.samhsa.gov/ResourceFiles/hrc_factsheet.pdf

Schatzberg, A.F., Cole, J.O., & Debattista, C. (2010). *Manual of clinical psychopharmacology* (7th ed.). Washington, DC: American Psychiatric Publishing.

Schoenen, J., Jacquy, J., & Lenaerts, M. (1998). Effectiveness of high-dose riboflavin in migraine prophylaxis: A randomized controlled trial. *Neurology, 50,* 466–469.

Schroeder, B. (2013). Getting started in home care. *Nurse.com Nursing CE Courses.* Retrieved from http://ce.nurse.com/course/60085/getting-started-in-home-care/

Schuster, P.M. (2012). *Concept mapping: A critical-thinking approach to care planning* (3rd ed.). Philadelphia: F.A. Davis.

Seligman, M. (1974). Depression and learned helplessness. In R. Friedman & M. Katz (Eds.), *The psychology of depression: Contemporary theory and research.* Washington, DC: V.H. Winston & Sons.

Selye, H. (1956). *The stress of life.* New York: McGraw-Hill.

Skinner, K. (1979, August). The therapeutic milieu: Making it work. *Journal of Psychiatric Nursing and Mental Health Services, 17,* 38–44.

Skodol, A.E. & Gunderson, J.G. (2008). Personality disorders. In R.E. Hales, S.C. Yudofsky, & G.O. Gabbard (Eds.), *Textbook of psychiatry*

(5th ed.). Washington, DC: American Psychiatric Publishing, pp. 821–860.

Smith, G. (2011). *Can a head injury cause or hasten Alzheimer's disease or other types of dementia?* The Mayo Clinic. Retrieved from www.mayoclinic.com/health/alzheimers-disease/AN01710

Soares, N. & Grossman, L. (2012, November 29). Conversion disorder. *eMedicine Pediatrics*. Retrieved from http://emedicine.medscape.com/article/917864-overview

Steinberg, L. (2002). Yoga. In M.A. Bright (Ed.), *Holistic health and healing*. Philadelphia: F.A. Davis, 285–304.

Sullivan, H.S. (1953). *The Interpersonal theory of psychiatry*. New York: W.W. Norton.

Sullivan, H.S. (1956). *Clinical studies in psychiatry*. New York: W.W. Norton.

Sullivan, H.S. (1962). *Schizophrenia as a human process*. New York: W.W. Norton.

Tardiff, K.J. (2003). Violence. In R.E. Hales & S.C. Yudofsky (Eds.), *Textbook of clinical psychiatry* (4th ed.). Washington, DC: The American Psychiatric Publishing, pp. 1485–1510.

The Joint Commission. (2010, January). *The comprehensive accreditation manual for hospitals: The official handbook*. Oakbrook Terrace, IL: Joint Commission Resources.

Townsend, M.C. (2014). *Essentials of psychiatric/mental health nursing* (6th ed.). Philadelphia: F. A. Davis.

Townsend, M.C. (2015). *Psychiatric mental health nursing: Concepts of care in evidence-based practice* (8th ed.). Philadelphia: F.A. Davis.

Trivieri, L. & Anderson, J.W. (2002). *Alternative medicine: The definitive guide*. Berkeley, CA: Celestial Arts.

Ulbricht, C. (2011). *Davis's pocket guide to herbs and supplements*. Philadelphia: F.A. Davis.

Ursano, A.M., Kartheiser, P.H., & Barnhill, L.J. (2008). Disorders usually first diagnosed in infancy, childhood, or adolescence. In R.E. Hales, S.C. Yudofsky, & G.O. Gabbard (Eds.), *Textbook of psychiatry* (5th ed.). Washington, DC: American Psychiatric Publishing, pp. 861–920.

USA.gov. (2013). Military personnel records and statistics. Retrieved from www.usa.gov/Federal-Employees/Active-Military-Records.shtml

U.S. Conference of Mayors (USCM). (2012). *A status report on hunger and homelessness in America's cities: 2012*. Washington, DC: U.S. Conference of Mayors.

U.S. Department of Agriculture & U.S. Department of Health and Human Services. (2010). *Dietary guidelines for Americans 2010* (7th ed.). Washington, DC: U.S. Government Printing Office.

Vallerand, A.H., Sanoski, C.A., & Deglin, J.H. (2013). *Davis's drug guide for nurses* (13th ed.). Philadelphia: F. A. Davis.

Vlahos, K.B. (2012). The rape of our military women. *Anti-War.Com*. Retrieved from http://original.antiwar.com/vlahos/2012/05/14/the-rape-of-our-military-women

Voeller, K.K.S. (2004). Attention-deficit hyperactivity disorder (ADHD). *Journal of Child Neurology, 19*(10), 798–814.

Wakefield, M. (2007). Guarding the military home front. *Counseling Today*. Retrieved from http://ct.counseling.org/2007/01/from-the-president-guarding-the-military-home-front

Wertsch, M.E. (1996). *Military brats: Legacies of childhood inside the fortress.* St. Louis, MO: Brightwell.

Whitaker, J. (2000). Pet owners are a healthy breed. *Health & Healing 10*(10), 1–8.

Wolfe, J., Sharkansky, E.J., Read, J.P., Dawson, R., Martin, J.A., & Oimette, P.C. (1998). Sexual harassment and assault as predictors of PTSD symptomatology among U.S. female Persian Gulf military personnel. *Journal of Interpersonal Violence, 13*(1), 40–57.

Wootton, J. (2008). Meditation and chronic pain. In J.F. Audette & A. Bailey (Eds.), *Integrative pain medicine.* New York: Springer-Vertag, 195–210.

Worden, J.W. (2009). *Grief counseling and grief therapy: A handbook for the mental health practitioner* (4th ed.). New York: Springer.

Yalom, I. (2005). *The theory and practice of group psychotherapy* (5th ed.). New York: Basic Books.

Yurkovich, E. & Smyer, T. (2000). Health maintenance behaviors of individuals with severe mental illness in a state prison. *Journal of Psychosocial Nursing and Mental Health Services, 38*(6), 20–31.

Yutzy, S.H. & Parish, B.S. (2008). Somatoform disorders. In R.E. Hales, S.C. Yudofsky, & G.O. Gabbard (Eds.), *Textbook of psychiatry* (5th ed.). Washington, DC: American Psychiatric Publishing, 609–664.

Zinner, S.H. (2004). Tourette syndrome—much more than tics. *Contemporary Pediatrics, 21*(8), 38–49.

Zucker, K.J., Bradley, S.J., Ben-Dat, D.N., Ho, C., Johnson, L., & Owen, A. (2003). Psychopathology in the parents of boys with gender identity disorder. *Journal of the American Academy of Child and Adolescent Psychiatry, 42*(1), 2–4.

Subject Index

Note: Page numbers followed by "f" indicate figures; those followed by "t" indicate tabular material.

Abilify, 460–461, 467–468, 492–494
Abnormal Involuntary Movement Scale (AIMS), 626–628
Abnormal thinking and sedative-hypnotics, 521
Abuse
  background assessment data, 302–305
  child, 302–303
    pedophilic disorder and, 231
  Internet resources, 310–311
  powerlessness and, 307–309
  rape-trauma syndrome and, 305–307
  risk for delayed development with, 309–310
  symptomatology, 304–305
Acceptance in stages of grief, 373, 551
Acceptance of reality of loss in stages of grief, 374–375
Acetazolamide, 450
Activity/rest domain in NANDA nursing diagnoses, 635–636
Acupressure and acupuncture, 355–356
Acute pain in premenstrual dysphoric disorder, 313–315
Acute stress disorder, 186, 187–188, 190
Adderall, 522, 524
Adderall XR, 522, 524
Addiction, substance
  background assessment data, 71
  chronic low self-esteem in, 98–100
  classification of substances, 72–75, 75–77t
  common patterns of use in, 78–86
  deficient knowledge in, 100–102
  defined, 71–72
  depressive disorder and, 134
  DSM-5 classification, 595–598
  dysfunctional family processes in, 102–105
  homelessness and, 322–323
  imbalanced nutrition: less than body requirements, 97–98
  ineffective coping in, 95–97
  ineffective denial in, 93–95
  Internet resources, 105–106
  in military families, 391–392
  NANDA nursing diagnoses corresponding to, 620
  nonsubstance-related disorder, 86–90, 598
  predisposing factors associated with, 78
  risk for injury in, 90–93
  substance-induced disorders, 72
  substance use disorders, 71–72
  substitution therapy for, 92–93, 348–349
  symptoms associated with intoxication and withdrawal from, 87–89t
Adjusting to a world without the lost entity in stages of grief, 375
Adjustment disorder, 186–187, 189–190

Adjustments, chiropractic, 360, 366
Adolescents
    concepts of death in, 381
    in military families, 393
Adrenergic blockers, 524
Adult(s)
    concept of death, 381
    physical abuse of, 303
    sexual abuse of, 303, 305
Advil, premenstrual dysphoric disorder and, 316t
Affect, 115–116
    in mental status assessment, 613–614
Affordable health care, 322
Affordable housing, 322
Age and homelessness, 321
Agitation, antidepressants and, 444
Agoraphobia, 170
Agranulocytosis and antipsychotic agents, 499
Akineton, 504, 506
Alcohol
    classification of, 72
    drug interactions, 405, 408, 412, 431, 434, 476, 479, 481, 490, 493, 513, 515,
        518, 530
    gambling disorder and, 92
    moderate consumption of, 358
    substitution therapy, 92–93, 348
Alcoholic cardiomyopathy, 79
Alcoholic hepatitis, 79
Alcohol-related disorders, 72, 595. *See also* Addiction, substance
    detoxification, 348
    patterns of use in, 78–80
    risk for injury and, 92
    symptomatology, 79–80
    symptoms associated with intoxication and withdrawal from, 87t
Aleve, premenstrual dysphoric disorder and, 316t
Almotriptan, premenstrual dysphoric disorder and, 316t
Alpha-adrenergic agonists, 529–531
Alprazolam, 406, 408
Alternative medicine, 350. *See also* Complementary therapies
Alzheimer's disease neurocognitive disorder due to, 55–56
Amantadine, 431, 507–509, 534
Ambien, 516, 519
Amenorrhea and antipsychotic agents, 498
Amerge, premenstrual dysphoric disorder and, 316t
American Botanical Council, 351
American Heart Association, 368
American Herbal Association, 351
American Massage Therapy Association, 367
American Medical Association (AMA), 351
American Nurses Association (ANA), 1
    on forensic nursing, 338
    on psychiatric home nursing care, 328
    Standards of Practice, 3
Amiodarone, 491
Amitriptyline, 416, 419
    posttraumatic stress disorder and, 395
Amnesia, dissociative, 220
Amobarbital, 514, 515
Amoxapine, 417, 422

Amphetamines
    for ADHD, 522–525
    interactions, 440
Amphetamine use disorder, 80–81
    symptoms associated with intoxication and withdrawal from, 87t
Anafranil, 416, 420
Anatomical abnormalities and schizophrenia, 111
Anergia, 116
Anesthetic agents, 440
Angel's trumpet, 405
Anger
    in borderline personality disorder, 275
    NANDA nursing diagnoses corresponding to, 618, 619
    in stages of grief, 372, 550
Anhedonia, 117
Animals and pet therapy, 368–369
Anorexia
    ADHD agents and, 536
    herbal remedies for, 353t
Anorexia nervosa, 251–252
    NANDA nursing diagnoses corresponding to, 618
    symptomatology, 251–252
Antianxiety agents
    antihistamines, 404–406
    for antisocial personality disorder, 292
    azaspirodecanediones, 412–413
    benzodiazepines, 406–411
    carbamate derivative, 411–412
    client/family education related to all, 414–415
    interactions, 405, 408, 412
    Internet resources, 415
    nursing diagnoses related to all, 413–414
    nursing implications for, 414
Antiarrhythmic agents, 481, 491
Anticholinergics, 476, 479, 480, 491, 504–506
Anticipatory grief, 377–378
Anticoagulants, 515
    interactions, 434, 476
Anticonvulsants, 451–459
Antidepressants
    client/family education related to all, 446–448
    interactions, 405, 431, 518, 530
    Internet resources, 448
    monoamine oxidase inhibitors, 439–441
    norepinephrine-dopamine reuptake inhibitors, 430–432
    nursing diagnoses related to all, 442
    nursing implications for, 442–446
    psychotherapeutic combinations, 441–442
    selective serotonin reuptake inhibitors, 422–429
    serotonin-2-antagonists/reuptake inhibitors, 436–438
    serotonin-norepinephrine reuptake inhibitors, 432–436
    in substitution therapy, 93, 349
    tricyclics and related, 416–422
Antihistamines, 404–406, 490, 518
Antihypertensives, 440, 479, 481, 491, 493, 523
Antimanics, 449–451
Antiparkinsonian agents
    anticholinergics, 504–506
    client/family education related to, 510–511

dopaminergic agonists, 507–509
 Internet resources, 511
 nursing diagnoses related to, 509
 nursing implications for, 509–510
Antipsychotic agents, 460–470
 benzisothiazolinone derivative, 494–495
 benzisoxazole derivatives, 489–492
 client/family education related to, 501–502
 dibenzepine derivatives, 482–489
 interactions, 431, 518
 Internet resources, 503
 nursing diagnoses related to all, 496
 nursing implications for, 496–501
 phenothiazines, 474–478
 phenylbutylpiperadines, 479–482
 quinolinones, 492–494
 thioxanthenes, 478–479
Antisocial personality disorder, 270, 288–290
 symptomatology, 290
Anxiety, 175–177
 adjustment disorder with, 187
 antianxiety agents
  antihistamines, 404–406
  for antisocial personality disorder, 292
  azaspirodecanediones, 412–413
  benzodiazepines, 406–411
  carbamate derivative, 411–412
  client/family education related to all, 414–415
  interactions, 405, 408, 412
  Internet resources, 415
  nursing diagnoses related to all, 413–414
  nursing implications for, 414
 disorder due to another medical condition, 172
 DSM-5 classification, 588–589
 herbal remedies for, 354t, 355t
 levels of, 547–548
 moderate to severe
  in disorders of infancy, childhood, and adolescence, 38–40
  in eating disorders, 261–262
  in trauma- and stressor-related disorders, 197–199
 NANDA nursing diagnoses corresponding to, 618
 severe
  in disorders of infancy, childhood, and adolescence, 49–50
  in personality disorders, 278–280
Anxious distress, depressive disorder with, 133
Apathy, 116
Aplenzin, 430, 431–432, 531, 534
Appearance in mental status assessment, 611
Application site reactions, antidepressants and, 446
Aripiprazole, 460–461, 462, 463–464, 467–468, 492–494
 interactions, 465, 484–485
Arrhythmias
 antidepressants and, 444
 mood-stabilizing agents and, 471
Asenapine, 461, 463, 465, 470, 482–483, 487
 interactions, 466, 486
Assertiveness training, 569–571
Assessment. *See also* Background assessment data
 Abnormal Involuntary Movement Scale (AIMS), 626–628
 brief mental status evaluation, 621–622

in correctional facilities, 343
cultural, 581–582
medication, 576–580
mental status, 610–617, 621–622
in nursing process, 2, 4–13
Associative looseness, 113–114
Ativan, 407, 410–411
Atomoxetine, 531, 533, 534–535
Atropine, 405
Attention-deficit/hyperactivity disorder, 26–27, 584
    medications for treatment of
        alpha-adrenergic agonists, 529–531
        client/family education related to, 537–538
        CNS stimulants (amphetamines), 522–525
        CNS stimulants (miscellaneous agents), 525–528
        Internet resources, 538
        miscellaneous, 531–535
        nursing diagnoses related to, 535
        nursing implications for, 535–537
Attention classification in NANDA nursing diagnoses, 636
Atypical antipsychotics, Tourette's disorder and, 45
Atypical features, depressive disorder with, 133
Auditory hallucinations, 114
Autism spectrum disorder, 20–21, 583–584
    disturbed personal identity with, 25–26
    impaired social interaction with, 22–23
    impaired verbal communication with, 23–24
    risk for self-mutilation with, 21–22
Autistic phase in theory of object relations, 273
Aventyl, 417, 421
Avoidant personality disorder, 271
Awareness
    development in stages of grief, 374
    training, 183
Axert, premenstrual dysphoric disorder and, 316t
Azaspirodecanediones, 412–413
Azole antifungals, 434, 481, 513, 518

Background assessment data. *See also* Assessment
    anxiety, obsessive-compulsive, and related disorders, 169–172
    bipolar and related disorders, 153–154
    depressive disorders, 132
    disorders of infancy, childhood, and adolescence, 14–15
    dissociative disorders, 220–221
    eating disorders, 251–255
    forensic nursing, 338–340
    homelessness, 321–323
    loss and bereavement, 371–382
    military families, 386–392
    neurocognitive disorders, 54–58
    personality disorders, 269–271
    premenstrual dysphoric disorder, 312–313
    problems related to abuse or neglect, 302–305
    psychiatric home nursing care, 328–330
    schizophrenia spectrum and other psychotic disorders, 107–117
    sexual disorders and gender dysphoria, 230–238
    somatic symptom disorders, 206–209
    substance-related and addictive disorders, 71
    trauma- and stressor-related disorders, 185–186
Barbiturates, 419, 514–516, 530

Bargaining in stages of grief, 372, 550
Behavioral theory and paraphilic disorders, 233
Behavior disorders, disruptive
  anxiety with, 39–40
  attention-deficit/hyperactivity disorder, 26–27
  conduct disorder, 27–29
  defensive coping with, 32–34
  impaired social interaction with, 34–35
  ineffective coping and, 35–37
  low self-esteem with, 37–38
  noncompliance with, 41–42
  oppositional defiant disorder, 29–30
  risk for self-directed or other-directed violence in, 30–32
Benadryl, 504–506
Benzisothiazolinone derivative, 494–495
Benzisoxazole derivatives, 489–492
Benzodiazepines, 406–411, 512–514
  for anxiety, 406–411
  interactions, 419, 425, 513
  posttraumatic stress disorder and, 395
  in substitution therapy, 92–93, 348, 349
Benztropine, 504, 506
Bereavement. *See* Loss and bereavement
Beta-blockers, 425, 440, 476, 505, 515, 530
Bethanechol, 505
Binge-eating disorder, 254, 255
Biochemical factors
  abuse, 303
  anxiety, obsessive-compulsive, and related disorders, 172–173
  attention-deficit/hyperactivity disorder, 26
  bipolar disorder, 154
  borderline personality disorder, 272
  depressive disorder, 134
  premenstrual dysphoric disorder, 312
  schizophrenia, 111
  somatic symptom disorders, 209
  substance-related disorders, 78
  Tourette's disorder, 43
Biofeedback, 568
Biological factors in paraphilic disorders, 232
Biological theory
  adjustment disorder and, 189
  trauma- and stressor-related disorders and, 187–188
Biperiden, 504, 506
Bipolar and related disorders
  background assessment data, 153–154
  disturbed sensory perception with, 163–165
  disturbed thought processes with, 162–163
  DSM-5 classification, 586–587
  imbalanced nutrition with, 160–162
  impaired social interaction with, 165–166
  insomnia with, 167–168
  Internet resources, 168
  medications (*See* Mood-stabilizing agents)
  predisposing factors to, 154–155
  risk for injury with, 156–158
  risk for self-directed or other-directed violence with, 158–160
  symptomatology, 155–156
  types, 153–154
Bipolar I disorder, 153
Bipolar II disorder, 153–154

Birth temperament, 28
Bite-mark injuries, 339
Black cohosh and premenstrual dysphoric disorder, 316t, 352t
Blaming of others, 372
Bland or flat affect, 116
Blood dyscrasias
 mood-stabilizing agents and, 471
 sedative-hypnotics and, 520
Blunt-force injuries, 339
Blurred vision
 antidepressants and, 443
 antiparkinsonian agents and, 509
 antipsychotic agents and, 496
Body dysmorphic disorder, 171
Body image, disturbed
 in anxiety, obsessive-compulsive, and related disorders, 180–182
 in eating disorders, 262–264, 266–267
 in NANDA nursing diagnoses, 618, 637
Body mass index (BMI), 254
Borderline personality disorder, 270, 272–275
 symptomatology, 274–275
Bowlby, John, 373–374
Bradycardia, mood-stabilizing agents and, 472
Breathing-related sleep disorders, DSM-5 classification, 592–593
Brief mental status evaluation, 621–622
Brief psychotic disorder, 108
Brintellix, 423, 429
Bromocriptine
 for Parkinson's disease, 507–509
 premenstrual dysphoric disorder and, 316t
Budeprion SR, 430, 431–432, 531, 534
Budeprion XL, 430, 531
Bugleweed and premenstrual dysphoric disorder, 316t
Bulimia nervosa, 252–254
Buprenorphine in substitution therapy, 92, 349
Bupropion, 426, 430, 431–432, 440, 531, 534–535
Buspirone HCL, 412–413, 426, 440
Butabarbital, 514, 515
Butisol, 514, 515

Caffeine-related disorders, 595
 symptoms associated with intoxication and withdrawal from, 87t
Calan, 459
Calcium channel blockers, 450, 459–460
Caloric balance, 357, 359t
Cannabinoids. See also Substance-related and addictive disorders
 classification of, 74, 77 (table)
 in substance-related and addictive disorders, 93
 in substitution therapy for substance withdrawal, 349
Cannabis-related disorders, 74, 77t, 595–596
 detoxification, 349
 pattern of use in, 81–82
 risk for injury, 93
 symptoms associated with intoxication and withdrawal from, 88t
Carbamate derivative, 411–412
Carbamazepine, 413, 419, 425, 431, 440, 450–456, 481, 490, 513, 515, 530, 534
Carbatrol, 451
Cardiovascular system
 arrhythmias
  antidepressants and, 419, 444
  mood-stabilizing agents and, 471

cardiovascular accident and depressive disorder, 135
cardiovascular/pulmonary responses in NANDA nursing diagnoses, 636
herbal remedies for, 353t
pet therapy and, 368–369
Caregiver role strain
in military families, 393, 401–403
NANDA nursing diagnoses corresponding to, 619
in neurocognitive disorders, 68–69
in psychiatric home nursing care, 335–337
Caregiving roles in NANDA nursing diagnoses, 637
Cascara sagrada, 352t
Catapres
ADHD and, 529, 530
Tourette's disorder and, 45
Catatonia
associated with another mental disorder, 109
depressive disorder with, 133
disorder due to another medical condition, 109–111
Celexa, 422, 425
Centrally-acting anticholinergics, 476
Chamomile, 352t
Chaste tree and premenstrual dysphoric disorder, 317t
Child abuse
physical, 302, 304
sexual, 302–303, 305
pedophilic disorder and, 231
Childhood trauma and personality disorders, 272–273
Child neglect, 303
symptomatology, 304
Children
borderline personality disorder and trauma in, 272–273
concepts of death in, 380–381
with gender dysphoria, 243
homeless, 323
of military members, 387–388, 393
risk for delayed development in, 309–310
theory of object relations and, 273–274
Chinese medicine, 351, 355–356, 366–367
Chiropractic medicine, 351, 360, 366
Chloral hydrate, 516–519
Chloramphenicol, 515
Chlordiazepoxide
for anxiety, 406, 409
in substitution therapy, 92–93, 348, 349
Chlordiazepoxide/amitriptyline, 441, 442
Chloroquine, 491
Chlorpromazine, 461, 462, 464, 468, 474, 476–477
interactions, 465, 491
Chronic confusion, 61–63
Chronic depression and borderline personality disorder, 274
Chronic low self-esteem
in personality disorders, 286–290, 295–297
in substance-related and addictive disorders, 98–100
Chronic or prolonged grieving, 379
Cigarette smoking and sedative-hypnotics, 513
Cimetidine, 408, 413, 419, 425, 431, 434, 513, 518, 534
Circumstantiality, 114
Cirrhosis of the liver, 79–80
Citalopram, 422, 425
CIV, 451

Clang associations, 114
Clarithromycin, 413, 518
Client behaviors and NANDA nursing diagnoses, 618–620
Client/family education
  related to ADHD agents, 537–538
  related to antianxiety agents, 414–415
  related to antidepressants, 446–448
  related to antiparkinsonian agents, 510–511
  related to antipsychotics, 501–502
  related to mood-stabilizing agents, 472–473
  related to sedative-hypnotics, 521
Clinging and distancing, 274–275
Clomipramine, 416, 420
Clonazepam, 406, 409, 451, 452, 454, 456, 515
Clonidine, 419, 529, 530
  posttraumatic stress disorder and, 395
  Tourette's disorder and, 45
Clopidogrel, 431, 534
Clorazepate, 409–410
Clozapine, 482, 483, 487
  interactions, 425, 434, 485, 486, 491
Clozaril, 482, 487
Cluster A personality, 269–270
Cluster B personality, 269, 270
Cluster C personality, 269, 271
CNS depressants. *See* Depressants, CNS
CNS stimulants. *See* Stimulants, CNS
Cocaine, 76 (table). *See also* Substance-related and addictive disorders
  symptoms associated with intoxication and withdrawal from, 88t
  use disorder, 76t, 82
Cogentin, 504, 506
Cognition domain in NANDA nursing diagnoses, 636
Cognitive ability and sensorium in mental status assessment, 616–617
Cognitive development stages, 541
Cognitive theory, 189
  anxiety, obsessive-compulsive, and related disorders and, 173–174
  depressive disorder and, 135
  trauma- and stressor-related disorders and, 189
Cognitive therapy, 571–572
Comfort domain in NANDA nursing diagnoses, 640
Communication disorders, DSM-5 classification, 583
Communication techniques
  in NANDA nursing diagnoses, 636
  nontherapeutic, 558–562
  therapeutic, 554–558
Compensation, 543
Competing response training, 183
Complementary therapies, 350
  acupressure and acupuncture, 355–356
  chiropractic medicine, 360, 366
  diet and nutrition, 357–358, 359–360t
  essential vitamins and minerals in, 361–365t
  herbal medicine, 351–352, 352–355t
  Internet resources, 369–370
  introduction to, 350–351
  pet therapy, 368–369
  therapeutic touch and massage, 366–367
  yoga, 367–368
Complicated grieving, 618. *See also* Loss and bereavement
  in depressive disorders, 139–141

in forensic nursing, 345–347
in military families, 399–401
in personality disorders, 280–282
risk for, 382–384
in trauma- and stressor-related disorders, 193–194
Concept mapping, 3–5
Concerta, 525, 527
Concrete thinking, 114
Conduct disorder, 27–29
adjustment disorder with, 187
Confusion, chronic, 61–63
NANDA nursing diagnoses corresponding to, 618
Consensual validation, 163
Constipation, 354t
ADHD agents and, 536
antidepressants and, 443
antiparkinsonian agents and, 509
antipsychotic agents and, 496
herbal remedies for, 352t
mood-stabilizing agents and, 472
Content of thought, 112–113
in mental status assessment, 615–616
Controlled substances schedules, DEA, 624–628
Conversion disorder, 207–208
Coping
defensive, 619
in disorders of infancy, childhood, and adolescence, 32–34
in forensic nursing, 343–345
in personality disorders, 293–295
ineffective, 620
in anxiety, obsessive-compulsive, and related disorders, 179–180
in disorders of infancy, childhood and adolescence, 35–37, 50–51
in dissociative disorders, 223–224
in premenstrual dysphoric disorder, 315–319
in schizophrenia spectrum and other psychotic disorders, 121–122
in somatic symptom and related disorders, 211–214
in substance-related and addictive disorders, 95–97
in trauma- and stressor-related disorders, 199–201
responses in NANDA nursing diagnoses, 638
and stress tolerance domain in NANDA nursing diagnoses, 638–639
Correctional facilities, forensic psychiatric nursing in, 343
complicated grieving and, 345–347
defensive coping and, 343–345
risk for injury and, 347–349
Corticosteroids, 515
Council for Responsible Nutrition, 351
Counseling and medical advice, DSM-5 classification, 609
Crime and legal system, DSM-5 classification, 608–609
Crisis intervention, 567
after sexual assault, 342
Cultural assessment tool, 581–582
Cyclobenzaprine, 440
Cyclosporine, 425
Cyclothymic disorder, 154
Cymbalta, 432–433, 435
Cyproheptadine, 426, 434

Dairy products, 358, 359t
Daytrana, 525, 527–528
DEA controlled substances schedules, 624–628

Death
  concepts of, 380–382
  in the emergency department, 339–340
  natural, 339
  risk and antipsychotic agents, 501
Decisional conflict, 618
Decreased sweating and antiparkinsonian agents, 510
Deep-breathing exercises, 568
Defense mechanisms, ego, 543–545
Defense wounds, 339
Defensive coping, 619
  in disorders of infancy, childhood, and adolescence, 32–34
  in forensic nursing, 343–345
  in personality disorders, 293–295
Deficient fluid volume, 257–259, 620
Deficient knowledge
  in personality disorders, 299–301
  in somatic symptom and related disorders, 216–217
  in substance-related and addictive disorders, 100–102
Dehydration, mood-stabilizing agents and, 471
Deinstitutionalization, 321–322
Delayed development risk, 309–310
Delayed ejaculation, 234–235
Delayed or inhibited grief, 378
Delirium, 54–55, 58
Delusional disorder, 107–108, 112–113
  NANDA nursing diagnoses corresponding to, 618
Delusions of grandeur, 155
Denial
  ego defense mechanism, 543
  ineffective, 620
    in eating disorders, 259–261
    in substance-related and addictive disorders, 93–95
  NANDA nursing diagnoses corresponding to, 618, 619
  in stages of grief, 372, 550
Depacon, 451
Depakene, 451, 456
Depakote, 451, 456
Department of Agriculture, U. S., 357
Department of Health and Human Services, U. S., 357
Dependence, physical and psychological
  on ADHD agents, 536
  on sedative-hypnotics, 520
Dependent personality disorder, 271
Depersonalization, 115
  -derealization disorder, 221
Deployment impact on military families, 388–389
Depressants, CNS, 73, 75t, 75 (table)
  antihistamines, 404–406
  diphenhydramine and, 505
  substance related and addictive disorders and, 92
  interactions, 419, 440, 476, 479, 481, 490, 493, 513, 515, 530
  risk for injury from, 92, 349
  sedative-hypnotics and, 520
  in substitution therapy, 93, 349
Depressive disorders
  adjustment disorder with, 186, 187
  antidepressants
    client/family education related to all, 446–448
    interactions, 405, 431, 518, 530

Internet resources, 448
monoamine oxidase inhibitors, 439–441
norepinephrine-dopamine reuptake inhibitors, 430–432
nursing diagnoses related to all, 442
nursing implications for, 442–446
psychotherapeutic combinations, 441–442
selective serotonin reuptake inhibitors, 422–429
serotonin-2-antagonists/reuptake inhibitors, 436–438
serotonin-norepinephrine reuptake inhibitors, 432–436
in substitution therapy, 93, 349
tricyclics and related, 416–422
background assessment data, 132
in borderline personality disorder, 274
complicated grieving and, 139–141
disturbed sleep pattern with, 150–151
disturbed thought processes in, 147–148
DSM-5 classification, 587–588
Hamilton Depression Rating Scale (HDRS), 629–631
herbal remedies for, 355t
imbalanced nutrition, less than body requirements, in, 135, 148–150
Internet resources, 151–152
low self-esteem with, 141–143
in military families, 391
NANDA nursing diagnoses corresponding to, 618
obesity and, 255
powerlessness with, 145–147
predisposing factors, 134–135
in response to loss, 381–382
risk for suicide, 136–139
sedative-hypnotics and, 520
social isolation/impaired social interaction with, 143–145
in stages of grief, 372–373, 381–382, 550–551
symptomatology, 135–136
types, 132–134
Desipramine, 416, 420, 431
Desoxyn, 522, 524
Despair in stages of grief, 373
Desvenlafaxine, 432, 435
Deteriorated appearance, 116
Detoxification, 348–349
NANDA nursing diagnoses corresponding to, 618 (*See also* Withdrawal, substance)
Developmental theories
Erikson's psychosocial theory, 540
Freud's stage of psychosexual development, 539
H. S. Sullivan's interpersonal theory, 540
Kohlberg's stages of moral development, 541
Mahler's theory of object relations, 541
Peplau's interpersonal theory, 541
Piaget's stages of cognitive development, 541
Dexamethasone, 413
Dexedrine, 522, 524
Dexmethylphenidate, 525, 526–527
Dextroamphetamine sulfate, 522, 524
Dextromethorphan, 440
Dextrostat, 522, 524
Diabetes
antipsychotic agents and, 501
depressive disorder and, 135
mood-stabilizing agents and, 472

Diagnoses
  assigned to client behaviors, 618–620
  DSM-5 classification, 583–609
  in nursing process, 2–3
  related to agents for ADHD, 535
  related to antianxiety agents, 413–414
  related to antidepressants, 442
  related to antiparkinsonian agents, 509
  related to antipsychotic agents, 496
  related to mood-stabilizing drugs, 470
  related to sedatives/hypnotics, 519–520
Diazepam
  for anxiety, 407, 410
  in substitution therapy, 92, 349
Dibenzepine derivatives, 482–489
Dibenzoxazepine, 417
Dicing injuries, 339
Dicumarol, 419
Diet and nutrition in complementary therapies, 357–358, 359–360t
Differentiation phase in theory of object relations, 273
Difficulty accepting new diagnosis, NANDA nursing diagnoses corresponding to, 618
Difficulty making important life decision, NANDA nursing diagnoses corresponding to, 618
Digitoxin, 515
Digoxin, 408, 426, 505, 513
Diltiazem, 413
Diphenhydramine, 504–506
Disbelief in stages of grief, 374
Discontinuation syndrome, 443
Discretionary calorie allowance, 360t
Disequilibrium in stages of grief, 373
Disorganization in stages of grief, 373
Displacement, 543–544
Disruptive, impulse-control, and conduct, DSM-5 classification, 594
Disruptive behavior disorders
  anxiety with, 39–40
  attention-deficit/hyperactivity disorder, 26–27
  conduct disorder, 27–29
  defensive coping with, 32–34
  impaired social interaction with, 34–35
  ineffective coping and, 35–37
  low self-esteem with, 37–38
  noncompliance with, 41–42
  oppositional defiant disorder, 29–30
  risk for self-directed or other-directed violence in, 30–32
Disruptive mood dysregulation disorder, 132
Dissociative disorders
  background assessment data, 220–221
  disturbed personal identity, 226–227
  disturbed sensory perception, 227–229
  DSM-5 classification, 590
  impaired memory, 224–226
  ineffective coping, 223–224
  Internet resources, 229
  predisposing factors, 221–222
  symptomatology, 222
Dissociative identity disorder (DID), 220–221
Distancing and clinging, 274–275

Distorted (exaggerated) grief response, 378–379
Disturbed body image
  in anxiety, obsessive-compulsive, and related disorders, 180–182
  in eating disorders, 262–264, 266–267
  in NANDA nursing diagnoses, 618, 637
Disturbed personal identity, 619
  in autism spectrum disorder, 25–26
  in borderline personality disorder, 284–286
  in dissociative disorders, 226–227
  in gender dysphoria, 245–247
Disturbed sensory perception, 619
  in bipolar and related disorders, 163–165
  in conversion disorder, 214–215
  in dissociative disorders, 227–229
  in neurocognitive disorders, 65–66
  in schizophrenia spectrum and other psychotic disorders, 123–124
Disturbed thought processes, 618
  in bipolar and related disorders, 162–163
  in depressive disorders, 147–148
  in military families, 396–398
  in schizophrenia spectrum and other psychotic disorders, 124–126
Disulfiram, 408, 513
Dizziness
  antiparkinsonian agents and, 510
  mood-stabilizing agents and, 471, 472
  sedative-hypnotics and, 520
Dolophine in substitution therapy, 92, 348
Domestic violence and homelessness, 322
Dopamine, 90, 440, 476, 479, 481
Dopaminergic agonists, 490, 507–509
Doral, 512, 514
Downward drift hypothesis, 112
Doxapram, 440
Doxepin, 417, 420–421
Doxorubicin, 515
Doxycycline, 515
Drowsiness. *See* Sedation
Dry mouth
  ADHD agents and, 536
  antidepressants and, 442
  antiparkinsonian agents and, 509
  antipsychotic agents and, 496
  mood-stabilizing agents and, 471, 472
  sedative-hypnotics and, 520
Duloxetine, 432–433, 435
Dysfunctional family processes in substance-related and addictive disorders,
    102–105
Dysphoria, gender, 242–245
  DSM-5 classification, 594
  NANDA nursing diagnoses corresponding to, 619
  symptomatology, 244–245
  transvestic disorder and, 232
Dysthymia, 133
Eating disorders
  anorexia nervosa, 251–252
  background assessment data, 251–255
  binge-eating disorder, 254, 255
  bulimia nervosa, 252–254
  deficient fluid volume, 257–259

    disturbed body image/low self-esteem, 262–264, 266–267
    DSM-5 classification, 591
    imbalanced nutrition, 255–257, 264–266
    ineffective denial, 259–261
    Internet resources, 267–268
    moderate to severe anxiety, 261–262
    NANDA nursing diagnoses corresponding to, 619
    obesity, 254–255
ECG changes
    antipsychotic agents and, 498–499
    mood-stabilizing agents and, 472
Echinacea, 352t
Echolalia, 115
Echopraxia, 115
Educational and occupational problems, DSM-5 classification, 608
Efavirenz, 431
Effexor, 433, 435–436
Ego defense mechanisms, 543–545
Eletriptan, premenstrual dysphoric disorder and, 316t
Electroconvulsive therapy (ECT), 573–575
Electrolyte disturbances and depressive disorder, 134
Eletriptan, premenstrual dysphoric disorder and, 316t
Elevated temperature and antiparkinsonian agents, 510
Elimination
    disorders, DSM-5 classification, 591–592
    and exchange, domain in NANDA nursing diagnoses, 635
Emergency department
    deaths in, 339–340
    forensic nurse examiners in, 338–339
Emotional ambivalence, 116
Emotional neglect, 303
Emotions in mental status assessment, 613–614
Emsam, 439, 441
Energy balance classification in NANDA nursing diagnoses, 636
Engel, George, 374
Environmental factors
    attention-deficit/hyperactivity disorder, 27
    autism spectrum disorder, 20
    schizophrenia, 111–112
    Tourette's disorder, 43
Epinephrine, 440, 476, 479, 481
Epitol, 451
Equetro, 451
Erectile disorder, 234
Erickson's psychosocial theory, 540
Erotomanic type delusional disorder, 108
Erythromycin, 413
Escitalopram, 422, 425–426
Esophageal varices, 79
Esophagitis, 79
Estazolam, 512, 513
Eszopiclone, 516, 517, 518, 519
Ethnicity and homelessness, 321
Etrafon, 442
Evaluation in nursing process, 2
Evening primrose and premenstrual dysphoric disorder, 317t
Evidence preservation, 339, 341, 342
Exacerbation of psychoses and antiparkinsonian agents, 510
Exhibitionistic disorder, 231

Extrapyramidal symptoms
 antipsychotic agents and, 500
 mood-stabilizing agents and, 472
Ezide, premenstrual dysphoric disorder and, 316t

Factitious disorder, 208–209
Failure to follow prescribed therapy, 619
Family dynamics, 29, 289
 antisocial personality disorder and, 289
 conduct disorder and, 28
 eating disorders and, 253–254
 gender dysphoria and, 244
 and homelessness, 321
 oppositional defiant disorder and, 29
 somatic symptom disorders and, 210
Family processes
 dysfunctional, in substance-related and addictive disorders,
  102–105
 interrupted, in military families, 398–399
 in NANDA nursing diagnoses, 637
 separation anxiety disorder and, 48
Family therapy, 564–565
Fanapt, 489, 492
Fast-force injuries, 339
FDA pregnancy categories, 623
Fear, 177–179, 619
 of having a serious illness, 217–219
Feeding and eating disorders, DSM-5 classification, 591
Feelings of unreality, 275
Felodipine, 515
Female orgasmic disorder, 234
Female sexual interest/arousal disorder, 233–234
Fennel, 353t
Fenoprofen, 515
Fetishistic disorder, 231
Fetzima, 433, 436
Feverfew, 353t
Fiber, dietary, 358
Finding enduring connection with the lost entity in stages of grief,
 376
Fine hand tremors and mood-stabilizing agents, 471
Flashbacks, 619
Flecainide, 431, 434
Flexibility, waxy, 116–117
Flight of ideas, 155, 619
Fluoxetine, 423, 426–427
 interactions, 408, 413, 426, 431, 434, 440, 450, 481, 490, 493
 premenstrual dysphoric disorder and, 316t
Fluphenazine, 474, 477
Flurazepam, 512, 513
Fluvoxamine, 413, 423, 427–428, 481, 518
Focalin, 525, 526–527
Focalin XR, 525, 526–527
Food and Drug Administration (FDA), 351
Forensic nurse examiners (FNEs), 338–339
Forensic nursing
 background assessment data, 338–340
 in correctional facilities, 343
  complicated grieving and, 345–347

defensive coping and, 343–345
risk for injury and, 347–349
Internet resources, 349
in trauma care, 338
post-trauma syndrome/rape-trauma
syndrome, 340–342
Form of thought, 113–114
in mental status assessment, 614–615
Freud's stages of psychosexual development, 539
Frontotemporal neurocognitive disorder, 56
Frotteuristic disorder, 231
Frova, premenstrual dysphoric disorder and, 316t
Frovatriptan, premenstrual dysphoric disorder and, 316t
Fruits, 358, 359t
Furazolidone, 523
Furosemide, premenstrual dysphoric disorder and, 316t

Gambling disorder, 86, 90
Gamma aminobutyric acid (GABA), 512
Gastritis, 79
Gastrointestinal function
classification in NANDA nursing diagnoses, 635
herbal remedies for, 352t, 353t, 354t
Gatifloxacin, 491
Gender and homelessness, 321
Gender dysphoria, 242–245
DSM-5 classification, 594
NANDA nursing diagnoses corresponding to, 619
symptomatology, 244–245
transvestic disorder and, 232
Gender identity, 242
General attitude in mental status assessment, 613
Generalized amnesia, 220
Generalized anxiety disorder, 170
General systems theory, 564–565
Genetic factors
abuse, 303
antisocial personality disorder, 288
anxiety, obsessive-compulsive, and related disorders, 173
attention-deficit/hyperactivity disorder, 26
autism spectrum disorder, 20
bipolar disorder, 154
borderline personality disorder, 272
conduct disorder and, 28
depressive disorder, 134
dissociative disorder, 221
eating disorders, 252–253
gambling disorder, 86, 90
gender dysphoria, 244
obesity, 254–255
schizophrenia, 111
separation anxiety disorder, 48
somatic symptom disorders, 209
substance-related disorders, 78
Tourette's disorder, 43
Genito-pelvic pain/penetration disorder, 235
Geodon, 461, 470, 489, 492
German Federal Health Agency, 351
Ginger, 353t

Ginkgo, 353t
Ginseng, 353t
Grains, refined and whole, 358, 359t
Grandiose type delusional disorder, 108, 155
Grieving, 619
    anticipatory, 377–378
    chronic or prolonged, 379
    complicated, 139–141, 193–194, 280–282, 345–347, 382–384, 399–401, 618
    delayed or inhibited, 378
    distorted (exaggerated) response, 378–379
    length of, 376–377
    normal versus maladaptive, 379–380
    stages of, 372–376, 550–551
Griseofulvin, 515
Group therapy, 563
Growth/development domain in NANDA nursing diagnoses, 640
Guanadrel, 440
Guanethidine, 419, 440, 476, 523
Guanfacine, 529, 530–531, 534
Gustatory hallucinations, 115

Habit Reversal Training (HRT), 183
Hair-pulling disorder (trichotillomania), 171
Halcion, 512, 514
Haldol, 479–482
    Tourette's disorder and, 44–45
Hallucinations, 114–115, 619
Hallucinogen-related disorders, 74, 77t, 596. *See also* Substance-related and addictive disorders
    detoxification, 349
    pattern of use in, 82–83
    risk for injury, 93
Hallucinogens
    classification of, 74, 77 (table)
    in substitution therapy for substance withdrawal, 349
    substance-related and addictive disorders and, 93
Haloperidol, 479–482
    diphenhydramine and, 505
    interactions, 413, 419, 426, 431, 434, 450
    Tourette's disorder and, 44–45
Hamilton Depression Rating Scale (HDRS), 629–631
Headache
    antidepressants and, 444
    herbal remedies for, 353t
    mood-stabilizing agents and, 471
Health awareness classification in NANDA nursing diagnoses, 634
Health behavior, risk-prone
    psychiatric home nursing care and, 332–334
    in trauma- and stressor-related disorders, 201–203
Health care
    access to affordable, 322
    holistic, 351
Healthy eating patterns, 358
Health maintenance, ineffective, 619
    homelessness and, 323–325
    psychiatric home nursing care and, 330–332
Health management classification in NANDA nursing diagnoses, 634

Health promotion domain in NANDA nursing diagnoses, 634
Hepatic failure, antidepressants and, 446
Hepatitis and depressive disorder, 135
Herbal medicines, 351–352, 352–355t
   drug interactions, 405, 408, 412, 413
   for symptoms of premenstrual syndrome, 317–318t, 352t
Hesitation wounds, 339
Histological changes and schizophrenia, 111
History and assessment tool, 4–13
Histrionic personality disorder, 270
HIV infection
   NANDA nursing diagnoses corresponding to, 619
   neurocognitive disorder due to, 56
Hoarding disorder, 171–172
Holistic health care, 351
Homelessness
   background assessment data, 321–323
   ineffective health maintenance, 323–325
   Internet resources, 326–327
   powerlessness and, 325–326
   symptomatology, 323
Home nursing care, psychiatric
   background assessment data, 328–330
   ineffective self-health management and, 330–332
   Internet resources, 337
   risk for caregiver role strain, 335–337
   risk-prone health behavior and, 332–334
   social isolation and, 334–335
Hops, 354t
Hormonal disorders and depressive disorder, 134–135
Hormonal effects and antipsychotic agents, 498
Housing and economic problems, DSM-5 classification, 608
Huntington's disease, neurocognitive disorder due to, 57
Hydantoins, 425
Hydration classification in NANDA nursing diagnoses, 635
Hydrochlorothiazide, premenstrual dysphoric disorder and, 316t
HydroDiuril, premenstrual dysphoric disorder and, 316t
Hydroxyzine, 404
Hypercholesterolemia, 355t
Hyperglycemia
   antipsychotic agents and, 501
   mood-stabilizing agents and, 472
Hypersalivation and antipsychotic agents, 499–500
Hypertensive crisis, antidepressants and, 440, 445
Hyperthermia, 509
Hyperventilation, 176–177
Hypoglycemic agents, 440
Hypotension, mood-stabilizing agents and, 471, 472

Ibuprofen, premenstrual dysphoric disorder and, 316t
Identification, 544
Identity, gender, 242. See also Gender dysphoria
Illness anxiety disorder, 207
Iloperidone, 489, 492
Imbalanced nutrition, 618, 619
   depressive disorder and, 135, 148–150
   less than body requirements
      in bipolar and related disorders, 160–162

in depressive disorders, 148–150
in eating disorders, 255–257
in substance-related and addictive disorders, 97–98
more than body requirements, in eating disorders, 264–266
premenstrual dysphoric disorder and, 312
Imipramine, 417, 421, 431
posttraumatic stress disorder and, 395
Imitrex, premenstrual dysphoric disorder and, 316t
Immune response and herbal remedies, 352t
Impaired social interaction, 618, 619
in bipolar and related disorders, 165–166
in depressive disorders, 143–145
in disorders of infancy, childhood, and adolescence, 19–20, 22–23, 34–35, 45–46, 51–52
in personality disorders, 282–284, 297–299
in schizophrenia spectrum and other psychotic disorders, 116
in sexual disorders and gender dysphoria, 247–248
Implementation in nursing process, 2
Impulse control
ineffective, 182–183
mental status assessment and, 617
Impulsivity, 275
Inability to be alone, 274
Inability to meet basic needs, 619
Inappropriate affect, 115
Inderal, premenstrual dysphoric disorder and, 316t
Indinavir, 434
Ineffective coping, 620
in anxiety, obsessive-compulsive, and related disorders, 179–180
in disorders of infancy, childhood, and adolescence, 35–37, 50–51
in dissociative disorders, 223–224
in premenstrual dysphoric disorder, 315–319
in schizophrenia spectrum and other psychotic disorders, 121–122
in somatic symptom and related disorders, 211–214
in substance-related and addictive disorders, 95–97
in trauma- and stressor-related disorders, 199–201
Ineffective denial
in eating disorders, 259–261
in substance-related and addictive disorders, 93–95
Ineffective health maintenance in homelessness, 323–325
Ineffective impulse control, 182–183
Ineffective protection, 619
Ineffective self-health management in psychiatric home nursing care, 330–332
Ineffective sexuality pattern, 240–245, 619
Infancy, childhood, or adolescence, disorders of
attention-deficit/hyperactivity disorder, 26–27
autism spectrum disorder, 20–21
background assessment data, 14–15
conduct disorder, 27–29
defensive coping, 32–34
disturbed personal identity, 25–26
impaired social interaction, 19–20, 22–23, 34–35, 45–46, 51–52
impaired verbal communication, 18–19, 23–24
ineffective coping, 35–37, 50–51
intellectual disability, 15–16
low self-esteem, 37–38, 47–48
moderate to severe anxiety, 38–40
noncompliance, 41–42
oppositional defiant disorder, 29–30

risk for injury, 16–17
risk for self-directed or other-directed violence, 30–32, 44–45
risk for self-mutilation, 21–22
self-care deficit, 17–18
separation anxiety disorder, 48–49
severe anxiety, 49–50
Tourette's disorder, 42–43
Infection risk classification in NANDA nursing diagnoses, 639
Ingestion classification in NANDA nursing diagnoses, 634
Inhalant-related disorders, 74, 596
    pattern of use in, 83
    symptoms associated with intoxication and withdrawal from, 88t
Inhalants, classification of, 74
Injury risk
    in bipolar and related disorders, 156–158
    in forensic nursing, 347–349
    in intellectual disability, 16–17
    in NANDA nursing diagnoses, 618, 639
    in substance-related and addictive disorders, 90–93
Insomnia
    ADHD agents and, 535
    antidepressants and, 444
    in bipolar and related disorders, 167–168
    herbal remedies for, 352t, 354t, 355t
    NANDA nursing diagnoses corresponding to, 618
    in schizophrenia spectrum and other psychotic disorders, 129–130
Insulin, 440, 524
Integumentary function classification in NANDA nursing diagnoses, 635
Intellectual disability, 15–16, 583
    impaired social interaction with, 19–20
    impaired verbal communication with, 18–19
    risk for injury with, 16–17
    self-care deficit with, 17–18
Intellectualization, 544
Intelligence quotient (IQ), 15–16
International Association of Forensic Nurses (IAFN), 338
Internet resources
    ADHD agents, 538
    antianxiety agents, 415
    antidepressants, 448
    antiparkinsonian agents, 511
    antipsychotic agents, 503
    anxiety, obsessive-compulsive, and related disorders, 183–184
    bipolar and related disorders, 168
    complementary therapies, 369–370
    depressive disorders, 151–152
    disorders of infancy, childhood, and adolescence, 53
    dissociative disorders, 229
    eating disorders, 267–268
    forensic nursing, 349
    homelessness, 326–327
    loss and bereavement, 385
    military families, 403
    mood-stabilizing agents, 473
    neurocognitive disorders, 69–70
    personality disorders, 301
    premenstrual dysphoric disorder, 320
    problems related to abuse or neglect, 310–311
    psychiatric home nursing care, 337

schizophrenia spectrum and other psychotic disorders, 130–131
sedative-hypnotics, 521
sexual disorders and gender dysphoria, 249–250
somatic symptom and related disorders, 219
substance-related and addictive disorders, 105–106
trauma- and stressor-related disorders, 205
Interpersonal functioning and relationship to the external world, 116
NANDA nursing diagnoses corresponding to difficulties with, 618
Interpersonal theory of development, 540, 541
Intoxication, substance, 72, 80–85
depressive disorder and, 134
Introjection, 544
Intuniv, 529, 530–531
Invega, 489, 492
Investigation of wound characteristics, 339
IQ, 15–16
Isocarboxazid, 439, 440–441
Isolation, social, 545, 620
in depressive disorders, 143–145
pet therapy for, 369
in psychiatric home nursing care, 334–335
in schizophrenia spectrum and other psychotic disorders, 116, 119–121
Isoniazid, 408, 513
Isoptin
for bipolar disorder, 459
premenstrual dysphoric disorder and, 316t
Itraconazole, 413, 518

Jealous type delusional disorder, 108
Jimson weed, 405
Judgment and insight in mental status assessment, 617

Kapvay, 529, 530
Kava-kava, 354t, 405
drug interactions, 413
Ketoconazole, 408, 413, 434, 491, 493, 518
Klonopin, 406, 409, 451, 456
Knowledge, deficient. *See* Deficient knowledge
Kohlberg's stages of moral development, 541
Kübler-Ross, Elisabeth, 372–373

Lamictal, 451–452, 457
Lamotrigine, 451–452, 453, 457
Lasix, premenstrual dysphoric disorder and, 316t
Latuda, 494–495
Learned helplessness, 135
Learning disorders, 584
Learning theory, 210, 304
abuse and, 304
anxiety, obsessive-compulsive, and related disorders and, 174
depressive disorder and, 135
somatic symptom disorders and, 210
Length of the grief process, 376–377
Levodopa, 408, 419, 431, 440, 490, 506, 530, 534
Levomethadyl, 491
Levomilnacipran, 433, 436
Levothyroxine, 419
Lewy bodies, neurocognitive disorder with, 56
Lexapro, 422, 425–426

Librium
  for anxiety, 406, 409
  in substitution therapy, 92–93, 348
Life experiences
  anxiety, obsessive-compulsive, and related disorders and, 174
  borderline personality disorder and, 272–273
  dissociative disorder and, 222
  somatic symptom disorders and, 210–211
Life principles domain in NANDA nursing diagnoses, 639
Lifestyle and obesity, 255
Limbitrol, 441, 442
Linezolid, 425, 431
Lisdexamfetamine, 522, 525
Lithium
  carbonate, 449
  citrate, 449
  interactions, 425
Lithobid, 449
Liver damage and ADHD agents, 536
Localized amnesia, 220
Loneliness, 369
Loop diuretics, 450
Loose associations, 619
Loquaciousness, 155
Lorazepam, 407, 410–411
Loss and bereavement. *See also* Complicated grieving
  anticipatory grief in, 377–378
  background assessment data, 371–382
  concepts of death and, 380–382
  Internet resources, 385
  length of grief in, 376–377
  maladaptive responses to, 378–379
  normal versus maladaptive grieving in, 379–380
  overload, 381
  risk for complicated grieving, 382–384
  risk for spiritual distress, 384–385
  stages of grief in, 372–376, 550–551
  symptomatology, 372–376
  of valued entity, NANDA nursing diagnoses corresponding to, 619
Loxapine, 482, 483, 484, 488
  interactions, 485, 486
Loxitane, 482, 488
L-tryptophan, 425, 440
Luminal, 514, 516
  in substitution therapy, 92, 349
Lunesta, 516, 519
Lurasidone, 494–495
Luvox, 423, 427–428

Macrolides, 481, 513
Magical thinking, 113
Mahler's theory of object relations, 541
Major depressive disorder (MDD), 132–133
Maladaptive responses to loss, 378–379
Male hypoactive sexual desire disorder, 234
Manic hyperactivity, 619
Manipulation, 275
  NANDA nursing diagnoses corresponding to, 619
Mapping, concept, 3–5

Maprotiline, 418, 419, 422
Marplan, 439, 440–441
Massage, 366–367
Maxalt, premenstrual dysphoric disorder and, 316t
MDD. *See* Major depressive disorder (MDD)
Meat and beans, 358, 359t
Medicaid, 329
Medicare, 329
Medication-induced movement disorders, DSM-5 classification, 603–604
Medications. *See also* Antianxiety agents; Antidepressants; Antiparkinsonian agents;
    Antipsychotic agents
    assessment tool, 576–580
    DEA controlled substances schedules, 624–628
    FDA pregnancy categories, 623
    for symptomatic relief of premenstrual dysphoric disorder, 316t
Meditation, 367, 568
Melancholic features, depressive disorder with, 133
Memory, impaired, 224–226
    herbal remedies for, 353t
    NANDA nursing diagnoses corresponding to, 618
Mental illness and homelessness, 321
Mental imagery, 568
Mental status assessment, 610–617
    brief evaluation, 621–622
    emotions, 613–614
    general description, 611–613
    identifying data, 610–611
    impulse control, 617
    judgment and insight, 617
    sensorium and cognitive ability, 616–617
    thought processes, 614–615
Meperidine, 440, 476
Meprobamate, 411
Meridians, 356, 367
Metabolism classification in NANDA nursing diagnoses, 634
Metadate CD, 525, 527
Metadate ER, 525
Methadone
    interactions, 425, 513
    in substitution therapy, 92, 348
Methamphetamine, 522, 524
Methoxyflurane, 515
Methyldopa, 440, 450
Methylin, 525, 527
Methylin ER, 525, 527
Methylphenidate, 440, 525, 527–528
Metoclopramide, 425
Metoprolol, 408, 431, 434
Metronidazole, 515
Mexiletine, 426
Midazolam, 434
Milieu therapy, 565–566
Military families
    background assessment data, 386–392
    caregiver role strain in, 401–403
    complicated grieving in, 399–401
    disturbed thought processes in, 396–398
    Internet resources, 403
    interrupted family processes in, 398–399
    posttrauma syndrome in, 393–395

risk for suicide in, 395–396
symptomatology, 392–393
veterans, 390–392
Milk products, 358, 359t
Minerals and vitamins, 361–365t
Mirtazepine, 418, 419, 422
Mixed features, depressive disorder with, 133
Mixed type delusional disorder, 108
Mixer (chiropractic medicine), 366
Monoamine oxidase inhibitors, 439–441
herbal, 355t
interactions, 413, 419, 425, 431, 434, 515, 523
Mood in mental status assessment, 613
Mood-stabilizing agents
anticonvulsants, 451–459
antimanic, 449–451
antipsychotics, 460–470
calcium channel blockers, 459–460
client/family education related to, 472–473
Internet resources, 473
nursing diagnoses related to all, 470
nursing implications for, 471–472
Moral development stages, 541
Motion sickness, 353t
Motor activity in mental status assessment, 611–612
Motor disorders, 584
Motrin, premenstrual dysphoric disorder and, 316t
Moxifloxacin, 491
Multiple personalities, 619
Mutism, 114

Nalmefene in substitution therapy, 92, 348
Naloxone in substitution therapy, 92, 348
Naltrexone in substitution therapy, 92, 348
NANDA nursing diagnoses, 618–620
taxonomy II, 634–640
Naproxen, premenstrual dysphoric disorder and, 316t
Naratriptan, premenstrual dysphoric disorder and, 316t
Narcan in substitution therapy, 92, 348
Narcissistic personality disorder, 270
Nardil, 439, 441
National Center for Complementary Medicine and Alternative Medicine, 350
National Certification Examination for Therapeutic Massage and Bodywork, 367
National Coalition for the Homeless, 322
National Council Licensure Examination for Registered Nurses, 2
National Council of State Boards of Nursing (NCSBN), 1–2
National Institutes of Health (NIH), 350
Natural death, 339
Nausea/vomiting
ADHD agents and, 536
antidepressants and, 443
antiparkinsonian agents and, 510
antipsychotic agents and, 496
mood-stabilizing agents and, 471, 472
NANDA nursing diagnoses corresponding to, 620
sedative-hypnotics and, 520
Navane, 478–479
Nefazodone, 413, 436, 438, 513, 518
Neglect, symptomatology, 304–305
Neglect of a child, 303

Nelfinavir, 518
Nembutal, 514, 516
Neologisms, 114
Neuroanatomical factors
  abuse and, 303–304
  anxiety, obsessive-compulsive, and related disorders, 173
  bipolar disorder, 155
  borderline personality disorder, 272
  schizophrenia, 111–112
  somatic symptom disorders, 209
  in Tourette's disorder, 43
Neurobehavioral stress classification in NANDA nursing diagnoses, 638–639
Neurobiological/neurochemical factors
  dissociative disorder and, 221
  eating disorders, 253
Neurocognitive disorders
  antipsychotic agents and, 501
  background assessment data, 54–58
  caregiver role strain and, 68–69
  chronic confusion in, 61–63
  defined, 55
  disturbed sensory perception in, 65–66
  DSM-5 classification, 599–602
  due to Alzheimer's disease, 55–56
  due to another medical condition, 57
  due to HIV infection, 56
  due to Huntington's disease, 57
  due to Parkinson's disease, 57
  due to prion disease, 56–57
  due to traumatic brain injury, 56
  frontotemporal, 56
  Internet resources, 69–70
  with Lewy bodies, 56
  low self-esteem in, 66–68
  risk for self-directed or other-directed violence, 60–61
  risk for trauma, 58–59
  self-care deficit in, 63–64
  substance/medication-induced, 57
  vascular, 56
Neurodevelopmental disorders, DSM-5 classification, 583–585
Neuroendocrine abnormalities, 253
  depressive disorder and, 134
  eating disorders and, 253
Neuroleptic malignant syndrome and antipsychotic agents, 500–501
Neurological factors, autism spectrum disorder, 20
Neuromuscular blocking agents, 450
Nicotine replacement agents, 431
Nightmares, 619
Nihilistic delusion, 113
Noncompliance, in disorders of infancy, childhood, and adolescence, 41–42
Nonsteroidal anti-inflammatory drugs (NSAIDs), 450
Nonsubstance-related disorders, 86–90, 598
Norepinephrine, 440
Norepinephrine-dopamine reuptake inhibitors, 430–432
Norpramin, 416, 420
Nortriptyline, 417, 421, 431
Numbness in stages of grief, 373
Nurse Practice Acts, 3
Nursing diagnoses. *See* Diagnoses

Nursing history and assessment tool, 4–13
Nursing process, 1–2
    concept mapping and, 3–5
    diagnosis in, 2–3
Nutrition
    and diet in complementary therapies, 357–358, 359–360t
    domain in NANDA nursing diagnoses, 634–635
    essential vitamins and minerals, 361–365t
    imbalanced nutrition, 618, 619
        in bipolar and related disorders, 160–162
        in depressive disorders, 135, 148–150
        in eating disorders, 255–257, 264–266
        in premenstrual dysphoric disorder, 312
        in substance-related and addictive disorders, 97–98

Obesity, 254–255, 357
Object loss theory, 135
Object relations theory, borderline personality disorder and, 273–274
Obsessive-compulsive and related disorders, DSM-5 classification, 589
    background assessment data, 169–172
    disturbed body image, 180–182
    fear, 177–179
    ineffective coping, 179–180
    ineffective impulse control, 182–183
    Internet resources, 183–184
    predisposing factors to, 172–174
    symptomatology, 174–175
Obsessive-compulsive personality disorder, 271
Office of Alternative Medicine (OAM), 350
Oils, 357, 358, 359–360t
Olanzapine, 460, 461–462, 463, 467, 482, 483, 484, 488
    and fluoxetine, 460, 467
    interactions, 425, 465, 485, 486
Olanzapine/fluoxetine, 441, 442
Older adults, concept of death in, 381–382
Oleptro ER, 436
Olfactory hallucinations, 115
On the way to object constancy phase in theory of object relations, 273
Opioid-related disorders, 72–73, 76t, 596–597
    detoxification, 348–349
    pattern of use in, 84
    symptoms associated with intoxication and withdrawal from, 89t
Opioids
    classification of, 72–73, 76 (table)
    detoxification, 348–349
    interactions, 405, 408, 412, 440, 490, 518, 530
    trauma- and stressor-related disorders and, 187–188
Oppositional defiant disorder, 29–30
Oral anticoagulants, 476
Oral contraceptives
    drug interactions, 408, 513, 515
    efficacy and mood-stabilizing agents, 471
Orap, 45, 482
Orgasmic disorders
    delayed ejaculation, 234–235
    female orgasmic disorder, 234
    predisposing factors, 236, 237
    premature ejaculation, 235
Orientation classification in NANDA nursing diagnoses, 636

Orientation phase in nurse-client relationship, 553
Orthostatic hypotension
    antidepressants and, 443
    antiparkinsonian agents and, 510
    antipsychotic agents and, 498
    sedative-hypnotics and, 520
Osmotic diuretics, 450
Other-directed or self-directed violence, risk for, 620
    in bipolar and related disorders, 158–160
    in disorders of infancy, childhood, and adolescence, 30–32, 44–45
    in neurocognitive disorders, 60–61
    in personality disorders, 276–278, 290–293
    in schizophrenia spectrum and other psychotic disorders, 117–119
    in trauma- and stressor-related disorders, 194–197
Outcome identification in nursing process, 2
Overstimulation and ADHD agents, 535
Overweight, 357
Oxazepam
    for anxiety, 407, 411
    in substitution therapy, 92, 348, 349
Oxcarbazepine, 452, 453, 455, 458–459

Pacing and rocking, 117
Pain
    acute, in premenstrual dysphoric disorder, 313–315
    chiropractic medicine for, 366
    massage for, 367
    sexual pain disorders
        genito-pelvic pain/penetration disorder, 235
        substance/medication-induced sexual dysfunction, 235
Paliperidone, 489, 492
Palpitations
    ADHD agents and, 535
    sedative-hypnotics and, 520
Pamelor, 417, 421
Pancreatitis, 79
Panic disorder, 169–170
Paralytic ileus and antiparkinsonian agents, 509
Paranoia, 113
Paranoid personality disorder, 269
Paraphilic disorders
    background assessment data, 230–233
    DSM-5 classification, 603
    symptomatology, 233, 235–236
Parasomnias, DSM-5 classification, 593
Paradoxical excitement and sedative-hypnotics, 520
Parkinson's disease
    anticholinergics for, 504–506
    dopaminergic agonists for, 507–509
    neurocognitive disorder due to, 57
Parlodel
    for Parkinson's disease, 507–509
    premenstrual dysphoric disorder and, 316t
Parnate, 439, 441
Paroxetine, 423, 428–429
    interactions, 426, 431, 434, 476, 490, 493
    premenstrual dysphoric disorder and, 316t
Passion flower, 354t
Past experience with physical illness. *See* Life experiences

Patterned injuries, 339
Paxil, 423, 428–429
    premenstrual dysphoric disorder and, 316t
Pedophilic disorder, 231
Peer relationships, 28
Penetration disorder, 235
Pentamidine, 491
Pentobarbital, 514, 516
Pen Tsao, 351
Peplau's interpersonal theory of development, 541
Peppermint, 354t
Perception, 114–115
    domain in NANDA nursing diagnoses, 636
Perceptual disturbances in mental status assessment, 616
Peripartum onset, depressive disorder with, 133
Peripheral neuropathy, 79
Perphenazine, 474, 477
Perphenazine/amitriptyline HCL, 441, 442
Persecutory type delusional disorder, 108, 156
Perseveration, 114
Persistent depressive disorder, 133
Personal history, DSM-5 classification, 609
Personal identity, disturbed, 619
    in disorders of infancy, childhood, and adolescence, 25–26
    in dissociative disorders, 226–227
    in personality disorders, 284–286
    in sexual disorders and gender dysphoria, 245–247
Personality clusters, 269
Personality disorders
    antisocial personality disorder, 270, 288–290
    background assessment data, 269–271
    borderline personality disorder, 270, 272–275
    chronic low self-esteem, 286–290, 295–297
    complicated grieving, 280–282
    defensive coping, 293–295
    deficient knowledge, 299–301
    disturbed personal identity, 284–286
    DSM-5 classification, 602–603
    impaired social interaction, 282–284, 297–299
    Internet resources, 301
    risk for other-directed violence in, 276–278, 290–293
    risk for self-mutilation/risk for self-directed or other-directed violence, 276–278
    severe to panic anxiety, 278–280
    types of, 269–271
Pet therapy, 368–369
Phencyclidine (PCP) use disorder, 85
    symptoms associated with intoxication and withdrawal from, 89t
Phenelzine, 439, 441
    posttraumatic stress disorder and, 395
Phenobarbital, 514, 516
    interactions, 413, 431
    in substitution therapy, 349
Phenothiazines, 419, 426, 434, 450, 474–478, 481
    diphenhydramine and, 506
Phenylbutazone, 515
Phenylbutylpiperadines, 479–482
Phenytoin, 413, 425, 513, 530
    interactions, 431, 476

Phobia
  NANDA nursing diagnoses corresponding to, 619
  social, 170
  specific, 170–171
Photosensitivity
  antidepressants and, 444
  antipsychotic agents and, 498
Physical abuse
  of an adult, 303
  of a child, 303
  symptomatology, 304
Physical neglect, 303
Piaget's stages of cognitive development, 541
Pimozide, 45, 426, 479–482
Planning in nursing process, 2
PMDD. *See* Premenstrual dysphoric disorder
Polyuria, mood-stabilizing agents and, 471
Posttrauma syndrome, 619
  in forensic nursing, 340–343
  in military families, 393–395
  in NANDA nursing diagnoses, 638
  in trauma- and stressor-related disorders, 191–192
Posttraumatic stress disorder, 186, 187–188, 190
  in military families, 391, 392
Posturing, 117
Potentilla and premenstrual dysphoric disorder, 317t
Poverty and homelessness, 322
Powerlessness, 145–147, 619
  behaviors indicating, 619
  homelessness and, 325–326
  problems related to abuse or neglect, 307–309
Practicing phase in theory of object relations, 273
Prazosin, 530
Pregnancy
  attention-deficit/hyperactivity disorder and, 26–27
  categories, FDA, 623
  risk evaluation and prevention after sexual assault, 341–342
Pre-interaction phase in nurse-client relationship, 552–553
Premature ejaculation, 235
Premenstrual dysphoric disorder, 133–134
  acute pain, 313–315
  background assessment data, 312–313
  herbals for symptoms of, 317–318t, 352t
  ineffective coping, 315–319
  Internet resources, 320
  medications for symptomatic relief of, 316t
  symptomatology, 313
Prenatal, perinatal, and postnatal factors, attention-deficit/hyperactivity disorder and, 26–27
Preparatory depression, 373
Preservation of evidence, 339, 341, 342
Prion disease, neurocognitive disorder due to, 56–57
Priapism, antidepressants and, 446
Pristiq, 432, 435
Probenecid, 513
Procainamide, 491
Processing the pain of grief in stages of grief, 375
Prochlorperazine, 474, 477–478
Procyclidine, 425

Progressive relaxation, 568
Projection, 545
    NANDA nursing diagnoses corresponding to, 619
Prolonged bleeding time and valproic acid, 471
Prolonged grief, 379
Propafenone, 425, 431, 434
Propoxyphene, 408
Propranolol
    interactions, 408
    posttraumatic stress disorder and, 395
    premenstrual dysphoric disorder and, 316t
Protection, ineffective, 619
Proteins, 358, 359t
Protest in stages of grief, 373
Protriptyline, 417, 421
Prozac, 423, 426–427
Psychiatric home nursing care
    background assessment data, 328–330
    ineffective self-health management and, 330–332
    Internet resources, 337
    risk for caregiver role strain, 335–337
    risk-prone health behavior and, 332–334
    social isolation and, 334–335
Psychoanalytic theory, 232, 255
    depressive disorder and, 135
    gender dysphoria and, 244
    obesity and, 255
    paraphilic disorders and, 232
Psychodrama, 564
Psychodynamic theory, 78, 253, 304
    abuse and, 304
    anxiety, obsessive-compulsive, and related disorders
        and, 173
    dissociative disorder, 221–222
    eating disorders and, 253
    somatic symptom disorders and, 209–210
    substance-related disorders and, 78
Psychological factors
    affecting other medical conditions, 208
    gambling disorder, 90
Psychological trauma, 222
Psychomotor behavior, 116–117
Psychosexual development stages, 539
Psychosocial theory, 540
    trauma- and stressor-related disorders and, 189
Psychosocial therapies
    assertiveness training, 569–571
    cognitive therapy, 571–572
    crisis intervention, 567
    family therapy, 564–565
    group therapy, 563
    milieu therapy, 565–566
    psychodrama, 564
    relaxation therapy, 567–568
Psychotherapeutic combinations, 441–442
Psychotic disorder due to another medical condition, 109
Psychotic features, depressive disorder with, 133
Psyllium, 354t
Pulse irregularities and mood-stabilizing agents, 471

Qi, 356, 367
Quazepam, 512, 514
Quetiapine, 461, 462, 464, 468–469, 482, 483, 484, 488–489
   interactions, 466, 485, 487
Quinidine, 426, 434, 491, 493, 515
Quinolinones, 492–494

Rage reactions, 275
Ramelteon, 516, 517, 518, 519
Rape-trauma syndrome, 305–307
   in forensic nursing, 340–343
Rapprochement phase in theory of object relations, 273
Rationalization, 543
   NANDA nursing diagnoses corresponding to, 619
Reaction formation, 543
Reactive depression, 373
Rebound syndrome and alpha-adrenergic agonists, 537
Recovery in stages of grief, 374
Refined grains, 358, 359t
Regression, 117, 543–544
   in stages of grief, 375
Relational problems, DSM-5 classification, 604–608
Relaxation therapy, 567–568
Religiosity, 113
Relocation stress syndrome, 203–205, 619
Relpax, premenstrual dysphoric disorder and, 316t
Remeron, 418, 422
Reorganization in stages of grief, 373–374
Repression, 544
Reproduction classification in NANDA nursing diagnoses, 638
Research Center for Human-Animal Interaction (ReCHAI), 368–369
Reserpine, 440
Resolution of the loss in stages of grief, 374
Respiratory function classification in NANDA nursing diagnoses, 635
Restitution in stages of grief, 374
Restlessness and ADHD agents, 535
Restoril, 512, 514
Revex in substitution therapy, 92, 348
ReVia in substitution therapy, 92, 348
Rifabutin, 413
Rifampicin, 425
Rifampin, 408, 413, 431, 513, 530
Rifamycins, 419, 481
Risk-prone health behavior, 618
Risperidal, 461, 469–470, 489, 491–492
Risperidone, 425, 461, 462–463, 464, 469–470, 489, 491–492
   interactions, 431, 466
Ritalin, 525, 527
Ritalin LA, 525, 527
Ritalin SR, 525, 527
Ritonavir, 413, 431, 518, 534
Ritualistic behaviors, 619
Rizatriptan, premenstrual dysphoric disorder and, 316t
Rocking and pacing, 117
Role performance in NANDA nursing diagnoses, 618, 637
Role-playing
   for risk-prone health behavior, 202
   for somatic symptom disorders, 219
Role relationships domain in NANDA nursing diagnoses, 637–638

Role strain, caregiver, 335–337
  in military families, 401–403
  NANDA nursing diagnoses corresponding to, 619
  in neurocognitive disorders, 68–69
  in psychiatric home nursing care, 335–337
Ropivacaine, 425
Rozerem, 516, 519

Safety/protection domain in NANDA nursing diagnoses, 639–640
Saphris, 461, 470, 482, 487
Sarafem, 423, 426–427
  premenstrual dysphoric disorder and, 316t
Saturated fatty acids, 357
Scarcity of affordable housing, 322
Schizoaffective disorder, 109
Schizoid personality disorder, 270
Schizophrenia spectrum and other psychotic disorders, 108–109
  antipsychotic agents, 460–470
    benzisothiazolinone derivative, 494–495
    benzisoxazole derivatives, 489–492
    client/family education related to, 501–502
    dibenzepine derivatives, 482–489
    interactions, 518
    Internet resources, 503
    nursing diagnoses related to all, 496
    nursing implications for, 496–501
    phenothiazines, 474–478
    phenylbutylpiperadines, 479–482
    quinolinones, 492–494
    thioxanthenes, 478–479
  background assessment data, 107–117
  disturbed sensory perception in, 123–124
  disturbed thought processes in, 124–126
  DSM-5 classification, 585–586
  and homelessness, 321
  impaired verbal communication in, 126–128
  ineffective coping in, 121–122
  insomnia in, 129–130
  Internet resources, 130–131
  risk for self-directed or other-directed violence in, 117–119
  self-care deficit in, 128–129
  social isolation in, 116, 119–121
  substance/medication-induced, 109, 110t
Schizophreniform disorder, 108
Schizotypal personality disorder, 270
Seasonal pattern, depressive disorder with, 133, 432
Secobarbital, 514, 516
Seconal, 514, 516
Sedation
  ADHD agents and, 536
  antidepressants and, 443
  antiparkinsonian agents and, 510
  antipsychotic agents and, 498
  herbal remedies for, 354t, 355t
  mood-stabilizing agents and, 471, 472
  sedative-hypnotics and, 520
Sedative-, hypnotic-, or anxiolytic-related disorders
  DSM-5 classification, 597
  pattern of use in, 85–86
  symptoms associated with intoxication and withdrawal from, 89t

Sedative-hypnotics, 406–411
  barbiturates, 514–516
  benzodiazepines, 512–514
  client/family education related to, 521
  interactions, 405, 408, 412, 490, 530
  Internet resources, 521
  miscellaneous (nonbarbiturate), 516–519
  nursing diagnoses related to, 519–520
  nursing implications for, 520–521
Seizures
  ADHD agents and, 536
  antidepressants and, 431, 444
  antipsychotic agents and, 431, 499
Selective amnesia, 220
Selective serotonin reuptake inhibitors (SSRIs), 422–429
  eating disorders and, 253
  interactions, 419, 425, 518, 523
  for posttraumatic stress disorder, 395
Selegiline transdermal system, 439, 441
Self-blame, 372
Self-care deficit
  in disorders of infancy, childhood, and adolescence, 17–18
  in NANDA nursing diagnoses, 619, 636
  in neurocognitive disorders, 63–64
  in personality disorders, 299–301
  in schizophrenia spectrum and other psychotic disorders, 128–129
Self-concept classification in NANDA nursing diagnoses, 637
Self-destructive behaviors, 275
Self-directed or other-directed violence, risk for, 620
  in bipolar and related disorders, 158–160
  in disorders of infancy, childhood, and adolescence, 30–32, 44–45
  in neurocognitive disorders, 60–61
  in personality disorders, 276–278, 290–293
  in schizophrenia spectrum and other psychotic disorders, 117–119
  in trauma- and stressor-related disorders, 194–197
Selfemra, 423, 426–427
Self-esteem, low
  chronic, 619
    in personality disorders, 286–290, 295–297
    in substance-related and addictive disorders, 98–100
  in depressive disorders, 141–143
  in disorders of infancy, childhood, and adolescence, 37–38, 47–48
  in eating disorders, 262–264, 266–267
  in neurocognitive disorders, 66–68
  in sexual disorders and gender dysphoria, 248–249
Self-mutilation risk, 619
  in autism spectrum disorder, 21–22
  in borderline personality disorder, 276–278
Self-perception domain in NANDA nursing diagnoses, 637
Sensation/perception classification in NANDA nursing diagnoses, 636
Sense of self, 115
Sensorium and cognitive ability in mental status assessment, 616–617
Sensory perception, disturbed, 619. See Disturbed sensory perception
  in bipolar and related disorders, 163–165
  in dissociative disorders, 227–229
  in neurocognitive disorders, 65–66
  in schizophrenia spectrum and other psychotic disorders, 123–124
  in somatic symptom and related disorders, 214–215

Separation anxiety disorder, 48–49
  impaired social interaction and, 51–52
  ineffective coping in, 50–51
  severe anxiety in, 49–50
Serax in substitution therapy, 92, 348, 349
Seroquel, 468–469, 482, 488–489
Serotonin-2-antagonists/reuptake inhibitors, 436–438
Serotonin-5-HT1 receptor agonists, 425
Serotonin-norepinephrine reuptake inhibitors, 432–436
  herbal, 355t
Serotonin syndrome, antidepressants and, 444–445
Sertraline, 423, 429, 431
  premenstrual dysphoric disorder and, 316t
Sexual abuse
  of an adult, 303, 305–306, 340–343
  of a child, 302–303, 305
Sexual assault
  forensic examination after, 341–342
  in the military, 389
  rape-trauma syndrome and, 305–306, 340–343
Sexual disorders and gender dysphoria
  background assessment data, 230–238
  disturbed personal identity, 245–247
  impaired social interaction, 247–248
  ineffective sexuality pattern, 240–245
  Internet resources, 249–250
  low self-esteem, 248–249
  in NANDA nursing diagnoses, 637
  sexual dysfunction, 238–240
Sexual dysfunctions, 238–240, 619
  antidepressants and, 444
  antipsychotic agents and, 498
  background assessment data, 233–238
  DSM-5 classification, 593–594
  symptomatology, 233, 235–236
Sexual harassment, 389
Sexual interest/arousal disorders
  erectile disorder, 234
  female sexual interest/arousal disorder, 233–234
  male hypoactive sexual desire disorder, 234
  predisposing factors, 235–237
Sexually transmitted diseases (STDs) and sexual assault, 341
Sexual masochism disorder, 231
Sexual pain disorders
  genito-pelvic pain/penetration disorder, 235
  predisposing factors, 236–237
  substance/medication-induced sexual dysfunction, 235
Sexual sadism disorder, 231–232
Sharp-force injuries, 339
Shepherd's purse and premenstrual dysphoric disorder, 317t
Shock in stages of grief, 374
Sibutramine, 425, 434
Sinequan, 417, 420–421
Single-room-occupancy (SRO) hotels, 322
Skin rash
  antipsychotic agents and, 496, 498
  mood-stabilizing agents and, 471
Skullcap, 355t

Sleep/rest
  classification in NANDA nursing diagnoses, 635
  difficulty, NANDA nursing diagnoses corresponding to, 618
Sleep-wake disorders, 618. *See also* Insomnia
  in bipolar and related disorders, 167–168
  in depressive disorders, 150–151
  DSM-5 classification, 592–593
  in schizophrenia spectrum and other psychotic disorders, 129–130
Smoking and sedative-hypnotics, 513
Social anxiety disorder, 170
Social interaction, impaired, 618, 619
  in bipolar and related disorders, 165–166
  in depressive disorders, 143–145
  in disorders of infancy, childhood, and adolescence, 19–20, 22–23, 34–35, 45–46,
    51–52
  in personality disorders, 282–284, 297–299
  in schizophrenia spectrum and other psychotic disorders, 116
  in sexual disorders and gender dysphoria, 247–248
Social isolation, 545, 620
  in depressive disorders, 143–145
  pet therapy for, 369
  in psychiatric home nursing care, 334–335
  in schizophrenia spectrum and other psychotic disorders, 116, 119–121
Social learning theory, 78
  substance-related disorders and, 78
Social phobia, 170
Social support in Habit Reversal Training (HRT), 183
Societal influences in problems related to abuse or neglect, 304
Sociocultural factors in schizophrenia, 111–112
Sodium intake, 357
Solfoton, 514, 516
Somatic delusion, 113
Somatic symptom and related disorders
  background assessment data, 206–209
    deficient knowledge, 216–217
    disturbed sensory perception, 214–215
    DSM-5 classification, 590–591
    fear of having a serious illness, 217–219
    ineffective coping, 211–214
    Internet resources, 219
    predisposing factors, 209–210
    symptomatology, 211
Somatic type delusional disorder, 108
Sonata, 516, 519
Sotalol, 491
Specific phobia, 170–171
Speech patterns in mental status assessment, 612
Spinal anesthesia, 440
Spiritual distress, risk for, 384–385, 619
Splitting, 275
Spouses and children in military families, 387–388, 393
SSRIs. *See* Selective serotonin reuptake inhibitors (SSRIs)
St. John's wort, 355t
  drug interactions, 408, 425, 434, 440, 513
Stavzor, 451
Stimulants, CNS, 73, 75–76t
  amphetamines, 522–525
  miscellaneous agents, 525–528
  -related disorders, DSM-5 classification, 597–598

risk for injury from, 92, 349
in substitution therapy, 92, 349
Strategic model, 565
Strattera, 531, 534–535
Stress-adaptation model, 189–190
Stressful life events
schizophrenia and, 112
separation anxiety disorder and, 48
Structural model, 565
Sublimation, 544
Subluxation, 360
Substance Abuse and Mental Health Services Administration, 390
Substance/medication-induced disorders
anxiety, obsessive-compulsive, and related disorders, 173
bipolar disorder, 154
classification of substances, 72–74, 75–77 (table)
depressive disorder, 134
neurocognitive disorder, 57
psychotic disorder, 109, 110t
sexual dysfunction, 235
substance intoxication, 72
substance withdrawal, 72
Substance-related and addictive disorders
background assessment data, 71
chronic low self-esteem in, 98–100
classification of substances, 72–75, 75–77t
common patterns of use in, 78–86
deficient knowledge in, 100–102
defined, 71–72
depressive disorder and, 134
detoxification, 348–349
DSM-5 classification, 595–598
dysfunctional family processes in, 102–105
homelessness and, 322–323
imbalanced nutrition: less than body requirements, 97–98
ineffective coping in, 95–97
ineffective denial in, 93–95
Internet resources, 105–106
in military families, 391–392
NANDA nursing diagnoses corresponding to, 620
nonsubstance-related disorder, 86–90, 598
predisposing factors associated with, 78
risk for injury in, 90–93
substance-induced disorders, 72
substance use disorders, 71–72
substitution therapy for, 92–93, 348–349
symptoms associated with intoxication and withdrawal from, 87–89t
Substitution therapy, 92–93, 348–349
Sugars, 358
Suicide risk
in depressive disorders, 136–139
in military families, 391, 395–396
mood-stabilizing agents and, 472
NANDA nursing diagnoses corresponding to behaviors indicating, 620
Sullivan's interpersonal theory, 540
Sumatriptan
interactions, 425
premenstrual dysphoric disorder and, 316t
Suppression, 544

Surmontil, 417, 421–422
Suspiciousness, 620
Swedish massage, 367
Symbiotic phase in theory of object relations, 273
Symbyax, 441, 442, 460, 467
Symmetrel, 507–509
Sympathomimetics, 419, 425, 440, 450
Symptomatology
    abuse, 304–305
    anorexia nervosa, 251–252
    antisocial personality disorder, 290
    anxiety, obsessive-compulsive, and related disorders, 174–175
    attention-deficit/hyperactivity disorder, 27
    autism spectrum disorder, 20–21
    bipolar disorder, 155–156
    borderline personality disorder, 274–275
    bulimia nervosa, 252
    conduct disorder, 28–29
    delirium, 55
    depressive disorder, 135–136
    dissociative disorder, 222
    gender dysphoria, 244–245
    homelessness, 323
    intellectual disability, 15–16
    loss and bereavement, 372–376
    in military families, 392–393
    neurocognitive disorder, 57–58
    oppositional defiant disorder, 29
    paraphilic disorders, 233, 237–238
    premenstrual dysphoric disorder, 313
    psychiatric home nursing care, 329–330
    schizophrenia, 112–117
    separation anxiety disorder, 48–49
    somatic symptom disorders, 211
    substance-related disorders, 78–86
    Tourette's disorder, 43
    trauma- and stressor-related disorders, 190
Synthetic stimulants, 76t
Systemic lupus erythematosus, 135
Systemic steroids, 431

Tachycardia
    ADHD agents and, 535
    antidepressants and, 444
    antiparkinsonian agents and, 510
    sedative-hypnotics and, 520
Tactile hallucinations, 115
Tangentiality, 114
Tardive dyskinesia
    antipsychotic agents and, 500
Tegretol, 451, 455
Tegretol-XR, 451
Temazepam, 512, 514
Temperament
    antisocial personality disorder and, 289
    gender dysphoria and, 244
    separation anxiety disorder and, 48
Temperature, antiparkinsonian agents and body, 510
Tenex, 529, 530–531
Terbinafine, 434

Teril, 451

Termination phase in nurse-client relationship, 553–554

Tetracyclics, 418

Theophylline, 408, 425, 431, 450, 513, 515

Theory of family dynamics
  antisocial personality disorder and, 289
  conduct disorder and, 28
  eating disorders and, 253–254
  gender dysphoria and, 244
  oppositional defiant disorder and, 29
  somatic symptom disorders and, 210

Theory of object relations, 273–274, 541

Therapeutic nurse-client relationship phases, 552–562

Therapeutic touch and massage, 366–367

Thiazide diuretics, 440, 450

Thioridazine, 431, 434, 474, 478, 491

Thiothixene, 478–479

Thioxanthenes, 478–479

Thought processes, disturbed, 618
  in bipolar and related disorders, 162–163
  in depressive disorders, 147–148
  in schizophrenia spectrum and other psychotic disorders, 124–126
  in veterans of military combat, 396–398

Thyroid hormones, 419

Tic disorders, 42–43, 584–585

Ticlopidine, 431, 534

Tobacco-related disorders
  DSM-5 classification, 598
  pattern of use in, 83–84
  symptoms associated with intoxication and withdrawal from, 88t

Tofranil, 417, 421

Tolerance
  of ADHD agents, 536
  of sedative-hypnotics, 520

Topamax, 452, 457–458

Topiramate, 452, 453, 454–455, 457–458

Touch, therapeutic, 366–367

Tourette's disorder, 42–43, 531, 584–585
  impaired social interaction with, 45–46
  low self-esteem with, 47–48
  medications for, 479–482
  risk for self-directed or other-directed violence with, 44–45

Tramadol, 425, 431, 491

Trans-fatty acids, 357

Transvestic disorder, 232

Tranxene, 409–410

Tranylcypromine, 439, 441

Trauma- and stressor-related disorders
  background assessment data, 185–186
  complicated grieving, 193–194
  DSM-5 classification, 590
  ineffective coping, 199–201
  Internet resources, 205
  moderate to severe anxiety, 197–199
  posttrauma syndrome, 191–192
  predisposing factors, 187–190
  relocation stress syndrome, 203–205
  risk for self-directed or other-directed violence, 194–197
  risk-prone health behavior, 201–203
  stress-adaptation theory and, 189–190

symptomatology, 190
types, 186–187
Trauma care, clinical forensic nursing in, 338–342
Trauma risk, in neurocognitive disorders, 58–59
Traumatic brain injury, 390, 392
military veterans and, 390
neurocognitive disorder due to, 56
Trazodone, 436–437, 438
interactions, 425, 434
posttraumatic stress disorder and, 395
Triazolam, 512–513, 514
Trichotillomania (hair-pulling disorder), 171
Tricyclic antidepressants, 416–422
interactions, 419, 425, 434, 450, 481, 524, 530
Trifluoperazine, 474, 478
Trihexyphenidyl, 504, 506
Trileptal, 452, 458–459
Trimipramine, 417, 421–422
Triptans, 434, 440
Tyramine, 440

Undoing, 545
Unreality, feelings of, 275
Urinary acidifiers, 523
Urinary alkalinizers, 450, 523
Urinary function classification in NANDA nursing diagnoses, 635
Urinary retention
antidepressants and, 443
antiparkinsonian agents and, 509
antipsychotic agents and, 496

Valerian, 355t, 405
drug interactions, 413
premenstrual dysphoric disorder and, 317t
Valium
for anxiety, 407, 410
in substitution therapy, 92, 349
Valproate, 491
Valproic acid, 408, 419, 451–454, 456, 515, 530
Value/belief/action congruence classification in NANDA nursing diagnoses, 639
Vascular neurocognitive disorder, 56
Vasoconstrictors, 440
Vegetable, 358, 359t
Venlafaxine, 433, 435–436
Verapamil
for bipolar disorders, 459
interactions, 413, 515, 530
premenstrual dysphoric disorder and, 316t
Verbal communication, impaired
in disorders of infancy, childhood, and adolescence, 18–19, 23–24
in schizophrenia spectrum and other psychotic disorders, 126–128
Verelan, 459
Veterans, 390–392
pet therapy for, 368
Veterans Administration, 329
Viibryd, 423, 429
Vilazodone, 423, 429
Violence classification in NANDA nursing diagnoses, 640
Vistaril, 404

Visual hallucinations, 114
Vitamins and minerals, essential, 361–365t
Vivactil, 417, 421
Volition, 116
Vomiting. *See* Nausea/vomiting
Vortioxetine, 423, 429
Voyeuristic disorder, 232
Vyvanse, 522, 525
Warfarin, 425, 431, 434
Waxy flexibility, 116–117
Weight gain
 antidepressants and, 444
 mood-stabilizing agents and, 471, 472
Weight loss
 ADHD agents and, 536
 antidepressants and, 444
Wellbutrin, 430, 431–432, 531, 534–535
Wellbutrin SR, 430, 531, 534–535
Wellbutrin XL, 430, 531, 534–535
Wernicke-Korsakoff syndrome, 79
Whole grains, 358, 359t
Withdrawal, substance, 72, 80–86
 depressive disorder and, 134
 NANDA nursing diagnoses corresponding to, 618
 substitution therapy for, 92–93, 348–349
Withdrawn behavior, NANDA nursing diagnoses corresponding to, 620
Women
 domestic violence against, 322
 and homelessness, 321
 in the military, 389–390
 rape-trauma syndrome and, 305–307, 340–343
Worden, J. William, 374–376
Word salad, 114
Working phase in nurse-client relationship, 553
Wound characteristics, investigation of, 339

Xanax, 406, 408

Yoga, 367–368

Zaleplon, 516, 517, 518, 519
Ziprasidone, 461, 463, 464, 470, 489, 492
 interactions, 466
Zolmitriptan, premenstrual dysphoric disorder and, 316t
Zoloft, 423, 429
 premenstrual dysphoric disorder and, 316t
Zolpidem, 425, 516, 517, 519
Zomig, premenstrual dysphoric disorder and, 316t
Zyban, 430, 431–432, 531, 534
Zyprexa, 460, 467, 482, 488

Drug Index

Note: Page numbers followed by "t" indicate tabular material. Trade names appear in **bold**.

Abilify (aripiprazole), 158, 460–461t, 467, 492t, 493–494, 497t
Adderall/Adderall XR (amphetamine/dextroamphetamine), 522t, 524
Advil (ibuprofen), 316t
Akineton (biperiden), 504t, 506
Aleve (naproxen), 316t
Almotriptan (**Axert**), 316t
Alprazolam (**Xanax**), 32, 40, 92, 199, 262, 279, 406t, 408
Amantadine (**Symmetrel**), 431, 507–508, 507t, 508t, 533t
Ambien (zolpidem), 516t, 519
Amerge (naratriptan), 316t
Amitriptyline, 395, 416t, 419, 441t, 442, 455t
Amitriptyline-chlordiazepoxide (**Limbitrol**), 441t, 442
Amitriptyline HCL and perphenazine (**Etrafon**), 442
Amobarbital (**Amytal**), 75t, 514t, 515
Amoxapine, 417t, 422
Amphetamine/dextroamphetamine mixtures (**Adderall/Adderall XR**), 522t, 524
Amytal (amobarbital), 75t, 514t, 515
Anafranil (clomipramine), 416t, 420
Aripiprazole (**Abilify**), 158, 460–461t, 467, 492t, 493–494, 497t
Asenapine (**Saphris**), 158, 461t, 463, 465, 466t, 470, 473, 482–483, 482t, 486t, 487, 497t, 498, 501
Ativan (lorazepam), 407t, 410–411
Atomoxetine (**Strattera**), 531–532, 531t, 532–533t, 533, 535–537
Aventyl (nortriptyline), 417t, 421
Axert (almotriptan), 316t

Benadryl (diphenhydramine), 504t, 506
Benztropine (**Cogentin**), 500, 504t, 506
Biperiden (**Akineton**), 504t, 506
Black cohosh (*Cimicifuga racemosa*), 316t, 352t
Bromocriptine (**Parlodel**), 316t, 501, 504, 507, 507t, 508–509, 508t
Bugleweed (*Lycopus virginicus*), 316t
Buprenorphine (**Subutex**), 92, 349
Bupropion (**Wellbutrin/Wellbutrin SR/Wellbutrin XL/Zyban**), 419, 425, 430–431, 430t, 439, 440, 443–444, 447, 454t, 531–536, 531t, 533t
BuSpar (buspirone HCL), 412t, 413–415, 424, 425, 438, 439, 440, 460
Buspirone HCL (**BuSpar**), 412t, 413–415, 424, 425, 438, 439, 440, 460
Butabarbital (**Butisol**), 514t, 515
Butisol (butabarbital), 514t, 515

Calan (verapamil), 459–460, 459t
Capsella bursa-pastoris (shepherd's purse), 317t
Carbamazepine (**Tegretol/Epitol/Carbatrol/Equetro/Teril/Tegretol-XR**), 317t, 419, 425, 431, 437–438, 439, 440, 450, 451t, 452, 453, 454t, 455–456, 457, 460, 465t, 466t, 481, 486t, 490, 493, 495, 513, 515, 519t, 530, 533t

Carbatrol (carbamazepine), 451t
Cascara sagrada *(Rhamnus purshiana)*, 352t
Catapres (clonidine), 45, 92, 529t, 530
Celexa (citalopram), 422t, 425
Chamomile *(Matricaria chamomilla)*, 352t
Chaste tree *(Vitex agnus-castus)*, 317t
Chloral hydrate, 73, 516t, 517–518, 519
Chlordiazepoxide (**Librium**), 75t, 87t, 92, 93, 348, 406t, 409
Chlordiazepoxide-amitriptyline (**Limbitrol**), 441t, 442
Chlorpromazine, 158, 454t, 461t, 462, 464, 465t, 466t, 468, 474t, 476, 486t, 491, 498t
Cimicifuga racemosa (black cohosh), 316t, 352t
Citalopram (**Celexa**), 422t, 425
clomipramine (**Anafranil**), 416t, 420
clonazepam (**Klonopin**), 406t, 409, 451t, 452, 453, 454t, 456, 515
clonidine (**Catapres**), 45, 92, 529t, 530
clorazepate (**Tranxene**), 406t, 409–410
clozapine (**Clozaril**), 425, 434, 466t, 482t, 483–484, 485, 486t, 487, 490, 491, 497t, 498–499, 501, 502
Clozaril (clozapine), 425, 434, 466t, 482t, 483–484, 485, 486t, 487, 490, 491, 497t, 498–499, 501, 502
Cogentin (benztropine), 500, 504t, 506
Concerta (methylphenidate), 525t, 527–528
Cymbalta (duloxetine), 432–433t, 435

Dalmane (flurazepam), 512, 512t, 513
Darvon (propoxyphene), 408
Depakene (valproic acid), 451t, 456
Depakote (valproic acid), 451t, 456
desipramine (**Norpramin**), 93, 416t, 420, 431, 533t
Desoxyn (methamphetamine), 522t, 524
desvenlafaxine (**Pristiq**), 432t, 435
Dexedrine (dextroamphetamine sulfate), 75t, 522t, 524
dexmethylphenidate (**Focalin/Focalin XR**), 73, 75t, 525t, 526–527
dextroamphetamine sulfate (**Dexedrine/Dextrostat**), 75t, 522t, 524
diazepam (**Valium**), 73, 75t, 92, 93, 349, 407t, 410
diphenhydramine (**Benadryl**), 504t, 506
Dolophine (methadone), 73, 76t, 85, 89t, 92, 348–349, 425, 513
Doral (quazepam), 512t, 514
doxepin (**Sinequan**), 417t, 420–421
duloxetine (**Cymbalta**), 432–433t, 435

Echinacea *(Echinacea angustifolia; Echinacea purpurea)*, 352t
Effexor (venlafaxine), 433t, 435
Eletriptan (**Relpax**), 316t
Emsam (selegiline transdermal system), 439t, 441, 446
Epitol (carbamazepine), 451t, 453, 454, 454t
Equetro (carbamazepine), 451t, 455
Escitalopram (**Lexapro**), 421t, 425–426
Estazolam (**ProSom**), 512t, 513
Eszopiclone (**Lunesta**), 73, 516, 517, 518t, 519
Etrafon (perphenazine/amitriptyline HCL), 442
Evening primrose *(Oenothera biennis)*, 317t
Ezide (hydrochlorothiazide), 316t

Fanapt (iloperidone), 489t, 492, 497t
Fennel *(Foeniculum vulgare; Foeniculum officinale)*, 353t
Feverfew *(Tanacetum parthenium)*, 353t

Fluoxetine (**Prozac/Sarafem**), 266, 316t, 408, 413, 423t, 424, 425, 426–427, 431, 434, 440, 441t, 442, 443, 450, 454t, 460t, 465, 466t, 533t
Fluphenazine, 474t, 477, 497t
Flurazepam, 512, 512t, 513
Fluvoxamine (**Luvox**), 413, 423t, 424, 427–428, 434, 465t, 466t, 481, 486t, 517, 518t
Focalin/Focalin XR (dexmethylphenidate), 73, 75t, 525t, 526–527
Foeniculum vulgare; Foeniculum officinale (fennel), 353t
Frova (frovatriptan), 316t
Frovatriptan (**Frova**), 316t
Furosemide (**Lasix**), 316t

Geodon (ziprasidone), 461t, 470, 489t, 492, 497t
ginger *(Zingiber officinale)*, 353t
ginkgo *(Ginkgo biloba)*, 353t, 437
ginseng *(Panax ginseng)*, 353t
guanfacine (**Tenex, Intuniv**), 431, 529t, 530, 533t, 535, 536, 537

Halcion (triazolam), 512t, 514
Haldol (haloperidol), 44, 93, 479t, 481–482, 497t
Haloperidol (**Haldol**), 44, 93, 479t, 481–482, 497t
Hops *(Humulus iupulus)*, 354t
Humulus iupulus (hops), 354t
Hydrochlorothiazide (**Ezide/HydroDiuril**), 316t
HydroDiuril (hydrochlorothiazide), 316t
Hydroxyzine (**Vistaril**), 404t
Hypericum perforatum (St. John's wort), 355t, 408, 425, 434, 438, 440

Ibuprofen (**Advil/Motrin/Nuprin**), 316t
Iloperidone (**Fanapt**), 489t, 492, 497t
Imipramine (**Tofranil**), 395, 417t, 421, 431, 460, 466t, 486t, 533t
Imitrex (sumatriptan), 316t
Inderal (propranolol), 316t
Intuniv (guanfacine), 431, 529t, 530, 533t, 535, 536, 537
Invega (paliperidone), 489t, 492, 497t
Isocarboxazid (**Marplan**), 439t, 440–441
Isoptin (verapamil), 316t, 459–460, 459t

Kava-kava *(Piper methylsticum)*, 354t
Klonopin (clonazepam), 406t, 409, 451t, 452, 453, 454t, 456, 515

Lamictal (lamotrigine), 451t, 457
Lamotrigine (**Lamictal**), 451t, 457
Lasix (furosemide), 316t
Latuda (lurasidone), 494t, 495–496
Levomilnacipran (Fetzima), 433, 436
Lexapro (escitalopgram), 421t, 425–426
Librium (chlordiazepoxide), 75t, 87t, 92, 93, 348, 406t, 409
Limbitrol (amitriptyline-chlordiazepoxide), 441t, 442
Lisdexamfetamine (**Vyvanse**), 522t, 523, 525
Lithium carbonate (**Lithobid**), 449t
Lithium citrate, 449t
Lithobid (lithium carbonate), 449t
Lorazepam (**Ativan**), 407t, 410–411
Loxapine (**Loxitane**), 482t, 483, 484, 485, 486t, 488, 497t
Loxitane (loxapine), 482t, 483, 484, 485, 486t, 488, 497t
Luminal (phenobarbital), 92, 349, 514t, 516
Lunesta (eszopiclone), 73, 516, 517, 518t, 519
Lurasidone (**Latuda**), 494t, 495–496
Luvox (fluvoxamine), 413, 423t, 424, 427–428, 434, 465t, 466t, 481, 486t, 517, 518t
Lycopus virginicus (bugleweed), 316t

Maprotiline, 418, 419, 422
Marplan (isocarboxazid), 439t, 440–441
Matricaria chamomilla (Chamomile), 352t
Maxalt (rizatriptan), 316t
Mentha piperita (peppermint), 354t
Meprobamate, 73, 411t
Metadate ER/Metadate CD (methylphenidate), 525t, 527, 528
Methadone (**Dolophine**), 73, 76t, 85, 89t, 92, 348–349, 425, 513
Methamphetamine (**Desoxyn**), 522t, 524
Methylin/Methylin ER (methylphenidate), 525t, 527, 528
Methylphenidate (**Ritalin/Ritalin SR/Ritalin LA/Methylin/Methylin ER/Metadate ER/Metadate CD/Concerta**), 525t, 527–528
Mirtazapine (**Remeron**), 418t, 419, 422
Motrin (ibuprofen), 316t

Nalmefene (**Revex**), 92, 348
Naloxone (**Narcan**), 92, 253, 348
Naltrexone (**ReVia**), 92, 348
Naprosyn (naproxen), 316t
Naproxen (**Naprosyn/Aleve**), 316t
Naratriptan (**Amerge**), 316t
Narcan (naloxone), 92, 253, 348
Nardil (phenelzine), 439t, 441
Navane (thiothixene), 478t, 497t
Nefazodone, 413, 436–437, 436t, 438, 446, 454t, 512, 513, 518t
Nembutal (pentobarbital), 75t, 514t, 516
Norpramin (desipramine), 93, 416t, 420, 431, 533t
Nortriptyline (**Aventyl/Pamelor**), 417t, 421
Nuprin (ibuprofen), 316t

Oenothera biennis (evening primrose), 317t
olanzapine (**Zyprexa**), 460t, 467, 482t, 488, 497t
olanzapine and fluoxetine (**Symbyax**), 441t, 442, 460t, 467
Orap (pimozide), 45, 479t, 482, 497t
oxazepam (**Serax**), 92, 292, 348, 349, 407t, 411
oxcarbazepine (**Trileptal**), 452t, 453, 454–455t, 458

Paliperidone (**Invega**), 489t, 492, 497t
Pamelor (nortriptyline), 417t, 421
Panax ginseng (ginseng), 353t
Parlodel (bromocriptine), 316t, 501, 504, 507, 507t, 508–509, 508t
Parnate (tranylcypromine), 439t, 441
Paroxetine (**Paxil**), 316t, 423t, 424, 425, 428, 431, 434, 465t, 466t, 476, 486t, 490, 493, 532t, 533
Passion flower (*Passiflora incarnata*), 354t
Paxil (paroxetine), 316t, 423t, 424, 425, 428, 431, 434, 465t, 466t, 476, 486t, 490, 493, 532t, 533
Pentobarbital (**Nembutal**), 75t, 514t, 516
Peppermint *(mentha piperita)*, 354t
Perphenazine, 474t, 477, 497t
Perphenazine-amitryptyline HCl (**Etrafon**), 441t, 442
Phenelzine (**Nardil**), 439t, 441
Phenobarbital (**Luminal**), 92, 349, 514t, 516
Pimozide (**Orap**), 45, 479t, 482, 497t
Piper methylsticum (Kava-Kava), 354t
Plantago ovata (psyllium), 354t
Potentilla *(Potentilla anserine)*, 317t
Pristiq (desvenlafaxine), 432t, 435
Prochlorperazine, 474t, 477, 497t

propoxyphene, 408
Propranolol (**Inderal**), 316t
ProSom (estazolam), 512t, 513
Protriptyline (**Vivactil**), 417t, 421
Prozac (fluoxetine), 423t, 426–427
Psyllium *(plantago ovata)*, 354t

quazepam (**Doral**), 512t, 514
quetiapine (**Seroquel**), 158, 461t, 462, 464, 466t, 468–469, 482t, 483, 484, 485, 487t, 488, 497t, 501

Ramelteon (**Rozerem**), 73, 516t, 517, 518t, 519, 520
Relpax (eletriptan), 316t
Remeron (mirtazapine), 418t, 419, 422
Restoril (temazepam), 512t, 514
Revex (nalmefene), 92, 348
ReVia (naltrexone), 92, 348
Rhamnus purshiana (cascara sagrada), 352t
Risperidal (risperidone), 45, 158, 425, 431, 455t, 461t, 462–463, 464, 466t, 469–470, 486t, 489t, 490–491, 497t, 501, 533t
Risperidone (**Risperdal**), 45, 158, 425, 431, 455t, 461t, 462–463, 464, 466t, 469–470, 486t, 489t, 490–491, 497t, 501, 533t
Ritalin/Ritalin-SR/Ritalin LA (methylphenidate), 75t, 525t, 527–528
Rizatriptan (**Maxalt**), 316t
Rozerem (ramelteon), 73, 516t, 517, 518t, 519, 520

Saphris (asenapine), 158, 461t, 463, 465, 466t, 470, 473, 482–483, 482t, 486t, 487, 497t, 498, 501
Sarafem (fluoxetine), 316t, 423t, 426–427
Scutellaria lateriflora (skullcap), 355t
secobarbital (**Seconal**), 73, 514t, 516
Seconal (secobarbital), 73, 514t, 516
selegiline transdermal system (**Emsam**), 439t, 441, 446
Serax (oxazepam), 92, 292, 348, 349, 407t, 411
Seroquel (quetiapine), 158, 461t, 462, 464, 466t, 468–469, 482t, 483, 484, 485, 487t, 488, 497t, 501
sertraline (**Zoloft**), 316t, 423t, 424, 429, 431, 486t, 533t
Shepherd's purse *(Capsella bursa-pastoris)*, 317t
Sinequan (doxepin), 417t, 420–421
Skullcap *(Scutellaria lateriflora)*, 355t
Sonata (zaleplon), 516t, 519
St. John's wort *(Hypericum perforatum)*, 355t, 408, 425, 434, 438, 440
Strattera (atomoxetine), 531–532, 531t, 532–533t, 533, 535–537
Subutex (buprenorphine), 92, 349
Sumatriptan (**Imitrex**), 316t
Surmontil (trimipramine), 417t, 421–422
Symbyax (olanzapine and fluoxetine), 441t, 442, 460t, 467
Symmetrel (amantadine), 431, 507–508, 507t, 508t, 533t

Tanacetum parthenium (feverfew), 353t
Tegretol/Tegretol-XR (carbamazepine), 451t, 455–456
Temazepam (**Restoril**), 512t, 514
Tenex (guanfacine), 431, 529t, 530, 533t, 535, 536, 537
Teril (carbamazepine), 451t
thioridazine, 424, 431, 434, 466t, 474t, 475, 478, 486–487t, 491, 497t, 498, 508t, 533t
thiothixene (**Navane**), 478t, 497t
Tofranil (imipramine), 395, 417t, 421, 431, 460, 466t, 486t, 533t
Topamax (topiramate), 452t, 457–458

Topiramate (**Topamax**), 452t, 457–458
Tranxene (clorazepate), 406t, 409–410
tranylcypromine (**Parnate**), 439t, 441
trazodone, 395, 425, 433t, 434, 437–438, 446, 447
triazolam (**Halcion**), 512t, 514
trifluoperazine, 474t, 478, 497t
trihexyphenidyl, 504t, 506
Trileptal (oxcarbazepine), 452t, 453, 454–455t, 458
trimipramine (**Surmontil**), 417t, 421–422

valerian (*Valeriana officinalis*), 317t, 355t, 405, 408, 412
Valium (diazepam), 73, 75t, 92, 93, 349, 407t, 410
valproic acid (**Depakene/Depakote**), 451t, 456
venlafaxine (**Effexor**), 433t, 435
verapamil (**Calan/Isoptin**), 316t, 459–460, 459t
Vilazodone (Viibryd), 423, 429
Vistaril (hydroxyzine), 404t
Vitex agnus-castus (chaste tree), 317t
Vivactil (protriptyline), 417t, 421
Vortioxetine (Brintellix), 423, 429
Vyvanse (lisdexamfetamine), 522t, 523, 525

Wellbutrin/Wellbutrin SR/Wellbutrin XL (bupropion), 430t, 431–432, 444,
447, 531t, 534–535

Xanax (alprazolam), 32, 40, 92, 199, 262, 279, 406t, 408

Zaleplon (**Sonata**), 516t, 519
Zingiber officinale (ginger), 353t
Ziprasidone (**Geodon**), 461t, 470, 489t, 492, 497t
Zolmitriptan (**Zomig**), 316t
Zoloft (sertraline), 316t, 423t, 424, 429, 431, 486t, 533t
Zolpidem (**Ambien**), 516t, 519
Zomig (zolmitriptan), 316t
Zyprexa (olanzapine), 460t, 467, 482t, 488, 497t

Nursing Diagnoses Index

Activity intolerance, risk for
   antianxiety agents and, 413
   antiparkinsonian agents and, 509
   CNS stimulants and, 535
   mood-stabilizing drugs and, 470
   sedative-hypnotics and, 520
Anxiety
   moderate to severe
      in adjustment disorder, 187
      client behavior leading to diagnosis of, 39–40, 197–198, 261–262, 618
      in disruptive behavior disorders, 29
      in eating disorders, 261–262
   panic in disorders of, 169–170
   severe
      client behavior leading to diagnosis of, 49–50, 278–279, 618
      in separation anxiety disorder, 48–49
   severe to panic, 278–280
      client behavior leading to diagnosis of, 278–279, 618

Body image, disturbed
   client behavior leading to diagnosis of, 181, 262–263, 266–267
   in eating disorders, 262–264
   in obesity, 266–267
   in obsessive-compulsive and related disorders, 180–181

Caregiver role strain, risk for
   client behavior leading to diagnosis of, 335–336
   in military families, 401–403
   in neurocognitive disorders, 68–69
   in psychiatric home nursing care, 335–336
Confusion, risk for
   antianxiety agents and, 413
   client behavior leading to diagnosis of, 618
   sedative-hypnotics and, 513, 515
Constipation and antidepressants, 443

Decisional conflict, client behavior leading to diagnosis of, 618
Defensive coping
   in antisocial personality disorder, 293–295
   client behavior leading to diagnosis of, 618
   in correctional facilities, 343–345
   in disruptive behavior disorders, 32–34
Denial, ineffective
   client behavior leading to diagnosis of, 618
   in substance-related disorders, 93–95

Family processes
dysfunctional, in alcoholism, 102–105
interrupted, in military families, 398–399
Fear
in anxiety disorders, 169–171
client behavior leading to diagnosis of, 619
Fluid volume, deficient
client behavior leading to diagnosis of, 620
in eating disorders, 257–259

Grieving, complicated
in borderline personality disorder, 280–282
client behavior leading to diagnosis of, 618, 619
in correctional facilities, 345–347
in loss and bereavement, 382–384
in major depressive disorder, 139–141
in military families, 399–401
Growth and development, delayed, in abuse and neglect, 309–311

Health maintenance, ineffective, in homelessness, 323–325
Hyperthermia and antiparkinsonian agents, 509

Ineffective coping
in adjustment disorders, 199–201
in anxiety disorders, 179–180
client behavior leading to diagnosis of, 619
in dissociative disorders, 223–224
in obsessive-compulsive and related disorders, 182–183
in premenstrual dysphoric disorder, 317–319
in psychotic disorders, 121–122
in separation anxiety disorders, 50–51
in somatic symptom disorders, 211–214
in substance-related disorders, 95–97
Injury, risk for
antianxiety agents and, 413
antidepressants and, 442
antiparkinsonian agents and, 509
antipsychotic agents and, 496
in bipolar disorder, 156–158
client behavior leading to diagnosis of, 618, 619
CNS stimulants and, 535
in correctional facilities, 347–349
in intellectual disability, 16–17
mood-stabilizing drugs and, 470
sedative-hypnotics and, 519–520
in substance-related disorders, 90–93
Insomnia
antianxiety agents and, 407t, 410, 414
in bipolar disorder, 167–168
client behavior leading to diagnosis of, 618
in psychotic disorders, 129–130
sedative-hypnotics and, 521

Knowledge, deficient
antianxiety agents and, 414
antiparkinsonian agents and, 509
in antisocial personality disorder, 299–301
in personality disorders, 299–301
in somatic symptom disorders, 216–217
in substance-related disorders, 100–102

Nausea, CNS stimulants and, 532, 535
Noncompliance
    antipsychotic agents and, 496
    in disruptive behavior disorders, 41–42
Nutrition
    imbalanced: less than body requirements
        in bipolar disorder, 160–162
        client behavior leading to diagnosis of, 618
        CNS stimulants and, 535
        in eating disorders, 255–257
        in major depressive disorder, 148–150
        in substance-related disorders, 97–98
    imbalanced: more than body requirements
        client behavior leading to diagnosis to, 619
        in obesity, 264–266

Pain
    acute, in premenstrual dysphoric disorder, 313–315, 316–317t
    in adjustment disorder, 190
    chronic, in somatoform disorders, 209
    CNS stimulants and, 535
Personal identity, disturbed
    in autistic disorder, 25–26
    in borderline personality disorder, 284–286
    client behavior leading to diagnosis of, 619
    in dissociative disorders, 226–227
    in gender dysphoria, 245–247
Post-trauma syndrome
    client behavior leading to diagnosis of, 619
    in forensic nursing, 340–343
    in military families, 393–395
    in trauma-related disorders, 191–192
Powerlessness
    in abuse and neglect, 307–309
    in anxiety disorders, 197–199
    client behavior leading to diagnosis of, 619
    in homelessness, 325–326
    in major depressive disorder, 145–147
Protection, client behavior leading to diagnosis of ineffective, 619

Rape-trauma syndrome, 305–307, 340–342
Relocation stress syndrome
    client behavior leading to diagnosis of, 619
    in trauma- and stressor-related disorders, 203–205
Risk-prone health behavior
    client behavior leading to diagnosis of, 618
    in psychiatric home nursing care, 332–334
    in trauma- and stressor-related disorders, 201–203
Role performance, ineffective
    client behavior leading to diagnosis of, 618
    in depressive disorders, 145, 147
    substance withdrawal and, 72

Self-care deficit
    in anxiety disorders, 181–182
    client behavior leading to diagnosis of, 619
    in intellectual disability, 17–18
    in psychotic disorders, 128–129
    in neurocognitive disorders, 63–64

Self-esteem, low
  in antisocial personality disorder, 295–297
  in avoidant personality disorder, 271
  in borderline personality disorder, 286–288
  chronic, in substance-related disorders, 98–100
  client behavior leading to diagnosis of, 619
  in disruptive behavior disorders, 28, 33, 35, 37–38
  in eating disorders, 262–264, 266–267
  in major depressive disorder, 141–143
  in maladaptive grieving, 379–380
  in neurocognitive disorders, 66–68
  in sexual disorders and gender dysphoria, 248–249
  in Tourette's disorder, 47–48
Self-health management, ineffective, in psychiatric home nursing care, 330–332
Self-mutilation, risk for
  in autism spectrum disorder, 21–22
  in borderline personality disorder, 276–278
  client behavior leading to diagnosis of, 619
Sensory perception, disturbed
  auditory/visual
    client behavior leading to diagnosis of, 619
    in psychotic disorders, 123–124
  in bipolar disorder, 163–165
  client behavior leading to diagnosis of, 618, 619
  in dissociative disorders, 227–229
  in neurocognitive disorders, 65–66
  in somatic symptom disorders, 214–215
Sexual dysfunction
  client behavior leading to diagnosis of, 619
  in sexual disorders and gender dysphoria, 238–240
Sexuality patterns, ineffective
  client behavior leading to diagnosis of, 619
  in sexual disorders and gender dysphoria, 240–242
Sleep pattern, disturbed, in major depressive disorder, 150–151
Social interaction, impaired
  in antisocial personality disorder, 297–299
  in autism spectrum disorder, 20–22
  in bipolar disorder, 165–166
  in borderline personality disorder, 282–284
  client behavior leading to diagnosis of, 618, 619
  in disruptive behavior disorders, 45–46
  in gender dysphoria, 247–248
  in intellectual disability, 19–20
  in major depressive disorder, 143–145
  in psychotic disorders, 116
  in separation anxiety disorder, 51–52
Social isolation
  in adjustment disorder, 190
  antidepressants and, 442
  client behavior leading to diagnosis of, 620
  in loss and bereavement, 373
  in major depressive disorder, 143–145
  in psychiatric home nursing care, 334–335
  in psychotic disorders, 116, 119–121, 270
  related to abuse or neglect, 304
Spiritual distress risk in loss and bereavement, 384–385
Suicide, risk for
  antidepressants and, 442
  client behavior leading to diagnosis of, 620

CNS stimulants and, 535
in major depressive disorder, 136–139
in military families, 395–396

Thought processes, disturbed
in bipolar disorder, 162–163
client behavior leading to diagnosis of, 618, 620
in major depressive disorder, 147–148
in military families, 396–398
in psychotic disorders, 124–126
Trauma risk in neurocognitive disorders , 58–59

Verbal communication, impaired
in autism spectrum disorder, 23–24
client behavior leading to diagnosis of, 619
in intellectual disability, 18–19
in psychotic disorders, 126–128
Violence, risk for self-/other-directed
antipsychotic agents and, 496
in antisocial personality disorder, 290–293
in bipolar disorder, 158–160
in borderline personality disorder, 276–278
client behavior leading to diagnosis of, 618, 620
in disruptive behavior disorders, 30–32
in neurocognitive disorder, 60–61
in psychotic disorders, 117–119
in Tourette's disorder, 44–45
in trauma- and stressor-related disorders, 194–197